MW00513386

Reference Textbook for
Anatomy & Physiology

Taken from:

Essentials of Human Anatomy & Physiology, Eighth Edition
by Elaine N. Marieb

Fundamentals of Anatomy & Physiology, Seventh Edition
by Frederic H. Martini

Human Anatomy & Physiology, Sixth Edition
by Elaine N. Marieb

Compiled by Janet L. Randall

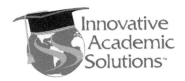

Innovative
Academic
Solutions™

Learning Solutions

New York Boston San Francisco
London Toronto Sydney Tokyo Singapore Madrid
Mexico City Munich Paris Cape Town Hong Kong Montreal

Pearson Learning Solutions, 501 Boylston Street, Suite 900, Boston, MA 02116
A Pearson Education Company
www.pearsoned.com

Printed in the United States of America

14 15 16 V0CR 16 15 14 13

000200010270594462

RG

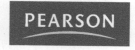

ISBN 10: 0-558-81919-2
ISBN 13: 978-0-558-81919-4

Contents

Unit 3   Dynamics of Support and Motion

3 Cells and Tissues   51

4 Skin and the Integumentary System   85

5 The Skeletal System   97

6 The Muscular System   145

Contents

Unit 4   Integration and Regulatory Mechanisms

7 The Nervous System   197

➤

Unit 5   Maintenance of the Human Body

10 The Cardiovascular System: The Blood   345

11 The Cardiovascular System: The Heart and Blood Vessels   361

➤

12 The Lymphatic System and Body Defenses   419

Unit 6   Urinary System
&
Unit 7   Fluid and Electrolyte Balance

15   The Urinary System   537

Unit 8   Reproduction and Development

16   The Reproductive System   579

➤

Unit 1

The Human Body:
An Overview

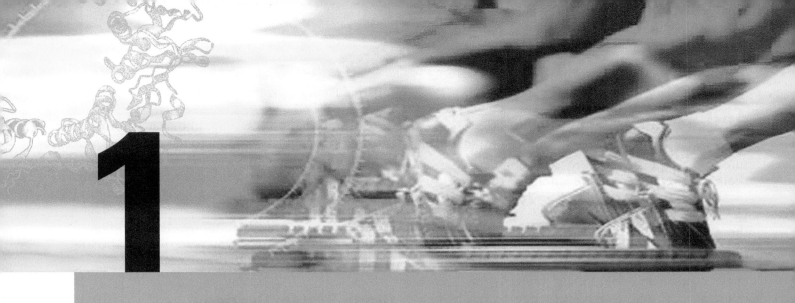

1

The Human Body:
An Orientation

KEY TERMS

An Overview of Anatomy and Physiology

Anatomy (ah-nat′o-me) is the study of the structure and shape of the body and body parts and their relationships to one another. **Physiology** (fiz″e-ol′o-je) is the study of how the body and its parts work or function (*physio* = nature; *ology* = the study of). In the real world, anatomy and physiology are always related. The parts of your body form a well-organized unit, and each of those parts has a job to do to make the body operate as a whole. Structure determines what functions can take place.

Levels of Structural Organization

From Atoms to Organisms

The human body exhibits many levels of structural complexity (Figure 1.1). The simplest level of the structural ladder is the *chemical level*. At this level, **atoms,** tiny building blocks of matter, combine to form *molecules* such as water, sugar, and proteins. Molecules, in turn, associate in specific ways to form microscopic **cells,** the smallest units of all living things. The *cellular level* is examined in Chapter 3. Individual cells vary widely in size and shape, reflecting their particular functions in the body.

The simplest living creatures are composed of single cells, but in complex organisms like trees or human beings, the structural ladder continues to the *tissue level*. **Tissues** consist of groups of similar cells that have a common function. Each of the four basic tissue types (epithelial, connective, muscular, and neural) plays a definite but different role in the body.

An **organ** is a structure that is composed of two or more tissue types and performs a specific function for the body. At the *organ level* of organization, extremely complex functions become possible. For example, the small intestine, which digests and absorbs food, is composed of all four tissue types. All the body's organs are grouped so that a number of organ systems are formed. An **organ system** is a group of organs that cooperate to accomplish a common purpose. For example, the digestive system includes the esophagus, the stomach, and the small and large intestines (to name a few of its

organs). Each organ has its own job to do, and, by working together, organs keep food moving through the digestive system so that it is properly broken down and absorbed into the blood, providing fuel for all the body's cells. In all, 11 organ systems make up the living body, or the **organism,** which represents the highest level of structural organization, the *organismal level*. The major organs of each of the systems are shown in Figure 1.2. Refer to the figure as you read through the following descriptions of the organ systems.

Organ System Overview

Integumentary System

The **integumentary** (in-teg″u-men′tar-e) **system** is the external covering of the body, or the skin. It waterproofs the body and cushions and protects the deeper tissues from injury. It also excretes salts and urea in perspiration and helps regulate body temperature. Temperature, pressure, and pain receptors located in the skin alert us to what is happening at the body surface.

Skeletal System

The **skeletal system** consists of bones, cartilages, ligaments, and joints. It supports the body and provides a framework that the skeletal muscles use to cause movement. It also has a protective function (for example, the skull encloses and protects the brain). *Hematopoiesis* (hem″ah-to-poi-e′sis), or formation of blood cells, goes on within the cavities of the skeleton. The hard substance of bones acts as a storehouse for minerals.

Muscular System

The muscles of the body have only one function—to *contract,* or shorten. When this happens, movement occurs. Hence, muscles can be viewed as the "machines" of the body. The mobility of the body as a whole reflects the activity of *skeletal muscles,* the large, fleshy muscles attached to bones. When these contract, you are able to stand erect, walk, leap, grasp, throw a ball, or smile. The skeletal muscles form the **muscular system.** These muscles are distinct from the muscles of the heart and of other hollow organs, which move fluids (blood, urine) or other substances (such as food) along definite pathways within the body.

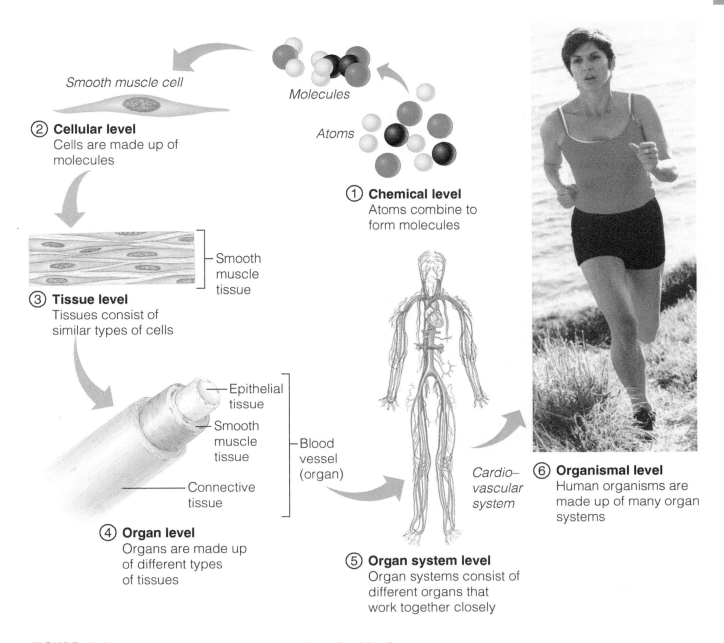

Smooth muscle cell

② **Cellular level**
Cells are made up of
molecules

Molecules

Atoms

① **Chemical level**
Atoms combine to
form molecules

— Smooth
muscle
tissue

③ **Tissue level**
Tissues consist of
similar types of cells

— Epithelial
tissue

— Smooth
muscle
tissue

— Connective
tissue

— Blood
vessel
(organ)

④ **Organ level**
Organs are made up
of different types
of tissues

*Cardio-
vascular
system*

⑤ **Organ system level**
Organ systems consist of
different organs that
work together closely

⑥ **Organismal level**
Human organisms are
made up of many organ
systems

FIGURE 1.1 Levels of structural organization. In this diagram,
components of the cardiovascular system are used to illustrate the various
levels of structural organization in a human being.

Nervous System

The **nervous system** is the body's fast-acting control system. It consists of the brain, spinal cord, nerves, and sensory receptors. The body must be able to respond to irritants or stimuli coming from outside the body (such as light, sound, or changes in temperature) and from inside the body (such as decreases in oxygen or stretching of tissue).

The sensory receptors detect these changes and send messages (via electrical signals called *nerve impulses*) to the central nervous system (brain and spinal cord) so that it is constantly informed about what is going on. The central nervous system then assesses this information and responds by activating the appropriate body effectors (muscles or glands).

Endocrine System

Like the nervous system, the **endocrine** (en' do-krin) **system** controls body activities, but it acts much more slowly. The endocrine glands produce chemical molecules called *hormones* and release them into the blood to travel to relatively distant target organs.

The endocrine glands include the pituitary, thyroid, parathyroids, adrenals, thymus, pancreas, pineal, ovaries (in the female), and testes (in the male). The endocrine glands are not connected anatomically in the same way that parts of the other organ systems are. What they have in common is that they all secrete hormones, which regulate other structures. The body functions controlled by hormones are many and varied, involving every cell in the body. Growth, reproduction, and food use by cells are all controlled (at least in part) by hormones.

Cardiovascular System

The primary organs of the **cardiovascular system** are the heart and blood vessels. Using blood as the transporting fluid, the cardiovascular system carries oxygen, nutrients, hormones, and other substances to and from the tissue cells where exchanges are made. White blood cells and chemicals in the blood help to protect the body from such foreign invaders as bacteria, toxins, and tumor cells. The heart acts as the blood pump, propelling blood through the blood vessels to all body tissues.

Lymphatic System

The role of the **lymphatic system** is complementary to that of the cardiovascular system. Its organs include lymphatic vessels, lymph nodes, and other lymphoid organs such as the spleen and tonsils. The lymphatic vessels return fluid leaked from the blood to the blood vessels so that blood can be kept continuously circulating through the body. The lymph nodes (and other lymphoid organs) help to cleanse the blood and house the cells involved in immunity.

Respiratory System

The job of the **respiratory system** is to keep the body constantly supplied with oxygen and to remove carbon dioxide. The respiratory system consists of the nasal passages, pharynx, larynx, trachea, bronchi, and lungs. Within the lungs are tiny air sacs. It is through the thin walls of these air sacs that gas exchanges are made to and from the blood.

Digestive System

The **digestive system** is basically a tube running through the body from mouth to anus. The organs of the digestive system include the oral cavity (mouth), esophagus, stomach, small and large intestines, and rectum. Their role is to break down food and deliver the products to the blood for dispersal to the body cells. The undigested food that remains in the tract leaves the body through the anus as feces. The breakdown activities that begin in the mouth are completed in the small intestine. From that point on, the major function of the digestive system is to reclaim water. The liver is considered to be a digestive organ because the bile it produces helps to break down fats. The pancreas, which delivers digestive enzymes to the small intestine, also is functionally a digestive organ.

Urinary System

The body produces wastes as by-products of its normal functions, and these wastes must be disposed of. One type of waste contains nitrogen (examples are urea and uric acid), which results from the breakdown of proteins and nucleic acids by the body cells. The **urinary system** removes the nitrogen-containing wastes from the blood and flushes them from the body in urine. This system, often called the *excretory system,* is composed of the kidneys, ureters, bladder, and urethra. Other important functions of this system include maintaining the body's water and salt (electrolyte) balance and regulating the acid-base balance of the blood.

Reproductive System

The **reproductive system** exists primarily to produce offspring. Sperm are produced by the testes of the male. Other male reproductive system structures are the scrotum, penis, accessory glands, and the duct system, which carries sperm to the outside of the body. The ovary of the female produces the eggs, or ova; the female duct system

THE INTEGUMENTARY SYSTEM

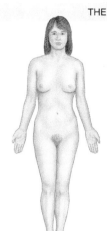

Major Organs:
- Skin
- Hair
- Sweat glands
- Nails

Functions:
- Protects against environmental hazards
- Helps regulate body temperature
- Provides sensory information

THE SKELETAL SYSTEM

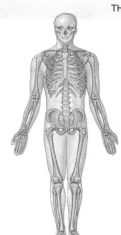

Major Organs:
- Bones
- Cartilages
- Associated ligaments
- Bone marrow

Functions:
- Provides support and protection for other tissues
- Stores calcium and other minerals
- Forms blood cells

THE MUSCULAR SYSTEM

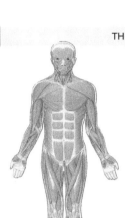

Major Organs:
- Skeletal muscles and associated tendons

Functions:
- Provides movement
- Provides protection and support for other tissues
- Generates heat that maintains body temperature

THE NERVOUS SYSTEM

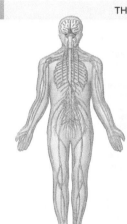

Major Organs:
- Brain
- Spinal cord
- Peripheral nerves
- Sense organs

Functions:
- Directs immediate responses to stimuli
- Coordinates or moderates activities of other organ systems
- Provides and interprets sensory information about external conditions

THE ENDOCRINE SYSTEM

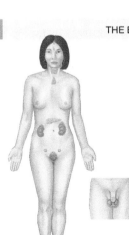

Major Organs:
- Pituitary gland
- Thyroid gland
- Pancreas
- Adrenal glands
- Gonads (testes and ovaries)
- Endocrine tissues in other systems

Functions:
- Directs long-term changes in the activities of other organ systems
- Adjusts metabolic activity and energy use by the body
- Controls many structural and functional changes during development

THE CARDIOVASCULAR SYSTEM

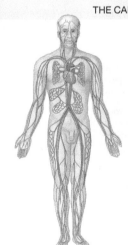

Major Organs:
- Heart
- Blood
- Blood vessels

Functions:
- Distributes blood cells, water, and dissolved materials, including nutrients, waste products, oxygen, and carbon dioxide
- Distributes heat and assists in control of body temperature

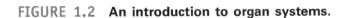

FIGURE 1.2   An introduction to organ systems.

(continued)

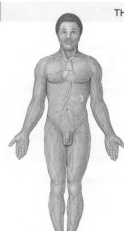

THE LYMPHATIC SYSTEM

Major Organs:
- Spleen
- Thymus
- Lymphatic vessels
- Lymph nodes
- Tonsils

Functions:
- Defends against infection and disease
- Returns tissue fluids to the bloodstream

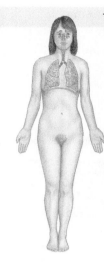
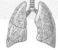

THE RESPIRATORY SYSTEM

Major Organs:
- Nasal cavities
- Sinuses
- Larynx
- Trachea
- Bronchi
- Lungs
- Alveoli

Functions:
- Delivers air to alveoli (sites in lungs where gas exchange occurs)
- Provides oxygen to bloodstream
- Removes carbon dioxide from bloodstream
- Produces sounds for communication

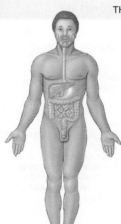

THE DIGESTIVE SYSTEM

Major Organs:
- Teeth
- Tongue
- Pharynx
- Esophagus
- Stomach
- Small Intestine
- Large intestine
- Liver
- Gallbladder
- Pancreas

Functions:
- Processes and digests food
- Absorbs and conserves water
- Absorbs nutrients (ions, water, and the breakdown products of dietary sugars, proteins, and fats)
- Stores energy reserves

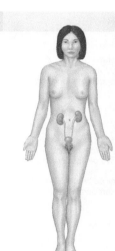
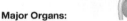

THE URINARY SYSTEM

Major Organs:
- Kidneys
- Ureters
- Urinary bladder
- Urethra

Functions:
- Excretes waste products from the blood
- Controls water balance by regulating volume of urine produced
- Stores urine prior to voluntary elimination
- Regulates blood ion concentrations and pH

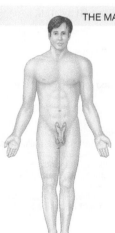
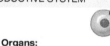

THE MALE REPRODUCTIVE SYSTEM

Major Organs:
- Testes
- Epididymis
- Ductus deferens
- Seminal vesicles
- Prostate gland
- Penis
- Scrotum

Functions:
- Produces male sex cells (sperm) and hormones

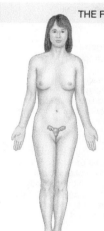

THE FEMALE REPRODUCTIVE SYSTEM

Major Organs:
- Ovaries
- Uterine tubes
- Uterus
- Vagina
- Labia
- Clitoris
- Mammary glands

Functions:
- Produces female sex cells (oocytes) and hormones
- Supports developing embryo from conception to delivery
- Provides milk to nourish newborn infant

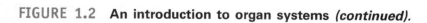

FIGURE 1.2   An introduction to organ systems *(continued).*

consists of the uterine tubes, uterus, and vagina. The uterus provides the site for the development of the fetus (immature infant) once fertilization has occurred.

Maintaining Life

Necessary Life Functions

Now that we have introduced the structural levels composing the human body, the question that naturally follows is: What does this highly organized human body do? Like all complex animals, human beings maintain their boundaries, move, respond to environmental changes, take in and digest nutrients, carry out metabolism, dispose of wastes, reproduce themselves, and grow. We will discuss each of these necessary life functions briefly here and in more detail in later chapters.

Organ systems do not work in isolation; instead, they work together to promote the well-being of the entire body. Because this theme will be emphasized throughout this book, it is worthwhile to identify the most important organ systems contributing to each of the necessary life functions (Figure 1.3). Also, as you read through this material, you may want to refer back to the more detailed descriptions of the organ systems provided in the previous sections and in Figure 1.2.

Maintaining Boundaries

Every living organism must be able to maintain its boundaries so that its "inside" remains distinct from its "outside." Every cell of the human body is surrounded by an external membrane that contains its contents and allows needed substances in while generally preventing the entry of potentially damaging or unnecessary substances. The body as a whole is also enclosed by the integumentary system, or skin. The integumentary system protects internal organs from drying out (which would be fatal), from bacteria, and from the damaging effects of heat, sunlight, and an unbelievable number of chemical substances in the external environment.

Movement

Movement includes all the activities promoted by the muscular system, such as propelling ourselves from one place to another by walking, swimming, and so forth, and manipulating the external environment with our fingers. The muscular system is aided by the skeletal system, which provides the bones that the muscles pull on as they work. Movement also occurs when substances such as blood, foodstuffs, and urine are propelled through the internal organs of the cardiovascular, digestive, and urinary systems, respectively.

Responsiveness

Responsiveness, or **irritability,** is the ability to sense changes (stimuli) in the environment and then to react to them. For example, if you cut your hand on broken glass, you involuntarily pull your hand away from the painful stimulus (the glass). It is not necessary to think about it—it just happens! Likewise, when the amount of carbon dioxide in your blood rises to dangerously high levels, the response is an increase in your breathing rate to blow off the excess carbon dioxide.

Because nerve cells are highly irritable and can communicate rapidly with each other by conducting electrical impulses, the nervous system bears the major responsibility for responsiveness. However, all body cells exhibit responsiveness to some extent.

Digestion

Digestion is the process of breaking down ingested food into simple molecules that can then be absorbed into the blood for delivery to all body cells by the cardiovascular system. In a simple, one-celled organism like an amoeba, the cell itself is the "digestion factory," but in the complex, multicellular human body, the digestive system performs this function for the entire body.

Metabolism

Metabolism is a broad term that refers to all chemical reactions that occur within body cells. It includes breaking down complex substances into simpler building blocks, making larger structures from smaller ones, and using nutrients and oxygen to produce ATP molecules, the energy-rich molecules that power cellular activities. Metabolism depends on the digestive and respiratory systems to make nutrients and oxygen available to the blood and on the cardiovascular system to distribute these substances throughout the body. Metabolism is regulated chiefly by hormones secreted by the glands of the endocrine system.

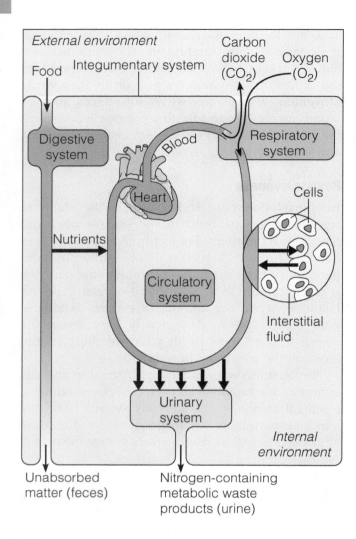

External environment

Food   Integumentary system   Carbon dioxide (CO$_2$)   Oxygen (O$_2$)

Digestive system   Blood   Respiratory system

Heart   Cells

Nutrients

Circulatory system   Interstitial fluid

Urinary system

Internal environment

Unabsorbed matter (feces)   Nitrogen-containing metabolic waste products (urine)

FIGURE 1.3 Examples of selected interrelationships among body organ systems. The integumentary system protects the body as a whole from the external environment. The digestive and respiratory systems, in contact with the external environment, take in nutrients and oxygen, respectively, which are then distributed by the blood to all body cells. Elimination from the body of metabolic wastes is accomplished by the urinary and respiratory systems.

Excretion

Excretion is the process of removing *excreta* (ek-skre'tah), or wastes, from the body. If the body is to continue to operate as we expect it to, it must get rid of the nonuseful substances produced during digestion and metabolism. Several organ systems participate in excretion. For example, the digestive system rids the body of indigestible food residues in feces, and the urinary system

disposes of nitrogen-containing metabolic wastes in urine.

Reproduction

Reproduction, the production of offspring, can occur on the cellular or organismal level. In cellular reproduction, the original cell divides, producing two identical daughter cells that may then be used for body growth or repair. Reproduction of the human organism, or making a whole new person, is the task of the organs of the reproductive system, which produce sperm and eggs. When a sperm unites with an egg, a fertilized egg forms, which then develops into a bouncing baby within the mother's body. The function of the reproductive system is exquisitely regulated by hormones of the endocrine system.

Growth

Growth is an increase in size, usually accomplished by an increase in the number of cells. For growth to occur, cell-constructing activities must occur at a faster rate than cell-destroying ones.

Survival Needs

The goal of nearly all body systems is to maintain life. However, life is extraordinarily fragile and requires that several factors be available. These factors, which we will call *survival needs,* include nutrients (food), oxygen, water, and appropriate temperature and atmospheric pressure.

Nutrients, taken in via the diet, contain the chemicals used for energy and cell building. Carbohydrates are the major energy-providing fuel for body cells. Proteins and, to a lesser extent, fats are essential for building cell structures. Fats also cushion body organs and provide reserve fuel. Minerals and vitamins are required for the chemical reactions that go on in cells and for oxygen transport in the blood.

All the nutrients in the world are useless unless **oxygen** is also available, because the chemical reactions that release energy from foods require oxygen. Approximately 20 percent of the air we breathe is oxygen. It is made available to the blood and body cells by the cooperative efforts of the respiratory and cardiovascular systems.

Water accounts for 60 to 80 percent of body weight. It is the single most abundant chemical substance in the body and provides the fluid base for body secretions and excretions. Water is obtained chiefly from ingested foods or liquids and is lost from the body by evaporation from the lungs and skin and in body excretions.

For good health, **body temperature** must be maintained at around 37°C (98°F). As body temperature drops below this point, metabolic reactions become slower and slower and finally stop. When body temperature is too high, chemical reactions proceed too rapidly, and body proteins begin to break down. At either extreme, death occurs. Most body heat is generated by the activity of the skeletal muscles.

The force exerted on the surface of the body by the weight of air is referred to as **atmospheric pressure.** Breathing and the exchange of oxygen and carbon dioxide in the lungs depend on appropriate atmospheric pressure. At high altitudes, where the air is thin and atmospheric pressure is lower, gas exchange may be too low to support cellular metabolism.

The mere presence of these survival factors is not sufficient to maintain life. They must be present in appropriate amounts as well; excesses and deficits may be equally harmful. For example, the food ingested must be of high quality and in proper amounts; otherwise, nutritional disease, obesity, or starvation is likely.

Homeostasis

When you really think about the fact that your body contains trillions of cells in nearly constant activity, and that remarkably little usually goes wrong with it, you begin to appreciate what a marvelous machine your body really is. The word **homeostasis** (ho″me-o-sta′sis) describes the body's ability to maintain relatively stable internal conditions even though the outside world is continuously changing. Although the literal translation of *homeostasis* is "unchanging" (*homeo* = the same; *stasis* = standing still), the term does not really mean an unchanging state. Instead, it indicates a *dynamic* state of equilibrium, or a balance in which internal conditions change and vary but always within relatively narrow limits.

In general, the body demonstrates homeostasis when its needs are being adequately met and it is functioning smoothly. Virtually every organ system plays a role in maintaining the constancy of the internal environment. Adequate blood levels of vital nutrients must be continuously present, and heart activity and blood pressure must be constantly monitored and adjusted so that the blood is propelled with adequate force to reach all body tissues. Additionally, wastes must not be allowed to accumulate, and body temperature must be precisely controlled.

Homeostatic Control Mechanisms

Communication within the body is essential for homeostasis and is accomplished chiefly by the nervous and endocrine systems, which use electrical signals delivered by nerves or bloodborne hormones, respectively, as information carriers. The details of how these two regulating systems operate are the subjects of later chapters, but the basic characteristics of the neural and hormonal control systems that promote homeostasis will be explained here.

Regardless of the factor or event being regulated (this is called the *variable*), all homeostatic control mechanisms have at least three components (Figure 1.4). The first component is a **receptor.** Essentially, it is some type of sensor that monitors and responds to changes in the environment. It responds to such changes, called *stimuli,* by sending information (input) to the second element, the *control center.* Information flows from the receptor to the control center along the *afferent pathway.* (It may help to remember that information traveling along the *afferent* pathway *approaches* the control center.)

The **control center,** which determines the level (set point) at which a variable is to be maintained, analyzes the information it receives and then determines the appropriate response or course of action.

The third component is the **effector,** which provides the means for the control center's response (output) to the stimulus. Information flows from the control center to the effector along the *efferent pathway.* (*Efferent* information *exits* from the control center.) The results of the response then *feed back* to influence the stimulus, either by depressing it (negative feedback) so that the whole control mechanism is shut off or by enhancing it (positive feedback) so that the reaction continues at an even faster rate.

Most homeostatic control mechanisms are **negative feedback mechanisms.** In such systems, the

Q *If this control system were regulating room temperature, what apparatus would be the effector?*

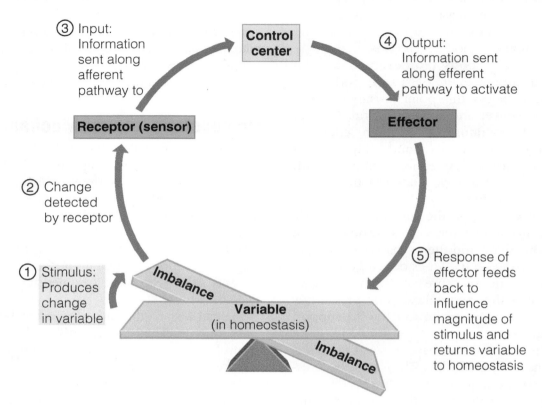

FIGURE 1.4 **The elements of a homeostatic control system.** Communication between the receptor, control center, and effector is essential for normal operation of the system.

net effect of the response to the stimulus is to shut off the original stimulus or reduce its intensity. A frequently used example of a negative feedback system is a home heating system connected to a thermostat. In this situation, the thermostat contains both the receptor and the control center. If the thermostat is set at 20°C (68°F), the heating system (effector) will be triggered ON when the house temperature drops below that setting. As the furnace produces heat, the air is warmed. When the temperature reaches 20°C or slightly higher, the thermostat sends a signal to shut off the furnace. Your body "thermostat," located in a part of your brain called the *hypothalamus*, operates in a similar way to regulate body temperature. Other negative feedback mechanisms regulate heart rate, blood pressure,

breathing rate, and blood levels of glucose, oxygen, carbon dioxide, and minerals.

Because they tend to increase the original disturbance (stimulus) and to push the variable *farther* from its original value, **positive feedback mechanisms** are rare in the body. Typically these mechanisms control infrequent events that occur explosively and do not require continuous adjustments. Blood clotting and the birth of a baby are the most familiar examples of positive feedback mechanisms.

Homeostatic Imbalance

Homeostasis is so important that most disease can be regarded as a result of its disturbance, a condition called **homeostatic imbalance.** As we age, our body organs become less efficient, and our internal conditions become less and less stable. These events place us at an increasing risk for illness and produce the changes we associate with aging.

A   *The heat-generating furnace or oil burner.*

Examples of homeostatic imbalance will be provided throughout this book to enhance your understanding of normal physiological mechanisms. These homeostatic imbalance sections are preceded by the symbol ▲ to alert you that an abnormal condition is being described. ▲

The Language of Anatomy

Learning about the body is exciting, but our interest sometimes dwindles when we are confronted with the terminology of anatomy and physiology. Let's face it. You can't just pick up an anatomy and physiology book and read it as though it were a novel. Unfortunately, confusion is inevitable without specialized terminology. For example, if you are looking at a ball, "above" always means the area over the top of the ball. Other directional terms can also be used consistently because the ball is a sphere. All sides and surfaces are equal. The human body, of course, has many protrusions and bends. Thus, the question becomes: Above what? To prevent misunderstanding, anatomists have accepted a set of terms that allow body structures to be located and identified clearly with just a few words. This language of anatomy is presented and explained next.

Anatomical Position

To accurately describe body parts and position, we must have an initial reference point and use directional terms. To avoid confusion, it is always assumed that the body is in a standard position called the **anatomical position.** It is important to understand this position because most body terminology used in this book refers to this body positioning *regardless* of the position the body happens to be in. The face-front diagrams in Figure 1.5 and Table 1.1 illustrate the anatomical position. As you can see, the body is erect with the feet parallel and the arms hanging at the sides with the palms facing forward.

- Stand up and assume the anatomical position. Notice that it is similar to "standing at attention" but is less comfortable because the palms are held unnaturally forward with thumbs pointing away from the body rather than hanging cupped toward the thighs.

Regions of the Body

There are many visible landmarks on the surface of the body. Once you know their proper anatomical names, you can be specific in referring to different regions of the body.

Anterior Body Landmarks

Look at Figure 1.5a to find the following body regions. Once you have identified all the anterior body landmarks, cover the labels that describe what the structures are, and again go through the list, pointing out these areas on your own body.

- **abdominal** (ab-dom′ĭ-nal): anterior body trunk inferior to ribs
- **acromial** (ah-kro′me-ul): point of shoulder
- **antecubital** (an″te-ku′bĭ-tal): anterior surface of elbow
- **axillary** (ak′sĭ-lar″e): armpit
- **brachial** (bra′ke-al): arm
- **buccal** (buk′al): cheek area
- **carpal** (kar′pal): wrist
- **cervical** (ser′vĭ-kal): neck region
- **coxal** (kox′al): hip
- **crural** (kroo′ral): leg
- **digital** (dij′ĭ-tal): fingers, toes
- **femoral** (fem′or-al): thigh
- **fibular** (fib′u-lar): lateral part of leg
- **inguinal** (in′gwĭ-nal): area where thigh meets body trunk; groin
- **nasal** (na′zul): nose area
- **oral** (o′ral): mouth
- **orbital** (or′bĭ-tal): eye area
- **patellar** (pah-tel′er): anterior knee
- **pelvic** (pel′vik): area overlying the pelvis anteriorly
- **pubic** (pu′bik): genital region
- **sternal** (ster′nul): breastbone area
- **tarsal** (tar′sal): ankle region
- **thoracic** (tho-ras′ik): chest
- **umbilical** (um-bil′ĭ-kal): navel

Q *Study this figure for a moment to answer these two questions. Where would you hurt if you (1) pulled a groin muscle or (2) cracked a bone in your olecranal area?*

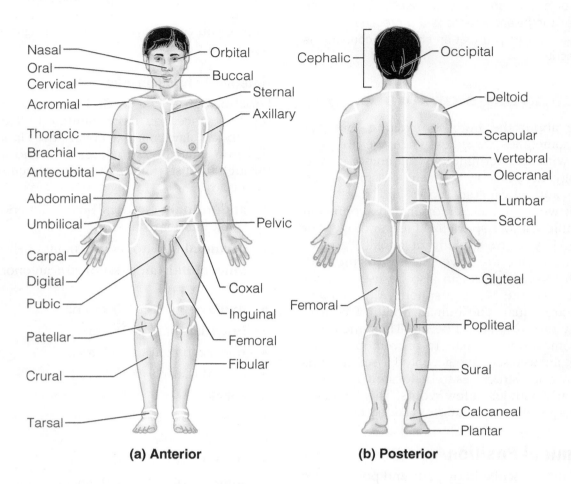

Nasal — — Orbital
Oral — — Buccal
Cervical —
Acromial — — Sternal
— Axillary
Thoracic —
Brachial —
Antecubital —
Abdominal —
Umbilical —
— Pelvic
Carpal —
Digital —
Pubic —
— Coxal
— Inguinal
Patellar —
— Femoral
— Fibular
Crural —

Tarsal —

Cephalic — — Occipital
— Deltoid
— Scapular
— Vertebral
— Olecranal
— Lumbar
— Sacral
Femoral —
— Gluteal
— Popliteal
— Sural
— Calcaneal
— Plantar

(a) Anterior　　　　　**(b) Posterior**

FIGURE 1.5   Surface anatomy: Regional terms. (a) Anterior body landmarks. **(b)** Posterior body landmarks. The heels are raised slightly to show the inferior plantar surface (sole) of the foot.

Posterior Body Landmarks

Identify the following body regions in Figure 1.5b, and then locate them on yourself without referring to this book.

- **calcaneal** (kal-ka′neul): heel of foot
- **cephalic** (seh-fǎ′lik): head
- **deltoid** (del′toyd): curve of shoulder formed by large deltoid muscle

- **femoral** (fem′or-al): thigh
- **gluteal** (gloo′te-al): buttock
- **lumbar** (lum′bar): area of back between ribs and hips
- **occipital** (ok-sip′ĭ-tal): posterior surface of head
- **olecranal** (ol-eh-cra′nel): posterior surface of elbow
- **popliteal** (pop-lit′e-al): posterior knee area
- **sacral** (sa′krul): area between hips
- **scapular** (skap′u-lar): shoulder blade region

A
(1) Your inguinal area. (2) Your posterior elbow region.

- **sural** (soo'ral): the posterior surface of lower leg; the calf
- **vertebral** (ver'tĕ-bral): area of spine

The **plantar** region, or the sole of the foot, actually on the inferior body surface, is illlustrated along with the posterior body landmarks in Figure 1.5b.

Directional Terms

Directional terms used by medical personnel and anatomists allow them to explain exactly where one body structure is in relation to another. For example, we can describe the relationship between the ears and the nose informally by saying, "The ears are located on each side of the head to the right and left of the nose." Using anatomical terminology, this condenses to, "The ears are lateral to the nose." Thus, using anatomical terminology saves a good deal of description and, once learned, is much clearer. Commonly used directional terms are defined and illustrated in Table 1.1. Although most of these terms are also used in everyday conversation, keep in mind that their anatomical meanings are very precise.

Before continuing, take a minute to check your understanding of what you have read in Table 1.1. Give the relationship between the following body parts using the correct anatomical terms.

The wrist is _____ to the hand.

The breastbone is _____ to the spine.

The brain is _____ to the spinal cord.

The lungs are _____ to the stomach.

The thumb is _____ to the fingers. (Be careful here. Remember the anatomical position.)

Body Planes and Sections

When preparing to look at the internal structures of the body, medical students find it necessary to make a **section,** or cut. When the section is made through the body wall or through an organ, it is made along an imaginary line called a **plane.** Since the body is three-dimensional, we can refer to three types of planes or sections that lie at right angles to one another (Figure 1.6).

A **sagittal** (saj'ĭ-tal) **section** is a cut made along the lengthwise, or longitudinal, plane of the body, dividing the body into right and left parts. If the cut is made down the median plane of the body and the right and left parts are equal in size, it is called a **midsagittal,** or **median, section.**

A **frontal section** is a cut made along a lengthwise plane that divides the body (or an organ) into anterior and posterior parts. It is also called a **coronal** (ko-ro'nal) **section.**

A **transverse section** is a cut made along a horizontal plane, dividing the body or organ into superior and inferior parts. It is also called a **cross section.**

Sectioning a body or one of its organs along different planes often results in very different views. For example, a transverse section of the body trunk at the level of the kidneys would show kidney structure in cross section very nicely; a frontal section of the body trunk would show a different view of kidney anatomy; and a midsagittal section would miss the kidneys completely. Information on body organ positioning that can be gained by taking magnetic resonance imaging (MRI) scans along different body planes is illustrated in Figure 1.6. (MRI scans are described further in the "A Closer Look" box on medical imaging later in this chapter.)

Body Cavities

Anatomy and physiology textbooks typically describe two sets of internal cavities that provide different degrees of protection to the organs within them (Figure 1.7). These cavities differ in their mode of embryological development and purpose and in their lining membranes. Consequently, the dorsal, or neural, body cavity is not named as an internal body cavity in many anatomical references. However, the idea of two major sets of internal body cavities is a useful learning concept and will continue to be used here.

Dorsal Body Cavity

The **dorsal body cavity** has two subdivisions, which are continuous with each other. The **cranial cavity** is the space inside the bony skull. The brain is well protected because it occupies the cranial cavity. The **spinal cavity** extends from the cranial cavity nearly to the end of the vertebral column. The spinal cord, which is a continuation of the brain, is protected by the vertebrae, which surround the spinal cavity.

| TABLE 1.1 | Orientation and Directional Terms | | |

Term	Definition	Illustration	Example
Superior (cranial or cephalad)	Toward the head end or upper part of a structure or the body; above		The forehead is superior to the nose.
Inferior (caudal)†	Away from the head end or toward the lower part of a structure or the body; below		The navel is inferior to the breastbone.
Anterior (ventral)*	Toward or at the front of the body; in front of		The breastbone is anterior to the spine.
Posterior (dorsal)*	Toward or at the backside of the body; behind		The heart is posterior to the breastbone.
Medial	Toward or at the midline of the body; on the inner side of		The heart is medial to the arm.
Lateral	Away from the midline of the body; on the outer side of		The arms are lateral to the chest.
Intermediate	Between a more medial and a more lateral structure		The armpit is intermediate between the breastbone and shoulder.
Proximal	Close to the origin of the body part or the point of attachment of a limb to the body trunk		The elbow is proximal to the wrist (meaning that the elbow is closer to the shoulder or attachment point of the arm than the wrist is).
Distal	Farther from the origin of a body part or the point of attachment of a limb to the body trunk		The knee is distal to the thigh.
Superficial (external)	Toward or at the body surface		The skin is superficial to the skeleton.
Deep (internal)	Away from the body surface; more internal		The lungs are deep to the rib cage.

†The term *caudal*, literally "toward the tail," is synonymous with *inferior* only to the inferior end of the spine.

Ventral and *anterior* are synonymous in humans; this is not the case in four-legged animals. *Ventral* refers to the "belly" of an animal and thus is the inferior surface of four-legged animals. Likewise, although the dorsal and posterior surfaces are the same in humans, the term *dorsal* refers to an animal's back. Thus, the dorsal surface of four-legged animals is their superior surface.

Q *Which section type would separate the two eyes?*

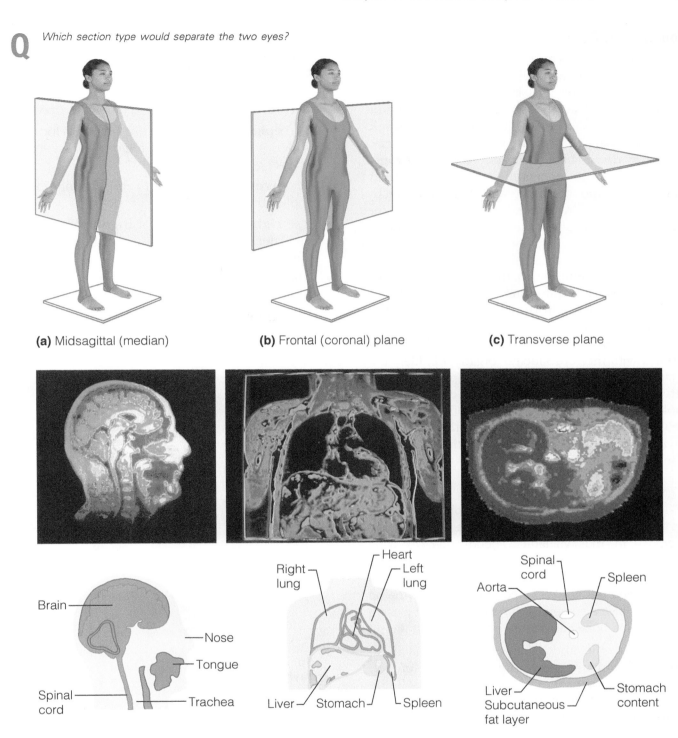

(a) Midsagittal (median)   **(b)** Frontal (coronal) plane   **(c)** Transverse plane

Brain
Nose
Tongue
Spinal cord
Trachea

Right lung
Heart
Left lung
Liver — Stomach — Spleen

Spinal cord
Aorta
Spleen
Liver
Subcutaneous fat layer
Stomach content

FIGURE 1.6 The anatomical position and planes of the body. The top row of the figure illustrates three major planes of space (midsagittal, frontal, and transverse) relative to humans in the anatomical position. Selected areas of the body, visualized using MRI scans taken at corresponding planes, are illustrated in the center row. Diagrams identifying body organs seen in the MRI scans are at the bottom.

A *A midsagittal section would separate the two eyes.*

Ventral Body Cavity

The **ventral body cavity** is much larger than the dorsal cavity. It contains all the structures within the chest and abdomen, that is, the visceral organs in those regions. Like the dorsal cavity, the ventral body cavity is subdivided. The superior **thoracic cavity** is separated from the rest of the ventral cavity by a dome-shaped muscle, the **diaphragm** (di'ah-fram). The organs in the thoracic cavity (lungs, heart, and others) are somewhat protected by the rib cage. A central region called the **mediastinum** separates the lungs into right and left cavities in the thoracic cavity. The mediastinum itself houses the heart, trachea, and other visceral organs.

The cavity inferior to the diaphragm is the **abdominopelvic** (ab-dom"ĭ-no-pel'vik) **cavity.** Some prefer to subdivide it into a superior **abdominal cavity,** containing the stomach, liver, intestines, and other organs, and an inferior **pelvic cavity,** with the reproductive organs, bladder, and rectum. However, there is no actual physical structure dividing the abdominopelvic cavity. If you look carefully at Figure 1.7, you will see that the pelvic cavity is not continuous with the abdominal cavity in a straight plane, but that it tips away from it in the posterior direction.

Homeostatic Imbalance

When the body is subjected to physical trauma (as often happens in an automobile accident, for example), the most vulnerable abdominopelvic organs are those within the abdominal cavity, because the cavity walls of that portion are formed only of trunk muscles and are not reinforced by bone. The pelvic organs receive a somewhat greater degree of protection from the bony pelvis in which they reside.

Because the abdominopelvic cavity is quite large and contains many organs, it is helpful to divide it up into smaller areas for study. A scheme commonly used by medical personnel divides the abdominopelvic cavity into four more or less equal regions called *quadrants*. The quadrants are then simply named according to their relative positions—that is, right upper quadrant, right lower quadrant, left upper quadrant, and left lower quadrant (Figure 1.8a).

Another system, used mainly by anatomists, divides the abdominopelvic cavity into nine separate *regions* by four planes, as shown in Figure 1.8b. Although the names of the nine regions are unfamiliar to you now, with a little patience and study,

they will become easier to remember. As you locate these regions in the figure, notice the organs they contain by referring to Figure 1.8c.

- The **umbilical region** is the centermost region, deep to and surrounding the umbilicus (navel).
- The **epigastric** (ep"ĭ-gas'trik) **region** is located superior to the umbilical region (*epi* = upon, above; *gastric* = stomach).
- The **hypogastric (pubic) region** is inferior to the umbilical region (*hypo* = below).
- The **right** and **left iliac,** or **inguinal, regions** are lateral to the hypogastric region (*iliac* = superior part of the hip bone).
- The **right** and **left lumbar regions** lie lateral to the umbilical region (*lumbus* = loin).
- The **right** and **left hypochondriac** (hi"po-kon'dre-ak) **regions** flank the epigastric region and contain the lower ribs (*chondro* = cartilage).

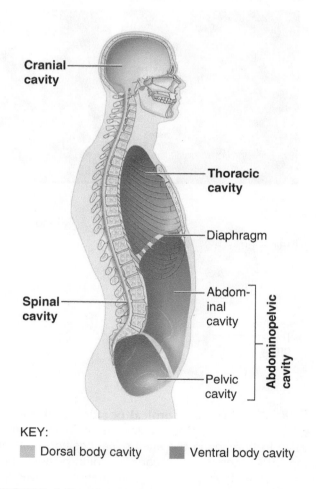

KEY:
▨ Dorsal body cavity   ▨ Ventral body cavity

FIGURE 1.7 Body cavities. Notice the angular relationship between the abdominal and pelvic cavities.

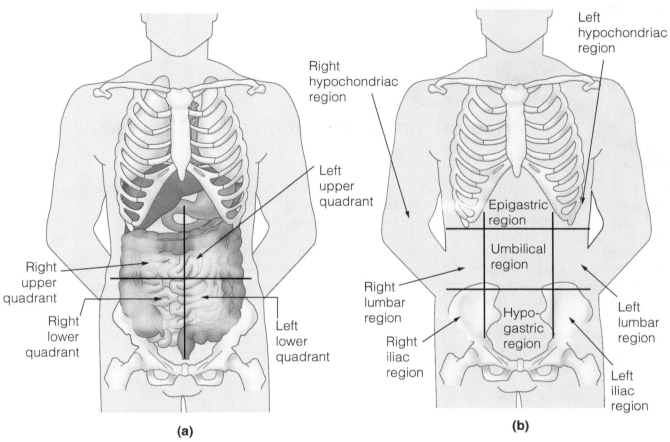

(a)

FIGURE 1.8 **Abdominopelvic surface and cavity.** **(a)** The four quadrants. **(b)** Nine regions delineated by four planes. The superior horizontal plane is at the inferior aspect of the ribs; the inferior horizontal plane is at the superior aspect of the hip bones, and the vertical planes are just medial to the nipples. **(c)** Anterior view of the ventral body cavity showing superficial organs.

(b)

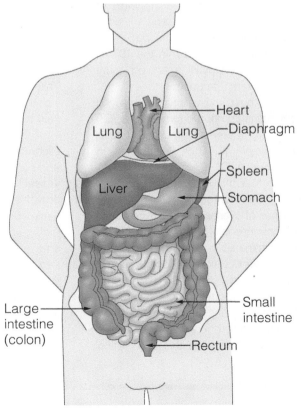

(c)

A Closer Look

Medical Imaging: Illuminating the Body

BY bombarding the body with energy, new scanning techniques can reveal the structure of internal organs and wring out information about the private and, until now, secret working of their molecules. These new imaging techniques are changing the face of medical diagnosis.

Until about 50 years ago, the magical but murky X-ray was the only means of peering into a living body. What X-rays did and still do best was visualize hard, bony structures and locate abnormally dense structures (tumors, tuberculosis nodules) in the lungs. The 1950s saw the birth of nuclear medicine, which uses radioisotopes to scan the body, and ultrasound techniques. In the 1970s, CT, PET, and MRI scanning techniques were introduced.

The best known of new imaging devices is *computed tomography (CT)* (formerly called *computerized axial tomography [CAT]*), a refined version of X-ray. A CT scanner confines its beam to a thin slice of the body and ends the confusion resulting from images of overlapping structures seen in conventional X-ray. CT's clarity has all but eliminated exploratory surgery. As the patient is slowly moved through the doughnut-shaped CT machine, its X-ray tube rotates around the body. Different tissues absorb the radiation in varying amounts. The device's computer translates this information into a detailed, cross-sectional picture of the body region scanned. CT scans are at the forefront in evaluating most problems that affect the brain (see photo a), abdomen, and calcification of the coronary arteries in those at an elevated risk for heart disease. Special ultrafast CT scanners have produced a technique called *dynamic spatial reconstruction (DSR)*, which provides three-dimensional images of body organs from any angle. It also allows their movements and changes in their internal volumes to be observed at normal speed, in slow motion, and at a specific moment in time. Although DSR can be used to evaluate the lungs and certain other mobile organs, its greatest value has been to visualize the heart beating and blood flowing through blood vessels. This allows heart defects, constricted blood vessels, and the status of coronary bypass grafts to be assessed.

Another computer-assisted X-ray technique is *digital subtraction angiography (DSA)* (angiography = vessel pictures). This technique provides an unobstructed view of diseased blood vessels. Conventional radiographs are taken before and after a contrast medium is injected into an artery. Then the computer subtracts the "before" image from the "after" image, eliminating all traces of body structures that obscure the vessel. DSA is often used to identify blockages in the arteries that supply the heart wall and the brain (photo b).

Just as the X-ray spawned "new technologies," so did nuclear medicine in the form of *positron emission tomography (PET)*. PET excels in observing metabolic processes. PET's greatest clinical value has been its ability to provide insights into brain activity in those affected by mental illness, Alzheimer's disease, and epilepsy. One of its most exciting uses is to determine which areas of the healthy brain are most active during certain tasks (speaking, listening to music, and so on). The patient is given an injection of short-lived radioisotopes that have been tagged to biological molecules (such as glucose) and then positioned in the PET scanner. As the radioisotopes are absorbed by the most active brain cells, high-energy gamma rays are produced. The computer analyzes the gamma emission and produces a picture of the brain's biochemical activity in vivid colors.

Ultrasound imaging, or *ultrasonography*, has distinct advantages over the approaches described so far: the equipment is inexpensive and it employs high-frequency sound waves (ultrasound) as its energy source. Ultrasound, unlike ionizing forms of radiation, has no harmful effects on living tissues (as far as we know). The body is probed with pulses of sound waves, which cause

Medical Imaging: Illuminating the Body *(continued)*

echos when reflected and scattered by body tissues. The echoes are analyzed by computer to construct visual images of body organs of interest. Because of its safety, ultrasound is the imaging technique of choice for obstetrics, that is, for determining fetal age and position and locating the placenta. Because sound waves have very low penetrating power and are rapidly scattered in air, ultrasonography is of little value for looking at air-filled structures (the lungs) or those surrounded by bone (the brain and spinal cord).

Another technique that depends on nonionizing radiation is *magnetic resonance imaging (MRI)*, which uses magnetic fields up to 60,000 times stronger than the Earth's to pry information from the body's tissues. The patient lies in a chamber within a huge magnet. Hydrogen molecules spin like tops in the magnetic field, and their energy is enhanced by radio waves. When the radio waves are turned off, the energy is released and translated by the computer into a visual image. MRI is immensely popular because it can do many things a CT scan cannot. Dense structures do not show up in MRI, so bones of the skull and/or vertebral column do not impair the view of *soft tissues* such as the brain (see Figure 1.6a, p. 15). MRI is also particularly good at detecting degenerative disease of various kinds. Multiple sclerosis plaques, for example, do not show up well in CT scans but are dazzlingly

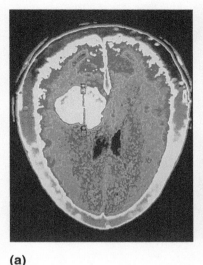

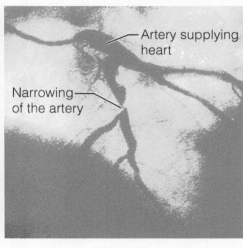

(a)   **(b)**

Two different methods for illuminating the body. **(a)** CT scan showing a brain tumor (oval area on right side of brain). **(b)** DSA image of arteries supplying the heart.

clear in MRI scans. A key issue being investigated by MRI studies is how brain development and behavior change with growth or experience.

A newer variation of MRI, called *magnetic resonance spectroscopy (MRS)*, maps the distribution of elements other than hydrogen to reveal more about how disease changes body chemistry. In 1992, MRI technology leaped forward with the development of the *functional MRI*, which allows tracking of blood flow into the brain in real time. Until then, matching thoughts, deeds, and disease to corresponding brain activity had been the sole domain of PET. Because functional MRI does not require injections of tracer elements, it provides another, perhaps more

desirable, alternative to such studies. Despite its advantages, the powerful magnets of the MRI present some problems. For example they can "suck" metal objects, such as implanted pacemakers and loose tooth fillings, through the body. Also, there is no convincing evidence that such magnetic fields are risk free.

As you can see, modern medical science has many remarkable tools at its disposal. CT and PET scans account for about 25 percent of all imaging. Ultrasonography, because of its safety and low cost, is the most widespread of the new techniques. Conventional X-rays remain the workhorse of diagnostic imaging techniques and still account for more than half of all imaging currently done.

Unit 2
Chemical Basis of Life

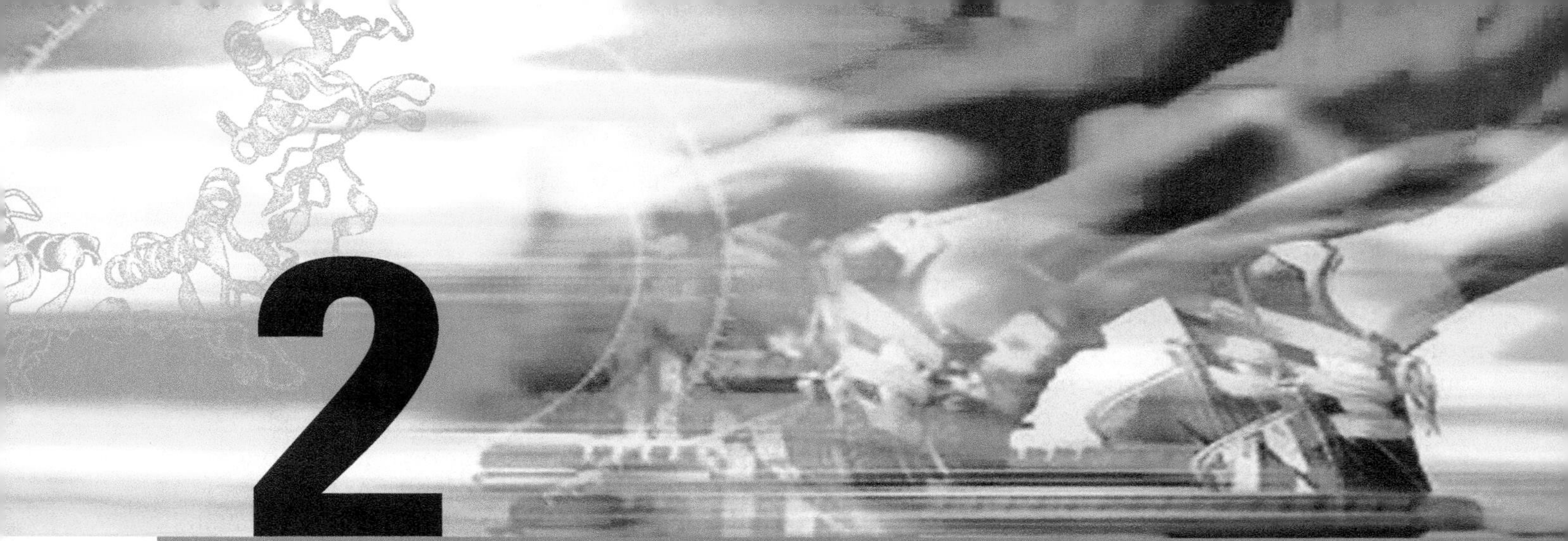

2

Basic Chemistry

KEY TERMS

- element, p. 22
- atom, p. 22
- isotope, p. 25
- compound, p. 26
- ion, p. 27
- salt, p. 27
- catalyst, p. 32
- inorganic compound, p. 32
- organic compound, p. 32
- solution, p. 33
- electrolyte, p. 33

Many short courses in anatomy and physiology lack the time to consider chemistry as a topic. So why include it here? Very simply, the food you eat and the medicines you take when you are ill are composed of chemicals. Indeed, your entire body is made up of chemicals—thousands of them—continuously interacting with one another at an incredible pace.

Although it is possible to study anatomy without much reference to chemistry, chemical reactions underlie all body processes—movement, digestion, the pumping of your heart, and even your thoughts. This chapter presents the basics of chemistry and biochemistry (the chemistry of living material), providing the background you will need to understand body functions.

Matter

Matter is the "stuff" of the universe. With some exceptions, it can be seen, smelled, and felt. More precisely, matter is anything that occupies space and has mass (weight). Chemistry studies the nature of matter—how its building blocks are put together and how they interact.

Energy

In contrast to matter, **energy** is weightless and does not take up space. It can only be measured by its effects on matter. Energy is commonly defined as the ability to do work or to put matter into motion.

Forms of Energy

- **Chemical energy** is stored in the bonds of chemical substances. When the bonds are broken, the (potential) stored energy is unleashed and becomes kinetic energy (energy in action). For example, when gasoline molecules are broken apart in your automobile engine, the energy released powers your car. In like manner, all body activities are "run" by the chemical energy harvested from the foods we eat.

- **Mechanical energy** is *directly* involved in moving matter. When you ride a bicycle, your legs provide the mechanical energy that moves the pedals. We can take this example one step further back: As the muscles in your legs shorten, they pull on your bones, causing

your limbs to move (so that you can pedal the bike).

Energy Form Conversions

With a few exceptions, energy is easily converted from one form to another. For example, an electrical current carried to a lamp socket is converted into light energy by the bulb. In the body, chemical energy of foods is trapped in the bonds of a high-energy chemical called ATP (adenosine triphosphate), and ATP's energy may ultimately be transformed into the electrical energy of a nerve impulse or mechanical energy of shortening muscles.

All energy conversions that occur in the body liberate heat. It is this heat that makes us warm-blooded animals and contributes to our relatively high body temperature, which has an important influence on body functioning.

Elements and Atomic Structure

All matter is composed of a limited number of substances called **elements,** unique substances (atoms) that cannot be broken down into simpler substances by ordinary chemical methods. Examples of elements include many commonly known substances, such as oxygen, carbon, gold, copper, and iron.

So far, 112 elements are known with certainty, and numbers 113 to 116 are alleged. Ninety-two of these occur naturally; the rest are produced artificially in accelerator devices. Four elements—carbon, oxygen, hydrogen, and nitrogen—make up about 96 percent of body weight, but several others are present in small or trace amounts. A complete listing of the elements appears in the **periodic table,** studied in chemistry classrooms the world over. The most abundant elements found in the body and their major roles are listed in Table 2.1.

The building block of an element, or the smallest particle that still retains its special properties, is called an **atom.** Because all elements are unique, the atoms of each element differ from those of all other elements. Each element is designated by a one- or two-letter chemical shorthand called an **atomic symbol.** In most cases, the atomic symbol is simply the first (or first two) letter(s) of the element's name. For example, C stands for carbon,

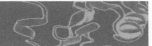

TABLE 2.1		Common Elements Making Up the Human Body	
Element	**Atomic symbol**	**Percentage of body mass**	**Role**
Major (96.1%)			
Oxygen	O	65.0	A major component of both organic and inorganic molecules; as a gas, essential to the oxidation of glucose and other food fuels, during which cellular energy (ATP) is produced.
Carbon	C	18.5	The primary elemental component of all organic molecules, including carbohydrates, lipids, proteins, and nucleic acids.
Hydrogen	H	9.5	A component of most organic molecules; in ionic form, influences the pH of body fluids.
Nitrogen	N	3.2	A component of proteins and nucleic acids (genetic material).
Lesser (3.9%)			
Calcium	Ca	1.5	Found as a salt in bones and teeth; in ionic form, required for muscle contraction, neural transmission, and blood clotting.
Phosphorus	P	1.0	Present as a salt, in combination with calcium, in bones and teeth; also present in nucleic acids and many proteins; forms part of the high-energy compound ATP.
Potassium	K	0.4	In its ionic form, the major intracellular cation; necessary for the conduction of nerve impulses and for muscle contraction.
Sulfur	S	0.3	A component of proteins (particularly contractile proteins of muscle).
Sodium	Na	0.2	As an ion, the major extracellular cation; important for water balance, conduction of nerve impulses, and muscle contraction.
Chlorine	Cl	0.2	In ionic form, a major extracellular anion.
Magnesium	Mg	0.1	Present in bone; also an important cofactor for enzyme activity in a number of metabolic reactions.
Iodine	I	0.1	Needed to make functional thyroid hormones.
Iron	Fe	0.1	A component of the functional hemoglobin molecule (which transports oxygen within red blood cells) and some enzymes.

Trace (less than 0.01%)*

Chromium (Cr), Cobalt (Co), Copper (Cu), Fluorine (F), Manganese (Mn), Molybdenum (Mo), Selenium (Se), Silicon (Si), Tin (Sn), Vanadium (V), Zinc (Zn)

*Referred to as the *trace elements* because are required in very minute amounts; many found as part of enzymes or required for enzyme activation.

O for oxygen, and Ca for calcium. In a few cases, the atomic symbol is taken from the Latin name for the element. For instance, sodium is indicated by Na (from the Latin word *natrium*).

Structure of Atoms

The word *atom* comes from the Greek word meaning "incapable of being divided," and historically this idea of an atom was accepted as a scientific truth. According to this notion, you could theoretically divide a pure element, such as a block of gold, into smaller and smaller particles until you got down to the individual atoms, and then could subdivide no further. We now know that atoms, although indescribably small, are clusters of even smaller (subatomic) particles and that, under very special circumstances, atoms can be split into these smaller particles. Even so, the old idea of atomic indivisibility is still very appropriate, because an atom loses the unique properties of its element when it is split into its subparticles.

The atoms representing the 112-plus elements are composed of different numbers and proportions of three basic subatomic particles, which differ in their mass, electrical charge, and location within the atom (Table 2.2). **Protons (p^+)** have a positive charge, whereas **neutrons (n^0)** are uncharged, or neutral. Protons and neutrons are heavy particles and have approximately the same mass (1 atomic mass unit, or 1 amu). The tiny **electrons (e^-)** bear a negative charge equal in strength to the positive charge of the protons, but their mass is so small that it is usually designated as 0 amu.

The electrical charge of a particle is a measure of its ability to attract or repel other charged particles. Particles with the same type of charge (+ to + or − to −) repel each other, but particles with unlike charges (+ to −) attract each other. Neutral particles are neither attracted to nor repelled by charged particles.

Because all atoms are electrically neutral, the number of protons an atom has must be precisely balanced by its number of electrons (the + and − charges will then cancel the effect of each other). Thus, hydrogen has one proton and one electron, and iron has 26 protons and 26 electrons. For any atom, the number of protons and electrons is always equal. Atoms that have gained or lost electrons are called *ions*, as discussed shortly.

Hydrogen is the simplest atom, with just one proton and one electron. You can visualize the spatial relationships within the hydrogen atom by imagining it enlarged until its diameter equals the length of a football field. In that case, the nucleus could be represented by a lead ball the size of a gumdrop in the exact center of the sphere and the lone electron pictured as a fly buzzing about unpredictably within the sphere. This mental picture should serve to remind you that most of the volume of an atom is empty space, and nearly all of the mass is concentrated in the central nucleus.

All protons are alike, regardless of the atom being considered. The same is true of all neutrons and all electrons. So what determines the unique properties of each element? The answer is that atoms of different elements are composed of *different numbers* of protons, neutrons, and electrons.

TABLE 2.2	Subatomic Particles		
Particle	**Position in atom**	**Mass (amu)**	**Charge**
Proton (p^+)	Nucleus	1	+
Neutron (n^0)	Nucleus	1	0
Electron (e^-)	Orbitals outside the nucleus	1/1800	−

Q *Which of these isotopes is the heaviest?*

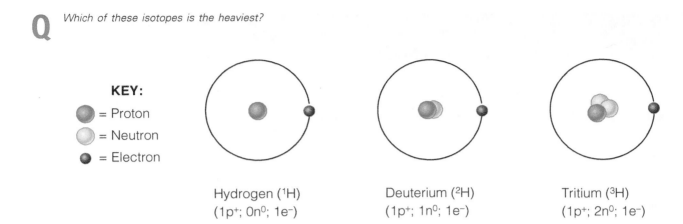

KEY:

● = Proton

○ = Neutron

● = Electron

Hydrogen (^{1}H)
($1p^+$; $0n^0$; $1e^-$)

Deuterium (^{2}H)
($1p^+$; $1n^0$; $1e^-$)

Tritium (^{3}H)
($1p^+$; $2n^0$; $1e^-$)

FIGURE 2.1   Isotopes of hydrogen.

All we need to know to identify a particular element is its atomic number, mass number, and atomic weight. Taken together, these indicators provide a fairly complete picture of each element.

Atomic Number

Each element is given a number, called its **atomic number,** that is equal to the number of protons its atoms contain. Atoms of each element contain a different number of protons than the atoms of any other element; hence, its atomic number is unique. Because the number of protons is always equal to the number of electrons, the atomic number *indirectly* also tells us the number of electrons that atom contains.

Atomic Mass Number and Atomic Weight

The **atomic mass number** of any atom is the sum of the protons and neutrons contained in its nucleus. (The mass of the electrons is so small that it is ignored.) Hydrogen has one bare proton and no neutrons in its nucleus; thus, its atomic number and atomic mass number are the same (1). Helium, with 2 protons and 2 neutrons, has a mass number of 4. The atomic mass number is written as a superscript to the left of the atomic symbol (see the examples in Figure 2.1).

Atomic Weight and Isotopes

At first glance, it would seem that the **atomic weight** of an atom should be equal to its atomic mass. This would be so if there were only one type of atom representing each element. However, the atoms of almost all elements exhibit two or more structural variations; these varieties are called **isotopes** (i′so-tōps). Isotopes have the same number of protons and electrons but vary in the number of *neutrons* they contain. Thus, the isotopes of an element have the same atomic number but have different atomic masses. The atomic numbers, mass numbers, and atomic weights for elements commonly found in the body are provided in Table 2.3.

The heavier isotopes of certain atoms are unstable and tend to decompose to become more stable; such isotopes are called **radioisotopes.**

Radioisotopes are used in minute amounts to tag biological molecules so that they can be followed, or traced, through the body and are valuable tools for medical diagnosis and treatment. For example, PET scans, which use radioisotopes, are used to study brain activity. Additionally, a radioisotope of iodine can be used to scan the thyroid gland of a patient suspected of having a thyroid tumor. Radium, cobalt, and certain other radioisotopes are used to destroy localized cancers.

Molecules and Compounds

When two or more atoms combine chemically, **molecules** are formed. If two or more atoms of

A   *Tritium.*

TABLE 2.3   Atomic Structures of the Most Abundant Elements in the Body

Element	Symbol	Atomic number (# of p)	Mass number (# of p + n)	Atomic weight	Electrons in valence shell
Calcium	Ca	20	40	40.08	2
Carbon	C	6	12	12.011	4
Chlorine	Cl	17	35	35.453	7
Hydrogen	H	1	1	1.008	1
Iodine	I	53	127	126.905	7
Iron	Fe	26	56	55.847	2
Magnesium	Mg	12	24	24.305	2
Nitrogen	N	7	14	14.007	5
Oxygen	O	8	16	15.999	6
Phosphorus	P	15	31	30.974	5
Sodium	Na	11	23	22.99	1
Sulfur	S	16	32	32.064	6

the same element bond together, a molecule of that element is produced. For example, when two hydrogen atoms bond, the product is a molecule of hydrogen gas:

$$2H \text{ (atom)} + O \text{ (atom)} \rightarrow H_2O \text{ (molecule)}^*$$

In the example given, the atoms taking part in the reaction are indicated by their atomic symbols, and the composition of the product is indicated by a *molecular formula* (H_2O) that shows its atomic makeup. The chemical reaction is shown by writing a *chemical equation:* $H + 2O = H_2O$.

When two or more *different* atoms bind together to form a molecule, the molecule is more specifically referred to as a molecule of a **compound.** For example, four hydrogen atoms and one carbon atom can interact chemically to form methane:

---

*Notice that when the number of atoms is written as a subscript, the subscript indicates that the atoms are joined by a chemical bond. Thus, 2H represents two unjoined atoms, but H_2 indicates that the two hydrogen atoms are bonded together to form a molecule.

$$4H + C = CH_4 \text{ (methane)}$$

It is important to understand that compounds always have properties quite different from those of the atoms making them up, and it would be next to impossible to determine the atoms making up a compound without analyzing it chemically. Notice that just as an atom is the smallest particle of an element that still retains that element's properties, a molecule is the smallest particle of a compound that still retains the properties of that compound. If you break the bonds between the atoms of the compound, properties of the atoms, rather than those of the compound, will be exhibited.

Chemical Bonds and Chemical Reactions

Chemical reactions occur whenever atoms combine with or dissociate from other atoms. When atoms unite chemically, chemical bonds are formed.

Bond Formation

It is important to understand that a chemical bond is not an actual physical structure, like a pair of handcuffs linking two people together. Instead, it is an energy relationship that involves interactions between the electrons of the reacting atoms.

Types of Chemical Bonds

Ionic Bonds   **Ionic** (i-on′ik) **bonds** form when electrons are completely transferred from one atom to another. Atoms are electrically neutral, but when they gain or lose electrons during bonding, their positive and negative charges are no longer balanced, and charged particles, called **ions,** result. When an atom gains an electron, it acquires a net negative charge because it now has more electrons than protons. Negatively charged ions are more specifically called *anions*. When an atom loses an electron, it becomes a positively charged ion, a *cation,* because it now possesses more protons than electrons. (It may help you to remember that a cation is a positively charged ion by thinking of its "t" as a plus [+] sign.) Both anions and cations result when an ionic bond is formed. Since opposite charges attract, the newly created ions tend to stay close together.

The formation of sodium chloride (NaCl), common table salt, provides a good example of ionic bonding. As illustrated in Figure 2.2, sodium's valence shell contains only 1 electron and so is incomplete. However, if this single electron is "lost" to another atom, shell 2, which contains 8 electrons, becomes the valence shell; thus sodium becomes a cation (Na^+) and achieves stability. Chlorine needs only 1 electron to fill its valence shell, and it is much easier to gain 1 electron (forming Cl^-) than it is to try to "give away" 7. Thus, the ideal situation is for sodium to donate its valence-shell electron to chlorine, and this is exactly what happens in the interaction between these two atoms. Sodium chloride and most other compounds formed by ionic bonding fall into the general category of chemicals called **salts.**

Covalent Bonds   Electrons do not have to be completely lost or gained for atoms to become stable. Instead, they can be shared in such a way that each atom is able to fill its valence shell at least part of the time.

Molecules in which atoms share electrons are called *covalent molecules,* and their bonds are **covalent bonds** (*co* = with; *valent* = having power). For example, hydrogen, with its single electron, can become stable if it fills its valence shell (energy level 1) by sharing a pair of electrons—its own and one from another atom. As shown in Figure 2.3a, a hydrogen atom can share an electron pair with another hydrogen atom to

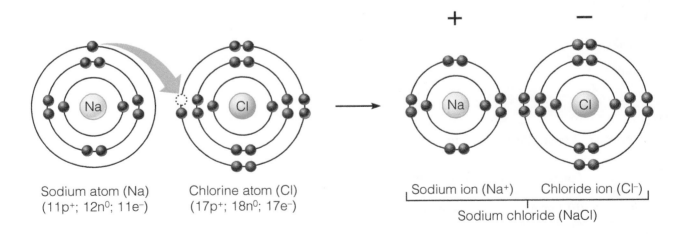

Sodium atom (Na)
(11p+; 12n0; 11e−)

Chlorine atom (Cl)
(17p+; 18n0; 17e−)

Sodium ion (Na+)   Chloride ion (Cl-)

Sodium chloride (NaCl)

FIGURE 2.2   Formation of an ionic bond. Both sodium and chlorine atoms are chemically reactive because their valence shells are incompletely filled. Sodium gains stability by losing one electron, whereas chlorine becomes stable by gaining one electron. After electron transfer, sodium becomes a sodium ion (Na+), and chlorine becomes a chloride ion (Cl−). The oppositely charged ions attract each other.

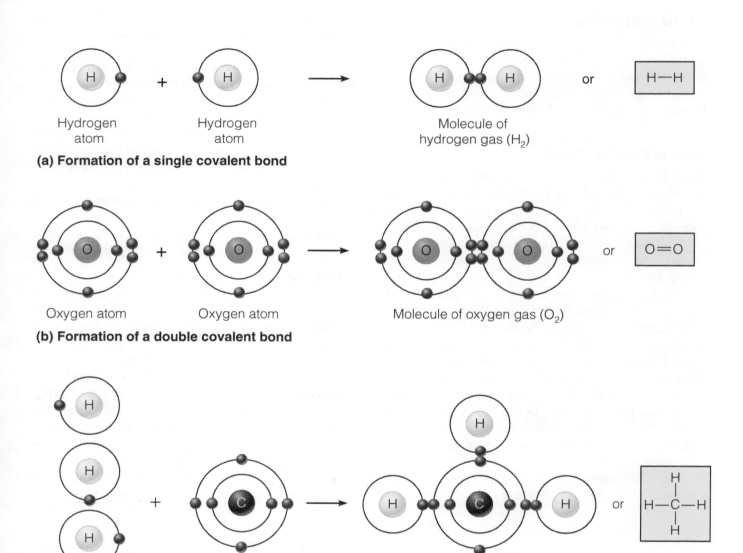

(a) **Formation of a single covalent bond**

(b) **Formation of a double covalent bond**

(c) **Formation of four single covalent bonds**

FIGURE 2.3 **Formation of covalent bonds. (a)** Formation of a single covalent bond between two hydrogen atoms to form a molecule of hydrogen gas. **(b)** Formation of a molecule of oxygen gas. Each oxygen atom shares two electron pairs with its partner; thus, a double covalent bond is formed. **(c)** Formation of a molecule of methane. A carbon atom shares four electron pairs with four hydrogen atoms. In the diagrams of molecules shown in the colored boxes at the far right, each pair of shared electrons is indicated by a single line between the sharing atoms.

form a molecule of hydrogen gas. The shared electron pair orbits the whole molecule and satisfies the stability needs of both hydrogen atoms. Likewise, 2 oxygen atoms, each with 6 valence-shell electrons, can share 2 pairs of electrons (form double bonds) with each other (Figure 2.3b) to form a molecule of oxygen gas (O_2).

A hydrogen atom may also share its electron with an atom of a different element. Carbon has 4 valence-shell electrons but needs 8 to achieve stability. As shown in Figure 2.3c, when methane (CH_4) is formed, carbon shares 4 electron pairs with 4 hydrogen atoms (1 pair with each hydrogen atom). Because the shared electrons orbit and "belong to" the whole molecule, each atom has a full valence shell enough of the time to satisfy its stability needs.

In the covalent molecules described thus far, electrons have been shared *equally* between the atoms of the molecule. Such molecules are called *nonpolar covalently bonded molecules*. However, electrons are not shared equally in all cases. When covalent bonds are made, the molecule formed always has a definite three-dimensional shape. A molecule's shape plays a major role in determining just what other molecules (or atoms) it can interact with; the shape may also result in unequal electron-pair sharing. The following two examples illustrate this principle (Figure 2.4).

Carbon dioxide is formed when a carbon atom shares its 4 valence-shell electrons with 2 oxygen atoms. Oxygen is a very electron-hungry atom and

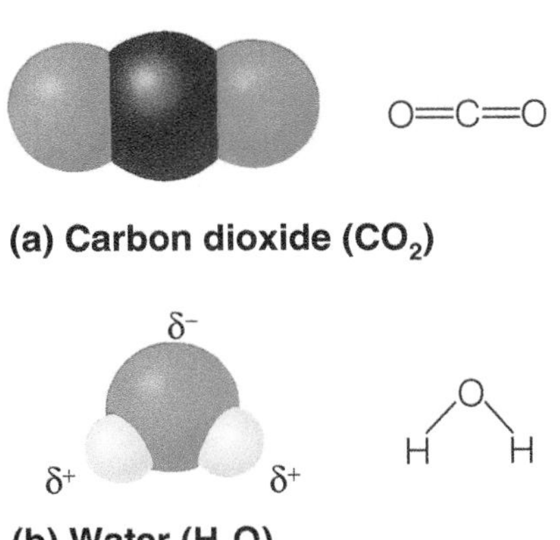

(a) Carbon dioxide (CO_2)

(b) Water (H_2O)

FIGURE 2.4 Molecular models illustrating the three-dimensional structure of carbon dioxide and water molecules.

attracts the shared electrons much more strongly than does carbon. However, because the carbon dioxide molecule is linear (O=C=O), the electron-pulling power of one oxygen atom is offset by that of the other, like a tug-of-war at a standoff. As a result, the electron pairs are shared equally and orbit the entire molecule, and carbon dioxide is a nonpolar molecule.

A water molecule is formed when 2 hydrogen atoms bind covalently to a single oxygen atom. Each hydrogen atom shares an electron pair with the oxygen atom, and again, the oxygen has the stronger electron-attracting ability. But in this case, the molecule formed is V-shaped (H\O/H). The two hydrogen atoms are located at one end of the molecule, and the oxygen atom is at the other. Consequently, the electron pairs are not shared equally and spend more time in the vicinity of the oxygen atom, causing that end of the molecule to become slightly more negative (indicated by δ^-) and the hydrogen end to become slightly more positive (indicated by δ^+). In other words, a *polar molecule,* a molecule with two charged *poles,* is formed.

Polar molecules orient themselves toward other polar molecules or charged particles (ions, proteins, and others), and they play an important role in chemical reactions that occur in body cells. Because body tissues are 60 to 80 percent water, the fact that water is a polar molecule is particularly significant, as will be described shortly.

Hydrogen Bonds **Hydrogen bonds** are extremely weak bonds formed when a hydrogen atom bound to one electron-hungry nitrogen or oxygen atom is attracted by another electron-hungry atom, and the hydrogen atom forms a "bridge" between them. Hydrogen bonding is common between water molecules (Figure 2.5a) and is reflected in water's surface tension. The surface tension of water causes it to "ball up," or form spheres, when it sits on a surface and allows some insects, such as water striders (Figure 2.5b), to walk on water as long as they tread lightly.

Hydrogen bonds are also important *intramolecular bonds;* that is, they help to bind different parts of the *same* molecule together into a special three-dimensional shape. These rather fragile bonds are very important in helping to maintain the structure of protein molecules, which are essential functional molecules and body-building materials.

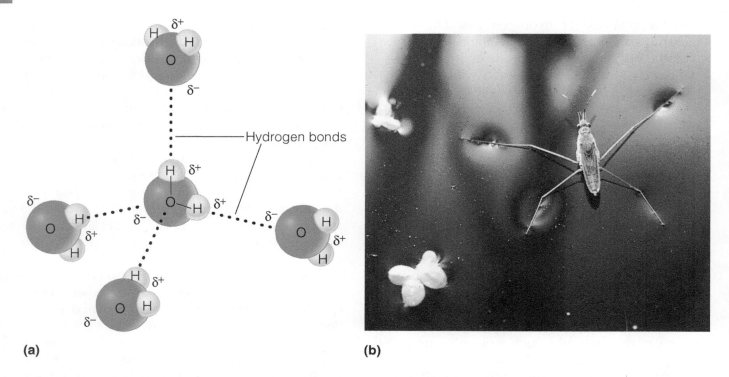

FIGURE 2.5 Hydrogen bonding between polar water molecules.
(a) The slightly positive ends (indicated by δ^+) of the water molecules
become aligned with the slightly negative ends (indicated by δ^-) of other
water molecules. **(b)** Water's high surface tension, a result of the combined
strength of its hydrogen bonds, allows a water strider to walk on a pond
without breaking the surface.

Patterns of Chemical Reactions

Chemical reactions involve the making or breaking
of bonds between atoms. The total number of
atoms remains the same, but the atoms appear
in new combinations. Most chemical reactions have
one of the three recognizable patterns described
next.

Synthesis Reactions

Synthesis reactions occur when two or more
atoms or molecules combine to form a larger, more
complex molecule, which can be simply represented as

$$A + B \rightarrow AB$$

Synthesis reactions always involve bond formation.
Because energy must be absorbed to make bonds,
synthesis reactions are energy-absorbing reactions.

Synthesis reactions underlie all anabolic or
constructive activities that occur in body cells.
They are particularly important for growth and for
repair of worn-out or damaged tissues. As shown
in Figure 2.6a, the formation of a protein molecule
by the joining of amino acids into long chains is a
synthesis reaction.

Decomposition Reactions

Decomposition reactions occur when a molecule is broken down into smaller molecules,
atoms, or ions and can be indicated by

$$AB \rightarrow A + B$$

Essentially, decomposition reactions are synthesis
reactions in reverse. Bonds are always broken, and
the products of these reactions are smaller and
simpler than the original molecules. As bonds are
broken, chemical energy is released.

Q *In all reactions shown, chemical bonds are being altered. What atomic subparticle is involved in these alterations?*

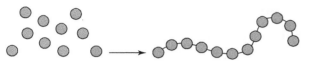

Amino acids   Protein molecule

(a) Example of a synthesis reaction: amino acids are joined to form a protein molecule

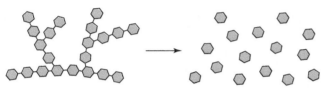

Glycogen   Glucose molecules

(b) Example of a decomposition reaction: breakdown of glycogen to release glucose units

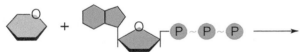

Glucose   Adenosine triphosphate (ATP)

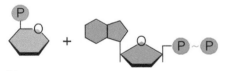

Glucose   Adenosine diphosphate (ADP)
phosphate

(c) Example of an exchange reaction: ATP transfers its terminal phosphate group to glucose to form glucose phosphate

FIGURE 2.6   Patterns of chemical reactions.
(a) In synthesis reactions, smaller particles (atoms, ions, or molecules) are bonded together to form larger, more complex molecules. **(b)** Decomposition reactions involve the breaking of bonds. **(c)** In exchange reactions, bonds are both made and broken.

Decomposition reactions underlie all catabolic or destructive processes that occur in body cells; that is, they are molecule-degrading reactions. Examples of decomposition reactions that occur in the body include the digestion of foods into their building blocks and the breakdown of glycogen (a large carbohydrate molecule stored in the liver) to release glucose (Figure 2.6b) when blood sugar levels start to decline.

Exchange Reactions

In an **exchange reaction,** parts of the reacting molecules are shuffled around to produce new products:

$$AB + CD \longrightarrow AD + CB$$

Although the reactants and products contain the same components (A, B, C, and D), those components are present in different combinations. In an exchange reaction, the reactant molecules AB and CD must break apart (a decomposition) before they can interact with each other to form AD and CB (a synthesis).

Reversible Reactions

Chemical reactions are (at least theoretically) reversible, so if $A + B \longrightarrow AB$, then $AB \longrightarrow A + B$. Many important biological reactions are freely reversible. Such reactions can be represented as an equation:

$$A + B \rightleftharpoons AB$$

This equation indicates that, in a sense, two reactions are occurring simultaneously, one a synthesis $(A + B \longrightarrow AB)$ and the other a decomposition $(AB \longrightarrow A + B)$. At equilibrium, the rates at which the two reactions proceed are in balance. As fast as one molecule of AB forms, another degrades into A + B.

The result of a disturbance in the equilibrium condition can be predicted. In our example, the rate at which the synthesis reaction proceeds is directly proportional to the frequency of encounters between A and B. In turn, the frequency of encounters depends on the degree of crowding: You are much more likely to run into another person in a crowded room than in a room that is almost empty. The addition of more AB molecules will increase the rate of conversion of AB to A and B. The amounts of A and B will then increase, leading to an increase in the rate of the reverse

A   *Electrons.*

reaction—the formation of AB from A and B. Eventually, an equilibrium is again established.

100 Keys | Things tend to even out, unless something prevents this from happening. Reversible reactions quickly reach equilibrium, in which opposing reaction rates are balanced. If reactants are added or removed, reaction rates change until a new equilibrium is established.

Enzymes, Energy, and Chemical Reactions

Most chemical reactions do not occur spontaneously, or they occur so slowly that they would be of little value to cells. Before a reaction can proceed, enough energy must be provided to activate the reactants. The amount of energy required to start a reaction is called the **activation energy.** Although many reactions can be activated by changes in temperature or acidity, such changes are deadly to cells. For example, every day your cells break down complex sugars as part of your normal metabolism. Yet to break down a complex sugar in a laboratory, you must boil it in an acidic solution. Your cells don't have that option; temperatures that high and solutions that corrosive would immediately destroy living tissues. Instead, your cells use special proteins called *enzymes* to perform most of the complex synthesis and decomposition reactions in your body.

Enzymes promote chemical reactions by lowering the activation energy requirements. In doing so, they make it possible for chemical reactions, such as the breakdown of sugars, to proceed under conditions compatible with life. Enzymes belong to a class of substances called **catalysts** (KAT-uh-lists; *katalysis,* dissolution), compounds that accelerate chemical reactions without themselves being permanently changed or consumed. A cell makes an enzyme molecule to promote a specific reaction. Enzymatic reactions, which are reversible, can be written as

$$A + B \underset{}{\overset{enzyme}{\rightleftharpoons}} AB$$

Although the presence of an appropriate enzyme can accelerate a reaction, an enzyme affects only the rate of the reaction, not its direction or the products that are formed. An enzyme cannot bring about a reaction that would otherwise be impossible. Enzymatic reactions are generally reversible, and they proceed until an equilibrium becomes established.

100 Keys | Most of the chemical reactions that sustain life cannot occur unless appropriate enzymes are present.

Inorganic Compounds

Although the human body is very complex, it contains relatively few elements. But knowing the identity and quantity of each element in the body will not help you understand the body any more than studying the alphabet will help you understand this textbook. Just as only 26 letters can be combined to form thousands of different words in this book, only about 26 elements combine to form thousands of different chemical compounds in our bodies. These compounds make up the living cells that constitute the framework of the body and carry on all its life processes. So it is impossible to understand the structure and functioning of the human body without learning about the major classes of chemical compounds.

We will next turn our attention to nutrients and metabolites. **Nutrients** are the essential elements and molecules normally obtained from the diet. **Metabolites** (me-TAB-ō-līts; *metabole,* change), a much larger group, include all the molecules (nutrients included) that can be synthesized or broken down by chemical reactions inside our bodies. Nutrients and metabolites can be broadly categorized as either inorganic or organic. **Inorganic compounds** generally do not contain carbon and hydrogen atoms as their primary structural ingredients, whereas carbon and hydrogen *always* form the basis for **organic compounds**.

The most important inorganic compounds in the body are (1) *carbon dioxide,* a by-product of cell metabolism; (2) *oxygen,* an atmospheric gas required in important metabolic reactions; (3) *water,* which accounts for most of our body weight; and (4) *inorganic acids, bases,* and *salts*—compounds held together partially or completely by ionic bonds. In this section, we will be concerned primarily with water, its properties, and how those properties establish the conditions necessary for life. Most of the other inorganic molecules and compounds in the body exist in association with water, the primary component of our body fluids. Both carbon dioxide and oxygen, for example, are gas molecules that are transported in body fluids, and all the inorganic acids, bases, and salts we will discuss are dissolved in body fluids.

Water and Its Properties

Water, H_2O, is the most important constituent of the body, accounting for up to two-thirds of total body weight. A change in the body's water content can have fatal consequences because virtually all physiological systems will be affected.

Although water is familiar to everyone, it has some highly unusual properties. These properties are a direct result of the hydrogen bonding that occurs between adjacent water molecules:

1. *Solubility.* A remarkable number of inorganic and organic molecules are soluble, meaning they will *dissolve* or break up in water. The individual molecules become distributed within the water, and the result is a **solution**—a uniform mixture of two or more substances. The medium in which other atoms, ions, or molecules are dispersed is called the **solvent;** the dispersed substances are the **solutes.** In **aqueous solutions,** water is the solvent. The solvent properties of water are so important that we will consider them further in the next section.

2. *Reactivity.* In our bodies, chemical reactions occur in water, and water molecules are also participants in some reactions. Hydrolysis and dehydration synthesis are two examples noted later in the chapter.

3. *High Heat Capacity. Heat capacity* is the ability to absorb and retain heat. Water has an unusually high heat capacity, because water molecules in the liquid state are attracted to one another through hydrogen bonding. Important consequences of this attraction include the following:

   - The temperature of water must be quite high before individual molecules have enough energy to break free and become water vapor, a gas. Consequently, water stays in the liquid state over a broad range of environmental temperatures, and the freezing and boiling points of water are far apart.

   - Water carries a great deal of heat away with it when it finally does change from a liquid to a gas. This feature accounts for the cooling effect of perspiration on the skin.

4. *Lubrication.* Water is an effective lubricant because there is little friction between water molecules. Thus, if two opposing surfaces are separated by even a thin layer of water, friction between those surfaces will be greatly reduced. (That is why driving on wet roads can be tricky; your tires may start sliding on a layer of water rather than maintaining contact with the road.) Within joints such as the knee, an aqueous solution prevents friction between the opposing surfaces. Similarly, a small amount of fluid in the ventral body cavities prevents friction between internal organs, such as the heart or lungs, and the body wall.

100 Keys | Water accounts for most of your body weight; proteins, the key structural and functional components of cells, and nucleic acids, which control cell structure and function, work only in solution.

The Properties of Aqueous Solutions

Water's chemical structure makes it an unusually effective solvent (Figure 2.7) The bonds in a water molecule are oriented such that the hydrogen atoms are relatively close together. As a result, the water molecule has positive and negative poles (Figure 2.7a). A water molecule is therefore called a *polar molecule,* or a *dipole.*

Many inorganic compounds are held together partially or completely by ionic bonds. In water, these compounds undergo *ionization* (ī-on-i-ZĀ-shun), or *dissociation* (di-sō-sē-Ā-shun). In this process, ionic bonds are broken as the individual ions interact with the positive or negative ends of polar water molecules (Figure 2.7b). The result is a mixture of cations and anions surrounded by water molecules. The water molecules around each ion form a *hydration sphere.*

An aqueous solution containing anions and cations will conduct an electrical current. Cations (+) move toward the negative side, or negative *terminal,* and anions (−) move toward the positive terminal. Electrical forces across cell membranes affect the functioning of all cells, and small electrical currents carried by ions are essential to muscle contraction and nerve function.

Electrolytes and Body Fluids   Soluble inorganic molecules whose ions will conduct an electrical current in solution are called **electrolytes** (e-LEK-trō-līts).

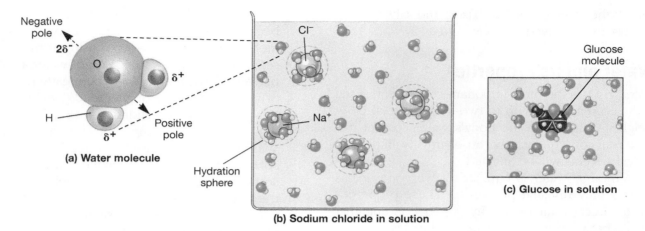

FIGURE 2.7   The activities of water molecules in aqueous solutions. (a) In a water molecule, oxygen forms polar covalent bonds with two hydrogen atoms. Because both hydrogen atoms are at one end of the molecule, it has an uneven distribution of charges, creating positive and negative poles. **(b)** Ionic compounds, such as sodium chloride, dissociate in water as the polar water molecules break the ionic bonds. Each ion in solution is surrounded by water molecules, creating hydration spheres. **(c)** Hydration spheres also form around an organic molecule containing polar covalent bonds. If the molecule binds water strongly, as does glucose, it will be carried into solution—in other words, it will dissolve.

TABLE 2.4	Important Electrolytes That Dissociate in Body Fluids	
Electrolyte		**Ions Released**
NaCl (sodium chloride)	$\longrightarrow$	$Na^+ + Cl^-$
KCl (potassium chloride)	$\longrightarrow$	$K^+ + Cl^-$
CaPo$_4$ (calcium phosphate)	$\longrightarrow$	$Ca2^+ + PO_4^{2-}$
NaHCO$_3$ (sodium bicarbonate)	$\longrightarrow$	$Na^+ + HCO_3^-$
MgCl$_2$ (magnesium chloride)	$\longrightarrow$	$Mg^{2+} + 2Cl^-$
Na$_2$HPO$_4$ (disodium phosphate)	$\longrightarrow$	$2Na^+ + HPO_4^{2-}$
Na$_2$SO$_4$ (sodium sulfate)	$\longrightarrow$	$2Na^+ + SO_4^{2-}$

Sodium chloride is an electrolyte. The dissociation of electrolytes in blood and other body fluids releases a variety of ions. Table 2.4 lists important electrolytes and the ions released by their dissociation.

Changes in the concentrations of electrolytes in body fluids will disturb almost every vital function. For example, declining potassium levels will lead to a general muscular paralysis, and rising concentrations will cause weak and irregular heartbeats. The concentrations of ions in body fluids are carefully regulated, primarily by the coordination of activities at the kidneys (ion excretion), the digestive tract (ion absorption), and the skeletal system (ion storage or release).

Hydrophilic and Hydrophobic Compounds Some organic molecules contain polar covalent bonds, which also attract water molecules. The hydration spheres that form may then carry these molecules

Clinical Note

Solute Concentrations

The concentration of a substance is the amount of that substance in a specified volume of solvent. Physiologists and clinicians often monitor inorganic and organic solute concentrations in body fluids such as blood or urine. Each solute has a normal range of values (see Appendix IV), and variations outside this range may indicate disease. Many solutes are participants in biochemical reactions, and as noted earlier, the concentrations of reactants and products in a chemical reaction directly affect reaction rates.

Solute concentrations can be expressed in several ways. In one method, we express the number of solute atoms, molecules, or ions in a specific volume of solution.

Values are reported in moles per liter (mol/L, or M) or millimoles per liter (mmol/L, or mM). A concentration expressed in these units is referred to as the *molarity* of the solution. (Recall that a mole is a quantity of any substance having a weight in grams equal to the atomic or molecular weight of that substance.) Physiological concentrations in clinical lab reports are most often reported in millimoles per liter.

You can report concentrations in terms of molarity only when you know the molecular weight of the ion or molecule in question. When the chemical structure is unknown or when you are dealing with a complex mixture of materials, concentration is expressed in terms of the weight of material dissolved in a unit volume of solution. Values are then reported in milligrams (mg) or grams (g) per deciliter (dl, or 100 ml). This is the method used, for example, in reporting the concentration of plasma proteins in a blood sample.

---

into solution (Figure 2.7c). Molecules such as *glucose,* an important soluble sugar, that interact readily with water molecules in this way are called **hydrophilic** (hī-drō-FIL-ik; *hydro-*, water + *philos,* loving).

Many other organic molecules either lack polar covalent bonds or have very few. Such molecules do not have positive and negative terminals, and are said to be *nonpolar.* When nonpolar molecules are exposed to water, hydration spheres do not form and the molecules do not dissolve. Molecules that do not readily interact with water are called **hydrophobic** (hī-drō-FŌ b-ik; *hydro-*, water + *phobos* fear). Among the most familiar hydrophobic molecules are fats and oils of all kinds. Body fat deposits, for example, consist of large, hydrophobic droplets trapped in the watery interior of cells. Gasoline and heating oil are hydrophobic molecules not found in the body; when accidentally discharged into lakes or oceans, they form tenacious oil slicks instead of dissolving.

Colloids and Suspensions

Body fluids may contain large and complex organic molecules, such as proteins and protein complexes, that are held in solution by their association with water molecules (Figure 2.7c). A solution containing dispersed proteins or other large molecules is called a **colloid**. Liquid Jell-O is a familiar viscous (thick) colloid.

The particles or molecules in a colloid will remain in solution indefinitely. A **suspension** contains even larger particles that will, if undisturbed, settle out of solution due to the force of gravity. Stirring beach sand into a bucket of water creates a temporary suspension that will last only until the sand settles to the bottom. Whole blood is another temporary suspension, because the blood cells are suspended in the blood plasma. If clotting is prevented, the cells in a blood sample will gradually settle to the bottom of the container. Measuring that settling rate, or "sedimentation rate," is a common laboratory test.

pH: The Concentration of Hydrogen Ions in Body Fluids

A hydrogen atom involved in a chemical bond or participating in a chemical reaction can easily lose its electron to become a hydrogen ion, H^+. Hydrogen ions are extremely reactive in solution. In excessive numbers, they will break chemical bonds, change the shapes of complex molecules, and generally disrupt cell and tissue functions. As a result, the concentration of hydrogen ions in body fluids must be regulated precisely.

A few hydrogen ions are normally present even in a sample of pure water, because some of the water molecules dissociate spontaneously, releasing cations and anions. The dissociation of water is a reversible reaction that can be represented as

$$H_2O \rightleftharpoons H^+ + OH^-.$$

The dissociation of one water molecule yields a hydrogen ion and a *hydroxide* (hī-DROK-sīd) *ion*, OH⁻.

The hydrogen ion concentration in body fluids is so important to physiological processes that a special shorthand is used to express it. The **pH** of a solution is defined as the negative logarithm of the hydrogen ion concentration in moles per liter.

The pH of blood normally ranges from 7.35 to 7.45. Abnormal fluctuations in pH can damage cells and tissues by breaking chemical bonds, changing the shapes of proteins, and altering cellular functions. *Acidosis* is an abnormal physiological state caused by low blood pH (below 7.35); a pH below 7 can produce coma. *Alkalosis* results from an abnormally high pH (above 7.45); a blood pH above 7.8 generally causes uncontrollable and sustained skeletal muscle contractions.

100 Keys | The pH of body fluids is an indication of how many free hydrogen ions are in solution. Hydrogen ions in excess (a low pH) can damage cells and tissues, change the shapes and functions of proteins, and interfere with normal physiological systems. A high pH also has adverse effects, but problems due to low pH are much more common.

Salts

The **salts** of many metal elements are commonly found in the body, but the most plentiful salts are those containing calcium and phosphorus, found chiefly in bones and teeth. When dissolved in body fluids, salts, which are ionic compounds, easily separate into their ions. This process, called *dissociation,* occurs rather easily because the ions have already been formed. All that remains is to pull the ions apart. This is accomplished by the polar water molecules, which orient themselves with their slightly negative ends toward the cations and their slightly positive ends toward the anions and thereby overcome the attraction between them (Figure 2.8).

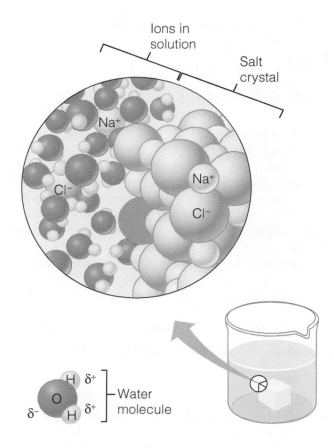

FIGURE 2.8 **Dissociation of a salt in water.** The slightly negative ends of the water molecules (δ^-) are attracted to Na⁺, whereas the slightly positive ends of water molecules (δ^+) orient toward Cl⁻, causing the ions of the salt crystal to be pulled apart.

Salts, both in their ionic forms and in combination with other elements, are vital to body functioning. For example, sodium and potassium ions are essential for nerve impulses, and iron forms part of the hemoglobin molecule that transports oxygen within red blood cells.

Because ions are charged particles, all salts are **electrolytes**—substances that conduct an electrical current in solution. When ionic (or electrolyte) balance is severely disturbed, virtually nothing in the body works. The functions of the elements found in body salts are summarized in Table 2.1.

Acids and Bases

Like salts, acids and bases are electrolytes. That is, they ionize and then dissociate in water and can then conduct an electrical current.

Characteristics of Acids   **Acids** have a sour taste and can dissolve many metals or "burn" a hole in your rug. But, the most useful definition of an acid is that it is a substance that can release *hydrogen ions (H⁺)* in detectable amounts. Because a hydrogen ion is essentially a hydrogen nucleus (a "naked proton"), acids are also defined as **proton donors.**

When acids are dissolved in water, they release hydrogen ions and some anions. The anions are unimportant; it is the release of the protons that determines an acid's effects on the environment. The ionization of hydrochloric acid (an acid produced by stomach cells that aids digestion) is shown in the following equation:

$$HCl \rightarrow H^+ + Cl^-$$
$$\text{(hydrochloric acid)} \quad \text{(proton)} \quad \text{(anion)}$$

Other acids found or produced in the body include acetic acid (the acidic component of vinegar) and carbonic acid.

Acids, like hydrochloric acid, that ionize completely and liberate all their protons are called *strong acids.* Acids that ionize incompletely, as do acetic and carbonic acid, are called *weak acids.* For example, when carbonic acid dissolves in water, only some of its molecules ionize to liberate H^+.

$$H_2CO_3 \rightarrow H^+ + HCO_3^- + H_2CO_3$$
$$\text{(carbonic acid)} \quad \text{(proton)} \quad \text{(anion)} \quad \text{(carbonic acid)}$$

Characteristics of Bases   **Bases** have a bitter taste, feel slippery, and are **proton acceptors.** The hydroxides are common inorganic bases. Like acids, the hydroxides ionize and dissociate in water; but in this case, the *hydroxyl ion (OH⁻)* and some cations are released. The ionization of sodium hydroxide (NaOH), commonly known as lye, is shown as

$$NaOH \rightarrow Na^+ + OH^-$$
$$\text{(sodium hydroxide)} \quad \text{(cation)} \quad \text{(hydroxyl ion)}$$

The hydroxyl ion is an avid proton (H^+) seeker, and any base containing this ion is considered a strong base. By contrast, *bicarbonate ion (HCO_3^-),* an important base in blood, is a fairly weak base.

When acids and bases are mixed, they react with each other (in an exchange reaction) to form water and a salt:

$$HCl + NaOH \rightarrow H_2O + NaCl$$
$$\text{(acid)} \quad \text{(base)} \quad \text{(water)} \quad \text{(salt)}$$

This type of exchange reaction, in which an acid and a base interact, is more specifically called a **neutralization reaction.**

pH: Acid-Base Concentrations   The relative concentration of hydrogen (and hydroxyl) ions in various body fluids is measured in concentration units called **pH** (pe-āch) **units.** The idea for a pH scale was devised in 1909 by a Danish biochemist (and part-time beer brewer) named Sørensen and is based on the number of protons in solution expressed in terms of moles per liter. (The *mole* is a concentration unit; its precise definition need not concern us here.) The pH scale runs from 0 to 14, and each successive change of 1 pH unit represents a tenfold change in hydrogen-ion concentration.

At a pH of 7, the scale midpoint, the number of hydrogen ions exactly equals the number of hydroxyl ions, and the solution is neutral; that is, neither acidic nor basic. Solutions with a pH lower than 7 are acidic: the hydrogen ions outnumber the hydroxyl ions. A solution with a pH of 6 has 10 times as many hydrogen ions as a solution with a pH of 7, and a pH of 3 indicates a 10,000-fold ($10 \times 10 \times 10 \times 10$) increase in hydrogen-ion concentration. Solutions with a pH number higher than 7 are alkaline, or basic, and solutions with a pH of 8 and 12 (respectively) have 1/10 and 1/100,000 the number of hydrogen ions present in a solution with a pH of 7.

Living cells are extraordinarily sensitive to even slight changes in pH; and acid-base balance is carefully regulated by the kidneys, lungs, and a number of chemicals called **buffers,** which are present in body fluids. Weak acids and weak bases are important components of the body's buffer systems, which act to maintain pH stability by taking up excess hydrogen or hydroxyl ions.

Because blood comes into close contact with nearly every body cell, regulation of blood pH is especially critical. Normally, blood pH varies in a narrow range, from 7.35 to 7.45. When blood pH changes more than a few tenths of a pH unit from these limits, death becomes a distinct possibility.

Although there are hundreds of examples that could be given to illustrate this point, we will provide just one very important one: when blood pH begins to dip into the acid range, the amount of life-sustaining oxygen that the hemoglobin in blood can carry to body cells begins to fall rapidly to dangerously low levels.

Organic Compounds

Organic compounds always contain the elements carbon and hydrogen, and generally oxygen as well. Many organic molecules are made up of long chains of carbon atoms linked by covalent bonds. The carbon atoms typically form additional covalent bonds with hydrogen or oxygen atoms and, less commonly, with nitrogen, phosphorus, sulfur, iron, or other elements.

Many organic molecules are soluble in water. Although the previous discussion focused on inorganic acids and bases, there are also important organic acids and bases. For example, *lactic acid* is an organic acid, generated by active muscle tissues, that must be neutralized by the carbonic acid–bicarbonate buffer system to prevent a potentially dangerous pH decline in body fluids.

In this discussion, we consider four major classes of organic compounds: *carbohydrates, lipids, proteins*, and *nucleic acids*. We also introduce *high-energy phosphate bonds*, which are vital to the survival and operation of our cells. In addition, the human body contains small quantities of many other organic compounds whose structures and functions we will consider in later chapters.

Although organic compounds are diverse, certain groupings of atoms occur again and again, even in very different types of molecules. These *functional groups* greatly influence the properties of any molecule they are part of. Table 2.5 details the functional groups you will encounter in this chapter.

Carbohydrates

Carbohydrates, which include sugars and starches, contain carbon, hydrogen, and oxygen. With slight variations, the hydrogen and oxygen atoms appear in the same ratio as in water; that is, 2 hydrogen atoms to 1 oxygen atom. This is reflected in the word *carbohydrate*, which means "hydrated carbon," and in the molecular formulas of sugars. For example, glucose is $C_6H_{12}O_6$, and ribose is $C_5H_{10}O_5$.

TABLE 2.5   Important Functional Groups of Organic Compounds

Functional Group	Structural Formula*	Importance	Examples
Carboxyl group, —COOH	R...—C=O with OH	Acts as an acid, releasing H^+ to become R—COO$^-$	Fatty acids, amino acids
Amino group, —NH₂	R—N with H, H	Can accept or release H^+, depending on pH; can form bonds with other molecules	Amino acids
Hydroxyl group, —OH	R—O—H	Strong bases dissociate to release hydroxide ions (OH$^-$); may link molecules through dehydration synthesis (condensation)	Carbohydrates, fatty acids, amino acids
Phosphate group, —PO₄	R—O—P—O$^-$ with O, O$^-$	May link other molecules to form larger structures; may store energy in high-energy bonds	Phospholipids, nucleic acids, high-energy compounds

*The term *R group* is used to denote the rest of the molecule, whatever that might be. The R group is also known as a *side chain*.

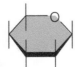

(a) Simple sugar (monosaccharide)

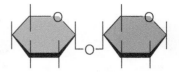

(b) Double sugar (disaccharide)

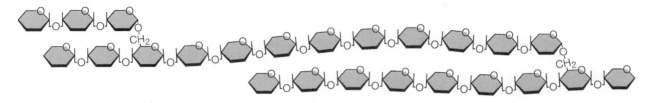

(c) Starch (polysaccharide)

FIGURE 2.9   Carbohydrates. (a) The generalized structure of a monosaccharide. **(b)** and **(c)** The basic structures of a disaccharide and a polysaccharide, respectively.

Carbohydrates are classified according to size as monosaccharides, disaccharides, or polysaccharides. Because monosaccharides are joined to form the molecules of the other two groups, they are the structural units, or building blocks, of carbohydrates.

Monosaccharides **Monosaccharide** means one (*mono*) sugar (*saccharide*), and thus monosaccharides are also referred to as *simple sugars*. They are single-chain or single-ring structures, containing from 3 to 7 carbon atoms (Figure 2.9a).

The most important monosaccharides in the body are glucose, fructose, galactose, ribose, and deoxyribose. **Glucose,** also called *blood sugar,* is the universal cellular fuel. *Fructose* and *galactose* are converted to glucose for use by body cells. *Ribose* and *deoxyribose* form part of the structure of nucleic acids, another group of organic molecules.

Disaccharides **Disaccharides,** or *double sugars* (Figure 2.9b) are formed when two simple sugars are joined by a synthesis reaction known as **dehydration synthesis.** In this reaction, a water molecule is lost as the bond forms (Figure 2.9c).

Some of the important disaccharides in the diet are *sucrose* (glucose-fructose), which is cane sugar; *lactose* (glucose-galactose), found in milk; and *maltose* (glucose-glucose), or malt sugar. Because the double sugars are too large to pass through cell membranes, they must be broken down (digested) to their monosaccharide units to be absorbed from the digestive tract into the blood. This is accomplished by **hydrolysis.** As a water molecule is added to each bond, the bond is broken, and the simple sugar units are released (Figure 2.10).

Polysaccharides **Polysaccharides** (literally, "many sugars") are long, branching chains of linked simple sugars (Figure 2.9c). Because they are large, insoluble molecules, they are ideal storage products. Another consequence of their large size is that they lack the sweetness of the simple and double sugars.

Only two polysaccharides, starch and glycogen, are of major importance to the body. *Starch* is the storage polysaccharide formed by plants. We ingest it in the form of "starchy" foods, such as grain products and root vegetables (potatoes and carrots, for example). *Glycogen* is a slightly smaller, but similar, polysaccharide found in animal tissues (largely in the muscles and the liver). Like starch, it is formed of linked glucose units.

Carbohydrates provide a ready, easily used source of food energy for cells, and glucose is at the top of the "cellular menu." When glucose is oxidized (combined with oxygen) in a complex set of chemical reactions, it is broken down into carbon dioxide and water. Some of the energy released as the glucose bonds are broken is trapped in the bonds of high-energy ATP molecules, the energy

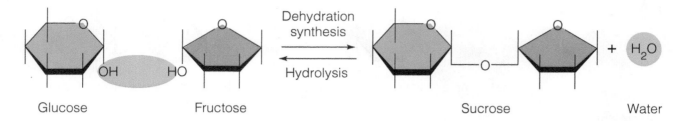

Glucose   Fructose   Sucrose   Water

FIGURE 2.10   Dehydration synthesis and hydrolysis of a molecule of sucrose. In the reaction going to the right (the dehydration synthesis reaction), glucose and fructose are joined through a process that involves the removal of a water molecule at the bond site. The resulting disaccharide is sucrose. Sucrose is broken down to its simple sugar units when the reaction is reversed (goes to the left). In this hydrolysis reaction, a water molecule must be added to the bond to release the monosaccharides.

"currency" of all body cells. If not immediately needed for ATP synthesis, dietary carbohydrates are converted to glycogen or fat and stored. Those of us who have gained weight from eating too many carbohydrate-rich snacks have a firsthand awareness of this conversion process!

Small amounts of carbohydrates are used for structural purposes and represent 1 to 2 percent of cell mass. Some sugars are found in our genes, and others are attached to outer surfaces of cell membranes, where they act as road signs to guide cellular interactions.

Lipids

Lipids are a large and diverse group of organic compounds (Table 2.6). They enter the body in the form of fat-marbled meats, egg yolks, milk products, and oils. The most abundant lipids in the body are triglycerides, phospholipids, and steroids. Like carbohydrates, all lipids contain carbon, hydrogen, and oxygen atoms, but in lipids, carbon and hydrogen atoms far outnumber oxygen atoms, as illustrated by the formula for a typical fat named tristearin: $C_{57}H_{110}O_6$. Most lipids are insoluble in water but readily dissolve in other lipids and in organic solvents such as alcohol and acetone.

Triglycerides   The **triglycerides** (tri-glis′er-īdz), or **neutral fats,** are composed of two types of building blocks, **fatty acids** and **glycerol.** Their synthesis involves the attachment of three fatty acids to a single glycerol molecule. The result is an E-shaped molecule that resembles the tines of a fork

(Figure 2.11a). Although the glycerol backbone is the same in all neutral fats, the fatty acid chains vary; this results in different kinds of neutral fats. Triglycerides may be solid (typical of animal fats) or liquid (plant oils). In general, animal fats tend to be *saturated,* whereas oils are *unsaturated.* In saturated fats, all carbons have single bonds. The carbons of unsaturated fats have some double (or triple) bonds and thus have the ability to bind with more hydrogen atoms or atoms of a different type.

Triglycerides represent the body's most abundant and concentrated source of usable energy. When they are oxidized, they yield large amounts of energy. They are stored chiefly in fat deposits beneath the skin and around body organs, where they help insulate the body and protect deeper body tissues from heat loss and bumps.

Phospholipids   **Phospholipids** (fos′fo-lip″idz) are very similar to the triglycerides. They differ in that a phosphorus-containing group is always part of the molecule and takes the place of one of the fatty acid chains. Thus, phospholipids have two instead of three attached fatty acids (Figure 2.11b).

Because the phosphorus-containing portion (the "head") bears an electrical charge, it gives phospholipids special chemical properties and polarity. For example, the charged region attracts and interacts with water and ions, but the fatty acid chains (the "tail") do not. The presence of phospholipids in cellular boundaries (membranes) allows cells to be selective about what may enter or leave.

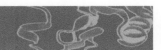

TABLE 2.6   Representative Lipids Found in the Body

Lipid type	Location/function
Neutral fats (Triglycerides)	Found in fat deposits (subcutaneous tissue and around organs); protect and insulate the body organs; the major source of stored energy in the body.
Phospholipids (Cephalin and others)	Found in cell membranes; participate in the transport of lipids in plasma; abundant in the brain and the nervous tissue in general, where they help to form insulating white matter.
Steroids	
Cholesterol	The basis of all body steroids.
Bile salts	A breakdown product of cholesterol; released by the liver into the digestive tract, where they aid in fat digestion and absorption.
Vitamin D	Produced in the skin, on exposure to UV (ultraviolet) radiation, from a modified cholesterol molecule; necessary for normal bone growth and function.
Sex hormones	Estrogen and progesterone (female hormones) and testosterone (male hormone) produced from cholesterol; necessary for normal reproductive function; deficits result in sterility.
Corticosteroids (adrenal cortical hormones)	Cortisol, a glucocorticoid, is a long-term antistress hormone that is necessary for life; aldosterone helps regulate salt and water balance in body fluids by targeting the kidneys.
Other lipoid substances	
Fat-soluble vitamins:	
A	Found in orange-pigmented vegetables (carrots) and fruits (tomatoes); part of the photoreceptor pigment involved in vision.
E	Taken in via plant products such as wheat germ and green leafy vegetables; may promote wound healing and contribute to fertility, but not proven in humans; an antioxidant; may help to neutralize free radicals (highly reactive particles believed to be involved in triggering some types of cancers).
K	Made available largely by the action of intestinal bacteria; also prevalent in a wide variety of foods; necessary for proper clotting of blood.
Prostaglandins	Derivatives of fatty acids found in cell membranes; various functions depending on the specific class, including stimulation of uterine contractions (thus inducing labor and abortions), regulation of blood pressure, and control of motility of the gastrointestinal tract; involved in inflammation.
Lipoproteins	Lipid and protein-based substances that transport fatty acids and cholesterol in the bloodstream; major varieties are high-density lipoproteins (HDLs) and low-density lipoproteins (LDLs).

Q Triglycerides and phospholipids are similar. What is the major structural difference between them?

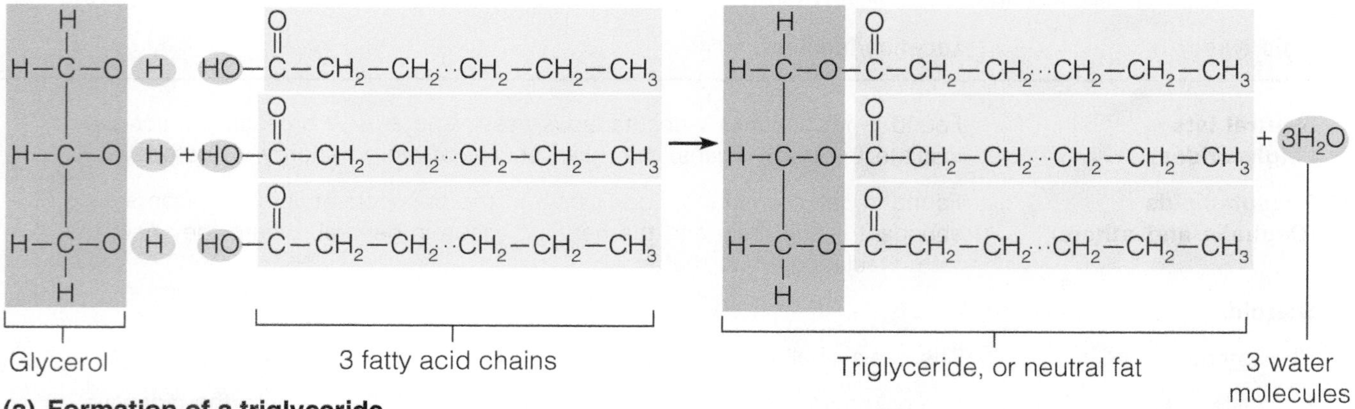

Glycerol   3 fatty acid chains

(a) Formation of a triglyceride

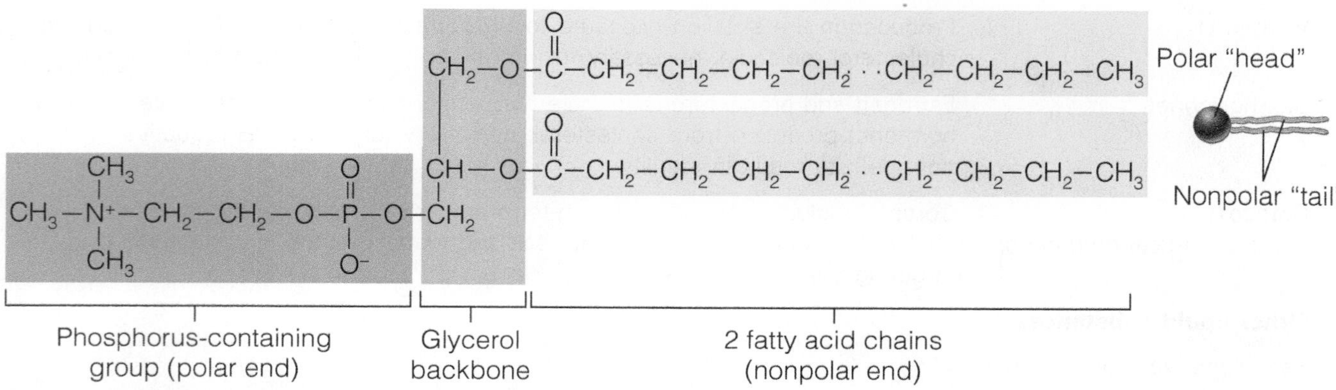

Triglyceride, or neutral fat   3 water molecules

+ 3H₂O

Polar "head"

Nonpolar "tail"

Phosphorus-containing group (polar end)

Glycerol backbone

2 fatty acid chains (nonpolar end)

(b) Phospholipid molecule (phosphatidylcholine)

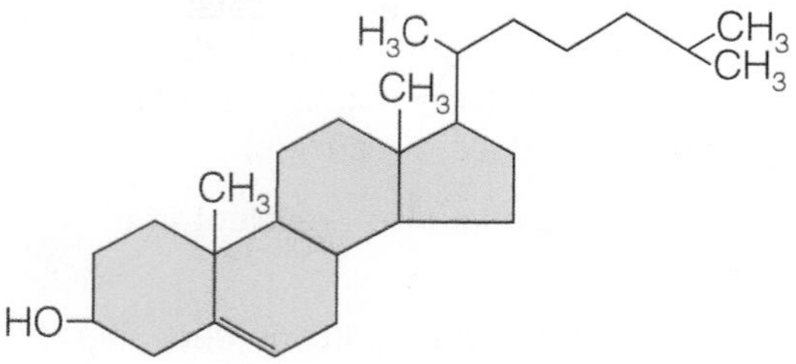

(c) Cholesterol

FIGURE 2.11 Lipids. (a) Triglycerides, or neutral fats, are synthesized by dehydration synthesis. In this process, three fatty acid chains are attached to a single glycerol molecule, and a water molecule is lost at each bond site. **(b)** Structure of a typical phospholipid molecule. Two fatty acid chains and a phosphorus-containing group are attached to the glycerol backbone. **(c)** The generalized structure of cholesterol. Cholesterol is the basis for all steroids made in the body.

A They both have a glycerol backbone and fatty acid chains. However, triglycerides have three attached fatty acid chains and phospholipids have only two; the third is replaced by a phosphorous-containing group.

Steroids **Steroids** are basically flat molecules formed of four interlocking rings (Figure 2.11c); thus their structure differs quite a bit from that of fats. However, like fats, steroids are made largely of hydrogen and carbon atoms and are fat-soluble.

The single most important steroid molecule is **cholesterol,** which enters the body in animal products such as meat, eggs, and cheese. A certain amount is also made by the liver, regardless of dietary intake. Cholesterol is found in all cell membranes, and it is particularly abundant in the brain. Cholesterol is the raw material used to form vitamin D, some hormones (sex hormones and cortisol), and bile salts.

Homeostatic Imbalance

Saturated fats, along with cholesterol, have been implicated as substances that encourage atherosclerosis (the deposit of fatty substances in artery walls) and eventual arteriosclerosis (hardening of the arteries). As a result, olive oil and liquid spreads made from polyunsaturated fats are being promoted as products that allow us to "have our cake and eat it too"—good-tasting substitutes that (unlike butter) do not damage our arteries. ▲

Proteins

Proteins account for over 50 percent of the organic matter in the body, and they have the most varied functions of the organic molecules. Some are construction materials; others play vital roles in cell function. Like carbohydrates and lipids, all proteins contain carbon, oxygen, and hydrogen. In addition, they contain nitrogen and sometimes sulfur atoms as well.

The building blocks of proteins are small molecules called **amino** (ah-me′no) **acids.** About 20 common varieties of amino acids are found in proteins. All amino acids have an *amine group* (NH_2), which gives them basic properties, and an *acid group* (COOH), which allows them to act as acids. In fact, all amino acids are identical except for a single group of atoms called their *R-group* (Figure 2.12). Hence, it is differences in the R-groups that make each amino acid chemically unique.

Amino acids are joined together in chains to form large, complex protein molecules that contain from 50 to thousands of amino acids. (Amino acid chains containing fewer than 50 amino acids are called *polypeptides*.) Because each type of amino acid has distinct properties, the sequence in which

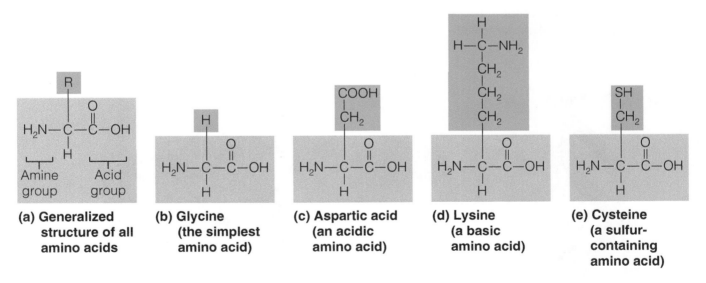

(a) Generalized structure of all amino acids

(b) Glycine (the simplest amino acid)

(c) Aspartic acid (an acidic amino acid)

(d) Lysine (a basic amino acid)

(e) Cysteine (a sulfur-containing amino acid)

FIGURE 2.12 Amino acid structures. (a) Generalized structure of amino acids. All amino acids have both an amine (—NH_2) group and an acid (—COOH) group; they differ only in the atomic makeup of their R-groups (green). **(b)–(e)** Specific structures of four amino acids. The simplest (glycine) has an R-group consisting of a single hydrogen atom. An acid in the R-group makes the amino acid (aspartic acid in this example) more acidic. An amine group in the R-group makes it more basic (as in lysine). The presence of sulfur (—SH) in the R-group of cysteine hints that this is an amino acid likely to take part in intramolecular bonding.

they are bound together produces proteins that vary widely both in structure and function. Perhaps this can be made more understandable if the 20 amino acids are compared to a 20-letter alphabet. The letters (amino acids) are then used in specific combinations to form words (a protein). Just as a change in one letter of any word can produce a word with an entirely different meaning (flour → floor) or is nonsensical (flour → fluur), changes in kinds of amino acids (letters) or in their positions in the protein allow literally thousands of different protein molecules to be made. The structure of proteins is specified by our genes.

Fibrous and Globular Proteins   Proteins are extremely versatile and have a variety of functions. The shape of a protein, determined by the sequence of amino acids, determines its functional properties. Based on their overall shape and structure, proteins are classed as either fibrous or globular proteins (Figure 2.13). The strandlike **fibrous proteins,** also called **structural proteins,** appear most often in body structures. They are very important in binding structures together and for providing strength in certain body tissues. For example, *collagen* (kol'ah-jen) is found in bones, cartilage, and tendons and is the most abundant protein in the body. *Keratin* (ker'ah-tin) is the structural protein of hair and nails and the material that makes skin tough.

Globular proteins are mobile, generally spherical molecules that play crucial roles in virtually all biological processes. Because they *do things* rather than just form structures, they are also called **functional proteins.** As noted in Table 2.7, the scope of their activities is remarkable. Some (antibodies) help to provide immunity; others (hormones) help to regulate growth and development. Still others, called *enzymes* (en'zīmz), are biological catalysts that regulate essentially every chemical reaction that goes on within the body.

The fibrous structural proteins are exceptionally stable; the globular functional proteins are quite the opposite. Hydrogen bonds are critically important in maintaining their structure, but hydrogen bonds are fragile and are easily broken by heat and excesses of pH. When their three-dimensional structures are destroyed, the proteins are said to be *denatured* and can no longer perform their physiological roles. This is because their function depends on their specific structure—most importantly, on the presence of particular collections of atoms called **active sites** on their surface that "fit" and interact chemically with other molecules of complementary shape and charge (Figure 2.14). As hinted earlier, hemoglobin becomes totally unable to bind and transport oxygen when blood pH becomes too acidic, and pepsin, a protein-digesting enzyme, is inactivated by

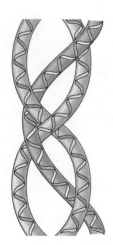

(a) Triple helix of collagen (a fibrous or structural protein).

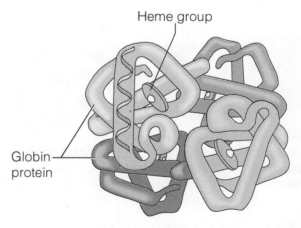

Heme group

Globin protein

(b) Hemoglobin molecule composed of the protein globin and attached heme groups. (Globin is a globular or functional protein.)

FIGURE 2.13   **General structure of (a) a fibrous protein and (b) a globular protein.**

TABLE **2.7**	Representative Groups of Functional Proteins
Functional group	**Role(s) in the body**
Antibodies (immunoglobulins)	Highly specialized proteins that recognize, bind with, and inactivate bacteria, toxins, and some viruses; function in the immune response, which helps protect the body from "invading" foreign substances.
Hormones	Help to regulate growth and development. Examples include • Growth hormone—an anabolic hormone necessary for optimal growth. • Insulin—helps regulate blood sugar levels. • Nerve growth factor—guides the growth of neurons in the development of the nervous system.
Transport proteins	Hemoglobin transports oxygen in the blood; other transport proteins in the blood carry iron, cholesterol, or other substances.
Catalysts (enzymes)	Essential to virtually every biochemical reaction in the body; increase the rates of chemical reactions by at least a millionfold; in their absence (or destruction), biochemical reactions cease.

alkaline pH. In each case, the structure needed for function has been destroyed by the improper pH.

Except for enzymes, most important types of functional proteins are described with the organ system or functional process to which they are closely related. For instance, protein hormones are discussed in Chapter 9 (Endocrine System), hemoglobin is considered in Chapter 10 (The Cadiovascular System: The Blood), and antibodies are described in Chapter 12 (The Lymphatic System and Body Defenses). However, enzymes are important in the functioning of all body cells, and so these incredibly complex molecules are considered here.

Enzymes and Enzyme Activity **Enzymes** are functional proteins that act as biological catalysts. A **catalyst** is a substance that increases the rate of a chemical reaction without becoming part of the product or being changed itself. Enzymes accomplish this feat by binding to and "holding" the reacting molecules (the substrates) in the proper position for chemical interaction. While the substrates are bound to the enzyme's active site (see Figure 2.14a), they undergo structural changes that result in a new product. Once the reaction has occurred, the enzyme releases the product. Because enzymes are not changed in doing their

job, they are reusable, and only small amounts of each enzyme are needed by the cells.

Enzymes are capable of catalyzing millions of reactions each minute. However, they do more than just increase the speed of chemical reactions; they also determine just which reactions are possible at a particular time. No enzyme, no reaction! Enzymes can be compared to a bellows used to fan a sluggish fire into flaming activity. Without enzymes, biochemical reactions would occur far too slowly to sustain life.

Although there are hundreds of different kinds of enzymes in body cells, they are very specific in their activities, each controlling only one (or a small group of) chemical reaction(s) and acting only on specific molecules. Most enzymes are named according to that specific type of reaction they catalyze. There are "hydrolases," which add water; "oxidases," which cause oxidation; and so on. (In most cases, an enzyme can be recognized by the suffix **-ase** forming part of its name.)

Many enzymes are produced in an inactive form and must be activated in some way before they can function. In other cases, enzymes are inactivated immediately after they have performed their catalytic function. Both events are true of enzymes that promote blood clotting when a

Q   *How does an enzyme recognize its substrate?*

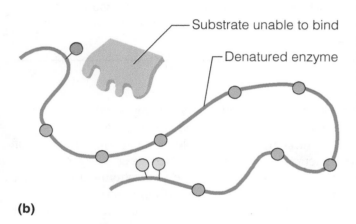

Substrate "fits" with active site

Active site

Enzyme (globular functional protein)

(a)

Substrate unable to bind

Denatured enzyme

(b)

FIGURE 2.14 Simple diagram illustrating denaturation of a functional protein molecule such as an enzyme. (a) The molecule's three-dimensional globular structure is maintained by intramolecular bonds. Atoms composing the active site of the enzyme are shown as stalked particles. The substrate, or molecule the enzyme acts on, has a corresponding binding site, and the two sites fit together very precisely. **(b)** Breaking the intramolecular bonds that maintain the three-dimensional structure of the enzyme results in a linear molecule, with the atoms of the former active site widely separated. Enzyme-substrate binding can no longer occur.

A   *The shape of the substrate and the enzyme's active site are complementary.*

blood vessel has been damaged. If this were not so, large numbers of unneeded and potentially lethal blood clots would be formed.

Prove It Yourself

Demonstrate the Presence of an Enzyme in Your Saliva

You can detect the presence of an enzyme (a catalytic protein) in one of your own body fluids, saliva, with the following demonstration.

Place a small cracker in your mouth. Don't swallow it, but move the cracker around in your mouth to moisten it with saliva. After a minute you will experience a sweet taste that was not present initially. This is because your saliva contains an enzyme that breaks the bonds in the starch of the cracker, producing the sweet-tasting disaccharide maltose. What you have just demonstrated is that the hydrolysis (digestion) of starch actually begins in your mouth, even before food reaches your stomach.

To prove that the starch was broken down by an enzyme and not by the watery component of your saliva, wet another cracker with tap water. Moisten it for the same length of time as the first cracker, and then place it in your mouth. It should not taste sweet.

Nucleic Acids

The role of **nucleic** (nu-kle′ik) **acids** is fundamental: they make up the genes, which provide the basic blueprint of life. Not only do they determine what type of organism you will be, but they also direct your growth and development—and they do this largely by dictating protein structure. (Remember that enzymes, which catalyze all the chemical reactions that occur in the body, are proteins.)

Nucleic acids, composed of carbon, oxygen, hydrogen, nitrogen, and phosphorus atoms, are the largest biological molecules in the body. Their building blocks, the **nucleotides** (nu′kle-o-tīdz), are quite complex. Each consists of three basic parts: (1) a nitrogen-containing base, (2) a pentose (5-carbon) sugar, and (3) a phosphate group (Figure 2.15a and 2.15b).

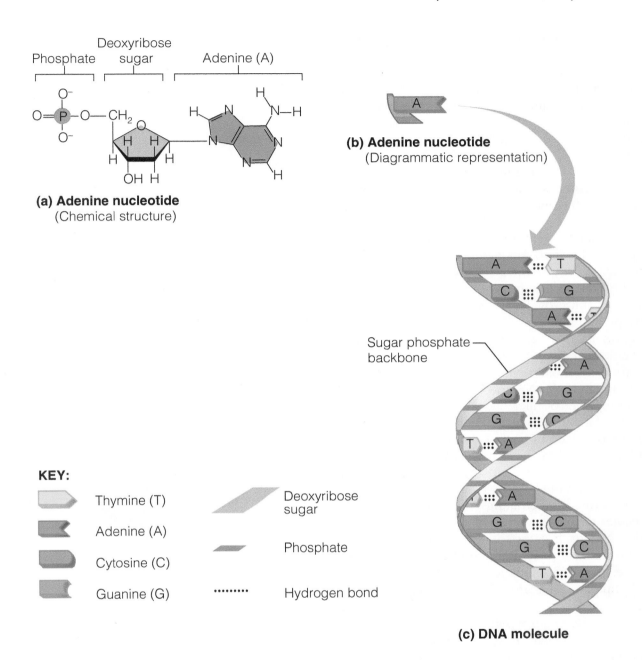

(a) Adenine nucleotide
(Chemical structure)

(b) Adenine nucleotide
(Diagrammatic representation)

Sugar phosphate backbone

KEY:

Thymine (T)

Adenine (A)

Cytosine (C)

Guanine (G)

Deoxyribose sugar

Phosphate

Hydrogen bond

(c) DNA molecule

FIGURE 2.15   Structure of DNA. (a) The unit of DNA (deoxyribonucleic acid) is the nucleotide, composed of a linked deoxyribose sugar molecule, a phosphate group, and a nitrogen-containing base (attached to the sugar). The nucleotide illustrated, both in its (a) chemical and (b) diagrammatic structures, contains the base adenine. (c) Structure of a DNA molecule—two nucleotide chains coiled into a double helix. The "backbones" of DNA are formed by alternating sugar and phosphate molecules. The "rungs" are formed by the binding together of complementary bases (A to T, G to C) by hydrogen bonds.

The bases come in five varieties: *adenine* (A), *guanine* (G), *cytosine* (C), *thymine* (T), and *uracil* (U). A and G are large, two-ring bases, whereas the others are smaller, single-ring structures. The nucleotides are named according to the base they contain: A-containing bases are adenine nucleotides, C-containing bases are cytosine nucleotides, and so on.

The two major kinds of nucleic acid are **deoxyribonucleic** (de-ok"sĭ-ri"bo-nu-kle'ik) **acid (DNA)** and **ribonucleic acid (RNA).** DNA and RNA differ in many respects. DNA is the genetic material found within the cell nucleus (the control center of the cell). It has two fundamental roles: (1) It replicates itself exactly before a cell divides, thus ensuring that the genetic information in every body cell is identical. (2) It provides the instructions for building every protein in the body. For the most part, RNA is located outside the nucleus and can be considered the "molecular slave" of DNA; that is, RNA carries out the orders for protein synthesis issued by DNA.

Although both RNA and DNA are formed by the joining together of nucleotides, their final structures are different. As shown in Figure 2.15c, DNA is a long double chain of nucleotides. Its bases are A, G, T, and C, and its sugar is *deoxyribose*. Its two nucleotide chains are held together by hydrogen bonds between the bases, so that a ladderlike molecule is formed. Alternating sugar and phosphate molecules form the "uprights," or backbones, of the ladder, and each "rung" is formed by two joined bases (one base pair). Binding of the bases is very specific: A always binds to T, and G always binds to C. Thus, A and T are said to be *complementary bases,* as are C and G. A base sequence of ATGA on one nucleotide chain would necessarily be bonded to the complementary base sequence TACT on the other nucleotide strand. The whole molecule is then coiled into a spiral-staircaselike structure called a *double helix.*

Whereas DNA is double-stranded, RNA molecules are single nucleotide strands. The RNA bases are A, G, C, and U (U replaces the T found in DNA), and its sugar is *ribose* instead of deoxyribose. Three major varieties of RNA exist— *messenger, ribosomal,* and *transfer RNA*—and each has a specific role to play in carrying out DNA's instructions for building proteins. Messenger RNA carries the information for building the protein from the DNA genes to the ribosomes, the

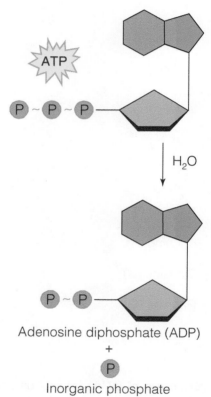

(a) Adenosine triphosphate (ATP)

(b) Hydrolysis of ATP

FIGURE 2.16   ATP. (a) The structure of ATP (adenosine triphosphate). **(b)** Hydrolysis of ATP to yield ADP (adenosine diphosphate) and inorganic phosphate. High-energy bonds are indicated by a red ~.

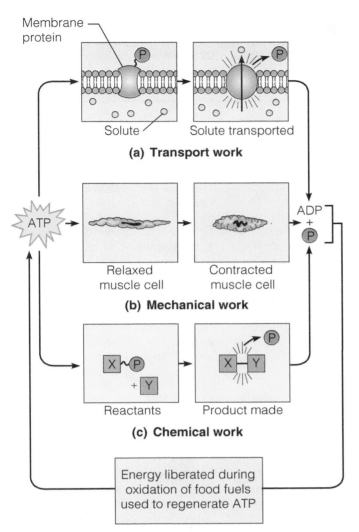

Membrane protein

Solute   Solute transported

(a) Transport work

ATP

Relaxed muscle cell   Contracted muscle cell

(b) Mechanical work

ADP + P

X~P + Y   X—Y + P

Reactants   Product made

(c) Chemical work

Energy liberated during oxidation of food fuels used to regenerate ATP

FIGURE 2.17   Three examples of how ATP drives cellular work. The high-energy bonds of ATP release energy for use by the cell when they are broken. **(a)** ATP drives the transport of certain solutes (amino acids, for example) across cell membranes. **(b)** ATP activates contractile proteins in muscle cells so that the cells can shorten and perform mechanical work. **(c)** ATP provides the energy needed to drive energy-absorbing chemical reactions. ATP is regenerated (phosphate is bound to ADP) as energy is released by the oxidation of food fuels and captured in the ADP– Ⓟ bond.

protein-synthesizing sites. Transfer RNA ferries amino acids to the ribosomes. Ribosomal RNA forms part of the ribosomes, where it oversees the translation of the message and the binding together of amino acids to form the proteins.

Adenosine Triphosphate (ATP)

The synthesis of **adenosine triphosphate** (ah-den′o-sēn tri-fos′fāt), or **ATP,** is all-important because it provides a form of chemical energy that is usable by all body cells. Without ATP, molecules cannot be made or broken down, cells cannot maintain their boundaries, and all life processes grind to a halt.

Although glucose is the most important fuel for body cells, none of the chemical energy contained in its bonds can be used directly to power cellular work. Instead, energy released as glucose is catabolized, captured, and stored in the bonds of ATP molecules as small packets of energy.

Structurally, ATP is a modified nucleotide; it consists of an adenine base, ribose sugar, and three phosphate groups (Figure 2.16a). The phosphate groups are attached by unique chemical bonds called *high-energy phosphate bonds*. When these bonds are ruptured by hydrolysis, energy that can be used immediately by the cell to do work or power a particular activity—such as synthesizing proteins, transporting substances across its membrane, or, in the case of muscle cells, contracting— is liberated (Figure 2.16b). ATP can be compared to a tightly coiled spring that is ready to uncoil with tremendous energy when the "catch" is released. The consequence of cleavage of its terminal phosphate bond can be represented as follows:

$$ATP \quad \rightarrow \quad ADP \quad + \quad Ⓟ \quad + \quad E$$

(adenosine   (adenosine   (inorganic   (energy) triphosphate)   diphosphate)   phosphate)

As ATP is used to provide cellular energy, **adenosine diphosphate (ADP)** accumulates, and ATP supplies are replenished by oxidation of food fuels (Figure 2.17). Essentially the same amount of energy must be captured and used to reattach a phosphate group to ADP (that is, to reverse the reaction) as is liberated when the terminal phosphate is cleaved off.

Table 2.8 summarizes the classes of inorganic and organic compounds.

TABLE 2.8	Classes of Inorganic and Organic Compounds		
Class	**Building Blocks**	**Sources**	**Functions**
INORGANIC			
Water	Hydrogen and oxygen atoms	Absorbed as liquid water or generated by metabolism	Solvent; transport medium for cooling through evaporation; medium for chemical dissolved materials and heat; reactions; reactant in hydrolysis
Acids, bases, salts	H^+, OH^- various and cations	Obtained from the diet or generated by metabolism	Structural components; buffers; sources of ions anions
Dissolved gases	O, C, N, and other atoms	Atmosphere	O_2: required for cellular metabolism O_2: generated by cells as a waste product
NO: chemical messenger in cardiovascular, nervous, and lymphatic systems
ORGANIC			
Carbohydrates	C, H, O, in some cases N; CHO in a 1:2:1 ratio	Obtained from the diet or manufactured in the body	Energy source; some structural role when attached to lipids or proteins; energy storage
Lipids	C, H, O, in some cases N or P; CHO not in 1:2:1 ratio	Obtained from the diet or manufactured in the body	Energy source; energy storage; insulation; structural components; chemical messengers; protection
Proteins	C, H, O, N, commonly S	20 common amino acids; roughly half can be manufactured in the body, others must be obtained from the diet	Catalysts for metabolic reactions; structural components; movement; transport; buffers;defense; control and coordination of activities
Nucleic acids	C, H, O, N, and P; nucleotides composed of phosphates, sugars, and nitrogenous bases	Obtained from the diet or manufactured in the body	Storage and processing of genetic information
High-energy phosphate bonds	Nucleotides joined to phosphates by high-energy bonds	Synthesized by all cells	Storage or transfer of energy

Unit 3

Dynamics of Support
and Motion

3

Cells and Tissues

PART I: CELLS

In the late 1600s, Robert Hooke was looking through a crude microscope at some plant tissue—cork. He saw some cubelike structures that reminded him of the long rows of monk's rooms (or cells) at the monastery, so he named these structures **cells.** The living cells that had formed the cork were long since dead. However, the name stuck and is still used to describe the smallest unit, or the building block, of all living things, plants and animals alike. Whatever its form, however it behaves, the cell contains all the parts necessary to survive in a changing world. The human body has trillions of these microscopic building blocks.

Overview of the Cellular Basis of Life

Perhaps the most striking thing about a cell is its organization. If we chemically analyze cells, we find that they are made up primarily of four elements—carbon, oxygen, hydrogen, and nitrogen—plus much smaller amounts of several other elements. Although the four major elements build most of the cell's structure (which is largely protein), the trace elements are very important for certain cell functions. For example, calcium is needed for blood clotting (among other things), and iron is necessary to make hemoglobin, which carries oxygen in the blood. Iodine is required to make the thyroid hormone that controls metabolism. In their ionic form, many of the metals (such as calcium, sodium, and potassium) can carry an electrical charge; when they do they are called *electrolytes* (e-lek′tro-līts). Sodium and potassium ions are essential if nerve impulses are to be transmitted and muscles are to contract.

Strange as it may seem, especially when we feel our firm muscles, living cells are about 60 percent water, which is one of the reasons water is essential for life. In addition to containing large amounts of water, all the body cells are constantly bathed in a dilute saltwater solution (something like seawater) called *interstitial fluid,* which is derived from the blood. All exchanges between cells and blood are made through this fluid.

Cells vary tremendously in length—ranging from 2 micrometers (1/12,000th of an inch) in the smallest cells to over a meter (3 feet) or more in the nerve cells that cause you to wiggle your toes. Furthermore, a cell's structure often reflects its function; this will become clear later in this chapter. Cells can have amazingly different shapes. Some are disk-shaped (red blood cells), some have threadlike extensions (nerve cells), others are like toothpicks pointed at each end (smooth muscle cells), and still others are cubelike (some types of epithelial cells).

Cells also vary dramatically in the functions, or roles, they play in the body. For example, white blood cells wander freely through the body tissues and protect the body by destroying bacteria and other foreign substances. Some cells make hormones or chemicals that regulate other body cells. Still others take part in gas exchanges in the lungs or cleanse the blood (kidney tubule cells).

Cell Structure

Although no one cell type is exactly like all others, cells *do* have the same basic parts, and there are certain functions common to *all* cells. Here we will talk about the **generalized cell,** which demonstrates these many typical features.

In general, all cells have three main regions or parts—a *nucleus* (nu′kle-us), *cytoplasm* (si′to-plazm″), and a *plasma membrane* (Figure 3.1). The nucleus is usually located near the center of the cell. It is surrounded by the semifluid cytoplasm, which in turn is enclosed by the plasma membrane, which forms the outer cell boundary. (Figure 3.3 shows the more detailed structure of the generalized cell as revealed by the electron microscope.)

The Nucleus

Anything that works, works best when it is controlled. For cells, "headquarters," or the control center, is the gene-containing **nucleus** (*nucle* = kernal). The genetic material, or *deoxyribonucleic acid (DNA),* is much like a blueprint that contains all the instructions needed for building the whole body; so, as one might expect, human DNA differs from that of a frog. More specifically, DNA has the instructions for building *proteins.* DNA is also absolutely necessary for cell reproduction. A cell that has lost or ejected its nucleus (for whatever reason) is programmed only to die.

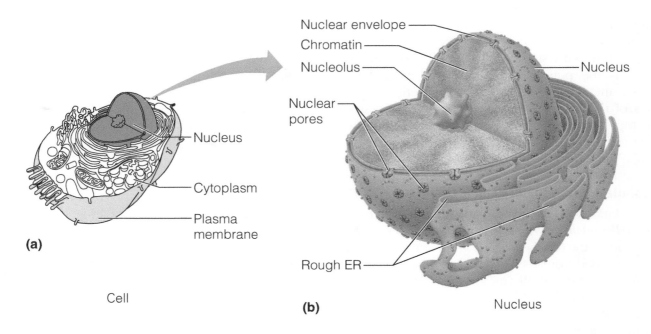

FIGURE 3.1 **Anatomy of the generalized animal cell nucleus.**
(a) Orientation diagram: The three main regions of the generalized cell.
(b) Structure of the nucleus.

While most often oval or spherical, the shape of the nucleus usually conforms to the shape of the cell. For example, if the cell is elongated, the nucleus is usually extended as well. The nucleus has three recognizable regions or structures: the nuclear envelope, nucleoli, and chromatin.

Nuclear Envelope

The nucleus is bound by a double membrane barrier called the **nuclear envelope,** or **nuclear membrane** (see Figure 3.1). Between the two membranes is a fluid-filled "moat," or space. At various points, the two layers of the nuclear envelope fuse, and **nuclear pores** penetrate through the fused regions. Like other cellular membranes, the nuclear envelope is selectively permeable, but passage of substances through it is much freer than elsewhere because of its relatively large pores. The nuclear membrane encloses a jellylike fluid called *nucleoplasm* (nu′kle-o-plazm″) in which other nuclear elements are suspended.

Nucleoli

The nucleus contains one or more small, dark-staining, essentially round bodies called **nucleoli** (nu-kle′o-li; "little nuclei"). Nucleoli are sites where ribosomes are assembled. The *ribosomes,* most of which eventually migrate into the cytoplasm, serve as the actual sites of protein synthesis, as described shortly.

Chromatin

When a cell is not dividing, its DNA is combined with protein and forms a loose network of bumpy threads called **chromatin** (kro′mah-tin) that is scattered throughout the nucleus. When a cell is dividing to form two daughter cells, the chromatin threads coil and condense to form dense, rodlike bodies called **chromosomes**—much the way a stretched spring becomes shorter and thicker when allowed to relax.

The Plasma Membrane Throughout the Cell

The flexible **plasma membrane** is a fragile, transparent barrier that contains the cell contents and separates them from the surrounding environment. (The term *cell membrane* is often used instead, but since nearly all cellular organelles are composed of membranes, we will specifically refer to the cell's surface or outer limiting membrane as the plasma membrane.) Although the plasma membrane is important in defining the limits of the cell, it is much more than a passive envelope, or "baggie." As you will see, its unique structure allows it to play a dynamic role in many cellular activities.

Specializations of the Plasma Membrane

Specializations of the plasma membrane—such as *microvilli* and *membrane junctions*—are commonly displayed by the (epithelial) cells that form the linings of hollow body organs, such as the small intestine (Figure 3.2). **Microvilli** (mi"kro-vil'i; "little shaggy hairs") are tiny fingerlike projections that greatly increase the cell's surface area for absorption so that the process occurs more quickly.

The **membrane junctions** vary structurally depending on their roles.

- **Tight junctions** are impermeable junctions that bind cells together into leakproof sheets that prevent substances from passing through the extracellular space between cells. In tight junctions, adjacent plasma membranes fuse together tightly like a zipper. In the small intestine, for example, these junctions prevent digestive enzymes from seeping into the bloodstream.

- **Desmosomes** (des'mo-somz) are anchoring junctions that prevent cells subjected to mechanical stress (such as skin cells) from being pulled apart. Structurally, these junctions are plaques, buttonlike thickenings of adjacent plasma membranes, which are connected by fine protein filaments. Thicker protein filaments extend from the plaques inside the cells to the plaques on the cells' opposite sides, thus forming an internal system of strong guy wires.

- **Gap junctions,** commonly seen in the heart and between embryonic cells, function mainly to allow communication. Chemical molecules, such as nutrients or ions, can pass directly from one cell to another through them. In gap junctions, the neighboring cells are connected by **connexons,** which are hollow cylinders composed of proteins that span the entire width of the abutting membranes.

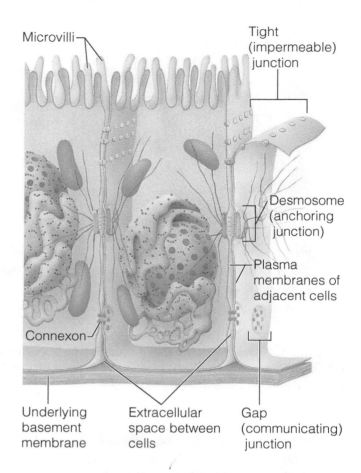

Microvilli

Tight (impermeable) junction

Desmosome (anchoring junction)

Plasma membranes of adjacent cells

Connexon

Underlying basement membrane

Extracellular space between cells

Gap (communicating) junction

FIGURE 3.2 Cell junctions. An epithelial cell is shown joined to adjacent cells by the three common types of cell junctions: tight junctions, desmosomes, and gap junctions. Also illustrated are microvilli (seen projecting from the free cell surface).

The Cytoplasm

The **cytoplasm** is the cellular material outside the nucleus and inside the plasma membrane. It is the site of most cellular activities, so it can be thought of as the "factory area" of the cell. Although early scientists believed that the cytoplasm was a structureless gel, the electron microscope has revealed that it has three major elements: the *cytosol, organelles,* and *inclusions.* The **cytosol** is semitransparent fluid that suspends the other elements. Dissolved in the cytosol, which is largely water, are nutrients and a variety of other solutes (dissolved substances).

The **organelles** (or"gah-nelz'), described in detail shortly, are the metabolic machinery of the cell. Each type of organelle is specialized to carry out a specific function for the cell as a whole. Some synthesize proteins, others package those proteins, and so on.

Inclusions are not functioning units, but instead are chemical substances that may or may not be present, depending on the specific cell type. Most inclusions are stored nutrients or cell products. They include the lipid droplets common in fat cells, glycogen granules abundant in liver and muscle cells, pigments such as melanin seen in skin and hair cells, mucus and other secretory products, and various kinds of crystals.

Cytoplasmic Organelles

The cytoplasmic organelles, literally "little organs," are specialized cellular compartments (Figure 3.3), each performing its own job to maintain the life of the cell. Many organelles are bounded by a membrane similar to the plasma membrane. The membrane boundaries of such organelles allow them to maintain an internal environment quite different from that of the surrounding cytosol. This compartmentalization is crucial to their ability to perform their specialized functions for the cell. Let us consider what goes on in each of the workshops of our cellular factory.

Mitochondria **Mitochondria** (mi″to-kon′dre-ah) are usually depicted as tiny threadlike (*mitos* = thread) or sausage-shaped organelles (see Figure 3.3), but in living cells they squirm, lengthen, and change shape almost continuously. The mitochondrial wall consists of a double membrane, equal to *two* plasma membranes, placed side by side. The outer membrane is smooth and featureless, but the inner membrane has shelflike protrusions called *cristae* (kris′te; crests). Enzymes dissolved in the fluid within the mitochondria, as well as enzymes that form part of the cristae membranes, carry out the reactions in which oxygen is used to break down foods. As the foods are broken down, energy is released. Much of this energy escapes as heat, but some is captured and used to form *ATP molecules*. ATP provides the energy for all cellular work, and every living cell requires a constant supply of ATP for its many activities. Because the mitochondria supply most of this ATP, they are referred to as the "powerhouses" of the cell.

Metabolically "busy" cells, like liver and muscle cells, use huge amounts of ATP and have hundreds of mitochondria. By contrast, cells that are relatively inactive (an unfertilized egg, for instance) have just a few.

Ribosomes **Ribosomes** (ri′bo-sōmz) are tiny, bilobed, dark bodies made of proteins and one variety of RNA called *ribosomal RNA*. Ribosomes are the actual sites of protein synthesis in the cell. Some ribosomes float free in the cytoplasm where they manufacture proteins that function in the cytoplasm. Others attach to membranes and the whole ribosome-membrane combination is called the *rough endoplasmic reticulum.*

Endoplasmic Reticulum The **endoplasmic reticulum** (en″do-plas′mik rĕ-tik′u-lum; "network within the cytoplasm") **(ER)** is a system of fluid-filled cisterns (tubules, or canals) that coil and twist through the cytoplasm. It accounts for about half of a cell's membranes. It serves as a minicirculatory system for the cell because it provides a network of channels for carrying substances (primarily proteins) from one part of the cell to another. There are two forms of ER; a particular cell may have both forms or only one, depending on its specific functions.

The **rough ER** is so called because it is studded with ribosomes. Because essentially all of the building materials of cellular membranes are formed either in it or on it, the rough ER can be thought of as the cell's membrane factory. The proteins made on its ribosomes migrate into the tubules of the rough ER where they fold into their functional three-dimensional shapes and then are dispatched to other areas of the cell in *transport vesicles* (Figure 3.4). In general the amount of rough ER a cell has is a good clue to the amount of protein that cell makes. Rough ER is especially abundant in cells that export protein products—for example, pancreas cells, which produce digestive enzymes to be delivered to the small intestine. The enzymes that catalyze the synthesis of membrane lipids reside on the external face of the rough ER, where the needed building blocks are readily available.

Although the **smooth ER** communicates with the rough variety, it plays no role in protein synthesis. Instead it functions in lipid metabolism (cholesterol and fat synthesis and breakdown), and detoxification of drugs and pesticides. Hence it is not surprising that the liver cells are chock-full of smooth ER. So too are body cells that produce steroid-based hormones—for instance, cells of the male testes that manufacture testosterone.

Q *Which nuclear component contains your genes?*

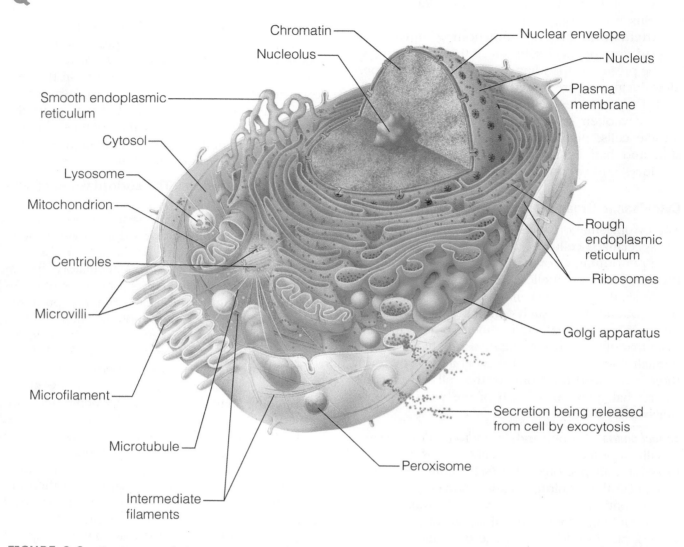

FIGURE 3.3 **Structure of the generalized cell.** No cell is exactly like this
one, but this generalized cell drawing illustrates features common to many
human cells.

Golgi Apparatus   The **Golgi** (gol′je) **apparatus**
appears as a stack of flattened membranous sacs,
associated with swarms of tiny vesicles. It is generally found close to the nucleus and is the principal
"traffic director" for cellular proteins. Its major
function is to modify and package proteins (sent to
it by the rough ER via **transport vesicles**) in
specific ways, depending on their final destination
(Figure 3.5).

As proteins "tagged" for export accumulate in
the Golgi apparatus, the sacs swell. Then their
swollen ends, filled with protein, pinch off and
form **secretory vesicles** (ves′ĭ-kuls), which travel
to the plasma membrane. When the vesicles reach
the plasma membrane, they fuse with it, the membrane ruptures, and the contents of the sac are
ejected to the outside of the cell (pathway 1 in
Figure 3.5). Mucus is packaged this way, as are
digestive enzymes made by pancreas cells.

In addition to its packaging-for-release functions,
the Golgi apparatus pinches off sacs containing

A   *The nucleus.*

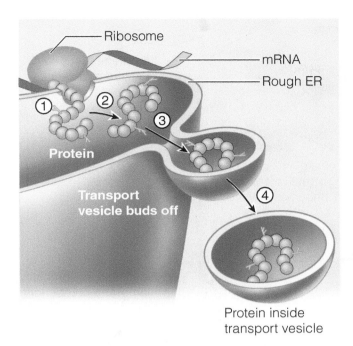

Protein inside
transport vesicle

FIGURE 3.4 Synthesis and export of a protein by the rough ER. ⟨1⟩ As the protein is synthesized on the ribosome, it migrates into the rough ER cisterna. ⟨2⟩ In the cisterna, short sugar chains may be attached to the protein (forming a glycoprotein) and the protein folds into its functional shape. ⟨3⟩ The protein is then packaged in a tiny membranous sac called a transport vesicle. ⟨4⟩ The transport vesicle buds from the rough ER and travels to the Golgi apparatus for further processing or directly to the plasma membrane where its contents are secreted.

proteins and phospholipids destined to become part of the plasma membrane (pathway 2 in Figure 3.5) and packages hydrolytic enzymes into membranous sacs called *lysosomes* that remain in the cell (pathway 3 in Figure 3.5).

Lysosomes **Lysosomes** (li′so-sōmz; "breakdown bodies"), which appear in different sizes, are membranous "bags" containing powerful digestive enzymes. Because lysosomal enzymes are capable of digesting worn-out or nonusable cell structures and most foreign substances that enter the cell, lysosomes function as the cell's demolition sites. Lysosomes are especially abundant in white blood cells that engulf bacteria and other potentially harmful substances because they digest and rid the body of such foreign invaders.

As described above, the enzymes they contain are formed by ribosomes and packaged by the Golgi apparatus.

Peroxisomes **Peroxisomes** (per-ok′sih-sōmz) are membranous sacs containing powerful oxidase (ok′sĭ-dāz) enzymes that use molecular oxygen (O_2) to detoxify a number of harmful or poisonous substances, including alcohol and formaldehyde. However, their most important function is to "disarm" dangerous free radicals. **Free radicals** are highly reactive chemicals with unpaired electrons that can scramble the structure of proteins and nucleic acids. Although free radicals are normal by-products of cellular metabolism, if allowed to accumulate, they can have devastating effects on cells. Peroxisomes convert free radicals to hydrogen peroxide (H_2O_2), a function indicated in their naming (*peroxisomes* = "peroxide bodies"). The enzyme *catalase* (kat′ah-lās) then converts excess hydrogen peroxide to water. Peroxisomes are especially numerous in liver and kidney cells, which are very active in detoxification.

Although peroxisomes look like small lysosomes (see Figure 3.3), they do not arise by budding from the Golgi apparatus. Instead, they appear to replicate themselves by simply pinching in half, as do mitochondria.

Cytoskeleton An elaborate network of protein structures extends throughout the cytoplasm. This network, or **cytoskeleton,** acts as a cell's "bones and muscles" by furnishing an internal framework that determines cell shape, supports other organelles, and provides the machinery needed for intracellular transport and various types of cellular movements. From its largest to its smallest elements, the cytoskeleton is made up of microtubules, intermediate filaments, and microfilaments (Figures 3.3 and 3.6). Although there is some overlap in roles, generally speaking the strong, stable ropelike **intermediate filaments** help form desmosomes (see Figure 3.2) and provide internal guy wires to resist pulling forces on the cell. **Microfilaments** (such as *actin* and *myosin*) are most involved in cell motility and in producing changes in cell shape. You could say that cells move when they get their act(in) together. The tubelike **microtubules** determine the overall shape of a cell and the distribution of organelles. They are very important during cell division.

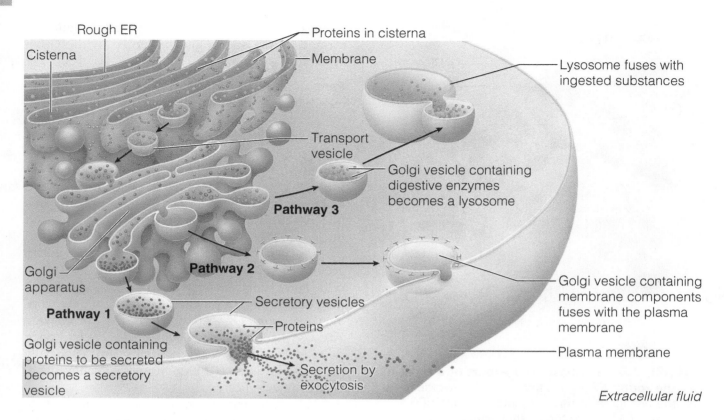

FIGURE 3.5 **Role of the Golgi apparatus in packaging the products of the rough ER.** Protein-containing transport vesicles pinch off the rough ER and migrate to fuse with the Golgi apparatus. As it passes through the Golgi apparatus, the protein product is sorted (and slightly modified). The product is then packaged within vesicles, which leave the Golgi apparatus and head for various destinations (pathways 1–3), as shown.

Centrioles The paired **centrioles** (sen′tre-ōlz) lie close to the nucleus (see Figure 3.3). They are rod-shaped bodies that lie at right angles to each other; internally they are made up of fine microtubules. During cell division, the centrioles direct the formation of the *mitotic spindle.*

In addition to the cell structures described above, some cells have projections called **cilia** (sil′e-ah; "eyelashes"), whiplike cellular extensions that move substances along the cell surface. For example, the ciliated cells of the respiratory system lining move mucus up and away from the lungs. Where cilia appear, there are usually many of them projecting from the exposed cell surface. When a cell is about to make cilia, its centrioles multiply and then line up beneath the plasma membrane at the free cell surface. Microtubules then begin to "sprout" from the centrioles and put pressure on the membrane, forming the projections. If the projections formed by the centrioles

are substantially longer, they are called **flagella** (flah-jel′ah). The only example of a flagellated cell in the human body is the sperm, which has a single propulsive flagellum called its *tail. Notice that cilia propel other substances across a cell's surface, whereas a flagellum propels the cell itself.*

Table 3.1 summarizes the organelles of a representative cell.

The Plasma Membrane's Structure

The structure of the plasma membrane consists of two lipid (fat) layers arranged "tail to tail" in which protein molecules float (Figure 3.7). Although most of the lipid portion is *phospholipids* (some with attached sugar groups), a substantial amount of *cholesterol* is also found in plasma membranes. The olive oil–like lipid bilayer forms the basic "fabric" of the membrane. The polar "heads" of the lollipop-shaped phospholipid molecules are

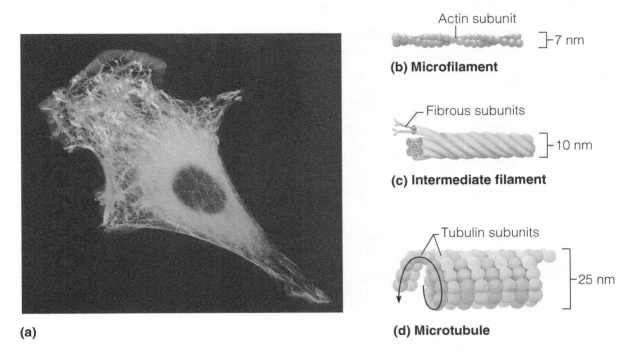

Actin subunit
]-7 nm
(b) Microfilament

Fibrous subunits
]-10 nm
(c) Intermediate filament

Tubulin subunits
-25 nm
(d) Microtubule

(a)

FIGURE 3.6 **The cytoskeleton. (a)** In this light micrograph of the cytoskeleton of a nerve cell, the microtubules appear green; the microfilaments are blue. Intermediate filaments form most of the rest of the network. **(b–d)** Diagrammatic views of the three types of cytoskeletal elements.

hydrophilic ("water loving") and are attracted to water, the main component of both the intercellular and extracellular fluids, and so they lie on both the inner and outer surfaces of the membrane. Their nonpolar "tails" are *hydrophobic* ("water hating") and avoid water, lining up in the center of the membrane. It is the hydrophobic makeup of the membrane interior that makes the plasma membrane relatively impermeable to most water-soluble molecules. The cholesterol has a stabilizing effect and helps keep the membrane fluid.

The proteins scattered in the lipid bilayer are responsible for most of the specialized functions of the membrane. Some proteins are enzymes. Many of the proteins mounted on the cell exterior are **receptor sites** for hormones or other chemical messengers or are binding sites for anchoring the cell to fibers or to other extracellular structures. Most proteins that span the membrane are involved in transport functions. For example, some cluster together to form protein channels (tiny *pores*) through which water and small water-soluble molecules or ions can move; others act as

carriers that bind to a substance and move it through the membrane. Branching sugar groups are attached to most of the proteins abutting the extracellular space. Such "sugar-proteins" are called *glycoproteins,* and because of their presence, the cell surface is a fuzzy, sticky, sugar-rich area. (You can think of your cells as being sugar-coated.) Among other things, these glycoproteins determine your blood type, act as *receptors* that certain bacteria, viruses, or toxins can bind to, and play a role in cell-to-cell interactions. Definite changes in glycoproteins occur in cells that are being transformed into cancer cells.

Membrane Transport

The fluid environment on both sides of the plasma membrane is an example of a solution. It is important that you really understand solutions before we dive into an explanation of membrane transport. In the most basic sense, a **solution** is a homogeneous mixture of two or more components. Examples include the air we breathe (a mixture of

TABLE 3.1   Organelles of a Representative Cell
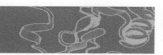

Appearance	Structure	Composition	Function
	CELL MEMBRANE	Lipid bilayer, containing phospholipids, steroids, and proteins	Isolation; protection; sensitivity; support; controls entrance/exit of materials
	CYTOSOL	Fluid component of cytoplasm	Distributes materials by diffusion
	NONMEMBRANOUS ORGANELLES		
	Cytoskeleton *Microtubule* *Microfilament*	Proteins organized in fine filaments or slender tubes	Strength and support; movement of cellular structures and materials; cell movement
	Microvilli	Membrane extensions containing microfilaments	Increase surface area to facilitate absorption of extracellular materials
	Cilia	Membrane extensions containing microtubule doublets	Movement of materials over cell surface
	Centrosome *Centriole*	Cytoplasm containing two centrioles at right angles; each centriole is composed of 9 microtubule triplets	Essential for movement of chromosomes during cell division; organization of microtubules in cytoskeleton
	Ribosomes	RNA + proteins; fixed ribosomes bound to rough ER, free ribosomes scattered in cytoplasm	Protein synthesis
	Proteasomes	Hollow cylinder of proteolytic enzymes with regulatory proteins at ends	Breakdown and recycling of intracellular proteins
	MEMBRANOUS ORGANELLES		
	Mitochondria	Double membrane, with inner membrane folds (cristae) enclosing important metabolic enzymes	Produce 95% of the ATP required by the cell
	Endoplasmic reticulum (ER)	Network of membranous channels extending throughout the cytoplasm	Synthesis of secretory products; intracellular storage and transport
	Rough ER	Has ribosomes bound to membranes	Modification and packaging of newly synthesized proteins
	Smooth ER	Lacks attached ribosomes	Lipid and carbohydrate synthesis
	Golgi apparatus	Stacks of flattened membranes (cisternae) containing chambers	Storage, alteration, and packaging of secretory products and lysosomal enzymes
	Lysosomes	Vesicles containing powerful digestive enzymes	Intracellular removal of damaged organelles or of pathogens
	Peroxisomes	Vesicles containing degradative enzymes	Neutralization of toxic compounds
	NUCLEUS *Nuclear envelope* *Nuclear pore*	Nucleoplasm containing nucleotides, enzymes, nucleoproteins, and chromatin; surrounded by a doublemembrane (nuclear envelope)	Control of metabolism; storage and processing of genetic information; control of protein synthesis
	Nucleolus	Dense region in nucleoplasm containing DNA and RNA	Site of rRNA synthesis and assembly of ribosomal subunits

Q *Why do the phospholipids organize into a bilayer, tail to tail, in an aqueous environment?*

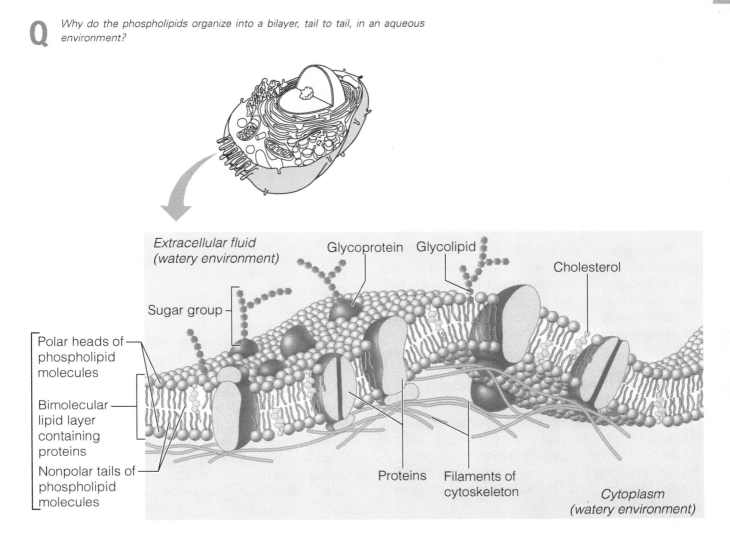

Extracellular fluid *(watery environment)*

Glycoprotein Glycolipid

Cholesterol

Sugar group

Polar heads of phospholipid molecules

Bimolecular lipid layer containing proteins

Nonpolar tails of phospholipid molecules

Proteins Filaments of cytoskeleton

Cytoplasm (watery environment)

FIGURE 3.7   Structure of the plasma membrane.

gases), seawater (a mixture of water and salts), and rubbing alcohol (a mixture of water and alcohol). The substance present in the largest amount in a solution is called the **solvent** (or dissolving medium). Water is the body's chief solvent. Components or substances present in smaller amounts are called **solutes.** The solutes in a solution are so tiny, they do not settle out.

Intracellular fluid (collectively, the nucleoplasm and the cytosol) is a solution containing small amounts of gases (oxygen and carbon

dioxide), nutrients, and salts, dissolved in water. So too is **interstitial fluid,** the fluid that continuously bathes the exterior of our cells. Interstitial fluid can be thought of as a rich, nutritious, and rather unusual "soup." It contains thousands of ingredients, including nutrients (amino acids, sugars, fatty acids, vitamins), regulatory substances such as hormones and neurotransmitters, salts, and waste products. To remain healthy, each cell must extract from this soup the exact amounts of the substances it needs at specific times and reject the rest.

The plasma membrane is a selectively permeable barrier. **Selective permeability** means that a barrier allows some substances to pass through it while excluding others. Thus, it allows nutrients to enter the cell but keeps many undesirable

A *The phospholipids have hydrophilic and hydrophobic regions. The hydrophobic (tail) regions shun water and form the inner portion of the membrane in an aqueous environment.*

substances out. At the same time, valuable cell proteins and other substances are kept within the cell, and wastes are allowed to pass out of it.

⚠ Homeostatic Imbalance

The property of selective permeability is typical only of healthy, unharmed cells. When a cell dies or is badly damaged, its plasma membrane can no longer be selective and becomes permeable to nearly everything. This phenomenon is evident when someone has been severely burned. Precious fluids, proteins, and ions "weep" (leak out) from the dead and damaged cells of the burned areas. ▲

Movement of substances through the plasma membrane happens in basically two ways—passively or actively. In **passive transport processes,** substances are transported across the membrane without any energy input from the cell. In **active transport processes,** the cell provides the metabolic energy (ATP) that drives the transport process.

Celluar Fluid Dynamics: Passive Transport Diffusion and Filtration

Diffusion (dĭ-fu′zhun) is an important means of passive membrane transport for every cell of the body. The other passive transport process, *filtration,* generally occurs only across capillary walls. Let us examine how these two types of passive transport differ.

Diffusion **Diffusion** is the process by which molecules (and ions) tend to scatter themselves throughout the available space. All molecules possess *kinetic energy* (energy of motion). As the molecules move about randomly at high speeds, they collide and change direction with each collision. Since the overall effect of this erratic movement is that molecules move away from a region where they are more concentrated (more numerous) to a region where they are less concentrated (fewer of them), we say that molecules move *down* their **concentration gradient.** Because the driving force (source of energy) is the kinetic energy of the molecules themselves, the speed of diffusion is affected by the size of the molecules (the smaller the faster) and temperature (the warmer the faster).

An example should help you understand diffusion. Picture yourself pouring a cup of coffee, and then adding a cube of sugar (but not stirring the cup). After adding the sugar, the phone rings, and you are called in to work. You never do get to

drink the coffee. Upon returning that evening, you find that the coffee tastes sweet even though it was never stirred. This is because the sugar molecules moved around all day and eventually, as a result of their activity, became sufficiently distributed throughout the coffee to sweeten the entire cup. A laboratory example that might be familiar to some students is illustrated in Figure 3.8.

The plasma membrane is a physical barrier to diffusion. Molecules will move *passively* through the plasma membrane by diffusion if (1) they are small enough to pass through its pores or (2) they can dissolve in the fatty portion of the membrane (Figure 3.9). The unassisted diffusion of solutes through the plasma membrane (or any selectively permeable membrane) is called **simple diffusion** (Figure 3.9a). Solutes transported this way are either lipid-soluble (fats, fat-soluble vitamins, oxygen, carbon dioxide) or small enough to pass through the membrane pores (some small ions such as chloride ions, for example).

Diffusion of water through a selectively permeable membrane such as the plasma membrane is specifically called **osmosis** (oz-mo′sis). Because water is highly polar, it is repelled by the (nonpolar) lipid core of the plasma membrane, but it can and does pass easily through special pores called *aquaporins* ("water pores") created by the proteins in the membrane. Osmosis into and out of cells is

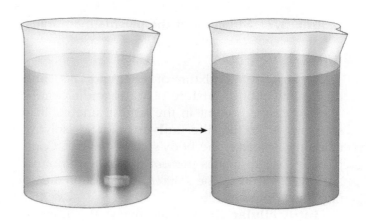

FIGURE 3.8 Diffusion. Particles in solution move continuously and collide constantly with other particles. As a result, particles tend to move away from areas where they are most highly concentrated and to become evenly distributed, as illustrated by the diffusion of dye molecules in a beaker of water.

Q *What "facilitates" facilitated diffusion?*

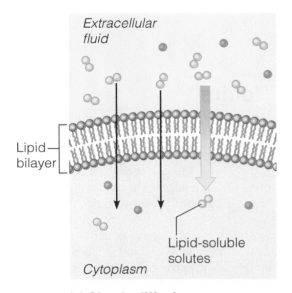

(a) Simple diffusion

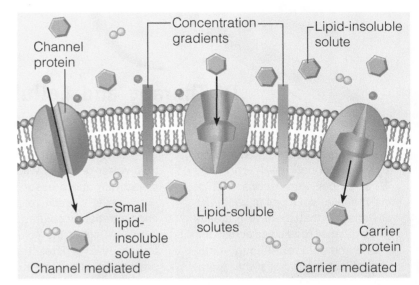

(b) Facilitated diffusion

FIGURE 3.9   Diffusion through the plasma membrane. (a) Simple diffusion. Lipid-soluble molecules diffuse directly through the lipid bilayer of the plasma membrane, in which they can dissolve. **(b)** Facilitated diffusion. On the left, small lipid-insoluble substances (water molecules or small ions) are shown diffusing through channels constructed by membrane proteins. On the right, facilitated diffusion moves large, lipid-insoluble molecules (e.g., glucose) across the membrane. The substance to be transported binds to a transmembrane protein carrier in this example.

occurring all the time as water moves down its concentration gradient.

Still another example of diffusion is **facilitated diffusion** (see Figure 3.9b). Facilitated diffusion provides passage for certain needed substances (notably glucose) that are both lipid-insoluble and too large to pass through the membrane pores. Although facilitated diffusion follows the laws of diffusion—that is, the substances move down their own concentration gradient—a protein membrane channel is used or a protein molecule that acts as a carrier is needed as a transport vehicle. Hence, some of the proteins in the plasma membrane form channels or act as carriers to move glucose and certain other solutes passively across the membrane and make it available for cell use.

Substances that pass into and out of cells by diffusion save the cell a great deal of energy. When you consider how vitally important water, glucose, and oxygen are to cells, it becomes apparent just how necessary these passive transport processes really are. Glucose and oxygen continually move into the cells (where they are in lower concentration because the cells keep using them up), and carbon dioxide (a waste product of cellular activity) continually moves out of the cells into the blood (where it is in lower concentration).

Filtration   **Filtration** is the process by which water and solutes are forced through a membrane (or capillary wall) by *fluid,* or *hydrostatic, pressure.* In the body, hydrostatic pressure is usually exerted by the blood. Like diffusion, filtration is a passive process, and a gradient is involved. In filtration, however, the gradient is a **pressure gradient** that actually pushes solute-containing fluid (*filtrate*) from the higher-pressure area to the lower-pressure area. Filtration is

A   *Carrier proteins or protein channels.*

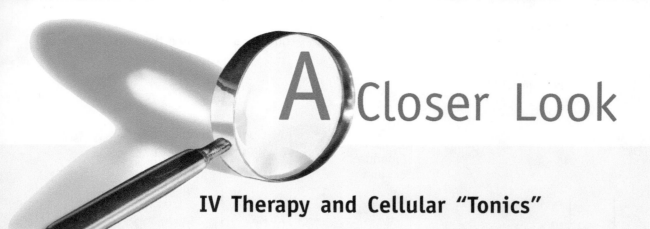

A Closer Look

IV Therapy and Cellular "Tonics"

WHY is it essential that medical personnel give only the proper *intravenous (IV)*, or into-the-vein, *solutions* to patients?

Consider that there is a steady traffic of small molecules across the plasma membrane. Although diffusion of solutes across the membrane is rather slow, osmosis, which moves water across the membrane, occurs very quickly. Anyone administering an IV must use the correct solution to protect the patient's cells from life-threatening dehydration or rupture due to excessive water entry.

The tendency of a solution to hold water or "pull" water into it is called osmotic pressure. Osmotic pressure is directly related to the concentration of solutes in the solution. The higher the solute concentration, the greater the osmotic pressure and the greater the tendency of water to move into the solution. Many molecules, particularly proteins and some ions, are prevented from diffusing through the plasma membrane. Consequently, any change in their concentration on one side of the membrane forces water to move from one side of the

membrane to the other, causing cells to lose or gain water. The ability of a solution to change the size and shape of cells by altering the amount of water they contain is called *tonicity* (ton-is'i-te; *ton* = strength).

Isotonic (i"so-ton'ik; "same tonicity") solutions (such as Ringer's lactate, 5 percent dextrose, and 0.9 percent saline) have the same solute and water concentrations as cells do. Isotonic solutions cause no visible changes in cells, and when such solutions are infused into the bloodstream, red blood cells retain their normal size and disclike shape

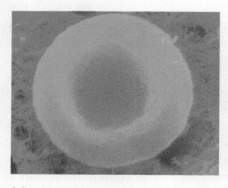
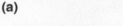

(a)

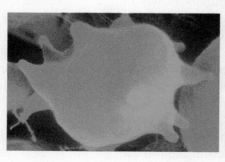

(b)

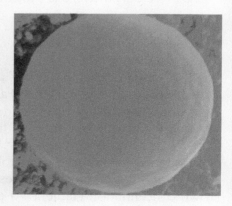

(c)

The effect of IV solutions of varying tonicity on living red blood cells.

IV Therapy and Cellular "Tonics" (continued)

(Photo a). As you might guess, interstitial fluid and most intravenous solutions are isotonic solutions.

If red blood cells are exposed to a *hypertonic* (hi"per-ton'ik) solution—a solution that contains more solutes, or dissolved substances, than there are inside the cells—the cells will begin to shrink, or *crenate* (kre'nāt). This is because water is in higher concentration inside the cell than outside, so it follows its concentration gradient and leaves the cell (Photo b). Hypertonic solutions are sometimes given to patients who have *edema* (swollen feet and hands because of fluid retention). Such solutions draw water out of the tissue spaces into the bloodstream so that excess fluid can be eliminated by the kidneys.

When a solution contains fewer solutes (and therefore more water) than the cell does, it is said to be *hypotonic* (hi"po-ton'ik) to the cell. Cells placed in hypotonic solutions plump up rapidly as water rushes into them (Photo c). Distilled water represents the most extreme example of a hypotonic fluid. Since it contains no solutes at all, water will enter cells until they finally burst, or *lyse*. Hypotonic solutions are sometimes infused intravenously (slowly and with care) to rehydrate the tissues of extremely dehydrated patients. In less extreme cases, drinking hypotonic fluids usually does the trick. (Many fluids that humans tend to drink regularly, such as tea, colas, apple juice, and sport drinks, are hypotonic.)

---

necessary for the kidneys to do their job properly. In the kidneys, water and small solutes filter out of the capillaries into the kidney tubules because the blood pressure in the capillaries is greater than the fluid pressure in the tubules. Part of the filtrate formed in this way eventually becomes urine. Filtration is not very selective. For the most part, only blood cells and protein molecules too large to pass through the membrane pores are held back.

Active Transport Processes

Whenever a cell uses some of its ATP supply to move substances across the membrane, the process is referred to as *active*. Substances moved actively are usually unable to pass in the desired direction by diffusion. They may be too large to pass through membrane channels or the membrane lacks special protein carriers for their transport, they may not be able to dissolve in the fat core, or they may have to move "uphill" *against* their concentration gradients. The two most important examples of active transport mechanisms, *solute pumping* and *bulk transport,* are described next.

Solute Pumping Solute pumping (more simply called *active transport* by some) is similar to the carrier-mediated facilitated diffusion described earlier in that both processes require protein carriers that combine reversibly with the substances to be transported across the membrane. However, facilitated diffusion is driven by the kinetic energy of the diffusing molecules, whereas solute pumping uses ATP to energize its protein carriers, which are called **solute pumps.** Amino acids, some sugars, and most ions are transported by solute pumps, and in most cases these substances move *against* concentration (or electrical) gradients. This is opposite to the direction in which substances would naturally flow by diffusion, which explains the need for energy in the form of ATP. Amino acids are needed to build cellular proteins but are too large to pass through the membrane channels and are not lipid-soluble. The **sodium-potassium pump** that simultaneously carries sodium ions out of and potassium ions into the cell is absolutely necessary for normal transmission of impulses by nerve cells. Sodium ions (Na$^+$) are moved out of cells by solute pumps (Figure 3.10). There are more sodium ions outside the cells than inside, so they tend to remain in the cell unless the cell uses ATP to force, or "pump," them out. Likewise, there are relatively more potassium ions inside cells than in the interstitial (extracellular) fluid, and potassium ions that leak out of cells must be

actively pumped back inside. Since each of the pumps in the plasma membrane transports only specific substances, solute pumping provides a way for the cell to be very selective in cases where substances cannot pass by diffusion. (No pump—no transport.)

Bulk Transport Some substances that cannot get through the plasma membrane in any other way are transported with the help of ATP out of or into cells by *bulk transport*. The two types of bulk transport are ***exocytosis*** and ***endocytosis***.

Exocytosis (ek"so-si-to'sis; "out of the cell") moves substances out of cells (Figure 3.11). It is the means by which cells actively secrete hormones, mucus, and other cell products or eject certain cellular wastes. The product to be released is first "packaged" (typically by the efforts of the Golgi apparatus) into a small membranous vesicle or sac.

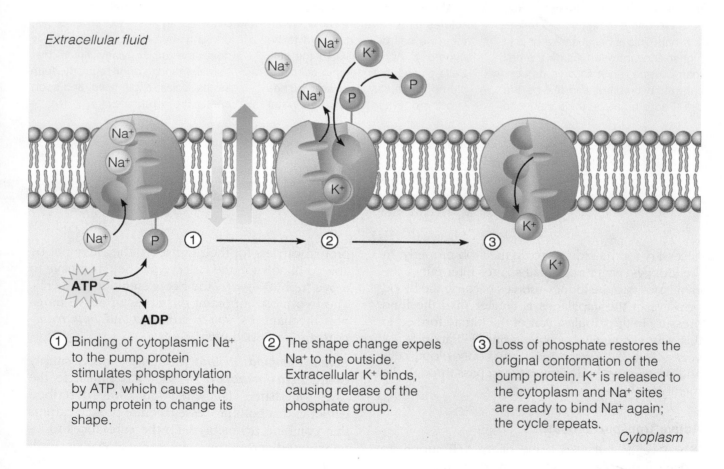

① Binding of cytoplasmic Na$^+$ to the pump protein stimulates phosphorylation by ATP, which causes the pump protein to change its shape.

② The shape change expels Na$^+$ to the outside. Extracellular K$^+$ binds, causing release of the phosphate group.

③ Loss of phosphate restores the original conformation of the pump protein. K$^+$ is released to the cytoplasm and Na$^+$ sites are ready to bind Na$^+$ again; the cycle repeats.

FIGURE 3.10 Operation of the sodium-potassium pump, a solute pump. ATP provides the energy for a "pump" protein to move three sodium ions out of the cell and two potassium ions into the cell. Both ions are moved against their concentration gradients.

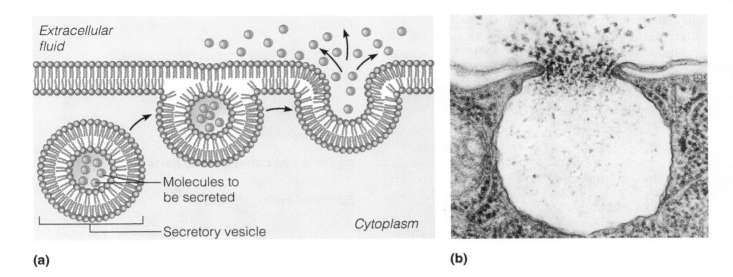

FIGURE 3.11   Exocytosis. (a) A secretory vesicle migrates to the plasma membrane, and the two membranes fuse. The fused site opens and releases the contents to the outside of the cell. **(b)** Electron micrograph of a vesicle in exocytosis (100,000×).

The sac migrates to the plasma membrane and fuses with it. The fused area then ruptures, spilling the sac contents out of the cell (also see Figure 3.5).

Endocytosis (en″do-si-to′sis; "into the cell") includes those ATP-requiring processes that take up, or engulf, extracellular substances by enclosing them in a small membranous vesicle. Once the vesicle, or sac, is formed, it detaches from the plasma membrane and moves into the cytoplasm, where it fuses with a lysosome and its contents are digested (by lysosomal enzymes). If the engulfed substances are relatively large particles such as bacteria or dead body cells, which are separated from the external environment by flowing cytoplasmic extensions called pseudopods, the endocytosis process is more specifically called **phagocytosis** (fag″o-si-to′sis), a term that means "cell eating." Certain white blood cells and other "professional" phagocytes of the body act as scavenger cells that police and protect the body by ingesting bacteria and other foreign debris as well as dead body cells. Hence, phagocytosis is a protective mechanism, not a means of getting nutrients.

If we say that cells can eat, we can also say that they can drink. This is **fluid-phase endocytosis,** also called **pinocytosis** (pi″no-si-to′sis; "cell drinking"). In this process, the plasma membrane invaginates to form a tiny pit and then its edges fuse around the droplet of extracellular fluid containing dissolved proteins or fats. Unlike phagocytosis, it is a routine activity of most cells. It is especially important in cells that function in absorption (for example, cells forming the lining of the small intestine and kidney tubule cells).

Receptor-mediated endocytosis is the main cellular mechanism for taking up specific target molecules. In this process, plasma membrane **receptor proteins** bind only with certain substances, and both the receptors and high concentrations of the attached target molecules are internalized in a vesicle and then the contents of the vesicle are dealt with in one of the following ways. Although phagocytosis and pinocytosis are important, compared to receptor-mediated endocytosis, they are pretty unselective. Substances encytosed by receptor-mediated endocytosis include enzymes, some hormones, cholesterol, and iron. Unfortunately, flu viruses also use this route to enter and attack our cells.

Cell Diversity

So far in this chapter, we have focused on an average human cell. However, the trillions of cells in the human body are made up of some 200 different cell types that vary greatly in size, shape, and function. They include sphere-shaped fat cells, disk-shaped red blood cells, branching nerve cells, and cube-shaped cells of kidney tubules. Figure 3.12 illustrates how the shapes of cells and the relative numbers of the various organelles they contain relate to specialized cell functions. Let's take a look at some of these cell specialists.

1. **Cells that connect body parts:**
   - *Fibroblast.* The elongated shape of this cell lies along the cable-like fibers that it secretes. It also has an abundant rough ER and a large Golgi apparatus to make and secrete the protein building blocks of these fibers.
   - *Erythrocyte (red blood cell).* This cell carries oxygen in the bloodstream. Its concave disk shape provides extra surface area for the uptake of oxygen and streamlines the cell so it flows easily through the bloodstream. So much oxygen-carrying pigment is packed in erythrocytes that all other organelles have been shed to make room.

2. **Cell that covers and lines body organs:**
   - *Epithelial cell.* The hexagonal shape of this cell is exactly like a "cell" in a honeycomb of a beehive. This shape allows epithelial cells to pack together in sheets. An epithelial cell has abundant intermediate filaments that resist tearing when the epithelium is rubbed or pulled.

3. **Cells that move organs and body parts:**
   - *Skeletal muscle* and *smooth muscle cells.* These cells are elongated and filled with abundant contractile filaments, so they can shorten forcefully and move the bones or change the size of internal organs.

4. **Cell that stores nutrients:**
   - *Fat cell.* The huge spherical shape of a fat cell is produced by a large lipid droplet in its cytoplasm.

5. **Cell that fights disease:**
   - *Macrophage (a phagocytic cell).* This cell extends long pseudopods ("false feet") to crawl through tissue to reach infection sites. The many lysosomes within the cell digest the infectious microorganisms it takes up.

FIGURE 3.12 Cell diversity. The shape of human cells and the relative abundances of their various organelles relate to their function in the body.

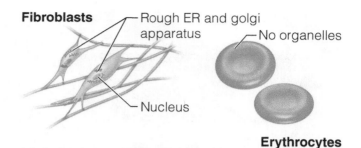

(a) Cells that connect body parts

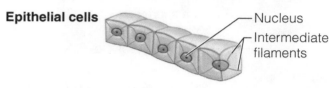

(b) Cells that cover and line body organs

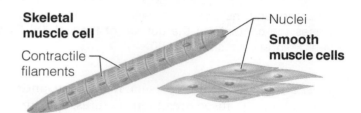

(c) Cells that move organs and body parts

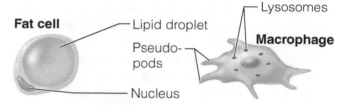

(d) Cell that stores nutrients

(e) Cell that fights disease

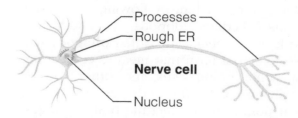

(f) Cell that gathers information and controls body functions

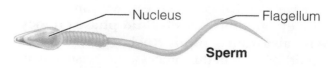

(g) Cell of reproduction

6. **Cell that gathers information and controls body functions:**
   - *Nerve cell (neuron).* This cell has long processes for receiving messages and transmitting them to other structures in the body. The processes are covered with an extensive plasma membrane, and a plentiful rough ER is present to synthesize membrane components.

7. **Cells of reproduction:**
   - *Oocyte (female).* The largest cell in the body, this egg cell contains many copies of all organelles, for distribution to the daughter cells that arise when the fertilized egg divides to become an embryo.
   - *Sperm (male).* This cell is long and streamlined, built for swimming to the egg for fertilization. Its flagellum acts as a motile whip to propel the sperm.

PART II: BODY TISSUES

The human body, complex as it is, starts out as a single cell, the fertilized egg, which divides almost endlessly. The millions of cells that result become specialized for particular functions. Some become muscle cells, others the transparent lens of the eye, still others skin cells, and so on. Thus, there is a division of labor in the body, with certain groups of highly specialized cells performing functions that benefit the organism as a whole.

Cell specialization carries with it certain hazards. When a small group of cells is indispensable, its loss can disable or even destroy the body. For example, the action of the heart depends on a very specialized cell group in the heart muscle that controls its contractions. If those particular cells are damaged or stop functioning, the heart will no longer work efficiently, and the whole body will suffer or die from lack of oxygen.

Groups of cells that are similar in structure and function are called **tissues.** The four primary tissue types—epithelium, connective tissue, nervous tissue, and muscle—interweave to form the fabric of the body. If we had to assign a single term to each primary tissue type that would best describe its overall role, the terms would most likely be *covering* (epithelium), *support* (connective), *movement* (muscle), and *control* (nervous). However, these terms reflect only a tiny fraction of the functions that each of these tissues performs.

Tissues are organized into *organs* such as the heart, kidneys, and lungs. Most organs contain several tissue types, and the arrangement of the tissues determines each organ's structure and what it is able to do. Thus, a study of tissues should be helpful in your later study of the body's organs and how they work.

Epithelial Tissue

Epithelial tissue, or **epithelium** (ep″ĭ-the′le-um; *epithe* = laid on, covering) is the *lining, covering,* and *glandular tissue* of the body. Glandular epithelium forms various glands in the body. Covering and lining epithelium covers all free body surfaces and contains versatile cells. One type forms the outer layer of the skin. Others dip into the body to line its cavities. Since epithelium forms the boundaries that separate us from the outside world, nearly all substances given off or received by the body must pass through epithelium.

Epithelial functions include *protection, absorption, filtration,* and *secretion.* For example, the epithelium of the skin protects against bacterial and chemical damage and that lining the respiratory tract has cilia, which sweep dust and other debris away from the lungs. Epithelium specialized to absorb substances lines some digestive system organs such as the stomach and small intestine, which absorb food into the body. In the kidneys, epithelium both absorbs and filters. Secretion is a specialty of the glands, which produce such substances as perspiration, oil, digestive enzymes, and mucus.

Special Characteristics of Epithelium

Epithelium generally has the characteristics listed below:

- Except for glandular epithelium, epithelial cells fit closely together to form continuous sheets. Neighboring cells are bound together at many points by cell junctions, including desmosomes and tight junctions.

- The membranes always have one free (unattached) surface or edge. This so-called **apical surface** is exposed to the body's exterior or to the cavity of an internal organ. The exposed surfaces of some epithelia are slick and smooth, but others exhibit cell surface modifications, such as microvilli or cilia.

- The lower surface of an epithelium rests on a **basement membrane,** a structureless material secreted by the cells.

- Epithelial tissues have no blood supply of their own (that is, they are *avascular*) and depend on diffusion from the capillaries in the underlying connective tissue for food and oxygen.

- If well nourished, epithelial cells regenerate themselves easily.

Classification of Epithelium

Each epithelium is given two names. The first indicates the relative number of cell layers it has (Figure 3.13a). The classifications by cell arrangement (layers) are **simple epithelium** (one layer of cells) and **stratified epithelium** (more than one cell layer). The second describes the shape of its cells (Figure 3.13b). On this basis there are *squamous* (skwa'mus) *cells,* flattened like fish scales (*squam* = scale), *cuboidal* (ku-boi'dal) *cells,* which are cube-shaped like dice, and *columnar cells,* shaped like columns. The terms describing the shape and arrangement are then combined to describe the epithelium fully. Stratified epithelia are named for the cells at the *free surface* of the epithelial membrane, not those resting on the basement membrane.

Simple Epithelia

The simple epithelia are most concerned with absorption, secretion, and filtration. Because simple epithelia are usually very thin, protection is not one of their specialties.

Simple Squamous Epithelium **Simple squamous epithelium** is a single layer of thin squamous cells resting on a basement membrane. The cells fit closely together, much like floor tiles. This type of epithelium usually forms membranes where filtration or exchange of substances by rapid diffusion occurs. It is in the air sacs of the lungs, where oxygen and carbon dioxide are exchanged (Figure 3.14a), and it forms the walls of capillaries, where nutrients and gases pass between the tissue cells and the blood in the capillaries. Simple squamous epithelium also forms **serous membranes,** or **serosae** (se-ro'se), the slick membranes that line the ventral body cavity and cover the organs in that cavity.

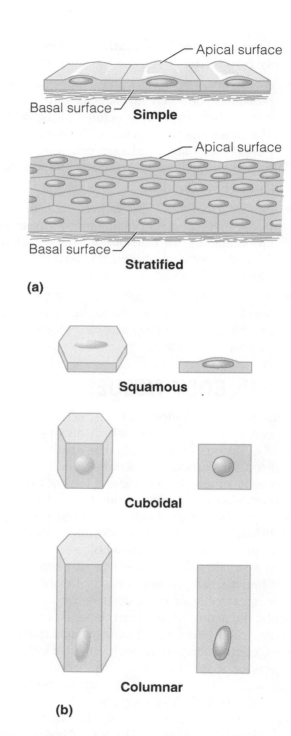

(a)

(b)

FIGURE 3.13 Classification of epithelia. (a) Classification on the basis of arrangement (layers). **(b)** Classification on the basis of cell shape; for each category, a whole cell is shown on the left and a longitudinal section is shown on the right.

Simple Cuboidal Epithelium **Simple cuboidal epithelium,** which is one layer of cuboidal cells resting on a basement membrane, is common in glands and their ducts (for example, the salivary glands and pancreas). It also forms the walls of the kidney tubules and covers the surface of the ovaries (Figure 3.14b).

Simple Columnar Epithelium **Simple columnar epithelium** is made up of a single layer of tall cells that fit closely together. **Goblet cells,** which produce a lubricating mucus, are often seen in this type of epithelium. Simple columnar epithelium lines the entire length of the digestive tract from the stomach to the anus (Figure 3.14c). Epithelial membranes that line body cavities open to the body exterior are called **mucosae** (mu-ko′se) or **mucous membranes.**

Pseudostratified Columnar Epithelium All of the cells of **pseudostratified** (soo″do-stră′tĭ-fĭd) **columnar epithelium** rest on a basement membrane. However, some of its cells are shorter than others, and their nuclei appear at different heights above the basement membrane. As a result, this epithelium gives the false (*pseudo*) impression that it is stratified; hence its name. Like simple columnar epithelium, this variety mainly functions in absorption and secretion. A ciliated variety (more precisely called *pseudostratified ciliated columnar epithelium*) lines most of the respiratory tract (Figure 3.14d). The mucus produced by the goblet cells in this epithelium traps dust and other debris, and the cilia propel the mucus upward and away from the lungs.

Stratified Epithelia

Stratified epithelia consist of two or more cell layers. Being considerably more durable than the simple epithelia, these epithelia function primarily to protect.

Stratified Squamous Epithelium **Stratified squamous epithelium** is the most common stratified epithelium in the body. It usually consists of several layers of cells. The cells at the free edge are squamous cells, whereas those close to the basement membrane are cuboidal or columnar. Stratified squamous epithelium is found in sites that receive a good deal of abuse or friction, such as the esophagus, the mouth, and the outer portion of the skin (Figure 3.14e).

Stratified Cuboidal and Stratified Columnar Epithelia **Stratified cuboidal epithelium** typically has just two cell layers with (at least) the surface cells being cuboidal in shape. The surface cells of **stratified columnar epithelium** are columnar cells, but its basal cells vary in size and shape. Both of these epithelia are fairly rare in the body, being found mainly in the ducts of large glands. (Because the distribution of these two epithelia is extremely limited, they are not illustrated in Figure 3.14. They are described here only to provide a complete listing of the epithelial tissues.)

Transitional Epithelium **Transitional epithelium** is a highly modified, stratified squamous epithelium that forms the lining of only a few organs—the urinary bladder, the ureters, and part of the urethra. *All* these organs are part of the urinary system and are subject to considerable stretching (Figure 3.14f). Cells of the basal layer are cuboidal or columnar; those at the free surface vary in appearance. When the organ is not stretched, the membrane is many-layered, and the superficial cells are rounded and domelike. When the organ is distended with urine, the epithelium thins, and the surface cells flatten and become squamous-like. This ability of transitional cells to slide past one another and change their shape (undergo "transitions") allows the ureter wall to stretch as a greater volume of urine flows through that tube-like organ. In the bladder, it allows more urine to be stored.

Glandular Epithelium

A **gland** consists of one or more cells that make and secrete a particular product. This product, called a **secretion,** typically contains protein molecules in an aqueous (water-based) fluid. The term *secretion* also indicates an active *process* in which the glandular cells obtain needed materials from the blood and use them to make their secretion, which they then discharge.

Two major types of glands develop from epithelial sheets. **Endocrine** (en′do-krin) **glands** lose their connection to the surface (duct); thus they are often called *ductless* glands. Their secretions (all hormones) diffuse directly into the blood vessels that weave through the glands. Examples of endocrine glands include the thyroid, adrenals, and pituitary.

Exocrine (ek′so-krin) **glands** retain their ducts, and their secretions empty through the ducts to the epithelial surface. Exocrine glands, which include the sweat and oil glands, liver, and pancreas,

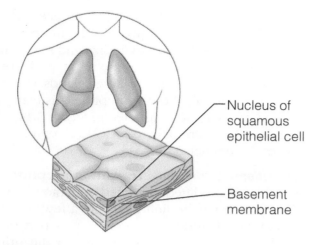

Nucleus of squamous epithelial cell

Basement membrane

(a) Diagram: Simple squamous

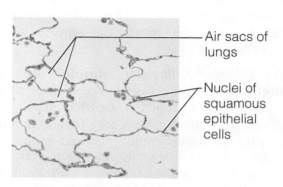

Air sacs of lungs

Nuclei of squamous epithelial cells

Photomicrograph: Simple squamous epithelium forming part of the alveolar (air sac) walls (400×).

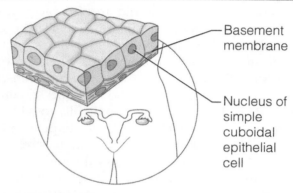

Basement membrane

Nucleus of simple cuboidal epithelial cell

(b) Diagram: Simple cuboidal

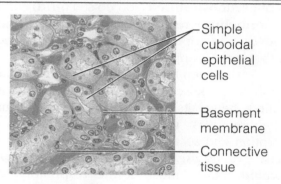

Simple cuboidal epithelial cells

Basement membrane

Connective tissue

Photomicrograph: Simple cuboidal epithelium in kidney tubules (400×).

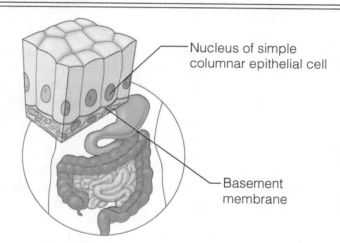

Nucleus of simple columnar epithelial cell

Basement membrane

(c) Diagram: Simple columnar

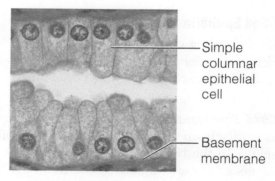

Simple columnar epithelial cell

Basement membrane

Photomicrograph: Simple columnar epithelium of the stomach lining (1300×).

FIGURE 3.14   Types of epithelia and their common locations in the body.

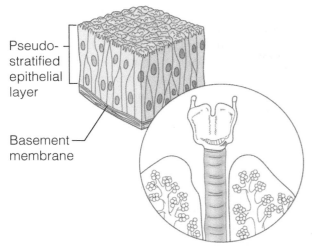

(d) Diagram: Pseudostratified (ciliated) columnar

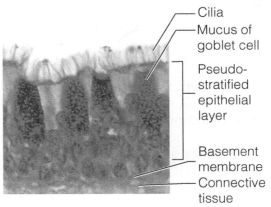

Photomicrograph: Pseudostratified ciliated columnar epithelium lining the human trachea (400×).

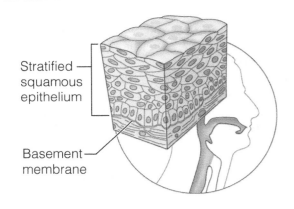

(e) Diagram: Stratified squamous

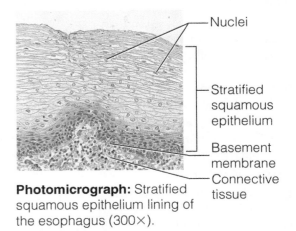

Photomicrograph: Stratified squamous epithelium lining of the esophagus (300×).

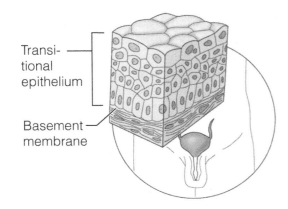

(f) Diagram: Transitional

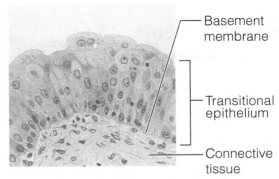

Photomicrograph: Transitional epithelium lining of the bladder, relaxed state (500×); note the bulbous, or rounded, appearance of the cells at the surface; these cells flatten and become elongated when the bladder is filled with urine.

are both internal and external. They are discussed with the organ systems to which their products are related.

Connective Tissue

Connective tissue, as its name suggests, connects body parts. It is found everywhere in the body. It is the most abundant and widely distributed of the tissue types. Connective tissues perform many functions but they are primarily involved in *protecting, supporting,* and *binding together* other body tissues.

Common Characteristics of Connective Tissue

The characteristics of connective tissue include the following:

- Variations in blood supply. Most connective tissues are well *vascularized* (that is, they have a good blood supply), but there are exceptions. Tendons and ligaments have a poor blood supply, and cartilages are avascular. Consequently, all these structures heal very slowly when injured. (This is why some people say that, given a choice, they would rather have a broken bone than a torn ligament.)

- Extracellular matrix. Connective tissues are made up of many different types of cells plus varying amounts of a nonliving substance found outside the cells, called the extracellular matrix.

Extracellular Matrix

The **extracellular matrix** deserves a bit more explanation because it is what makes connective tissue so different from the other tissue types. The matrix, which is produced by the connective tissue cells and then secreted to their exterior, has two main elements, a structureless ground substance and fibers. The *ground substance* of the matrix is composed largely of water plus some adhesion proteins and large, charged polysaccharide molecules. The cell adhesion proteins serve as a glue that allows the connective tissue cells to attach themselves to the matrix fibers embedded in the ground substance. The charged polysaccharide molecules trap water as they intertwine. As the relative abundance of these polysaccharides increases, they

cause the matrix to vary from fluid to gel-like to firm to rock-hard in its consistency. The ability of the ground substance to absorb large amounts of water allow it to serve as a water reservoir for the body. Various types and amounts of fibers are deposited in the matrix and form part of it. These include collagen (white) fibers distinguished by their high tensile strength, elastic (yellow) fibers (the key characteristic of which is an ability to be stretched and then recoil), and reticular fibers (fine collagen fibers that form the internal "skeleton" of soft organs such as the spleen), depending on the connective tissue type. The building blocks, or monomers, of these fibers are made by the connective tissue cells and secreted into the ground substance in the extracellular space, where they spontaneously join together to form the various fiber types.

Because of its extracellular matrix, connective tissue is able to form a soft packing tissue around other organs, to bear weight, and to withstand stretching and other abuses, such as abrasion, that no other tissue could endure. But there is variation. At one extreme, fat tissue is composed mostly of cells, and the matrix is soft. At the opposite extreme, bone and cartilage have very few cells and large amounts of hard matrix, which makes them extremely strong. Find the various types of connective tissues in Figure 3.15 as you read their descriptions that follow.

Types of Connective Tissue

As noted above, all connective tissues consist of living cells surrounded by a matrix. Their major differences reflect fiber type and the number of fibers in the matrix. From most rigid to softest, the major connective tissue classes are *bone, cartilage, dense connective tissue, loose connective tissue,* and *blood.*

Bone

Bone, sometimes called *osseous* (os'e-us) *tissue,* is composed of bone cells sitting in cavities called *lacunae* (lah-ku'ne) and surrounded by layers of a very hard matrix that contains calcium salts in addition to large numbers of collagen fibers (Figure 3.15a). Because of its rocklike hardness, bone has an exceptional ability to protect and support other body organs (for example, the skull protects the brain).

Cartilage

Cartilage is less hard and more flexible than bone. It is found in only a few places in the body. Most widespread is **hyaline** (hi'ah-lin) **cartilage,** which has abundant collagen fibers hidden by a rubbery matrix with a glassy (*hyalin* = glass), blue-white appearance (Figure 3.15b). It forms the supporting structures of the larynx, or voice box, attaches the ribs to the breastbone, and covers the ends of bones where they form joints. The skeleton of a fetus is made largely of hyaline cartilage; but, by the time the baby is born, most of that cartilage has been replaced by bone.

Although hyaline cartilage is the most abundant type of cartilage in the body, there are others. Highly compressible **fibrocartilage** forms the cushionlike disks between the vertebrae of the spinal column (Figure 3.15c). **Elastic cartilage** is found where a structure with elasticity is desired. For example, it supports the external ear. (Elastic cartilage is not illustrated in Figure 3.15.)

Dense Connective Tissue

Dense connective tissue, also called **dense fibrous tissue,** has collagen fibers as its main matrix element (Figure 3.15d). Crowded between the collagen fibers are rows of *fibroblasts* (fiber-forming cells) that manufacture the building blocks of the fibers. Dense connective tissue forms strong, ropelike structures such as tendons and ligaments. **Tendons** attach skeletal muscles to bones; **ligaments** connect bones to bones at joints. Ligaments are more stretchy and contain more elastic fibers than tendons. Dense connective tissue also makes up the lower layers of the skin (dermis), where it is arranged in sheets.

Loose Connective Tissue

Relatively speaking, the **loose connective tissues** are softer and have more cells and fewer fibers than any other connective tissue type except blood.

Areolar Tissue **Areolar** (ah-re'o-lar) **tissue,** the most widely distributed connective tissue variety in the body, is a soft, pliable, "cobwebby" tissue that cushions and protects the body organs it wraps (Figure 3.15e). It functions as a universal packing tissue and connective tissue "glue" because it helps to hold the internal organs together and in their proper positions. A soft layer of areolar connective tissue called the *lamina propria* (lah'mĭ-nah pro'pre-ah) underlies all mucous membranes. Its fluid matrix contains all types of fibers, which form a loose network. In fact, when viewed through a microscope, most of the matrix appears to be empty space, which explains the name of this tissue type (*areola* = small open space). Because of its loose and fluid nature, areolar connective tissue provides a reservoir of water and salts for the surrounding tissues, and essentially all body cells obtain their nutrients from and release their wastes into this "tissue fluid." When a body region is inflamed, the areolar tissue in the area soaks up the excess fluid like a sponge, and the area swells and becomes puffy, a condition called **edema.** Many types of *phagocytes* wander through this tissue, scavenging for bacteria, dead cells, and other debris, which they destroy.

Adipose Tissue **Adipose** (ad'ĭ-pōs) **tissue** is commonly called *fat.* Basically, it is an areolar tissue in which fat cells predominate (Figure 3.15f). A glistening droplet of stored oil occupies most of a fat cell's volume and compresses the nucleus, displacing it to one side. Since the oil-containing region looks empty and the thin rim of cytoplasm containing the bulging nucleus looks like a ring with a seal, fat cells are sometimes called *signet ring cells.*

Adipose tissue forms the subcutaneous tissue beneath the skin, where it insulates the body and protects it from extremes of both heat and cold. Adipose tissue also protects some organs individually. For example, the kidneys are surrounded by a capsule of fat, and adipose tissue cushions the eyeballs in their sockets. There are also fat "depots" in the body, such as the hips and breasts, where fat is stored and available for fuel if needed.

Reticular Connective Tissue **Reticular connective tissue** consists of a delicate network of interwoven reticular fibers associated with *reticular cells,* which resemble fibroblasts (Figure 3.15g). Reticular tissue is limited to certain sites: it forms the **stroma** (literally, "bed" or "mattress"), or internal framework, which can support many free blood cells (largely lymphocytes) in lymphoid organs such as lymph nodes, the spleen, and bone marrow.

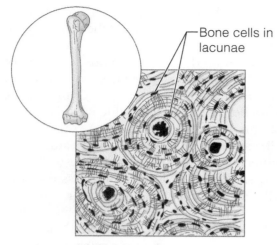

Bone cells in lacunae

(a) Diagram: Bone

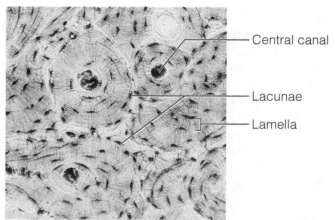

Central canal

Lacunae

Lamella

Photomicrograph: Cross-sectional view of ground bone (70×).

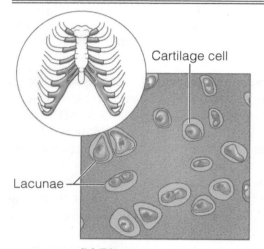

Cartilage cell

Lacunae

(b) Diagram: Hyaline cartilage

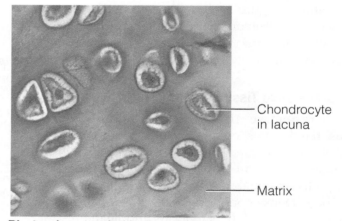

Chondrocyte in lacuna

Matrix

Photomicrograph: Hyaline cartilage from the trachea (300×).

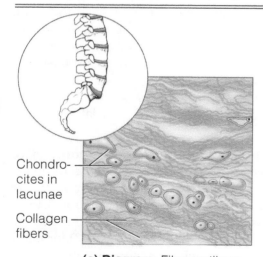

Chondrocites in lacunae

Collagen fibers

(c) Diagram: Fibrocartilage

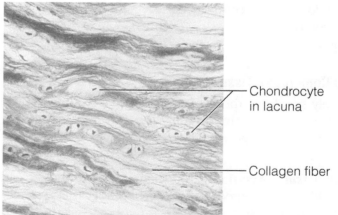

Chondrocyte in lacuna

Collagen fiber

Photomicrograph: Fibrocartilage of an intervertebral disc (200×).

FIGURE 3.15   Connective tissues and their common body locations.
(**e, f,** and **g** are subclasses of loose connective tissues.)

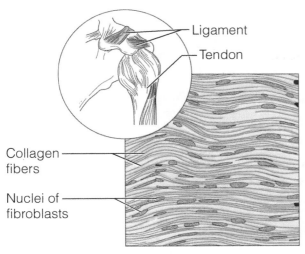

Ligament

Tendon

Collagen fibers

Nuclei of fibroblasts

(d) Diagram: Dense fibrous

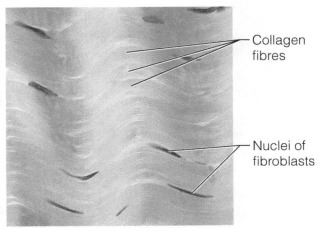

Collagen fibres

Nuclei of fibroblasts

Photomicrograph: Dense fibrous connective tissue from a tendon (1000×).

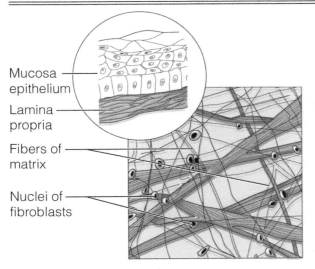

Mucosa epithelium

Lamina propria

Fibers of matrix

Nuclei of fibroblasts

(e) Diagram: Areolar

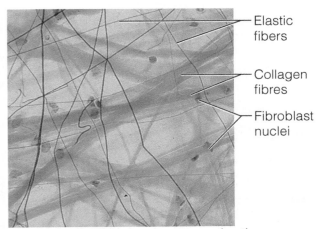

Elastic fibers

Collagen fibres

Fibroblast nuclei

Photomicrograph: Areolar connective tissue, a soft packaging tissue of the body (400×).

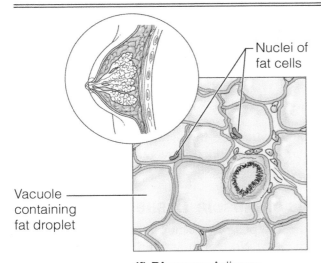

Nuclei of fat cells

Vacuole containing fat droplet

(f) Diagram: Adipose

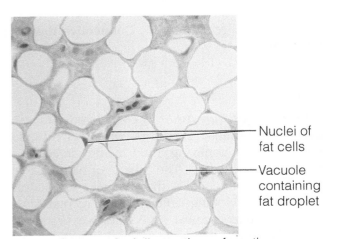

Nuclei of fat cells

Vacuole containing fat droplet

Photomicrograph: Adipose tissue from the subcutaneous layer beneath the skin (600×).

(Continues on page 78)

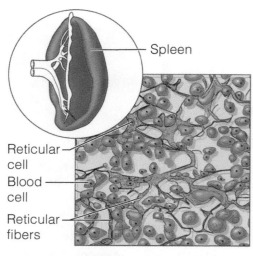

Spleen

Reticular cell

Blood cell

Reticular fibers

(g) Diagram: Reticular

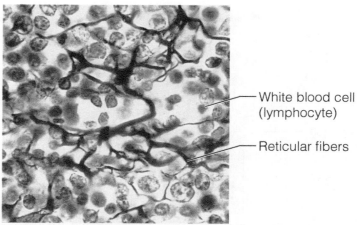

White blood cell (lymphocyte)

Reticular fibers

Photomicrograph: Dark-staining network of reticular connective tissue (350×).

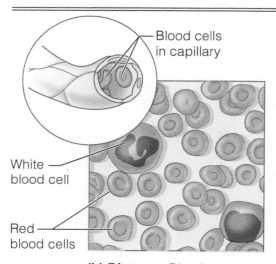

Blood cells in capillary

White blood cell

Red blood cells

(h) Diagram: Blood

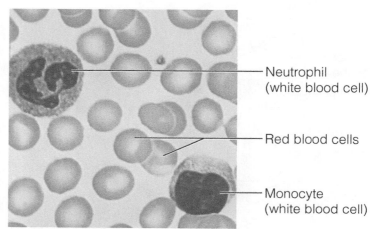

Neutrophil (white blood cell)

Red blood cells

Monocyte (white blood cell)

Photomicrograph: Smear of human blood (1500×); two white blood cells are seen among the red blood cells.

FIGURE 3.15 (*continued*)   **Connective tissues and their common body locations.**

Blood

Blood, or *vascular tissue*, is considered a connective tissue because it consists of *blood cells*, surrounded by a nonliving, fluid matrix called *blood plasma* (Figure 3.15h). The "fibers" of blood are soluble protein molecules that become visible only during blood clotting. Still, we must recognize that blood is quite atypical as connective tissues go. Blood is the transport vehicle for the cardiovascular system, carrying nutrients, wastes, respiratory gases, and many other substances throughout the body.

Muscle Tissue

Muscle tissues are highly specialized to *contract*, or *shorten*, to produce movement.

Types of Muscle Tissue

The three types of muscle tissue are illustrated in Figure 3.16. Notice their similarities and differences as you read through the descriptions that follow.

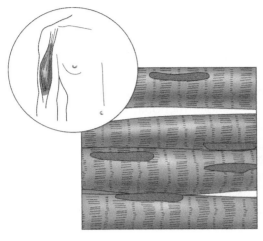 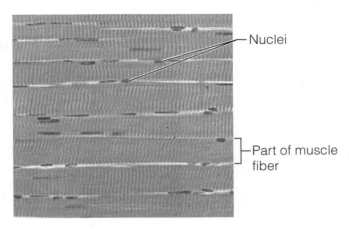

(a) Diagram: Skeletal muscle   **Photomicrograph:** Skeletal muscle (approx. 300×).

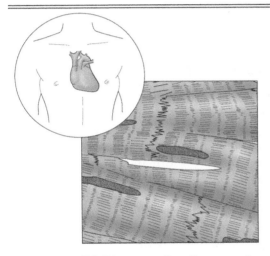 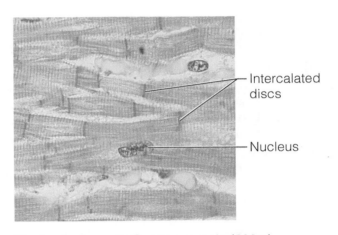

(b) Diagram: Cardiac muscle   **Photomicrograph:** Cardiac muscle (800×).

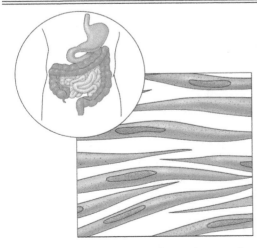 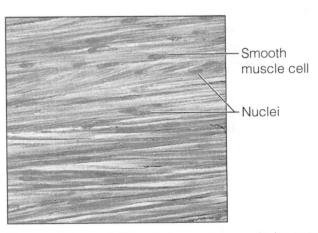

(c) Diagram: Smooth muscle   **Photomicrograph:** Sheet of smooth muscle (approx. 600×).

FIGURE 3.16   Types of muscle tissue and their common locations in the body.

Skeletal Muscle

Skeletal muscle tissue is packaged by connective tissue sheets into organs called *skeletal muscles,* which are attached to the skeleton. These muscles, which can be controlled *voluntarily* (or consciously), form the flesh of the body, the so-called muscular system. When the skeletal muscles contract, they pull on bones or skin. The result of their action is gross body movements or changes in our facial expressions. The cells of skeletal muscle are long, cylindrical, multinucleate, and they have obvious *striations* (stripes). Because skeletal muscle cells are elongated to provide a long axis for contraction, they are often called *muscle fibers.*

Cardiac Muscle

Cardiac muscle is found only in the heart. As it contracts, the heart acts as a pump and propels blood through the blood vessels. Like skeletal muscle, cardiac muscle has striations, but cardiac cells are uninucleate, relatively short, branching cells that fit tightly together (like clasped fingers) at junctions called **intercalated disks.** These intercalated disks contain gap junctions that allow ions to pass freely from cell to cell, resulting in rapid conduction of the exciting electrical impulse across the heart. Cardiac muscle is under *involuntary control,* which means that we cannot consciously control the activity of the heart. (There are, however, rare individuals who claim they have such an ability.)

Smooth Muscle

Smooth, or **visceral, muscle** is so called because no striations are visible. The individual cells have a single nucleus and are spindle-shaped (pointed at each end). Smooth muscle is found in the walls of hollow organs such as the stomach, bladder, uterus, and blood vessels. As smooth muscle contracts, the cavity of an organ alternately becomes smaller (constricts on smooth muscle contraction) or enlarges (dilates on smooth muscle relaxation) so that substances are propelled through the organ along a specific pathway. Smooth muscle contracts much more slowly than the other two muscle types. *Peristalsis* (per"ĭ-stal'sis), a wavelike motion that keeps food moving through the small intestine, is typical of its activity.

Nervous Tissue

When we think of **nervous tissue,** we think of cells called **neurons.** All neurons receive and conduct electrochemical impulses from one part of the body to another; thus *irritability* and *conductivity* are their two major functional characteristics. The structure of neurons is unique (Figure 3.17). Their cytoplasm is drawn out into long processes (extensions), as much as 3 feet or more in the leg, which allows a single neuron to conduct an impulse over long distances in the body. Neurons, along with a special group of **supporting cells** that insulate, support, and protect the delicate neurons, make up the structures of the nervous system—the brain, spinal cord, and nerves.

PART III: DEVELOPMENTAL ASPECTS OF CELLS AND TISSUES

We all begin life as a single cell, which divides thousands of times to form our multicellular embryonic body. Very early in embryonic development, the cells begin to specialize to form the primary tissues, and by birth, most organs are well formed and functioning. The body continues to grow and enlarge by forming new tissue throughout childhood and adolescence.

Cell division is extremely important during the body's growth period. Most cells (except neurons) undergo mitosis until the end of puberty, when adult body size is reached and overall body growth ends. After this time, only certain cells routinely divide—for example, cells exposed to abrasion that continually wear away, such as skin and intestinal cells. Liver cells stop dividing; but they retain this ability should some of them die or become damaged and need to be replaced. Still other cell groups (for example, heart muscle and nervous tissue) almost completely lose their ability to divide when they are fully mature; that is, they become *amitotic* (am"ĭ-tot'ik). Amitotic tissues are severely handicapped by injury because the lost cells cannot be replaced by the same type of cells. This is why the heart of an individual who has had several severe heart attacks becomes weaker and weaker. Damaged cardiac muscle does not regenerate and is replaced by scar tissue that cannot contract, so the heart becomes less

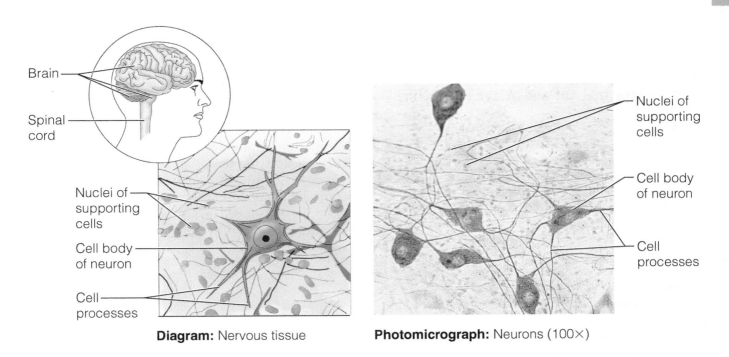

Diagram: Nervous tissue   **Photomicrograph:** Neurons (100×)

FIGURE 3.17   Nervous tissue. Neurons and supporting cells form the brain, spinal cord, and nerves.

and less capable of acting as an efficient blood pump.

The aging process begins once maturity has been reached. (Some believe it begins at birth.) No one has been able to explain just *what* causes aging, but there have been many suggestions. Some believe it is a result of little "chemical insults" which occur continually through life—for example, the presence of toxic chemicals (such as alcohol, certain drugs, or carbon monoxide) in the blood, or the temporary absence of needed substances such as glucose or oxygen. Perhaps the effect of these chemical insults is cumulative and finally succeeds in upsetting the delicate chemical balance of the body cells. Others think that external physical factors such as radiation (X-rays or ultraviolet waves) contribute to the aging process. Several believe that the aging "clock" is genetically programmed, or built into our genes. We all know of cases like the radiant woman of 50 who looks about 35 or the barely-out-of-adolescence man of 24 who looks 40. It appears that such traits can run in families.

There is no question that certain events are part of the aging process. For example, with age, epithelial membranes thin and are more easily damaged, and the skin loses its elasticity and begins to sag. The exocrine glands of the body (epithelial tissue) become less active and we begin to "dry out" as less oil, mucus, and sweat are produced. Some endocrine glands produce decreasing amounts of hormones, and the body processes that they control (such as metabolism and reproduction) become less efficient or stop altogether.

Connective tissue structures also show changes with age. Bones become porous and weaken, and the repair of tissue injuries slows. Muscles begin to atrophy. Although a poor diet may contribute to some of these changes, there is little doubt that decreased efficiency of the circulatory system, which reduces nutrient and oxygen delivery to body tissues, is a major factor.

Besides the tissue changes associated with aging, which accelerate in the later years of life, other modifications of cells and tissues may occur at any time. For example, when cells fail to honor normal controls on cell division and multiply wildly, an abnormal mass of proliferating cells, known as a **neoplasm** (ne′o-plazm″; "new growth"), results. Neoplasms may be benign or malignant (cancerous).

Prove It Yourself

Demonstrate that Oil and Water Don't Mix

Place water and cooking oil in a jar and shake it. Notice that the oil separates from the water, first as small droplets, then as larger drops that join together, and finally as a single layer of oil on top.

Water is a polar molecule, and oils are uncharged, nonpolar molecules. When water and oil mingle, the water molecules are attracted to each other and join together, excluding oil from the regions they occupy. Over time, the oil is forced into ever-larger droplets until it is completely separated from the water. It rises to the top because oil is less dense than water.

Although you probably don't have any phospholipids available, you would get a different result if you repeated this experiment with phospholipids because they do not separate from water. On microscopic examination, you would see numerous small spheres, each comprised of a bilayer of phospholipids enclosing a small volume of water. In effect, this is a nonliving version of a cell's outer membrane and internal contents.

However, not all increases in cell number involve neoplasms. Certain body tissues (or organs) may enlarge because there is some local irritant or condition that stimulates the cells. This is called **hyperplasia** (hī-per-pla′ze-ah). For example, a woman's breasts enlarge during pregnancy in response to increased hormones; this is a normal but temporary situation that doesn't have to be treated. On the other hand, **atrophy** (at′ro-fe), or decrease in size, can occur in an organ or body area that loses its normal stimulation. For example, muscles that are not used or that have lost their nerve supply begin to atrophy and waste away rapidly.

A Closer Look

Cancer—The Intimate Enemy

THE word *cancer* elicits dread in nearly everyone. Why does cancer strike some and not others? Before attempting to answer that question, let's define some terms. An abnormal cell mass that develops when controls of the cell cycle and cell division malfunction is called a *neoplasm* ("new growth") or *tumor.* However, not all neoplasms are cancerous. *Benign* (be-nīn': "kindly") neoplasms are strictly local affairs. They tend to be surrounded by a capsule, grow slowly, and seldom kill their hosts if they are removed before they compress vital organs. In contrast, *malignant* ("bad") neoplasms (cancers) are nonencapsulated masses that grow more relentlessly and may become killers. Their cells resemble immature cells, and they invade their surroundings rather than pushing them aside, as reflected in the name *cancer,* from the Latin word for "crab." Malignant cells also tend to break away from the parent mass and spread via the blood to distant parts of the body, where they form new masses. This last capability is called *metastasis* (mĕ-tas'tă-sis).

What causes transformation— the changes that convert a normal cell into a cancerous one? It is well known that radiation, mechanical trauma, certain viral infections, and many chemicals (tobacco tars, saccharine) can act as carcinogens (cancer-causers). What all of these factors have in common is that they all cause *mutations*—changes in DNA that alter the expression of certain genes. However, most carcinogens are eliminated by peroxisomal or lysosomal enzymes or the immune system. Furthermore, one mutation doesn't do it—apparently it takes a sequence of several genetic changes to change a normal cell to a full-fledged cancer cell (Figure a).

Clues to the role of genes were provided by the discovery of *oncogenes* (cancer-causing [*onco* = tumor] genes), and then *proto-oncogenes.* Proto-oncogenes code for proteins that are needed for normal cell division and growth. However, many have fragile sites that break when they are exposed to carcinogens, and this event converts them into oncogenes. An example of a problem that might result from this conversion is the switching on of dormant genes that allow cells to become invasive (an ability of embryonic cells—and cancer cells—but not normal adult cells).

However, oncogenes have been discovered in only 15 to 20 percent of human cancers, so the more recent discovery of *tumor suppressor genes,* which work to suppress or prevent cancer, was not too surprising. The tumor suppressor genes (such as *p*53) aid DNA repair, put the "brakes" on cell division, help to inactivate carcinogens, or enhance the ability of the immune system to destroy cancer cells. When the tumor suppressor genes are damaged or changed in some way, the oncogenes are free to "do their thing." One of the best-understood of human cancers, colon cancer, illustrates this principle (Figure b). The first sign of colon cancer is a polyp (benign tumor), due to an unusual increase in the division rate of apparently normal cells of the colon lining. In time, a malignant neoplasm makes its appearance at the site. In most cases, these changes parallel cellular changes at the DNA level and include activation of an oncogene and inactivation of two tumor suppressor genes. Whatever the precise genetic factor at work, the seeds of cancer do appear to be in our own genes. Thus, as you can see, cancer is an intimate enemy indeed.

Cancer—The Intimate Enemy *(continued)*

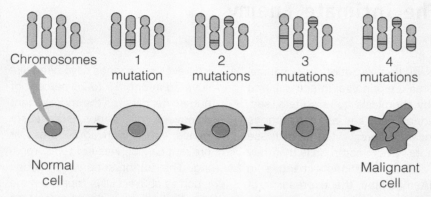

(a) **Accumulation of mutations in the development of a cancer cell.**

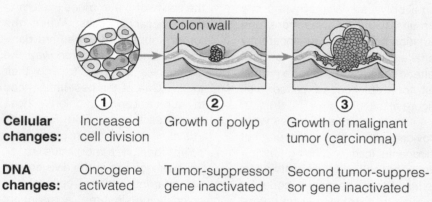

(b) **Stepwise development of a typical colon cancer.**

symptoms (pain, bloody discharge, lump, etc.), and the diagnostic method most used is the biopsy. In a biopsy, a sample of the primary tumor is removed surgically (or by scraping) and examined microscopically for structural changes typical of malignant cells.

The treatment of choice for either type of neoplasm is surgical removal. If surgery is not possible—as in cases where the cancer has spread widely or is inoperable—radiation and drugs (chemotherapy) are used. Anticancer drugs have unpleasant side effects because most target *all* rapidly dividing cells, including normal ones. The side effects include nausea, vomiting, and loss of hair. X-rays, even if highly localized, also have side effects because, in passing through the body, they kill healthy cells that lie in the path to the cancer cells.

Current cancer treatments— "cut, burn, and poison"—are recognized as crude and painful. Promising new methods focus on delivering anticancer drugs more precisely to the cancer (via monoclonal antibodies that respond to one type of protein on a cancer cell) and on increasing the immune system's ability to fend off cancer. The most recent research focuses on starving tumors by inhibiting their ability to attract a rich blood supply.

Almost half of all Americans develop cancer in their lifetime, and a fifth of us will die of it. Cancer can arise from almost any cell type, but the most common cancers originate in the skin, lung, colon, breast, and male prostate gland.

Screening procedures, such as self-examination of one's breasts or testicles for lumps and checking fecal samples for blood, aid in early detection of cancers. However, most cancers are diagnosed only after they have begun to cause

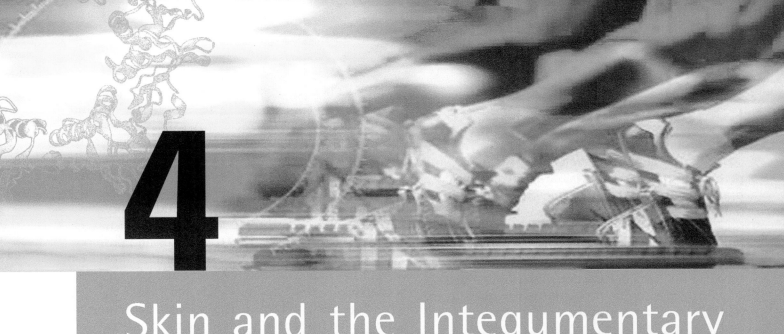

4

Skin and the Integumentary System

Integumentary System (Skin)

Would you be enticed by an advertisement for a coat that is waterproof, stretchable, washable, and permanent-press, that invisibly repairs small cuts, rips, and burns, and that is guaranteed to last a lifetime with reasonable care? Sounds too good to be true, but you already have such a coat—your *cutaneous membrane,* or **skin.** The skin and its derivatives (sweat and oil glands, hair, and nails) serve a number of functions, mostly protective. Together, these organs are called the **integumentary** (in-teg″u-men′ta-re) **system.**

Basic Skin Functions

Also called the **integument** (in-teg′u-ment), which simply means "covering," the skin is much more than an external body covering. It is absolutely essential because it keeps water and other precious molecules in the body. It also keeps water (and other things) out. (This is why one can swim for hours without becoming waterlogged.) Structurally, the skin is a marvel. It is pliable yet tough, which allows it to take constant punishment from external agents. Without our skin, we would quickly fall prey to bacteria and perish from water and heat loss.

The skin has many functions; most, but not all, are protective (Table 4.1). It insulates and cushions the deeper body organs and protects the entire body from mechanical damage (bumps and cuts), chemical damage (such as from acids and bases), thermal damage (heat and cold), ultraviolet radiation (in sunlight), and bacteria. The uppermost layer of the skin is full of **keratin** and *cornified,* or hardened, in order to prevent water loss from the body surface.

The skin's rich capillary network and sweat glands (both controlled by the nervous system) play an important role in regulating heat loss from

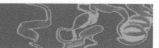

TABLE 4.1	Functions of the Skin
Functions	**How accomplished**
Protects deeper tissues from	
• Mechanical damage (bumps)	Physical barrier contains keratin, which toughens cells, and pressure receptors, which alert the nervous system to possible damage.
• Chemical damage (acids and bases)	Has relatively impermeable keratinized cells; contains pain receptors, which alert the nervous system to possible damage.
• Bacterial damage	Has an unbroken surface and "acid mantle" (skin secretions are acidic, and thus inhibit bacteria). Phagocytes ingest foreign substances and pathogens, preventing them from penetrating into deeper body tissues.
• Ultraviolet radiation (damaging effects of sunlight)	Melanin produced by melanocytes offers protection from UV damage.
• Thermal (heat or cold) damage	Contains heat/cold/pain receptors.
• Desiccation (drying out)	Contains a waterproofing glycolipid and keratin.
Aids in body heat loss or heat retention (controlled by the nervous system)	*Heat loss:* By activating sweat glands and allowing blood to flush into skin capillary beds. *Heat retention:* By not allowing blood to flush into skin capillary beds.
Aids in excretion of urea and uric acid	Contained in perspiration produced by sweat glands.
Synthesizes vitamin D	Modified cholesterol molecules in skin converted to vitamin D by sunlight.

the body surface. The skin acts as a mini-excretory system; urea, salts, and water are lost when we sweat. The skin also manufactures several proteins important to immunity and synthesizes vitamin D. (Modified cholesterol molecules located in the skin are converted to vitamin D by sunlight.) Finally, the *cutaneous sensory receptors,* which are actually part of the nervous system, are located in the skin. These tiny sensors, which include touch, pressure, temperature, and pain receptors, provide us with a great deal of information about our external environment. They alert us to bumps and the presence of tissue-damaging factors as well as to the feel of wind in our hair and a caress.

Structure of the Skin

The skin is composed of two kinds of tissue. The outer **epidermis** (ep″ĭ-der′mis) is made up of stratified squamous epithelium that is capable of *keratinizing* (ker′ah-tin-īz-ing), or becoming hard and tough. The underlying **dermis** is mostly made up of dense connective tissue. The epidermis and dermis are firmly connected. However, a burn or friction (such as the rubbing of a poorly fitting shoe) may cause them to separate, allowing interstitial fluid to accumulate in the cavity between the layers, which results in a *blister.*

Deep to the dermis is the **subcutaneous tissue,** or **hypodermis,** which essentially is adipose tissue. It is not considered part of the skin, but it does anchor the skin to underlying organs. Subcutaneous tissue serves as a shock absorber and insulates the deeper tissues from extreme temperature changes occurring outside the body. It is also responsible for the curves that are more a part of a woman's anatomy than a man's. The main skin areas and structures are described next.

Epidermis

The epidermis is composed of up to five zones or layers called *strata* (strah′tah). From the inside out these are the stratum basale, spinosum, granulosum, lucidum, and corneum (see Figure 4.1).

Like all epithelial tissues, the epidermis is *avascular;* that is, it has no blood supply of its own. This explains why a man can shave daily and not bleed even though he is cutting off many cell layers each time he shaves.

Most cells of the epidermis are **keratinocytes** (keratin cells), which produce keratin, the fibrous

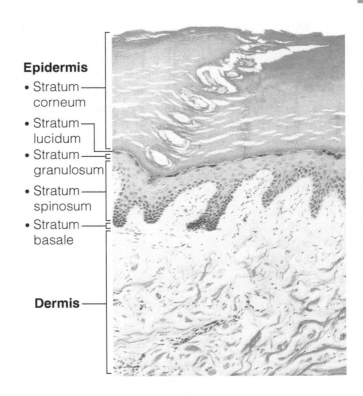

Epidermis
• Stratum corneum
• Stratum lucidum
• Stratum granulosum
• Stratum spinosum
• Stratum basale

Dermis

FIGURE 4.1 **The epidermis of thick skin** (150×). From *Gray's Anatomy,* Henry Gray. Churchill Livingstone, UK.

protein that makes the epidermis a tough protective layer. The deepest cell layer of the epidermis, the **stratum basale** (stra′tum bă-sah′le), lies closest to the dermis and contains epidermal cells that receive the most adequate nourishment via diffusion of nutrients from the dermis. These cells are constantly undergoing cell division, and millions of new cells are produced daily; hence its alternate name, *stratum germinativum* (jer″min-ah-tiv′um; "germinating layer"). The daughter cells are pushed upward, away from the source of nutrition, to become part of the epidermal layers closer to the skin surface. They move away from the dermis and become part of the more superficial layers, the **stratum spinosum** and then the **stratum granulosum.** Then they become flatter, increasingly full of keratin (keratinized), and finally die, forming the clear **stratum lucidum** (lu′sid-um). This latter epidermal layer is not seen in all skin regions; it occurs only where the skin is hairless and extra thick, that is, on the palms of the hands and soles of the feet. The combination of accumulating keratin inside them, secreting a water-repellent glycoprotein into the extracellular space, and their increasing distance from the blood supply (in the dermis) effectively dooms the stratum lucidum cells and the more superficial epidermal cells because they are unable to get adequate nutrients and oxygen.

The outermost layer, the **stratum corneum** (kor′ne-um), is 20 to 30 cell layers thick. It accounts for about three-quarters of the epidermal thickness. The shinglelike dead cell remnants, completely filled with keratin, are referred to as *cornified* or *horny cells* (*cornu* = horn). The common saying "Beauty is only skin deep" is especially interesting in light of the fact that nearly everything we see when we look at someone is dead! Keratin is an exceptionally tough protein. Its abundance in the stratum corneum allows that layer to provide a durable "overcoat" for the body, which protects deeper cells from the hostile external environment (air) and from water loss and helps the body resist biological, chemical, and physical assaults. The stratum corneum rubs and flakes off slowly and steadily and is replaced by cells produced by the division of the deeper stratum basale cells. Indeed, we have a totally "new" epidermis every 25 to 45 days.

Melanin (mel′ah-nin), a pigment that ranges in color from yellow to brown to black, is produced by special cells called **melanocytes** (mel′ah-no sītz), found chiefly in the stratum basale. When the skin is exposed to sunlight, which stimulates the melanocytes to produce more of the melanin pigment, tanning occurs. The stratum basale cells phagocytize (eat) the pigment, and as it accumulates within them, the melanin forms a protective pigment umbrella over the superficial, or "sunny," side of their nuclei that shields their genetic material (DNA) from the damaging effects of ultraviolet radiation in sunlight. *Freckles* and *moles* are seen where melanin is concentrated in one spot.

▲ Homeostatic Imbalance

Despite melanin's protective effects, excessive sun exposure eventually damages the skin. It causes the elastic fibers to clump, leading to leathery skin. It also depresses the immune system. This may help to explain why many people infected with the *herpes simplex,* or *cold sore,* virus are more likely to have an eruption after sunbathing. Overexposure to the sun can also alter the DNA of skin cells and in this way lead to skin cancer. Black people seldom have skin cancer, attesting to melanin's amazing effectiveness as a natural sunscreen. ▲

Dermis

The dermis is your "hide." It is a strong, stretchy envelope that helps to hold the body together. When you purchase leather goods (bags, belts, shoes, and the like), you are buying the treated dermis of animals.

The dense (fibrous) connective tissue making up the dermis consists of two major regions—the *papillary* and the *reticular* areas. Like the epidermis, the dermis varies in thickness. For example, it is particularly thick on the palms of the hands and soles of the feet but is quite thin on the eyelids.

The **papillary layer** is the upper dermal region. It is uneven and has fingerlike projections from its superior surface, called **dermal papillae** (pah-pil′e; *papill* = nipple), which indent the epidermis above. Many of the dermal papillae contain capillary loops, which furnish nutrients to the epidermis. Others house pain receptors (*free nerve endings*) and touch receptors called *Meissner's corpuscles* (mīs′nerz kor′puh-sulz). On the palms of the hands and soles of the feet, the papillae are arranged in definite patterns that form looped and whorled ridges on the epidermal surface that increase friction and enhance the gripping ability of the fingers and feet. Papillary patterns are genetically determined. The ridges of the fingertips are well provided with sweat pores and leave unique, identifying films of sweat called *fingerprints* on almost anything they touch.

The **reticular layer** is the deepest skin layer. It contains blood vessels, sweat and oil glands, and deep pressure receptors called *Pacinian* (pah-sin′e-an) *corpuscles* (see Figure 4.2). Phagocytes found here (and, in fact, throughout the dermis) act to prevent bacteria that have managed to get through the epidermis from penetrating any deeper into the body.

Both *collagen* and *elastic fibers* are found throughout the dermis. Collagen fibers are responsible for the toughness of the dermis; they also attract and bind water and thus help to keep the skin hydrated. Elastic fibers give the skin its elasticity when we are young. As we age, the number of collagen and elastic fibers decreases, and the subcutaneous tissue loses fat. As a result, the skin loses its elasticity and begins to sag and wrinkle.

The dermis is abundantly supplied with blood vessels that play a role in maintaining body temperature homeostasis. When body temperature is high, the capillaries of the dermis become

Q   *What component of the hypodermis makes it a good insulator and shock absorber?*

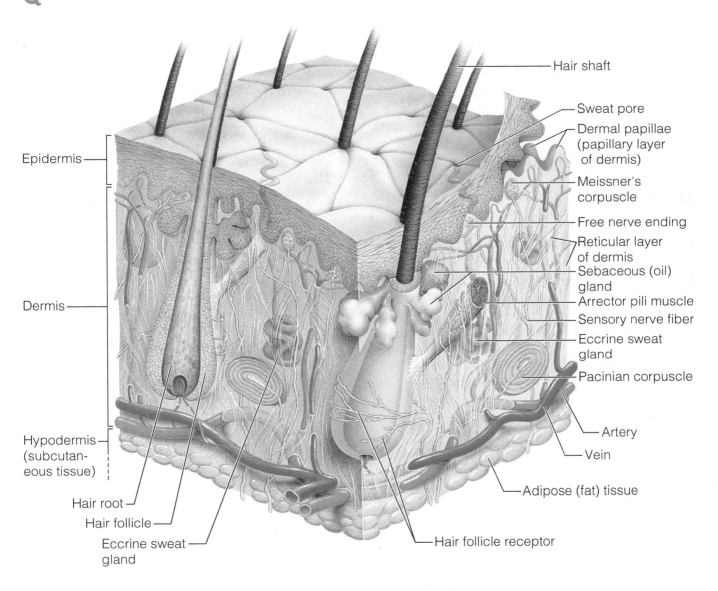

Epidermis

Dermis

Hypodermis (subcutaneous tissue)

Hair root

Hair follicle

Eccrine sweat gland

Hair shaft

Sweat pore

Dermal papillae (papillary layer of dermis)

Meissner's corpuscle

Free nerve ending

Reticular layer of dermis

Sebaceous (oil) gland

Arrector pili muscle

Sensory nerve fiber

Eccrine sweat gland

Pacinian corpuscle

Artery

Vein

Adipose (fat) tissue

Hair follicle receptor

FIGURE 4.2 Skin structure. Three-dimensional view of the skin and underlying subcutaneous tissue.

engorged, or swollen, with heated blood, and the skin becomes reddened and warm. This allows body heat to radiate from the skin surface. If the environment is cool and body heat must be conserved, blood bypasses the dermis capillaries temporarily, allowing internal body temperature to stay high.

A

Its fatty tissue.

Homeostatic Imbalance

Any restriction of the normal blood supply to the skin results in cell death and, if severe or prolonged enough, skin ulcers. *Decubitus* (de-ku'bĭ-tus) *ulcers* (bedsores) occur in bedridden patients who are not turned regularly or who are dragged or pulled across the bed repeatedly. The weight of the body puts pressure on the skin, especially over bony projections. Because this restricts the blood supply, the skin becomes pale or blanched at pressure points. At first, the skin reddens when pressure is released, but if the situation is not corrected, the cells begin to die, and typically small cracks or breaks in the skin appear at compressed sites. Permanent damage to the superficial blood vessels and tissue eventually results in degeneration and ulceration of the skin (Figure 4.3). ▲

The dermis also has a rich nerve supply. As mentioned earlier, many of the nerve endings have specialized receptor end-organs that send messages to the central nervous system for interpretation when they are stimulated by environmental factors (pressure, temperature, and the like).

Skin Color

Three pigments contribute to skin color:

1. The amount and kind (yellow, reddish brown, or black) of *melanin* in the epidermis.

2. The amount of *carotene* deposited in the stratum corneum and subcutaneous tissue. (Carotene is an orange-yellow pigment found in abundant amounts in carrots and other orange, deep yellow, or leafy green vegetables.) The skin tends to take on a yellow-orange cast when large amounts of carotene-rich foods are eaten.

3. The amount of *oxygen-rich hemoglobin* (pigment in red blood cells) in the dermal blood vessels.

People who produce a lot of melanin have brown-toned skin. In light-skinned (Caucasian) people, who have less melanin, the crimson color of oxygen-rich hemoglobin in the dermal blood supply flushes through the transparent cell layers above and gives the skin a rosy glow.

▲ Homeostatic Imbalance

When hemoglobin is poorly oxygenated, both the blood and the skin of Caucasians appear blue, a condition called *cyanosis* (si"ah-no'sis). Cyanosis is common during heart failure and severe breathing disorders. In black people, the skin does not appear cyanotic in the same situations because of the masking effects of melanin, but cyanosis is apparent in their mucous membranes and nail beds. ▲

Skin color is also influenced by emotional stimuli, and many alterations in skin color signal certain disease states:

- *Redness*, or *erythema* (er"ĭ-the'mah): Reddened skin may indicate embarrassment (blushing), fever, hypertension, inflammation, or allergy.

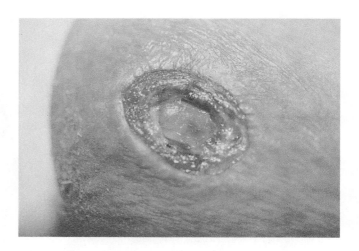

FIGURE 4.3   **Photograph of a deep (stage III) decubitus ulcer.**

- *Pallor*, or *blanching:* Under certain types of emotional stress (fear, anger, and others), some people become pale. Pale skin may also signify anemia, low blood pressure, or impaired blood flow into the area.

- *Jaundice* (jon'dis) or a *yellow cast:* An abnormal yellow skin tone usually signifies a liver disorder in which excess bile pigments are absorbed into the blood, circulated throughout the body, and deposited in body tissues.

- *Bruises* or *black-and-blue marks:* Black-and-blue marks reveal sites where blood has escaped from the circulation and has clotted in the tissue spaces. Such clotted blood masses are called *hematomas*. An unusual tendency to bruising may signify a deficiency of vitamin C in the diet or hemophilia (bleeder's disease).

Appendages of the Skin

The **skin appendages** include cutaneous glands, hair and hair follicles, and nails (see Figure 4.2). Each of these appendages arises from the epidermis and plays a unique role in maintaining body homeostasis.

Cutaneous Glands

The cutaneous glands are all **exocrine glands** that release their secretions to the skin surface via ducts. They fall into two groups: *sebaceous glands* and *sweat glands*. As these glands are formed by the cells of the stratum basale, they push into the

Q   *Which of these gland types can make your hair lank and oily?*

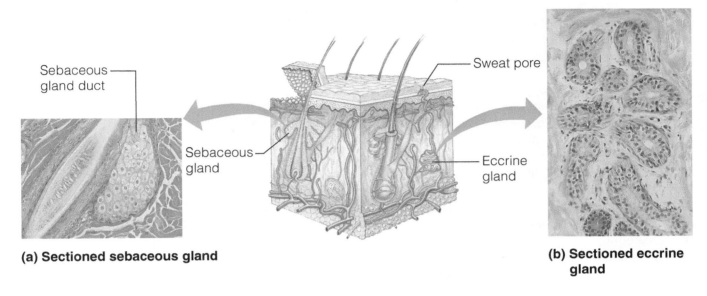

Sebaceous gland duct

Sebaceous gland

Sweat pore

Eccrine gland

(a) Sectioned sebaceous gland

(b) Sectioned eccrine gland

FIGURE 4.4   Cutaneous glands. (a) Photomicrograph of a sebaceous gland (104×). **(b)** Photomicrograph of eccrine sweat glands (148×).

deeper skin regions and ultimately reside almost entirely in the dermis.

Sebaceous (Oil) Glands   The **sebaceous** (seh-ba′shus) **glands,** or oil glands, are found all over the skin, except on the palms of the hands and the soles of the feet. Their ducts usually empty into a hair follicle (see Figures 4.2 and 4.4), but some open directly onto the skin surface.

The product of the sebaceous glands, **sebum** (se′bum; *seb* = grease), is a mixture of oily substances and fragmented cells. Sebum is a lubricant that keeps the skin soft and moist and prevents the hair from becoming brittle. Sebum also contains chemicals that *kill* bacteria, so it is important in preventing the bacteria present on the skin surface from invading the deeper skin regions. The sebaceous glands become very active when male sex hormones are produced in increased amounts (in both sexes) during adolescence. Thus, the skin tends to become oilier during this period of life.

Homeostatic Imbalance

If a sebaceous gland's duct becomes blocked by sebum, a *whitehead* appears on the skin surface. If

A   *The sebaceous glands, which produce oily secretions.*

the accumulated material oxidizes and dries, it darkens, forming a *blackhead. Acne* is an active infection of the sebaceous glands accompanied by pimples on the skin. It can be mild or extremely severe, leading to permanent scarring. *Seborrhea* (seb″o-re′ah), known as "cradle cap" in infants, is caused by overactivity of the sebaceous glands. It begins on the scalp as pink, raised lesions that gradually form a yellow to brown crust that sloughs off as oily dandruff. Careful washing to remove the excessive oil often helps. ▲

Sweat Glands   **Sweat glands,** also called **sudoriferous** (su″do-rif′er-us; *sudor* = sweat) **glands,** are widely distributed in the skin. Their number is staggering—more than 2.5 million per person. There are two types of sweat glands, *eccrine* and *apocrine.*

The **eccrine** (ek′rin) **glands** are far more numerous and are found all over the body. They produce **sweat,** a clear secretion that is primarily water plus some salts (sodium chloride), vitamin C, traces of metabolic wastes (ammonia, urea, uric acid), and lactic acid (a chemical that accumulates during vigorous muscle activity). Sweat is acidic (pH from 4 to 6), a characteristic that inhibits the growth of bacteria, which are always present on the skin surface. Typically, sweat reaches the skin surface via a duct that opens externally as a funnel-shaped *pore* (see Figures 4.2 and 4.4). Notice, however, that the facial "pores" commonly referred to when we talk about our complexion are *not* these sweat pores, but the external outlets of hair follicles.

The eccrine sweat glands are an important and highly efficient part of the body's heat-regulating equipment. They are supplied with nerve endings that cause them to secrete sweat when the external temperature or body temperature is high. When sweat evaporates off the skin surface, it carries large amounts of body heat with it. On a hot day, it is possible to lose up to 7 liters of body water in this way. The heat-regulating functions of the body are important—if internal temperature changes more than a few degrees from the normal 37°C (98.2°F), life-threatening changes occur in the body.

Apocrine (ap'o-krin) **glands** are largely confined to the axillary and genital areas of the body. They are usually larger than eccrine glands, and their ducts empty into hair follicles. Their secretion contains fatty acids and proteins, as well as all the substances present in eccrine secretion; consequently, it may have a milky or yellowish color. The secretion is odorless, but when bacteria that live on the skin use its proteins and fats as a source of nutrients for their growth, it takes on a musky, unpleasant odor.

Apocrine glands begin to function during puberty under the influence of *androgens* (male sex hormones). Although their secretion is produced almost continuously, apocrine glands play a minimal role in thermoregulation. Their precise function is not yet known, but they are activated by nerve fibers during pain and stress and during sexual foreplay.

Hair and Hair Follicles

There are millions of **hairs** scattered all over the body. But, other than serving a few minor protective functions—such as guarding the head against bumps, shielding the eyes (via eyelashes), and helping to keep foreign particles out of the respiratory tract (via nose hairs)—our body hair has lost much of its usefulness. Hair served early humans (and still serves hairy animals) by providing insulation in cold weather, but now we have other means of keeping warm.

A hair, produced by a *hair follicle,* is a flexible epithelial structure. That part of the hair enclosed in the follicle is called the *root.* The part projecting from the surface of the scalp or skin is called the *shaft* (Figure 4.5). A hair is formed by division

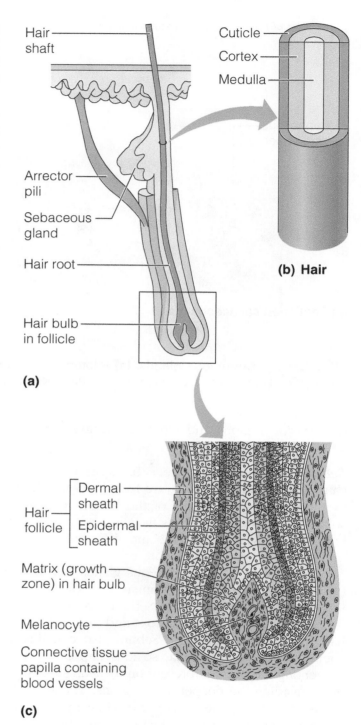

(b) Hair

(a)

(c)

FIGURE 4.5   Structure of a hair and hair follicle. **(a)** Longitudinal section of a hair within its follicle. **(b)** Enlarged longitudinal section of a hair. **(c)** Enlarged longitudinal view of the expanded hair bulb in the follicle showing the matrix, the region of actively dividing epithelial cells that produces the hair.

of the well-nourished stratum basale epithelial cells in the **matrix** (growth zone), of the hair bulb at the inferior end of the follicle. As the daughter cells are pushed farther away from the growing region, they become keratinized and die. Thus the bulk of the hair shaft, like the bulk of the epidermis, is dead material and almost entirely protein.

Each hair consists of a central core called the *medulla* (me-dul'ah) surrounded by a bulky *cortex* layer. The cortex is, in turn, enclosed by an outermost *cuticle* formed by a single layer of cells that overlap one another like shingles on a roof. This arrangement of the cuticle cells helps to keep the hairs apart and keeps them from matting (see Figures 4.5b and 4.6). The cuticle is the most heavily keratinized region; it provides strength and helps keep the inner hair layers tightly compacted. Because it is most subject to abrasion, the cuticle tends to wear away at the tip of the shaft, allowing the keratin fibrils in the inner hair regions to frizz out, a phenomenon called "split ends." Hair pigment is made by melanocytes in the hair bulb, and varying amounts of different types of melanin (yellow, rust, brown, and black) combine to produce *all* varieties of hair color from pale blond to pitch black.

Hairs come in a variety of sizes and shapes. They are short and stiff in the eyebrows, long and flexible on the head, and usually nearly invisible almost everywhere else. When the hair shaft is oval, hair is smooth and silky and the person has wavy hair. When the shaft is flat and ribbonlike, the hair is curly or kinky. If it is perfectly round, the hair is straight and tends to be coarse. Hairs are found all over the body surface except the palms of the hands, soles of the feet, nipples, and lips. Humans are born with as many hair follicles as they will ever have, and hairs are among the fastest growing tissues in the body. Hormones account for the development of hairy regions—the scalp and, in the adult, the pubic and axillary (armpit) areas.

Hair follicles are actually compound structures. The inner *epidermal sheath* is composed of epithelial tissue and forms the hair. The outer *dermal sheath* is actually dermal connective tissue. This dermal region supplies blood vessels to the epidermal portion and reinforces it. Its nipplelike *papilla* provides the blood supply to the matrix in the hair bulb.

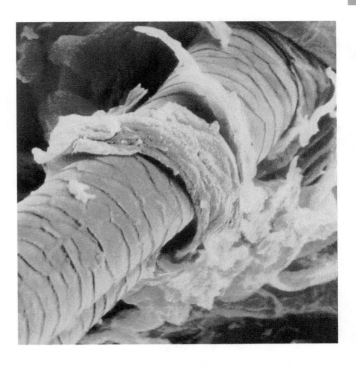

FIGURE 4.6 Scanning electron micrograph showing a hair shaft emerging from a follicle at the skin surface. Notice how the scalelike cells of the cuticle overlap one another (1500×).

Prove It Yourself

Plot the Distribution of Sweat Glands

For this experiment investigating the distribution of sweat glands in different body areas, you will need two squares of bond paper (each 1 cm by 1 cm), adhesive tape, an iodine solution, and a cotton-tipped swab.

First, paint an area of the medial aspect of your left palm (avoid the crease lines) and left forearm with the iodine solution, and let it dry thoroughly. Now have a friend tape a square of bond paper securely over each iodine-painted area, and leave the paper in place for 20 minutes.

After 20 minutes, remove the paper squares and count the number of blue-black dots on each square. Each blue-black dot indicates an active sweat gland. (The iodine in the pore dissolves in your sweat and reacts chemically with the starch in the bond paper to produce the blue-black color.) Thus, you have now produced "sweat maps" of two areas of your skin. Which region has the greater density of sweat glands?

Look carefully at the structure of the hair follicle at the front corner of Figure 4.2. Notice that it is slanted. Small bands of smooth muscle cells—**arrector pili** (ah-rek'tor pi'li)—connect each side of the hair follicle to the dermal tissue. When these muscles contract (as when we are cold or frightened), the hair is pulled upright, dimpling the skin surface with "goose bumps." This action helps keep animals warm in winter by adding a layer of insulating air to the fur. It is especially dramatic in a scared cat, whose fur actually stands on end to make it look larger to scare off its enemy. However, this hair-raising phenomenon is not very useful to human beings.

Nails

A **nail** is a scalelike modification of the epidermis that corresponds to the hoof or claw of other animals. Each nail has a *free edge,* a *body* (visible attached portion), and a *root* (embedded in the skin). The borders of the nail are overlapped by skin folds, called *nail folds.* The thick proximal nail fold is commonly called the *cuticle* (Figure 4.7).

The stratum basale of the epidermis extends beneath the nail as the *nail bed.* Its thickened proximal area, called the *nail matrix,* is responsible for nail growth. As the nail cells are produced by the matrix, they become heavily keratinized and die. Thus, nails, like hairs, are mostly nonliving material.

Nails are transparent and nearly colorless, but they look pink because of the rich blood supply in the underlying dermis. The exception to this is the region over the thickened nail matrix that appears as a white crescent and is called the *lunula* (loo'nyu-luh; *lunul* = crescent). As noted earlier, when the supply of oxygen in the blood is low, the nail beds take on a cyanotic (blue) cast.

Homeostatic Imbalances of Skin

It is difficult to scoff at anything that goes wrong with the skin because, when it rebels, it is quite a visible revolution. Loss of homeostasis in body cells and organs can reveal itself on the skin in ways that are sometimes almost unbelievable. The skin can develop more than 1000 different ailments. The most common skin disorders result from allergies or bacterial, viral, or fungal infections. Less common, but far more damaging, are burns and skin cancers. ▲

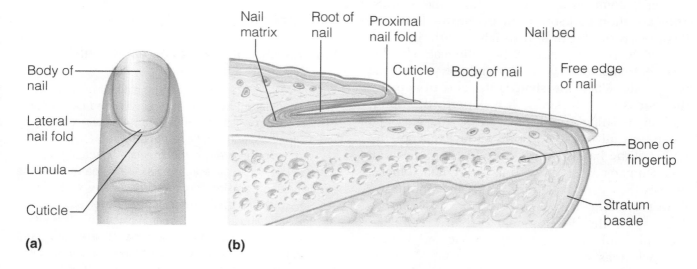

(a)   **(b)**

FIGURE 4.7   Structure of a nail. (a) Surface view. **(b)** Longitudinal section of the distal part of a finger, showing nail parts and the nail matrix that forms the nail.

Systems in Sync

Homeostatic Relationships between the Integumentary System and Other Body Systems

Nervous System
- Skin protects nervous system organs; cutaneous sensory receptors located in skin
- Nervous system regulates diameter of blood vessels in skin; activates sweat glands, contributing to thermoregulation; interprets cutaneous sensation; activates arrector pili muscles

Respiratory System
- Skin protects respiratory organs
- Respiratory system furnishes oxygen to skin cells and removes carbon dioxide via gas exchange with blood

Cardiovascular System
- Skin protects cardiovascular organs; prevents fluid loss from body surface; serves as blood reservoir
- Cardiovascular system transports oxygen and nutrients to skin and removes wastes from skin; provides substances needed by skin glands to make their secretions

Reproductive System
- Skin protects reproductive organs; highly modified sweat glands (mammary glands) produce milk. During pregnancy, skin stretches to accommodate growing fetus; changes in skin pigmentation may occur

Integumentary System (Skin)

Skeletal System
- Skin protects bones; skin synthesizes vitamin D bones need for normal calcium absorption and deposit of bone (calcium) salts which make bones hard
- Skeletal system provides support for the skin

Endocrine System
- Skin protects endocrine organs
- Androgens produced by the endocrine system activate sebaceous glands and help regulate hair growth; estrogen helps maintain skin hydration

Lymphatic System/Immunity
- Skin protects lymphatic organs; prevents pathogen invasion
- Lymphatic system prevents edema by picking up excessive leaked fluid; immune system protects skin cells

Digestive System
- Skin protects digestive organs; provides vitamin D needed for calcium absorption
- Digestive system provides needed nutrients for the skin

Urinary System
- Skin protects urinary organs; excretes salts and some nitrogenous wastes in sweat
- Urinary system activates vitamin D made by keratinocytes; disposes of nitrogenous wastes of skin metabolism

Muscular System
- Skin protects muscles
- Active muscles generate large amounts of heat which increase blood flow to the skin and may promote activation of sweat glands of skin

5

The Skeletal System

Although the word *skeleton* comes from the Greek word meaning "dried-up body," our internal framework is so beautifully designed and engineered that it puts any modern skyscraper to shame. Strong, yet light, it is perfectly adapted for its functions of body protection and motion. Shaped by an event that happened more than one million years ago—when a being first stood erect on hind legs—our skeleton is a tower of bones arranged so that we can stand upright and balance ourselves. No other animal has such relatively long legs (compared to the arms or forelimbs) or such a strange foot, and few have such remarkable grasping hands. Even though the infant's backbone is like an arch, it soon changes to the swayback, or S-shaped, structure that is required for the upright posture.

The skeleton is subdivided into two divisions: the **axial skeleton,** the bones that form the longitudinal axis of the body, and the **appendicular skeleton,** the bones of the limbs and girdles. In addition to bones, the **skeletal system** includes *joints, cartilages, tendons* (fibrous cords that attach muscle to bone), and *ligaments* (fibrous cords that bind the bones together at joints). The joints give the body flexibility and allow movement to occur.

Skeletal System Overview

At one time or another, all of us have heard the expressions "bone tired," "dry as a bone," or "bag of bones"—pretty unflattering and inaccurate images of some of our most phenomenal organs. Our brains, not our bones, convey feelings of fatigue, and bones are far from dry. As for "bag of bones," they are indeed more obvious in some of us, but without them to form our internal skeleton, we would creep along the ground like slugs. Let's examine how our bones contribute to overall body homeostasis.

Functions of the Bones

Besides contributing to body shape and form, our bones perform several important body functions:

1. **Support.** Bones, the "steel girders" and "reinforced concrete" of the body, form the internal framework that supports and anchors all soft organs. The bones of the legs act as pillars to support the body trunk when we stand, and the rib cage supports the thoracic wall.

2. **Protection.** Bones protect soft body organs. For example, the fused bones of the skull provide a snug enclosure for the brain, allowing one to head a soccer ball without worrying about injuring the brain. The vertebrae surround the spinal cord, and the rib cage helps protect the vital organs of the thorax.

3. **Movement.** Skeletal muscles, attached to bones by tendons, use the bones as levers to move the body and its parts. As a result, we can walk, swim, throw a ball, and breathe. Before continuing, take a moment to imagine that your bones have turned to putty. What if you were running when this change took place? Now imagine your bones forming a rigid metal framework inside your body, somewhat like a system of plumbing pipes. What problems could you envision with this arrangement? These images should help you understand how well our skeletal system provides support and protection while allowing movement.

4. **Storage.** Fat is stored in the internal cavities of bones. Bone itself serves as a storehouse for minerals, the most important being calcium and phosphorus, although others are also stored. A small amount of calcium in its ion form (Ca^{2+}) must be present in the blood at all times for the nervous system to transmit messages, for muscles to contract, and for blood to clot. Because most of the body's calcium is deposited in the bones as calcium salts, the bones are a convenient place to get more calcium ions for the blood as they are used up. Problems occur not only when there is too little calcium in the blood, but also when there is too much. Hormones control the movement of calcium to and from the bones and blood according to the needs of the body. Indeed, "deposits" and "withdrawals" of calcium (and other minerals) to and from bones go on almost all the time.

5. **Blood cell formation.** Blood cell formation, or hematopoiesis (hem"ah-to-poi-e'sis), occurs within the marrow cavities of certain bones.

Classification of Bones

The adult skeleton is composed of 206 bones. There are two basic types of osseous, or bone, tissue: **Compact bone** is dense and looks smooth and

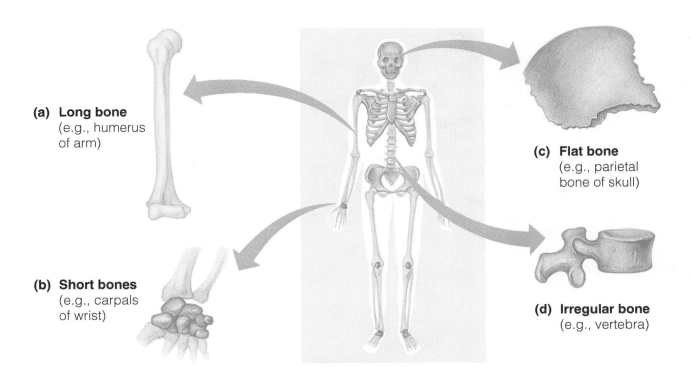

(a) Long bone
(e.g., humerus of arm)

(b) Short bones
(e.g., carpals of wrist)

(c) Flat bone
(e.g., parietal bone of skull)

(d) Irregular bone
(e.g., vertebra)

FIGURE 5.1   Classification of bones on the basis of shape.

homogeneous. **Spongy bone** is composed of small needlelike pieces of bone and lots of open space.

Bones come in many sizes and shapes (Figure 5.1). For example, the tiny pisiform bone of the wrist is the size and shape of a pea, whereas the femur, or thigh bone, is nearly 2 feet long and has a large, ball-shaped head. The unique shape of each bone fulfills a particular need. Bones are classified according to shape into four groups: long, short, flat, and irregular (Figure 5.1).

As their name suggests, **long bones** are typically longer than they are wide. As a rule they have a shaft with heads at both ends. Long bones are mostly compact bone. All the bones of the limbs, except the wrist and ankle bones, are long bones.

Short bones are generally cube-shaped and contain mostly spongy bone. The bones of the wrist and ankle are short bones. *Sesamoid* (ses′ah-moyd) *bones,* which form within tendons, are a special type of short bone. The best-known example is the patella, or kneecap.

Flat bones are thin, flattened, and usually curved. They have two thin layers of compact bone sandwiching a layer of spongy bone between them. Most bones of the skull, the ribs, and the sternum (breastbone) are flat bones.

Bones that do not fit one of the preceding categories are called **irregular bones.** The vertebrae, which make up the spinal column, and the hip bones fall into this group.

Gross Anatomy

The gross structure of a long bone is shown in Figure 5.2. The **diaphysis** (di-af′ĭ-sis), or shaft, makes up most of the bone's length and is composed of compact bone. The diaphysis is covered and protected by a fibrous connective tissue membrane, the **periosteum** (per-e-ŏs′te-um). Hundreds of connective tissue fibers, called **perforating,** or **Sharpey's, fibers,** secure the periosteum to the underlying bone. The **epiphyses** (ĕ-pif′ĭ-sēz) are the ends of the long bone. Each epiphysis consists of a thin layer of compact bone enclosing an area filled with spongy bone. **Articular cartilage,** instead of a periosteum, covers its external surface. Because the articular cartilage is glassy hyaline cartilage, it provides a smooth, slippery surface that decreases friction at joint surfaces.

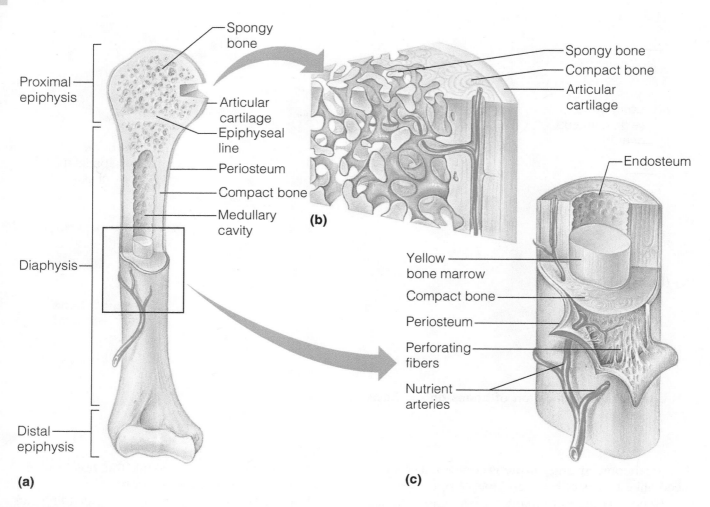

Proximal epiphysis

Spongy bone

Articular cartilage

Epiphyseal line

Periosteum

Compact bone

Medullary cavity

Diaphysis

Distal epiphysis

(a)

(b)

Spongy bone

Compact bone

Articular cartilage

Endosteum

Yellow bone marrow

Compact bone

Periosteum

Perforating fibers

Nutrient arteries

(c)

FIGURE 5.2   The structure of a long bone (humerus). (a) Anterior view with longitudinal section cut away at the proximal end. **(b)** Pie-shaped, three-dimensional view of spongy bone and compact bone of the epiphysis. **(c)** Cross section of the shaft (diaphysis). Note that the external surface of the diaphysis is covered by a periosteum, but the articular surface of the epiphysis (see b) is covered with hyaline cartilage.

In adult bones, there is a thin line of bony tissue spanning the epiphysis that looks a bit different from the rest of the bone in that area. This is the **epiphyseal line.** The epiphyseal line is a remnant of the **epiphyseal plate** (a flat plate of hyaline cartilage) seen in a young, growing bone. Epiphyseal plates cause the lengthwise growth of a long bone. By the end of puberty, when hormones inhibit long bone growth, epiphyseal plates have been completely replaced by bone, leaving only the epiphyseal lines to mark their previous location.

In adults the cavity of the shaft is primarily a storage area for adipose (fat) tissue. It is called the **yellow marrow,** or **medullary, cavity.** However, in infants this area forms blood cells, and **red marrow** is found there. In adult bones, red marrow is confined to the cavities of spongy bone of flat bones and the epiphyses of some long bones.

Even when looking casually at bones, one can see that their surfaces are not smooth but scarred with bumps, holes, and ridges. These **bone markings** reveal where muscles, tendons, and ligaments were attached and where blood vessels and nerves passed. There are two categories of bone markings: (a) *projections,* or *processes,* which grow out from the bone surface, and (b) *depressions,* or *cavities,* which are indentations in the bone. These terms do not have to be learned now, but they can help you remember some of the specific markings on bones to which you will be introduced later in this chapter.

Microscopic Anatomy

To the naked eye, spongy bone has a spiky, open appearance, whereas compact bone appears to be very dense. Looking at compact bone tissue through a microscope, however, one can see that it has a complex structure. It is riddled with passageways carrying nerves, blood vessels, and the like, which provide the living bone cells with nutrients and a route for waste disposal. The mature bone cells, **osteocytes** (os′te-o-sītz″), are found in tiny cavities within the matrix called **lacunae** (lah-ku′ne). The lacunae are arranged in concentric circles called **lamellae** (lah-mel′e) around **central (Haversian) canals.** Each complex consisting of central canal and matrix rings is called an **osteon,** or **Haversian system.** Central canals run lengthwise through the bony matrix, carrying blood vessels and nerves to all areas of the bone. Tiny canals, **canaliculi** (kan″ah-lik′u-li), radiate outward from the central canals to all lacunae. The canaliculi form a transportation system that connects all the bone cells to the nutrient supply through the hard bone matrix. Because of this elaborate network of canals, bone cells are well nourished in spite of the hardness of the matrix, and bone injuries heal quickly and well. The communication pathway from the outside of the bone to its interior (and the central canals) is completed by **perforating (Volkmann's) canals,** which run into the compact bone at right angles to the shaft.

Bone is one of the hardest materials in the body, and although relatively light in weight, it has a remarkable ability to resist tension and other forces acting on it. Nature has given us an extremely strong and exceptionally simple (almost crude) supporting system without giving up mobility. The calcium salts deposited in the matrix give bone its hardness, whereas the organic parts (especially the collagen fibers) provide for bone's flexibility and great tensile strength.

Cartilage

In addition to bone, there is another kind of supporting connective tissues in the body: cartilage.

The matrix of **cartilage** is a firm gel that cotains polysaccharide derivatives called **chondroitin sulfates** (kon-DROY-tin; *chondros,* cartilage). Chondroitin sulfates form complexes with proteins in the ground substance, producing proteoglycans. Cartilage cells, or **chondrocytes** (KON-drō-sīts), are the only cells in the cartilage matrix. They occupy small chambers known as **lacunae** (la-KOO-nē; *lacus,* pool). The physical properties of cartilage depend on the proteoglycans of the matrix, and on the type and abundance of extracellular fibers.

Unlike other connective tissues, cartilage is avascular, so all exchange of nutrients and waste products must occur by diffusion through the matrix. Blood vessels do not grow into cartilage because chondrocytes produce a chemical that discourages their formation. This chemical, named **antiangiogenesis factor** (*anti-,* against + *angeion,* vessel + *genno,* to produce), is now being tested as a potential anticancer agent.

A cartilage is generally set apart from surrounding tissues by a fibrous **perichondrium** (per-i-KON-drē-um); *peri-,* around). The perichondrium contains two distinct layers: an outer, fibrous region of dense irregular connective tissue, and an inner, cellular layer. The fibrous layer provides mechanical support and protection and attaches the cartilage to other structures. The cellular layer is important to the growth and maintenance of the cartilage.

Cartilage Growth   Cartilage grows by two mechanisms: *interstitial growth* and *appositional growth* (Figure 5.3).

In **interstitial growth,** chondrocytes in the cartilage matrix undergo cell division, and the daughter cells produce additional matrix (Figure 5.3a). This process enlarges the cartilage from within. Interstitial growth is most important during development. The process begins early in embryonic development and continues through adolescence.

In **appositional growth,** new layers of cartilage are added to the surface (Figure 5.3b). In this process, cells of the inner layer of the perichondrium undergo repeated cycles of division. The innermost cells then differentiate into immature chondrocytes, which begin producing cartilage matrix. As they become surrounded by and embedded in new matrix, they differentiate into mature chondrocytes. Appositional growth gradually increases the size of the cartilage by adding to its outer surface.

Both interstitial and appositional growth occur during development, although interstitial growth contributes more to the mass of the adult cartilage. Neither interstitial nor appositional growth occurs in the cartilages of normal adults. However, appositional growth may occur in unusual circumstances, such as after cartilage has been damaged or excessively stimulated by *growth hormone* from the pituitary gland. Minor damage to cartilage can be repaired by appositional growth at the damaged surface. After more severe damage, the injured portion of the cartilage will be replaced by a dense fibrous patch.

Types of Cartilage   The body contains three major types of cartilage: hyaline cartilage, elastic cartilage, and fibrocartilage.

1. **Hyaline cartilage** (hī-uh-lin; *hyalos,* glass) is the most common type of cartilage. Except inside joint cavities, a dense perichondrium surrounds hyaline cartilages. The matrix of hyaline cartilage contains closely packed collagen fibers, making it tough but somewhat flexible. Because the fibers are not in large bundles and do not stain darkly, they are not always apparent in light microscopy (Figure 5.4a). Examples in adults include the connections between the ribs and the sternum; the nasal cartilages and the supporting cartilages along the conducting passageways of the respiratory tract; and the *articular cartilages,* which cover opposing bone surfaces within many joints, such as the elbow and knee.

2. **Elastic cartilage** (Figure 5.4b) contains numerous elastic fibers that make it extremely resilient and flexible. These cartilages usually have a yellowish color on gross dissection. Elastic cartilage forms the external flap (the *auricle,* or *pinna*) of the outer ear, the epiglottis, a passageway to the middle ear cavity (the *auditory tube*), and small cartilages in the larynx (the *cuneiform cartilages*).

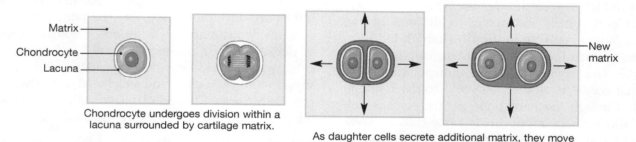

Matrix —
Chondrocyte —
Lacuna —

Chondrocyte undergoes division within a lacuna surrounded by cartilage matrix.

(a) Interstitial growth

New matrix

As daughter cells secrete additional matrix, they move apart, expanding the cartilage from within.

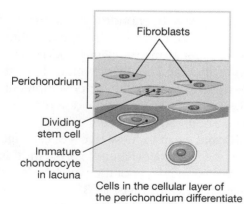

Fibroblasts

Perichondrium —

Dividing stem cell

Immature chondrocyte in lacuna

Cells in the cellular layer of the perichondrium differentiate into immature chondrocytes.

(b) Appositional growth

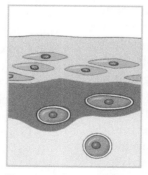

These immature chondrocytes secrete new matrix.

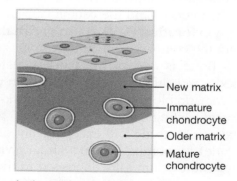

New matrix
Immature chondrocyte
Older matrix
Mature chondrocyte

As the matrix enlarges, more cells are incorporated; they are replaced by divisions of stem cells in the perichondrium.

FIGURE 5.3   The growth of cartilage. (a) In interstitial growth, the cartilage expands from within as chondrocytes in the matrix divide, grow, and produce new matrix. **(b)** In appositional growth, the cartilage grows at its external surface as fibroblasts in the cellular layer of the perichondrium differentiate into chondrocytes.

HYALINE CARTILAGE

LOCATIONS: Between tips of ribs and bones of sternum; covering bone surfaces at synovial joints; supporting larynx (voice box), trachea, and bronchi; forming part of nasal septum

FUNCTIONS: Provides stiff but somewhat flexible support; reduces friction between bony surfaces

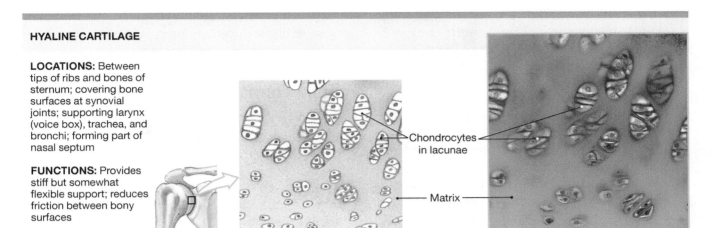

Chondrocytes in lacunae

Matrix

LM × 500

(a) Hyaline cartilage

ELASTIC CARTILAGE

LOCATIONS: Auricle of external ear; epiglottis; auditory canal; cuneiform cartilages of larynx

FUNCTIONS: Provides support, but tolerates distortion without damage and returns to original shape

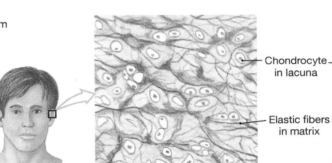
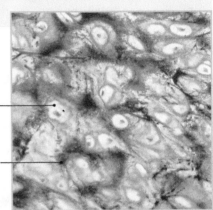

Chondrocyte in lacuna

Elastic fibers in matrix

LM × 358

(b) Elastic cartilage

FIBROCARTILAGE

LOCATIONS: Pads within knee joint; between pubic bones of pelvis; intervertebral discs

FUNCTIONS: Resists compression; prevents bone-to-bone contact; limits relative movement

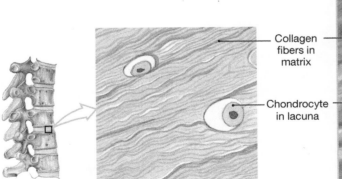
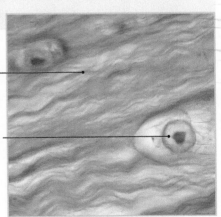

Collagen fibers in matrix

Chondrocyte in lacuna

LM × 750

(c) Fibrocartilage

FIGURE 5.4 The types of cartilage. (a) Hyaline cartilage. Note the translucent matrix and the absence of prominent fibers. **(b)** Elastic cartilage. The closely packed elastic fibers are visible between the chondrocytes. **(c)** Fibrocartilage. The collagen fibers are extremely dense, and the chondrocytes are relatively far apart.

3. Fibrocartilage has little ground substance, and its matrix is dominated by densely interwoven collagen fibers (Figure 5.4c), making this tissue extremely durable and tough. Fibrocartilaginous pads lie between the spinal vertebrae, between the pubic bones of the pelvis, and around tendons and within or around joints. In these positions, fibrocartilage resists compression, absorbs shocks, and prevents damaging bone-to-bone contact. Cartilage heals poorly, and damaged fibrocartilage in joints such as the knee can interfere with normal movements.

Several complex joints, including the knee, contain both hyaline cartilage and fibrocartilage. The hyaline cartilage covers bony surfaces, and fibrocartilage pads in the joint prevent contact between bones during movement. Injuries to these joints can produce tearing in the fibrocartilage pads that does not heal. Eventually, joint mobility is severely reduced. Surgery generally produces only a temporary or incomplete repair.

Bone Formation, Development, and Growth

The growth of the skeleton determines the size and proportions of your body. The bony skeleton begins to form about six weeks after fertilization, when the embryo is approximately 12 mm (0.5 in.) long. (At this stage, the existing skeletal elements are cartilaginous.) During subsequent development, the bones undergo a tremendous increase in size. Bone growth continues through adolescence, and portions of the skeleton generally do not stop growing until roughly age 25. Figure 5.5 shows the microscopic structure of a mature adult bone.

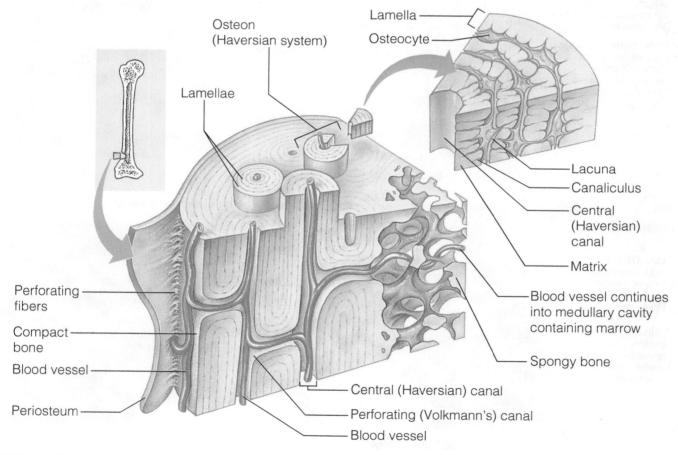

FIGURE 5.5 Microscopic structure of mature adult compact bone.
Diagram of a pie-shaped segment of compact bone. (The inset shows a more highly magnified view.) Notice the position of osteocytes in lacunae (cavities in the matrix).

In this section, we consider the physical process of osteogenesis (bone formation) and bone growth.

The process of replacing other tissues with bone is called **ossification** (os″ĭ-fĭ-ka′shun). The term refers specifically to the formation of bone. The process of **calcification**—the deposition of calcium salts—occurs during ossification, but it can also occur in other tissues. When calcification occurs in tissues other than bone, the result is a calcified tissue (such as calcified cartilage) that does not resemble bone. Two major forms of ossification exist: endochondral and intramembranous. In *endochondral ossification,* bone replaces existing cartilage. In *intramembranous ossification,* bone develops directly from mesenchyme or fibrous connective tissue.

Bone Formation, Growth, and Remodeling

The skeleton is formed from two of the strongest and most supportive tissues in the body—cartilage and bone. In embryos, the skeleton is primarily made of hyaline cartilage, but in the young child most of the cartilage has been replaced by bone. Cartilage remains only in isolated areas such as the bridge of the nose, parts of the ribs, and the joints.

Except for flat bones, which form on fibrous membranes, most bones develop using hyaline cartilage structures as their "models." Most simply, this process of bone formation, or **ossification,** involves two major phases. First, the hyaline cartilage model is completely covered with bone matrix (a bone "collar") by bone-forming cells called **osteoblasts.** So, for a short period, the fetus has cartilage "bones" enclosed by "bony" bones. Then, the enclosed hyaline cartilage model is digested away, opening up a medullary cavity within the newly formed bone.

By birth or shortly after, most hyaline cartilage models have been converted to bone except for two regions—the **articular cartilages** (that cover the bone ends) and the **epiphyseal plates.** The articular cartilages persist for life, reducing friction at the joint surfaces. The epiphyseal plates provide for longitudinal growth of the long bones during childhood (Figure 5.6a). New cartilage is formed continuously on the external face of the articular cartilage and on the epiphyseal plate surface that is farther away from the medullary cavity. At the same time, the old cartilage abutting the internal face of the articular cartilage and the medullary cavity is broken down and replaced by bony matrix. Growing bones also must widen as they lengthen. How do they widen? Simply, osteoblasts in the periosteum add bone tissue to the external face of the diaphysis as osteoclasts in the endosteum remove bone from the inner face of the diaphysis wall. Since these two processes occur at about the same rate, the circumference of the long bone expands and the bone widens. This process by which bones increase in diameter is called *appositional growth*. This process of long-bone growth is controlled by hormones, most importantly *growth hormone* and, during puberty, the *sex hormones*. It ends during adolescence, when the epiphyseal plates are completely converted to bone (Figure 5.6b).

Intramembranous Ossification

Intramembranous (in-tra-MEM-bra-nus) **ossification** begins when osteoblasts differentiate within a mesenchymal or fibrous connective tissue. This type of ossification is also called *dermal ossification* because it normally occurs in the deeper layers of the dermis. The bones that result are called **dermal bones.** Examples of dermal bones are the flat bones of the skull, the mandible (lower jaw), and the clavicle (collarbone). Figure 5.7 shows the steps in the process of intramembranous ossification.

Hormonal and Nutritional Effects on Bone

Normal bone growth and maintenance depend on a combination of nutritional and hormonal factors:

- Normal bone growth and maintenance cannot occur without a constant dietary source of calcium and phosphate salts. Lesser amounts of other minerals, such as magnesium, fluoride, iron, and manganese, are also required.

- The hormone *calcitriol,* synthesized in the kidneys, is essential for normal calcium and phosphate ion absorption in the digestive tract. Calcitriol synthesis is dependent on the availability of a related steroid, *cholecalciferol* (vitamin D_3), which may be synthesized in the skin or absorbed from the diet.

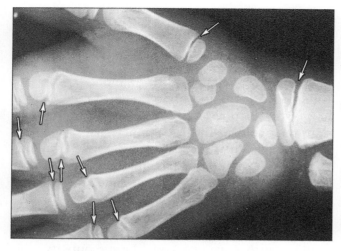

(a) Epiphyseal cartilages in child's hand

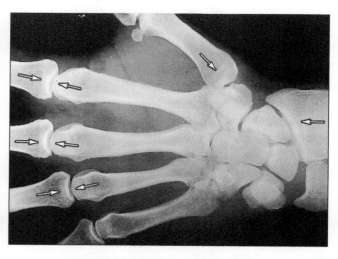

(b) Epiphyseal lines in adult hand

FIGURE 5.6 **Bone growth at an epiphyseal cartilage. (a)** An x-ray of growing epiphyseal cartilages (arrows). **(b)** Epiphyseal lines in an adult (arrows).

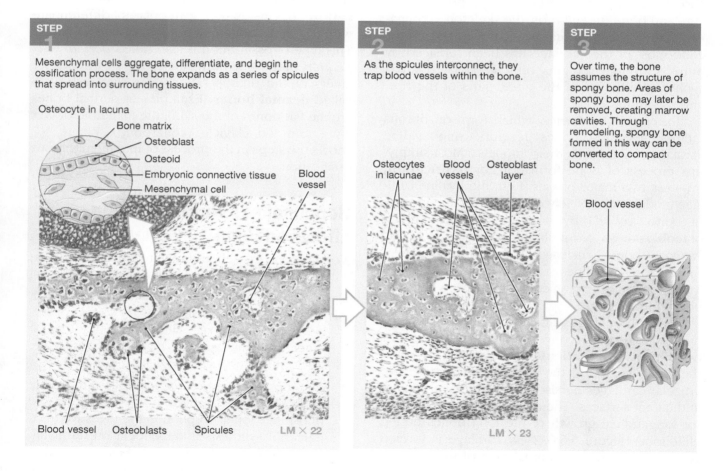

STEP 1

Mesenchymal cells aggregate, differentiate, and begin the ossification process. The bone expands as a series of spicules that spread into surrounding tissues.

Osteocyte in lacuna

Bone matrix

Osteoblast

Osteoid

Embryonic connective tissue

Mesenchymal cell

Blood vessel

Blood vessel   Osteoblasts   Spicules   LM × 22

STEP 2

As the spicules interconnect, they trap blood vessels within the bone.

Osteocytes in lacunae   Blood vessels   Osteoblast layer

LM × 23

STEP 3

Over time, the bone assumes the structure of spongy bone. Areas of spongy bone may later be removed, creating marrow cavities. Through remodeling, spongy bone formed in this way can be converted to compact bone.

Blood vessel

FIGURE 5.7 **Intramembranous Ossification.**

- Adequate levels of vitamin C must be present in the diet. This vitamin, which is required for certain key enzymatic reactions in collagen synthesis, also stimulates osteoblast differentiation. One of the signs of vitamin C deficiency—a condition called *scurvy*—is a loss of bone mass and strength.

- Three other vitamins have significant effects on bone structure. Vitamin A, which stimulates osteoblast activity, is particularly important for normal bone growth in children. Vitamins K and B_{12} are required for the synthesis of proteins in normal bone.

- *Growth hormone,* produced by the pituitary gland, and *thyroxine,* from the thyroid gland, stimulate bone growth. Growth hormone stimulates protein synthesis and cell growth throughout the body. Thyroxine stimulates cell metabolism and increases the rate of osteoblast activity. In proper balance, these hormones maintain normal activity at the epiphyseal cartilages until roughly the time of puberty.

- At puberty, rising levels of sex hormones (*estrogens* in females and *androgens* in males) stimulate osteoblasts to produce bone faster than the rate at which epiphyseal cartilage expands. Over time, the epiphyseal cartilages narrow and eventually close. The timing of epiphyseal closure differs from bone to bone and from individual to individual. The toes may complete ossification by age 11, but parts of the pelvis or the wrist may continue to enlarge until roughly age 25. Differences in male and female sex hormones account for significant variations in body size and proportions. Because estrogens cause faster epiphyseal closure than do androgens, women are generally shorter than men at maturity.

Two other hormones—*calcitonin* (kal-si-TŌ-nin), from the thyroid gland, and *parathyroid hormone,* from the parathyroid gland—are important in the homeostatic control of calcium and phosphate levels in body fluids. We consider the interactions of these hormones in the next section. The major hormones affecting the growth and maintenance of the skeletal system are summarized in Table 5.1.

The skeletal system is unique in that it persists after life, providing clues to the sex, lifestyle, and environmental conditions experienced by the individual. Not only do the bones reflect the physical stresses placed on the body, but they also provide clues concerning the person's health and diet. By using the appearance, strength, and composition of

TABLE 5.1   Hormones Involved in the Regulation of Bone Growth and Maintenance

Hormone	Primary Source	Effects on Skeletal System
Calcitriol	Kidneys	Promotes calcium and phosphate ion absorption along the digestive tract
Growth hormone	Pituitary gland	Stimulates osteoblast activity and the synthesis of bone matrix
Thyroxine	Thyroid gland (follicle cells)	With growth hormone, stimulates osteoblast activity and the synthesis of bone matrix
Sex hormones	Ovaries (estrogens) Testes (androgens)	Stimulate osteoblast activity and the synthesis of bone matrix
Parathyroid hormone	Parathyroid glands	Stimulates osteoclast (and osteoblast) activity; elevates calcium ion concentrations in body fluid
Calcitonin	Thyroid gland (C cells)	Inhibits osteoclast activity; promotes calcium loss at kidneys; reduces calcium ion concentrations in body fluids

bone, forensic scientists and physical anthropologists can detect features characteristic of hormonal deficiencies. Combining the physical clues provided by the skeleton with modern molecular techniques, such as DNA fingerprinting, can provide a wealth of information.

The Skeleton as a Calcium Reserve

The chemical analysis shown in Figure 5.8 reveals the importance of bones as mineral reservoirs. For the moment, we will focus on the homeostatic regulation of calcium ion concentration in body fluids. Calcium is the most abundant mineral in the human body. A typical human body contains 1–2 kg (2.2–4.4 lb) of calcium, with roughly 99 percent of it deposited in the skeleton.

Calcium ions play a role in a variety of physiological processes, so the body must tightly control calcium ion concentrations in order to prevent damage to essential physiological systems. Even small variations from the normal concentration affect cellular operations; larger changes can cause a clinical crisis. Calcium ions are particularly important to both the membranes and the intracellular activities of neurons and muscle cells, especially cardiac muscle cells. If the calcium concentration of body fluids increases by 30 percent, neurons and muscle cells become relatively unresponsive. If calcium levels decrease by 35 percent, neurons become so excitable that convulsions can occur. A 50 percent reduction in calcium concentration generally causes death. Calcium ion concentration is so closely regulated, however, that daily fluctuations of more than 10 percent are highly unusual.

Hormones and Calcium Balance

Calcium ion homeostasis is maintained by a pair of hormones with opposing effects. These hormones, parathyroid hormone and calcitonin, coordinate the storage, absorption, and excretion of calcium ions. Three target sites and functions are involved: (1) the bones (storage), (2) the digestive tract (absorption), and (3) the kidneys (excretion). Figure 5.9a indicates factors that elevate calcium levels in the blood; Figure 5.9b indicates factors that depress blood calcium levels.

When calcium ion concentrations in the blood fall below normal, cells of the **parathyroid glands,** embedded in the thyroid gland in the neck, release **parathyroid hormone (PTH)** into the bloodstream. Parathyroid hormone has three major effects, all of which increase blood calcium levels:

1. *Stimulating osteoclast activity* and enhancing the recycling of minerals by osteocytes. (PTH also stimulates osteoblast activity, but to a lesser degree.)

2. *Increasing the rate of intestinal absorption of calcium ions* by enhancing the action of calcitriol. Under normal circumstances, calcitriol is always present, and parathyroid hormone controls its effect on the intestinal epithelium.

3. *Decreasing the rate of excretion of calcium ions at the kidneys.*

Under these conditions, more calcium ions enter body fluids, and losses are restricted. The calcium ion concentration increases to normal levels, and homeostasis is restored.

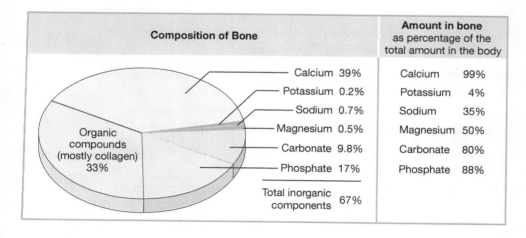

Composition of Bone		Amount in bone as percentage of the total amount in the body	
Calcium	39%	Calcium	99%
Potassium	0.2%	Potassium	4%
Sodium	0.7%	Sodium	35%
Magnesium	0.5%	Magnesium	50%
Carbonate	9.8%	Carbonate	80%
Phosphate	17%	Phosphate	88%
Total inorganic components	67%		

Organic compounds (mostly collagen) 33%

FIGURE 5.8   **A chemical analysis of bone.**

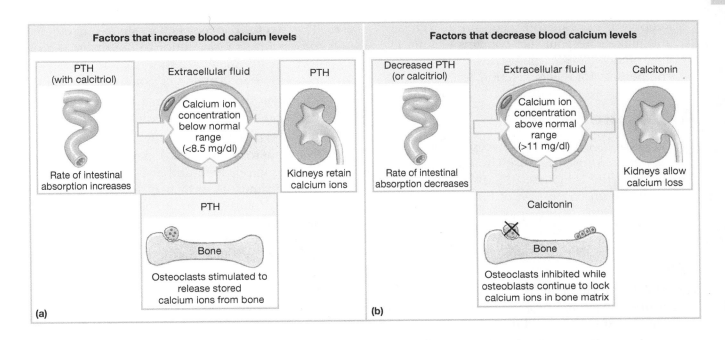

| Factors that increase blood calcium levels | Factors that decrease blood calcium levels |

PTH (with calcitriol) — Rate of intestinal absorption increases

Extracellular fluid — Calcium ion concentration below normal range (<8.5 mg/dl)

PTH — Kidneys retain calcium ions

PTH — Bone — Osteoclasts stimulated to release stored calcium ions from bone

(a)

Decreased PTH (or calcitriol) — Rate of intestinal absorption decreases

Extracellular fluid — Calcium ion concentration above normal range (>11 mg/dl)

Calcitonin — Kidneys allow calcium loss

Calcitonin — Bone — Osteoclasts inhibited while osteoblasts continue to lock calcium ions in bone matrix

(b)

FIGURE 5.9   Factors that alter the concentration of calcium ions in body Fluids.

If the calcium ion concentration of the blood instead rises above normal, special cells (*parafollicular cells,* or *C cells*) in the thyroid gland secrete **calcitonin.** This hormone has two major functions, which together act to decrease calcium ion concentrations in body fluids:

1. *Inhibiting osteoclast activity.*

2. *Increasing the rate of excretion of calcium ions at the kidneys.*

Under these conditions, less calcium *enters* body fluids because osteoclasts leave the mineral matrix alone. More calcium *leaves* body fluids because osteoblasts continue to produce new bone matrix while calcium ion excretion at the kidneys accelerates. The net result is a decline in the calcium ion concentration of body fluids, restoring homeostasis.

By providing a calcium reserve, the skeleton plays the primary role in the homeostatic maintenance of normal calcium ion concentrations of body fluids. This function can have a direct effect on the shape and strength of the bones in the skeleton. When large numbers of calcium ions are mobilized in body fluids, the bones become weaker; when calcium salts are deposited, the bones become denser and stronger.

Because the bone matrix contains protein fibers as well as mineral deposits, changes in mineral content do not necessarily affect the shape of the bone. In *osteomalacia* (os-tē-ō-ma-LĀ-shē-uh; *malakia,* softness), the bones appear normal, although they are weak and flexible owing to poor mineralization. *Rickets,* a form of osteomalacia affecting children, generally results from a vitamin D₃ deficiency caused by inadequate exposure to sunlight and an inadequate dietary supply of the vitamin. The bones of children with rickets are so poorly mineralized that they become very flexible. Because the walls of each femur can no longer resist the tension and compression forces applied by the body weight, the bones bend laterally and affected individuals develop a bowlegged appearance. In the United States, homogenized milk is fortified with vitamin D specifically to prevent rickets.

100 Keys | Each day, calcium and phosphate ions circulating in the blood are lost in the urine. To keep body fluid concentrations stable, those ions must be replaced; if they aren't obtained from the diet, they will be released from the skeleton, and the bones will become weaker as a result. If you want to keep your bones strong, you must exercise and make sure your diet contains vitamin D and plenty of calcium—at least enough to compensate for daily excretion.

Axial Skeleton

The skeleton is divided into two parts, the *axial* and *appendicular skeletons*. The axial skeleton, which forms the longitudinal axis of the body, is shown as the green portion of Figure 5.10. It can be divided into three parts—the *skull,* the *vertebral column,* and the *bony thorax*.

Skull

The **skull** is formed by two sets of bones. The **cranium** encloses and protects the fragile brain tissue. The **facial bones** hold the eyes in an anterior position and allow the facial muscles to show our feelings through smiles or frowns. All but one of the bones of the skull are joined together by *sutures,* which are interlocking, immovable joints. Only the mandible (jawbone) is attached to the rest of the skull by a freely movable joint.

In addition, each bone in the body has characteristic external and internal features, described in Table 5.2. As you study the descriptions of the bones that follow, review the distinctive surface features of these bones as well.

Cranium

The boxlike cranium is composed of eight large, flat bones. Except for two paired bones (the parietal and temporal), they are all single bones.

Frontal Bone   The frontal bone forms the forehead, the bony projections under the eyebrows, and the superior part of each eye's orbit (Figure 5.11).

Parietal Bones   The paired parietal bones form most of the superior and lateral walls of the cranium (see Figure 5.11). They meet in the midline of the skull at the **sagittal suture** and form the **coronal suture** where they meet the frontal bone.

Temporal Bones   The temporal bones lie inferior to the parietal bones; they join them at the **squamous sutures.** Several important bone markings appear on the temporal bone (see Figure 5.11):

- The **external acoustic (auditory) meatus** is a canal that leads to the eardrum and the middle ear.

- The **styloid process,** a sharp, needlelike projection, is just inferior to the external auditory meatus. Many neck muscles use the styloid process as an attachment point.

- The **zygomatic** (zi″go-mat′ik) **process** is a thin bridge of bone that joins with the cheekbone (zygomatic bone) anteriorly.

- The **mastoid** (mas′toid) **process** is a rough projection posterior and inferior to the external acoustic meatus, which is full of air cavities (mastoid sinuses). It provides an attachment site for some muscles of the neck. The mastoid sinuses are so close to the middle ear—a high-risk spot for infections—that they may become infected too, a condition called *mastoiditis.* Also, this area is so close to the brain, mastoiditis may spread to the brain itself.

- The **jugular foramen,** at the junction of the occipital and temporal bones (Figures 5.12 and 5.13), allows passage of the jugular vein, the largest vein of the head, which drains the brain. Just anterior to it in the cranial cavity is the **internal acoustic meatus** (Figure 5.12) which transmits cranial nerves VII and VIII (the facial and vestibulocochlear nerves). Anterior to the jugular foramen on the skull's inferior aspect is the **carotid canal** (see Figure 5.13), through which the internal carotid artery runs, supplying blood to most of the brain.

Occipital Bone   If you look at Figures 5.11, 5.12, and 5.13, you can see that the occipital (ok-sip′ĭ-tal) bone is the most posterior bone of the cranium. It forms the floor and back wall of the skull. The occipital bone joins the parietal bones anteriorly at the **lambdoid** (lam′doyd) **suture.** In the base of the occipital bone is a large opening, the **foramen magnum** (literally, "large hole"). The foramen magnum surrounds the lower part of the brain and allows the spinal cord to connect with the brain. Lateral to the foramen magnum on each side are the rockerlike **occipital condyles** (see Figure 5.13), which rest on the first vertebra of the spinal column.

Sphenoid Bone   The butterfly-shaped sphenoid (sfe′noid) bone spans the width of the skull and forms part of the floor of the cranial cavity (see Figure 5.12). In the midline of the sphenoid is a small depression, the **sella turcica** (sel′ah tur′sĭ-kah), or *Turk's saddle,* which holds the pituitary gland in place.

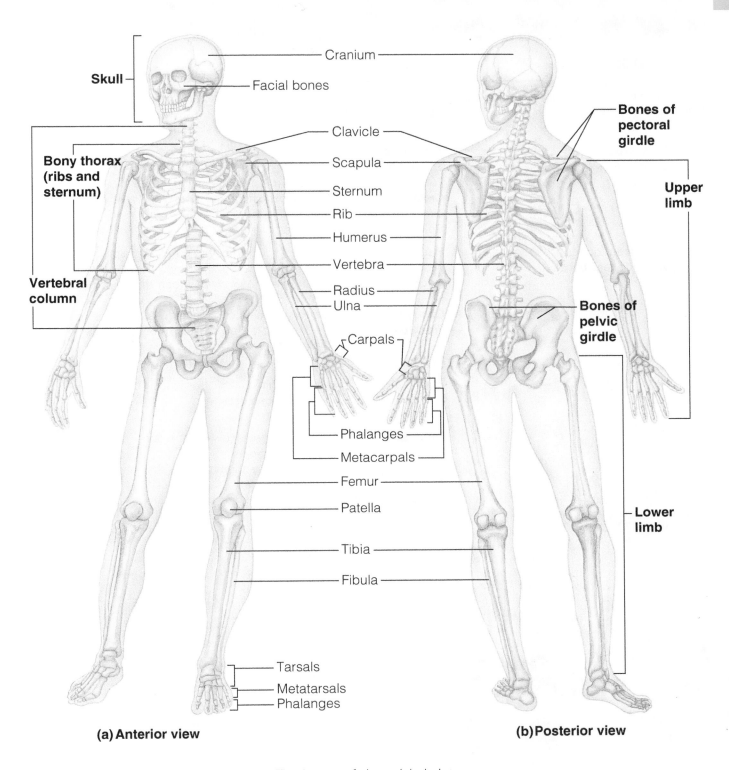

Skull — Cranium

Facial bones

Bony thorax (ribs and sternum)

Clavicle

Scapula

Sternum

Rib

Humerus

Vertebra

Vertebral column

Radius

Ulna

Carpals

Phalanges

Metacarpals

Femur

Patella

Tibia

Fibula

Tarsals

Metatarsals

Phalanges

Bones of pectoral girdle

Upper limb

Bones of pelvic girdle

Lower limb

(a) Anterior view

(b) Posterior view

FIGURE 5.10   The human skeleton. The bones of the axial skeleton are colored green to distinguish them from the bones of the appendicular skeleton.

General Description	Anatomical Term	Definition
Elevations and projections (general)	**Process**	Any projection or bump
	Ramus	An extension of a bone making an angle with the rest of the structure
Processes formed where tendons or ligaments attach	**Trochanter**	A large, rough projection
	Tuberosity	A smaller, rough projection
	Tubercle	A small, rounded projection
	Crest	A prominent ridge
	Line	A low ridge
	Spine	A pointed process
Processes formed for articulation with adjacent bones	**Head**	The expanded articular end of an epiphysis, separated from the shaft by a neck
	Neck	A narrow connection between the epiphysis and the diaphysis
	Condyle	A smooth, rounded articular process
	Trochlea	A smooth, grooved articular process shaped like a pulley
	Facet	A small, flat articular surface
Depressions	**Fova**	A narrow pit
	Fossa	A shallow depression
	Sulcus	A narrow groove
Openings	**Foramen**	A rounded passageway for blood vessels or nerves
	Canal	A passageway through the substance of a bone
	Fissure	An elongate cleft
	Sinus or antrum	A chamber within a bone, normally filled with air

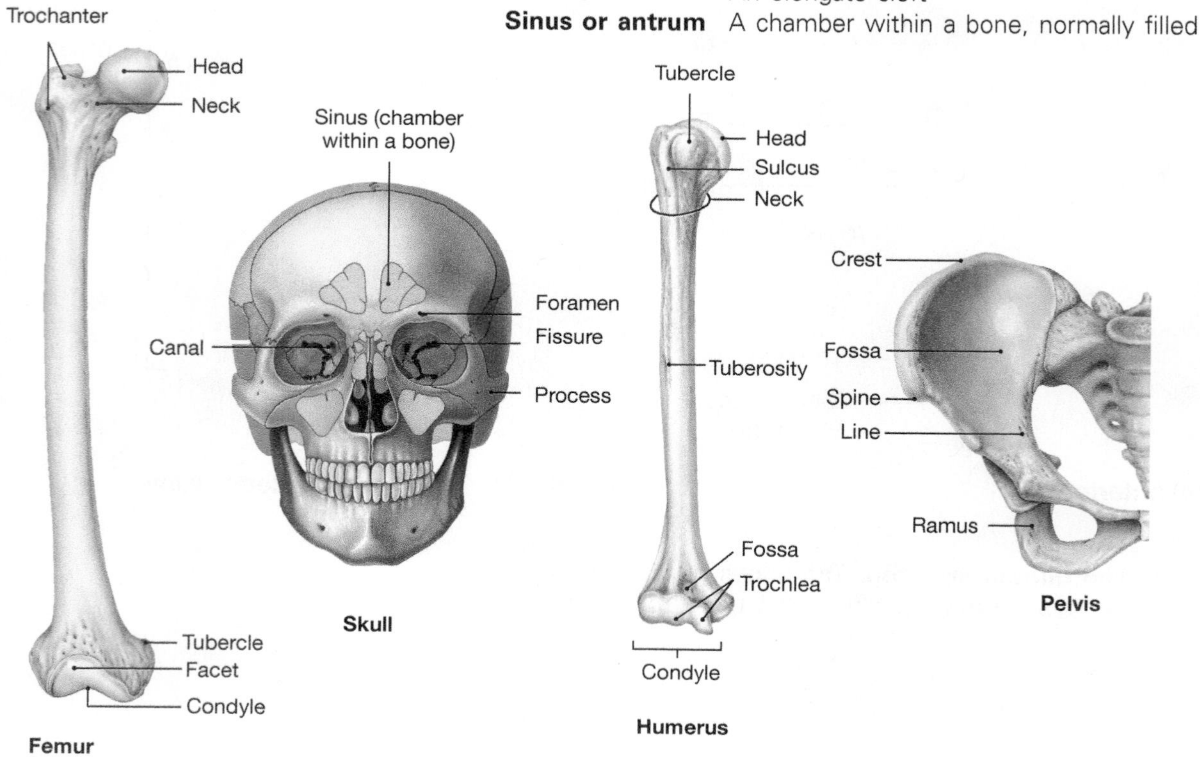

Trochanter — Head — Neck — Tubercle — Facet — Condyle

Femur

Sinus (chamber within a bone) — Foramen — Fissure — Process — Canal

Skull

Tubercle — Head — Sulcus — Neck — Tuberosity — Fossa — Trochlea — Condyle

Humerus

Crest — Fossa — Spine — Line — Ramus

Pelvis

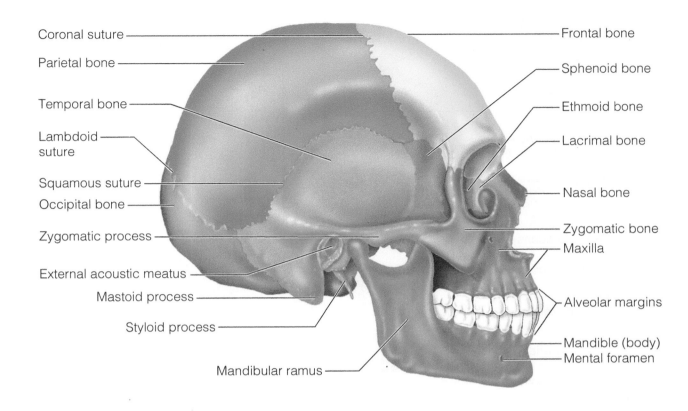

FIGURE 5.11   Human skull, lateral view.

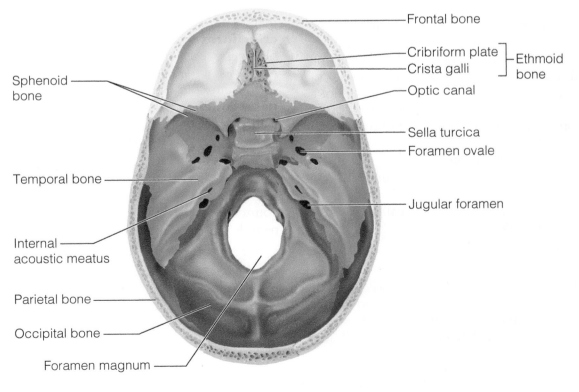

FIGURE 5.12   Human skull, superior view (top of cranium removed).

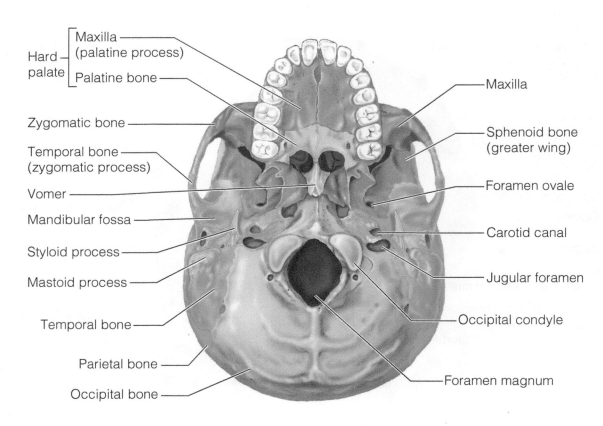

Maxilla
(palatine process)
Palatine bone
Hard palate

Zygomatic bone

Temporal bone
(zygomatic process)

Vomer

Mandibular fossa

Styloid process

Mastoid process

Temporal bone

Parietal bone

Occipital bone

Maxilla

Sphenoid bone
(greater wing)

Foramen ovale

Carotid canal

Jugular foramen

Occipital condyle

Foramen magnum

FIGURE 5.13   Human skull, inferior view (mandible removed).

The **foramen ovale,** a large oval opening in line with the posterior end of the sella turcica (Figure 5.12), allows fibers of cranial nerve V (the trigeminal nerve) to pass to the chewing muscles of the lower jaw (mandible). Parts of the sphenoid, seen exteriorly forming part of the eye orbits, have two important openings, the **optic canal** which allows the optic nerve to pass to the eye, and the slit-like **superior orbital fissure** through which the cranial nerves controlling eye movements (III, IV, and VI) pass (see Figures 5.11 and 5.15). The central part of the sphenoid bone is riddled with air cavities, the **sphenoid sinuses** (Figure 5.14).

Ethmoid Bone   The ethmoid (eth′moid) bone is very irregularly shaped and lies anterior to the sphenoid (see Figures 5.11, 5.12, and 5.15). It forms the roof of the nasal cavity and part of the medial walls of the orbits. Projecting from its superior surface is the **crista galli** (kris′tah gah′le), literally "cock's comb" (see Figure 5.12). The outermost covering of the brain attaches to this projection. On each side of the crista galli are

many small holes. These holey areas, the **cribriform** (krib′rĭ-form) **plates,** allow nerve fibers carrying impulses from the olfactory (smell) receptors of the nose to reach the brain. Extensions of the ethmoid bone, the **superior** and **middle nasal conchae** (see Figure 5.15), form part of the lateral walls of the nasal cavity and increase the turbulence of air flowing through the nasal passages.

Facial Bones

Fourteen bones compose the face. Twelve are paired; only the mandible and vomer are single. Figures 5.11 and 5.15 show most of the facial bones.

Maxillae   The two maxillae (mak-si′le), or **maxillary bones,** fuse to form the upper jaw. All facial bones except the mandible join the maxillae; thus they are the main, or "keystone," bones of the face. The maxillae carry the upper teeth in the **alveolar margin.**

Extensions of the maxillae called the **palatine** (pal′ah-tīn) **processes** form the anterior part of

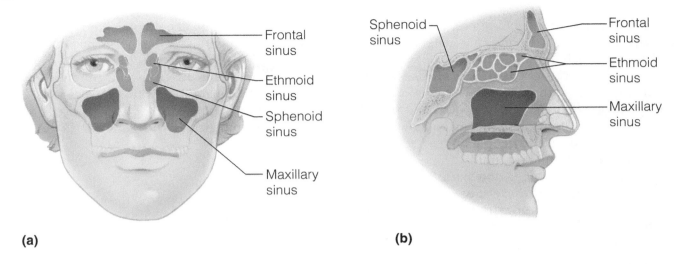

FIGURE 5.14   Paranasal sinuses. (a) Anterior view. **(b)** Medial view.

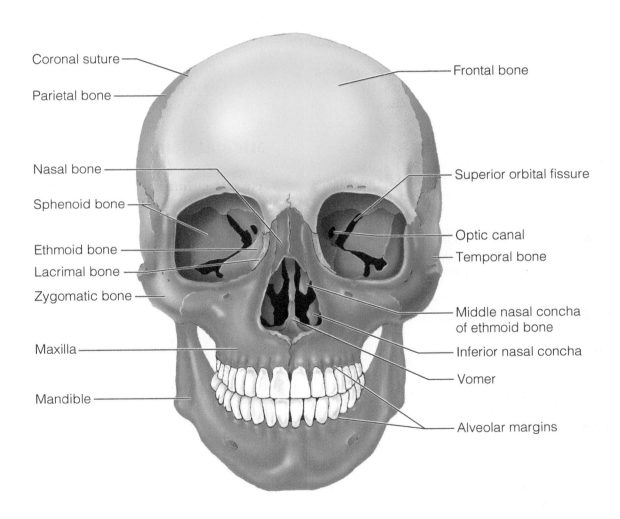

FIGURE 5.15   Human skull, anterior view.

the hard palate of the mouth (see Figure 5.8). Like many other facial bones, the maxillae contain **sinuses,** which drain into the nasal passages (see Figure 5.14). These **paranasal sinuses,** whose naming reveals their position surrounding the nasal cavity, lighten the skull bones and probably act to amplify the sounds we make as we speak. They also cause many people a great deal of misery. Since the mucosa lining these sinuses is continuous with that in the nasal passages and throat, infections in these areas tend to migrate into the sinuses, causing *sinusitis.* Depending on which sinuses are infected, a headache or upper jaw pain is the usual result.

Palatine Bones   The paired palatine bones lie posterior to the palatine processes of the maxillae. They form the posterior part of the hard palate (see Figure 5.13). Failure of these or the palatine processes to fuse medially results in *cleft palate.*

Zygomatic Bones   The zygomatic bones are commonly referred to as the cheekbones. They also form a good-sized portion of the lateral walls of the orbits, or eye sockets.

Lacrimal Bones   The lacrimal (lak′rĭ-mal) bones are fingernail-size bones forming part of the medial walls of each orbit. Each lacrimal bone has a groove that serves as a passageway for tears (*lacrima* = tear).

Nasal Bones   The small rectangular bones forming the bridge of the nose are the nasal bones. (The lower part of the skeleton of the nose is made up of cartilage.)

Vomer Bone   The single bone in the median line of the nasal cavity is the vomer. (*Vomer* means "plow," which refers to the bone's shape.) The vomer forms most of the nasal septum.

Inferior Nasal Conchae   The inferior nasal conchae (kong′ke) are thin, curved bones projecting from the lateral walls of the nasal cavity. (As mentioned earlier, the superior and middle conchae are similar but are parts of the ethmoid bone.)

Mandible   The mandible, or lower jaw, is the largest and strongest bone of the face. It joins the temporal bones on each side of the face, forming the only freely movable joints in the skull. You can find these joints on yourself by placing your fingers over your cheekbones and opening and closing your mouth. The horizontal part of the mandible (the *body*) forms the chin. Two upright bars of bone (the *rami*) extend from the body to connect the mandible with the temporal bone. The lower teeth lie in *alveoli* (sockets) in the **alveolar margin** at the superior edge of the mandibular body.

The Hyoid Bone

Though not really part of the skull, the **hyoid** (hi′oid) **bone** is closely related to the mandible and temporal bones. The hyoid bone is unique in that it is the only bone of the body that does not articulate directly with any other bone. Instead, it is suspended in the midneck region about 2 cm (1 inch) above the larynx, where it is anchored by ligaments to the styloid processes of the temporal bones. Horseshoe-shaped, with a *body* and two pairs of *horns,* or *cornua,* the hyoid bone serves as a movable base for the tongue and an attachment point for neck muscles that raise and lower the larynx when we swallow and speak.

Vertebral Column (Spine)

Serving as the axial support of the body, the **vertebral column,** or **spine,** extends from the skull, which it supports, to the pelvis, where it transmits the weight of the body to the lower limbs. Some people think of the vertebral column as a rigid supporting rod, but that picture is inaccurate. Instead, the spine is formed from 26 irregular bones connected and reinforced by ligaments in such a way that a flexible, curved structure results (Figure 5.16). Running through the central cavity of the vertebral column is the delicate spinal cord, which it surrounds and protects.

Before birth, the spine consists of 33 separate bones called **vertebrae,** but 9 of these eventually fuse to form the two composite bones, the *sacrum* and the *coccyx,* that construct the inferior portion of the vertebral column. Of the 24 single bones, the 7 vertebrae of the neck are *cervical vertebrae,* the next 12 are the *thoracic vertebrae,* and the remaining 5 supporting the lower back are *lumbar vertebrae.*

● Remembering common meal times, 7 AM, 12 noon, and 5 PM, may help you to recall the number of bones in these three regions of the vertebral column.

The single vertebrae are separated by pads of flexible fibrocartilage—**intervertebral discs**—which cushion the vertebrae and absorb shocks while allowing the spine flexibility. In a young person, the discs have a high water content (about 90 percent) and are spongy and compressible. But as a person ages, the water content of the discs decreases (as it does in other tissues throughout the body), and the discs become harder and less compressible.

Homeostatic Imbalance

Drying of the discs, along with a weakening of the ligaments of the vertebral column, predisposes older people to *herniated* ("slipped") *discs.* However, herniation also may result when the vertebral column is subjected to exceptional twisting forces. If the protruding disc presses on the spinal cord or the spinal nerves exiting from the cord, numbness and excruciating pain can result. ▲

The discs and the S-shaped structure of the vertebral column work together to prevent shock to the head when we walk or run. They also make the body trunk flexible. The spinal curvatures in the thoracic and sacral regions are referred to as **primary curvatures** because they are present when we are born. Later, the **secondary curvatures** develop. The cervical curvature appears when a baby begins to raise its head, and the lumbar curvature develops when the baby begins to walk.

Homeostatic Imbalance

Why do they do "spine checks" in middle school? The answer is that they are looking for abnormal spinal curvatures. There are several types of abnormal spinal curvatures. Figure 5.17 shows three of these—*scoliosis* (sko"le-o'sis), *kyphosis* (ki-fo'sis), and *lordosis* (lor-do'sis). These abnormalities may be congenital (present at birth) or result from disease,

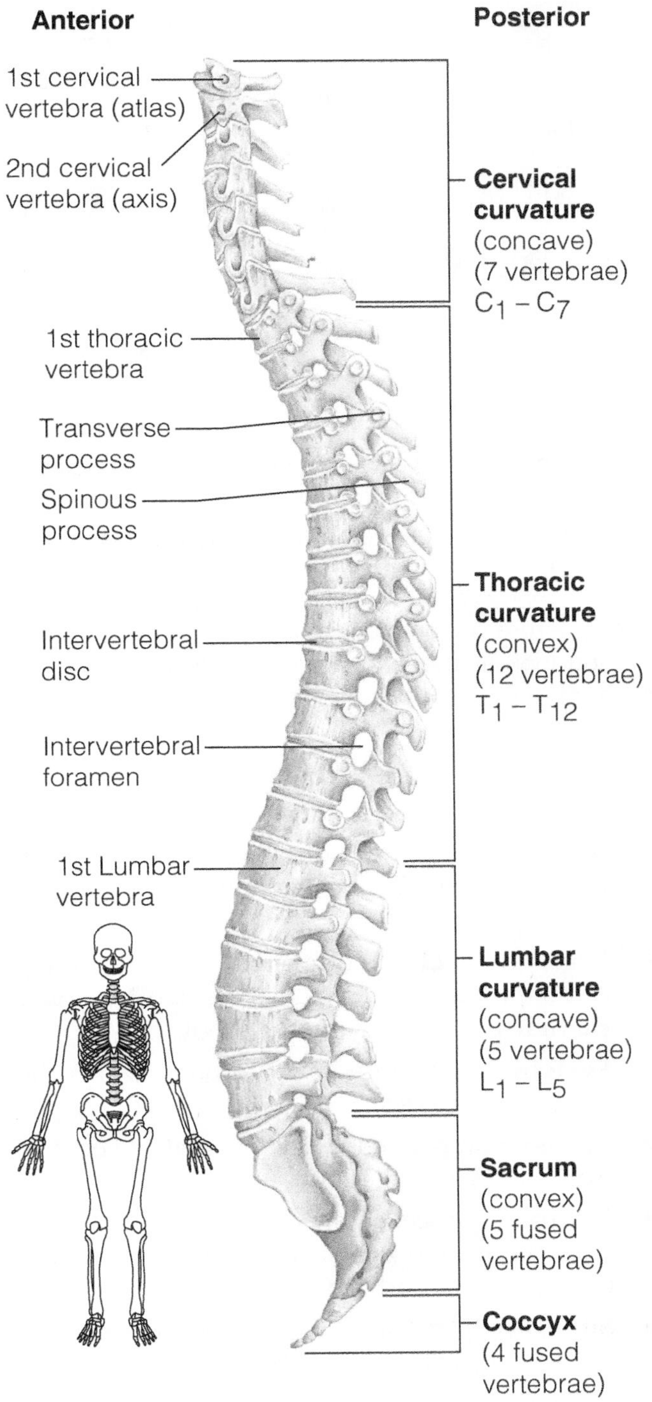

FIGURE 5.16 The vertebral column. Thin discs between the thoracic vertebrae allow great flexibility in the thoracic region; thick discs between the lumbar vertebrae reduce flexibility. Notice that the terms *convex* and *concave* refer to the curvature of the posterior aspect of the vertebral column.

Q *What is a slipped disc?*

A *A disc that protrudes outward from its normal position in the vertebral column and which may cause pain by pressing on adjacent nerves.*

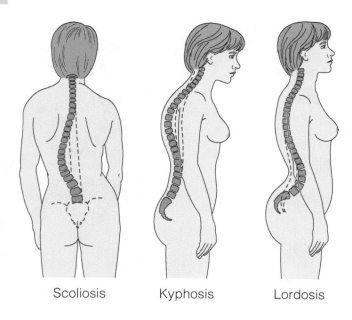

Scoliosis   Kyphosis   Lordosis

FIGURE 5.17 Abnormal spinal curvatures.

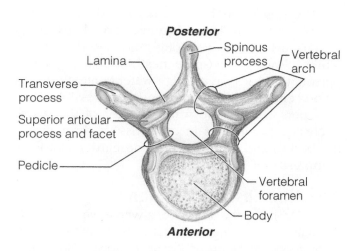

FIGURE 5.18 A typical vertebra, superior view. (Inferior articulating surfaces are not shown.)

poor posture, or unequal muscle pull on the spine. As you look at these diagrams, try to pinpoint how each of these conditions differs from the normal healthy spine. ▲

All vertebrae have a similar structural pattern (Figure 5.18). The common features are listed below:

- **Body** or **centrum:** disclike, weight-bearing part of the vertebra facing anteriorly in the vertebral column.

- **Vertebral arch:** arch formed from the joining of all posterior extensions, the **laminae** and **pedicles,** from the vertebral body.

- **Vertebral foramen:** canal through which the spinal cord passes.

- **Transverse processes:** two lateral projections from the vertebral arch.

- **Spinous process:** single projection arising from the posterior aspect of the vertebral arch (actually the fused laminae).

- **Superior and inferior articular processes:** paired projections lateral to the vertebral foramen, allowing a vertebra to form joints with adjacent vertebrae (see also Figure 5.19).

In addition to the common features just described, vertebrae in the different regions of the spine have very specific structural characteristics. These unique regional characteristics of the vertebrae are described next.

Cervical Vertebrae

The seven **cervical vertebrae** (identified as C_1 to C_7) form the neck region of the spine. The first two vertebrae (*atlas* and *axis*) are different because they perform functions not shared by the other cervical vertebrae. As you can see in Figure 5.19a, the **atlas** (C_1) has no body. The superior surfaces of its transverse processes contain large depressions that receive the occipital condyles of the skull. This joint allows you to nod "yes." The **axis** (C_2) acts as a pivot for the rotation of the atlas (and skull) above. It has a large upright process, the **dens,** or **odontoid** (o-don'toid) **process,** which acts as the pivot point. The joint between C_1 and C_2 allows you to rotate your head from side to side to indicate "no."

The "typical" cervical vertebrae (C_3 through C_7) are shown in Figure 5.19b. They are the smallest, lightest vertebrae, and most often their spinous processes are short and divided into two branches. The transverse processes of the cervical vertebrae contain foramina (openings) through which the vertebral arteries pass on their way to the brain above. Any time you see these foramina in a vertebra, you should know immediately that it is a cervical vertebra.

Thoracic Vertebrae

The 12 **thoracic vertebrae** (T_1 to T_{12}) are all typical. As seen in Figure 5.19c, they are larger

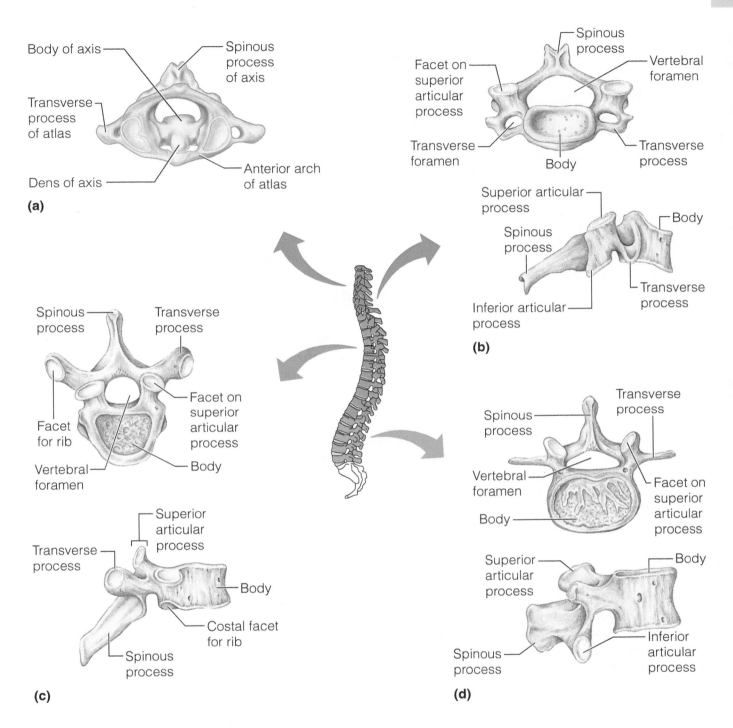

FIGURE 5.19 Regional characteristics of vertebrae. (a) Superior view of the articulated atlas and axis. **(b)** Cervical vertebrae; superior view above, lateral view below. **(c)** Thoracic vertebrae; superior view above, lateral view below. **(d)** Lumbar vertebrae; superior view above, lateral view below.

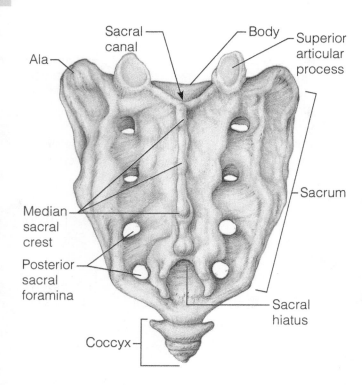

FIGURE 5.20   Sacrum and coccyx, posterior view.

than the cervical vertebrae. The body is somewhat heart-shaped and has two costal facets (articulating surfaces) on each side, which receive the heads of the ribs. The spinous process is long and hooks sharply downward, causing the vertebra to look like a giraffe's head viewed from the side.

Lumbar Vertebrae

The five **lumbar vertebrae** (L_1 to L_5) have massive, blocklike bodies. Their short, hatchet-shaped spinous processes (Figure 5.19d) make them look like a moose head from the lateral aspect. Since most of the stress on the vertebral column occurs in the lumbar region, these are the sturdiest of the vertebrae.

Sacrum

The **sacrum** (sa'krum) is formed by the fusion of five vertebrae (Figure 5.20). Superiorly it articulates with L_5, and inferiorly it connects with the coccyx. The winglike **alae** articulate laterally with the hip bones, forming the sacroiliac joints. The sacrum

forms the posterior wall of the pelvis. Its posterior midline surface is roughened by the **median sacral crest,** the fused spinous processes of the sacral vertebrae. This is flanked laterally by the posterior sacral foramina. The vertebral canal continues inside the sacrum as the **sacral canal** and terminates in a large inferior opening called the **sacral hiatus.**

Coccyx

The **coccyx** is formed from the fusion of three to five tiny, irregularly shaped vertebrae (Figure 5.20). It is the human "tailbone," a remnant of the tail that other vertebrate animals have.

Bony Thorax

The sternum, ribs, and thoracic vertebrae make up the **bony thorax.** The bony thorax is often called the **thoracic cage** because it forms a protective, cone-shaped cage of slender bones around the organs of the thoracic cavity (heart, lungs, and major blood vessels). The bony thorax is shown in Figure 5.21.

Sternum

The **sternum** (breastbone) is a typical flat bone and the result of the fusion of three bones—the **manubrium** (mah-nu'bre-um), **body,** and **xiphoid** (zif'oid) **process.** It is attached to the first seven pairs of ribs.

The sternum has three important bony landmarks—the jugular notch, the sternal angle, and the xiphisternal joint.

- The **jugular notch** (concave upper border of the manubrium) can be palpated easily; generally it is at the level of the third thoracic vertebra.

- The **sternal angle** results where the manubrium and body meet at a slight angle to each other, so that a transverse ridge is formed at the level of the second ribs. It provides a handy reference point for counting ribs to locate the second intercostal space for listening to certain heart valves.

- The **xiphisternal** (zi'fe-ster"nal) **joint,** the point where the sternal body and xiphoid process fuse, lies at the level of the ninth thoracic vertebra.

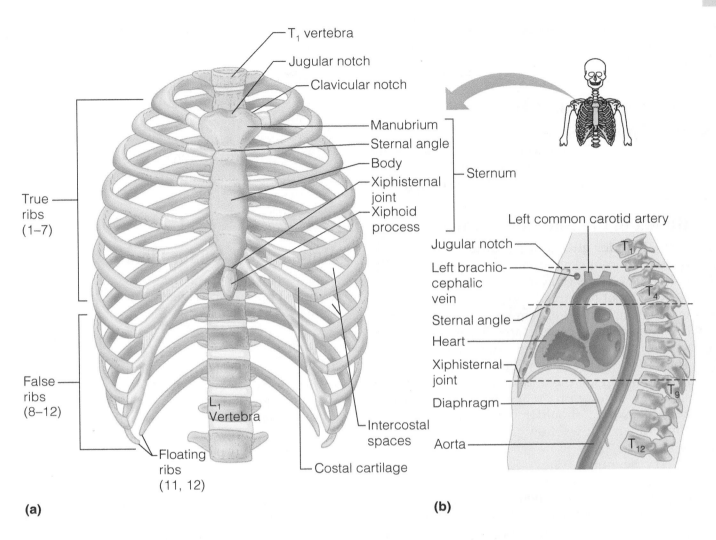

FIGURE 5.21 The bony thorax. (a) Skeleton of the bony thorax, anterior view (costal cartilages are shown in blue). **(b)** Left lateral view of the thorax, showing the relationship of the surface landmarks of the thorax to the vertebral column (thoracic portion).

Palpate your sternal angle and jugular notch.

Because the sternum is so close to the body surface, it is easy to obtain samples of blood-forming (hematopoietic) tissue for the diagnosis of suspected blood diseases from this bone. A needle is inserted into the marrow of the sternum, and the sample is withdrawn; this procedure is called a *sternal puncture*. Because the heart lies immediately posterior to the sternum, the physician must take extreme care not to penetrate through the sternum during this procedure.

Ribs

Twelve pairs of **ribs** form the walls of the bony thorax. (Contrary to popular misconception, males do *not* have one rib less than females!) All the ribs articulate with the vertebral column posteriorly and then curve downward and toward the anterior body surface. The **true ribs,** the first seven pairs, attach directly to the sternum by costal cartilages. **False ribs,** the next five pairs, either attach indirectly to the sternum or are not attached to the sternum at all. The last two pairs of false ribs lack the sternal attachments, and so they are also called **floating ribs.**

The intercostal spaces (spaces between the ribs) are filled with the intercostal muscles that aid in breathing.

Appendicular Skeleton

The *appendicular skeleton* is shaded gold in Figure 5.10. It is composed of 126 bones of the limbs (appendages) and the pectoral and pelvic girdles, which attach the limbs to the axial skeleton.

Bones of the Shoulder Girdle

Each **shoulder girdle,** or **pectoral girdle,** consists of two bones—a clavicle and a scapula (Figure 5.22).

The **clavicle** (klav′ĭ-kl), or *collarbone,* is a slender, doubly curved bone. It attaches to the manubrium of the sternum medially (at its sternal end) and to the scapula laterally, where it helps to form the shoulder joint (at its acromial end). The clavicle acts as a brace to hold the arm away from the top of the thorax and helps prevent shoulder dislocation. When the clavicle is broken, the whole shoulder region caves in medially, which shows how important its bracing function is.

The **scapulae** (skap′u-le), or *shoulder blades,* are triangular and are commonly called "wings" because they flare when we move our arms posteriorly. Each scapula has a flattened body and two important processes—the **acromion** (ah-kro′me-on), which is the enlarged end of the spine of the scapula, and the beaklike **coracoid** (kor′ah-koid) **process.** The acromion connects with the clavicle laterally at the **acromioclavicular joint.** The coracoid process points over the top of the shoulder and anchors some of the muscles of the arm. Just medial to the coracoid process is the large **suprascapular notch,** which serves as a nerve passageway. The scapula is not directly attached to the axial skeleton; it is loosely held in place by trunk muscles. The scapula has three borders—superior, medial (vertebral), and lateral (axillary). It also has three angles—superior, inferior, and lateral. The **glenoid cavity,** a shallow socket that receives the head of the arm bone, is in the lateral angle.

The shoulder girdle is very light and allows the upper limb to have exceptionally free movement. This is due to the following factors:

1. Each shoulder girdle attaches to the axial skeleton at only one point—the *sternoclavicular joint.*

2. The loose attachment of the scapula allows it to slide back and forth against the thorax as muscles act.

3. The glenoid cavity is shallow, and the shoulder joint is poorly reinforced by ligaments.

However, this exceptional flexibility also has a drawback; the shoulder girdle is very easily dislocated.

Bones of the Upper Limbs

Thirty separate bones form the skeletal framework of each upper limb (Figures 5.22 and 5.23). They form the foundations of the arm, forearm, and hand.

Arm

The arm is formed by a single bone, the **humerus** (hu′mer-us), which is a typical long bone (see Figure 5.23a and b). At its proximal end is a rounded head that fits into the shallow glenoid cavity of the scapula. Opposite the head are two bony projections—the **greater** and **lesser tubercles,** which are sites of muscle attachment. In the midpoint of the shaft is a roughened area called the **deltoid tuberosity,** where the large, fleshy deltoid muscle of the shoulder attaches. Nearby, the **radial groove** runs obliquely down the posterior aspect of the shaft. This groove marks the course of the radial nerve, an important nerve of the upper limb. At the distal end of the humerus is the medial **trochlea** (trok′le-ah), which looks somewhat like a spool, and the lateral ball-like **capitulum** (kah-pit′u-lum). Both of these processes articulate with bones of the forearm. Above the trochlea anteriorly is a depression, the **coronoid fossa;** on the posterior surface is the **olecranon** (o-lek′rah-non) **fossa.** These two depressions, which are flanked by **medial** and **lateral epicondyles,** allow the corresponding processes of the ulna to move freely when the elbow is bent and extended.

Forearm

Two bones, the radius and the ulna, form the skeleton of the forearm (see Figure 5.23c). When the

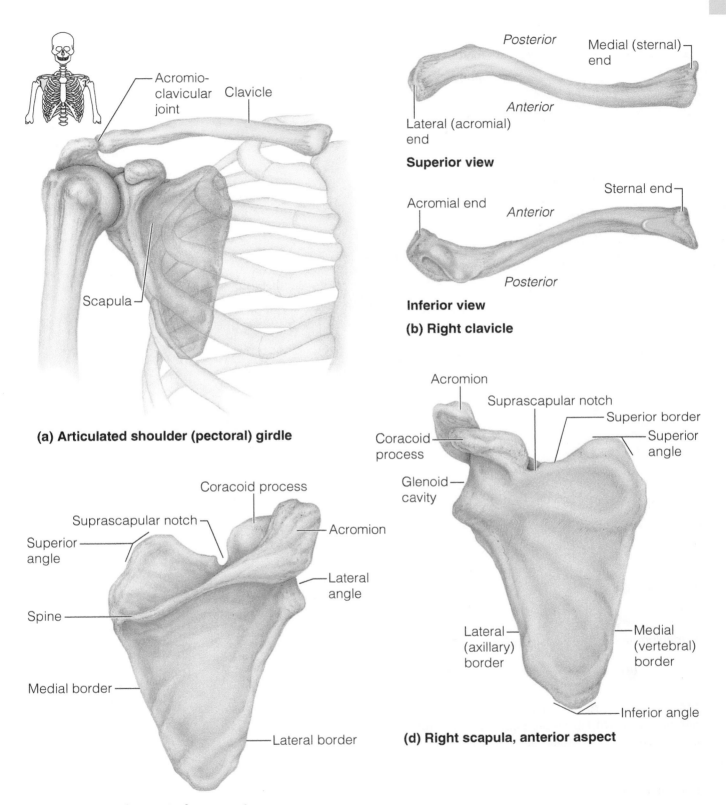

(a) Articulated shoulder (pectoral) girdle

Superior view

(b) Right clavicle

Inferior view

(c) Right scapula, posterior aspect

(d) Right scapula, anterior aspect

FIGURE 5.22   Bones of the shoulder girdle. (a) Relationship of the right shoulder girdle to the bones of the thorax and arm. **(b)** Right clavicle, superior and inferior views. **(c)** Right scapula, posterior view. **(d)** Right scapula, anterior view.

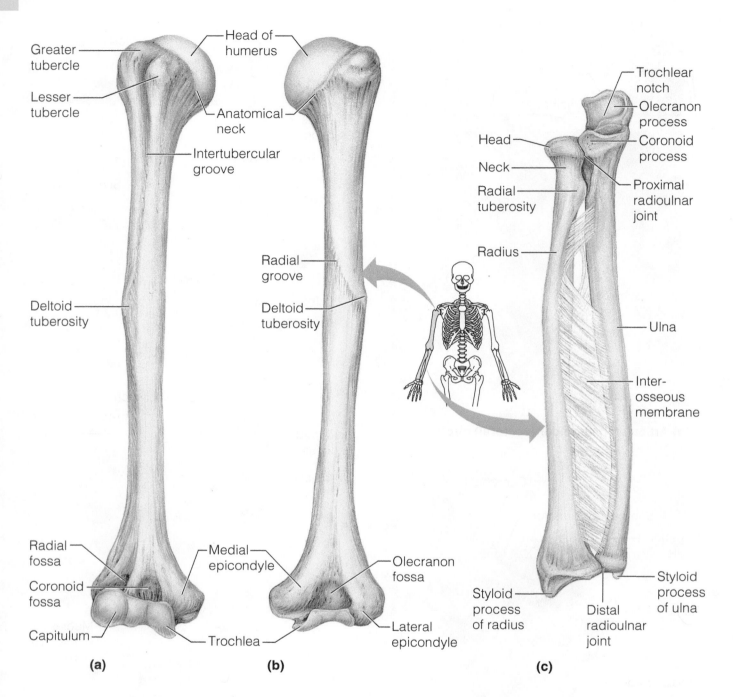

FIGURE 5.23 **Bones of the right arm and forearm. (a)** Humerus, anterior view. **(b)** Humerus, posterior view. **(c)** Anterior view of the bones of the forearm: the radius and the ulna.

body is in the anatomical position, the **radius** is the lateral bone; that is, it is on the thumb side of the forearm. When the hand is rotated so that the palm faces backward, the distal end of the radius crosses over and ends up medial to the ulna. Both proximally and distally the radius and ulna articulate at

small **radioulnar joints,** and the two bones are connected along their entire length by the flexible **interosseous membrane.** Both the ulna and the radius have a **styloid process** at their distal end.

The disc-shaped head of the radius also forms a joint with the capitulum of the humerus. Just below the head is the **radial tuberosity,** where the tendon of the biceps muscle attaches.

When the upper limb is in the anatomical position, the **ulna** is the medial bone (on the little-finger side) of the forearm. On its proximal end are the anterior **coronoid process** and the posterior **olecranon process,** which are separated by the **trochlear notch.** Together these two processes grip the trochlea of the humerus in a pliers-like joint.

Hand

The skeleton of the hand consists of the carpals, the metacarpals, and the phalanges (Figure 5.24). The eight **carpal bones,** arranged in two irregular rows of four bones each, form the part of the hand called the **carpus** or, more commonly, the *wrist.* The carpals are bound together by ligaments that restrict movements between them. (In case you need to learn their names, the individual carpal bones are identified in Figure 5.24.)

The palm of the hand consists of the **metacarpals.** The **phalanges** (fah-lan′jēz) are the

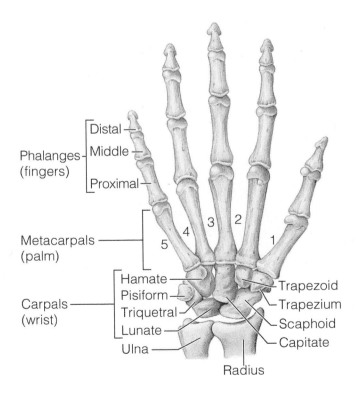

FIGURE 5.24   Bones of the right hand, anterior view.

Labels on figure:
Phalanges (fingers) — Distal, Middle, Proximal
Metacarpals (palm)
Carpals (wrist)
Hamate
Pisiform
Triquetral
Lunate
Ulna
Trapezoid
Trapezium
Scaphoid
Capitate
Radius
5 4 3 2 1

bones of the fingers. The metacarpals are numbered 1 to 5 from the thumb side of the hand toward the little finger. When the fist is clenched, the heads of the metacarpals become obvious as the "knuckles." Each hand contains 14 phalanges. There are three in each finger (proximal, middle, and distal), except in the thumb, which has only two (proximal and distal).

Bones of the Pelvic Girdle

The **pelvic girdle** is formed by two **coxal** (kok′sal) **bones,** or **ossa coxae,** commonly called **hip bones.** Together with the sacrum and the coccyx, the hip bones form the *bony pelvis* (Figure 5.25). Note that the terms *pelvic girdle* and *pelvis* have slightly different meanings.

The bones of the pelvic girdle are large and heavy, and they are attached securely to the axial skeleton. The sockets, which receive the thigh bones, are deep and heavily reinforced by ligaments that attach the limbs firmly to the girdle. Bearing weight is the most important function of this girdle; the total weight of the upper body rests on the pelvis. The reproductive organs, urinary bladder, and part of the large intestine lie within and are protected by the bony pelvis.

Each hip bone is formed by the fusion of three bones: the *ilium, ischium,* and *pubis.* The **ilium** (il′e-um), which connects posteriorly with the sacrum at the **sacroiliac** (sak″ro-il′e-ac) **joint,** is a large, flaring bone that forms most of the hip bone. When you put your hands on your hips, they are resting over the *alae* or winglike portions of the ilia. The upper edge of the alae, the **iliac crest,** is an important anatomical landmark that is always kept in mind by those who give injections. The iliac crest ends anteriorly in the **anterior superior iliac spine** and posteriorly in the **posterior superior iliac spine.** Small inferior spines are located below these.

The **ischium** (is′ke-um) is the "sit-down bone," since it forms the most inferior part of the coxal bone. The **ischial tuberosity** is a roughened area that receives body weight when you are sitting. The **ischial spine,** superior to the tuberosity, is another important anatomical landmark, particularly in the pregnant woman, because it narrows the outlet of the pelvis through which the baby must pass during the birth process. Another

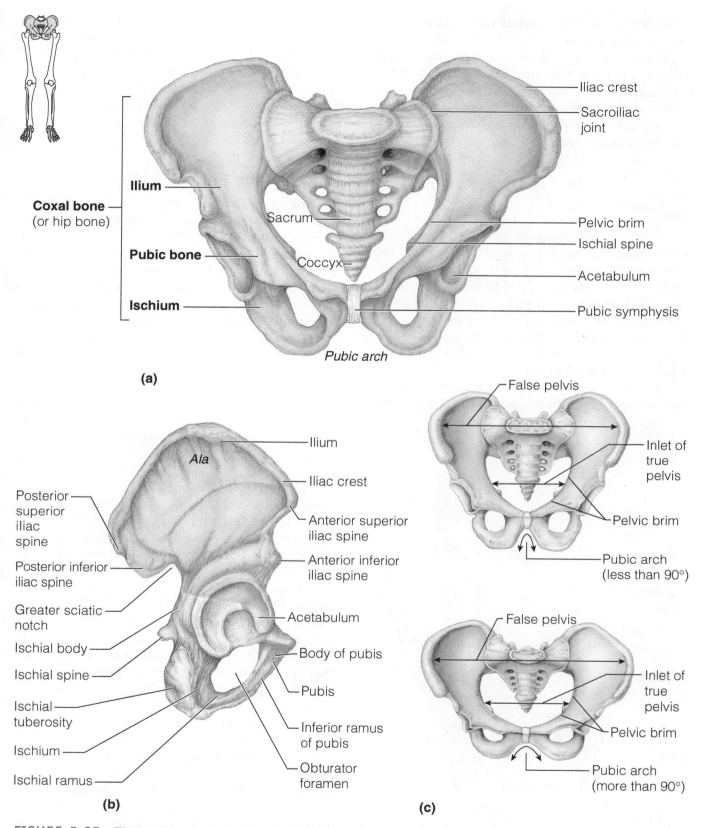

Coxal bone — Ilium
(or hip bone)

Ilium

Sacrum

Pubic bone

Coccyx

Ischium

Pubic arch

Iliac crest

Sacroiliac joint

Pelvic brim

Ischial spine

Acetabulum

Pubic symphysis

(a)

Ala

Posterior superior iliac spine

Posterior inferior iliac spine

Greater sciatic notch

Ischial body

Ischial spine

Ischial tuberosity

Ischium

Ischial ramus

Ilium

Iliac crest

Anterior superior iliac spine

Anterior inferior iliac spine

Acetabulum

Body of pubis

Pubis

Inferior ramus of pubis

Obturator foramen

(b)

False pelvis

Inlet of true pelvis

Pelvic brim

Pubic arch (less than 90°)

False pelvis

Inlet of true pelvis

Pelvic brim

Pubic arch (more than 90°)

(c)

FIGURE 5.25   The pelvis. (a) Articulated male pelvis. **(b)** Right coxal bone, showing the point of fusion of the ilium, ischium, and pubic bones. **(c)** Comparison of the male (above) and female (below) pelves.

important structural feature of the ischium is the **greater sciatic notch,** which allows blood vessels and the large sciatic nerve to pass from the pelvis posteriorly into the thigh. Injections in the buttock should always be given well away from this area.

The **pubis** (pu′bis), or **pubic bone,** is the most anterior part of a coxal bone. Fusion of the *rami* of the pubis anteriorly and the ischium posteriorly forms a bar of bone enclosing the **obturator** (ob′tu-ra″tor) **foramen,** an opening that allows blood vessels and nerves to pass into the anterior part of the thigh. The pubic bones of each hip bone fuse anteriorly to form a cartilaginous joint, the **pubic symphysis** (pu′bik sim′fĭ-sis).

The ilium, ischium, and pubis fuse at the deep socket called the **acetabulum** (as″ĕ-tab′u-lum), which means "vinegar cup." The acetabulum receives the head of the thigh bone.

The bony pelvis is divided into two regions. The **false pelvis** is superior to the true pelvis; it is the area medial to the flaring portions of the ilia. The **true pelvis** is surrounded by bone and lies inferior to the flaring parts of the ilia and the pelvic brim. The dimensions of the true pelvis of a woman are very important because they must be large enough to allow the infant's head (the largest part of the infant) to pass during childbirth. The dimensions of the cavity, particularly the **outlet** (the inferior opening of the pelvis), and the **inlet** (superior opening) are critical, and thus they are carefully measured by the obstetrician.

Of course, individual pelvic structures vary, but there are fairly consistent differences between a male and a female pelvis. Look at Figure 5.25c and notice the following characteristics that differ in the pelvis of the male and female.

- The female inlet is larger and more circular.
- The female pelvis as a whole is shallower, and the bones are lighter and thinner.
- The female ilia flare more laterally.
- The female sacrum is shorter and less curved.
- The female ischial spines are shorter and farther apart; thus the outlet is larger.
- The female pubic arch is more rounded because the angle of the pubic arch is greater.

Bones of the Lower Limbs

The lower limbs carry our total body weight when we are erect. Hence, it is not surprising that the bones forming the three segments of the lower limbs (thigh, leg, and foot) are much thicker and stronger than the comparable bones of the upper limb.

Thigh

The **femur** (fe′mur), or *thigh bone,* is the only bone in the thigh (Figure 5.26a and b). It is the heaviest, strongest bone in the body. Its proximal end has a ball-like head, a neck, and **greater** and **lesser trochanters** (separated anteriorly by the **intertrochanteric line** and posteriorly by the **intertrochanteric crest**). The trochanters, intertrochanteric crest, and the **gluteal tuberosity,** located on the shaft, all serve as sites for muscle attachment. The head of the femur articulates with the acetabulum of the hip bone in a deep, secure socket. However, the neck of the femur is a common fracture site, especially in old age.

The femur slants medially as it runs downward to join with the leg bones; this brings the knees in line with the body's center of gravity. The medial course of the femur is more noticeable in females because of the wider female pelvis. Distally on the femur are the **lateral** and **medial condyles,** which articulate with the tibia below. Posteriorly these condyles are separated by the deep **intercondylar fossa.** Anteriorly on the distal femur is the smooth **patellar surface,** which forms a joint with the patella, or kneecap.

Leg

Connected along their length by an **interosseous membrane,** two bones, the tibia and fibula, form the skeleton of the leg (see Figure 5.26c). The **tibia,** or *shinbone,* is larger and more medial. At the proximal end, the **medial** and **lateral condyles** (separated by the **intercondylar eminence**) articulate with the distal end of the femur to form the knee joint. The patellar (kneecap) ligament attaches to the **tibial tuberosity,** a roughened area on the anterior tibial surface. Distally, a process called the **medial malleolus** (mal-le′o-lus) forms the inner bulge of the ankle. The anterior surface of the tibia is a sharp ridge, the **anterior border,** that is unprotected by muscles; thus, it is easily felt beneath the skin.

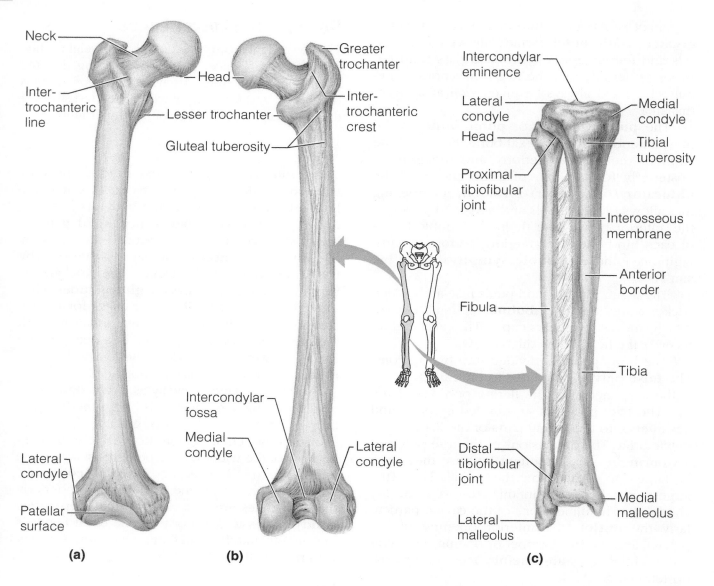

FIGURE 5.26 Bones of the right thigh and leg. (a) Femur (thigh bone), anterior view. **(b)** Femur, posterior view. **(c)** Tibia and fibula of the leg, anterior view.

The **fibula,** which lies alongside the tibia and forms joints with it both proximally and distally, is thin and sticklike. The fibula has no part in forming the knee joint. Its distal end, the **lateral malleolus,** forms the outer part of the ankle.

Foot

The foot, composed of the tarsals, metatarsals, and phalanges, has two important functions. It supports our body weight and serves as a lever that allows us to propel our bodies forward when we walk and run.

The **tarsus,** forming the posterior half of the foot, is composed of seven **tarsal bones** (Figure 5.27). Body weight is mostly carried by the two largest tarsals, the **calcaneus** (kal-ka′ne-us), or heelbone, and the **talus** (ta′lus; "ankle"), which lies between the tibia and the calcaneus. Five **metatarsals** form the sole, and 14 **phalanges** form the toes. Like the fingers of the hand, each toe has three phalanges, except the great toe, which has two.

The bones in the foot are arranged to form three strong arches: two longitudinal (medial and lateral) and one transverse (Figure 5.28). *Ligaments,* which bind the foot bones together, and *tendons* of the foot muscles help to hold the bones firmly in the arched position but still allow a certain amount of give or springiness. Weak arches are referred to as "fallen arches" or "flat feet."

Joints

With one exception (the hyoid bone of the neck), every bone in the body forms a joint with at least one other bone. **Joints,** also called **articulations,** have two functions: they hold the bones together securely but also give the rigid skeleton mobility.

The graceful movements of a ballet dancer and the rough-and-tumble grapplings of a football player illustrate the great variety of motion allowed by joints, the sites where two or more bones meet.

With fewer joints, we would move like robots. Nevertheless, the bone-binding function of joints is just as important as their role in providing mobility. The immovable joints of the skull, for instance, form a snug enclosure for our vital brain.

Joints are classified in two ways—functionally and structurally. The functional classification focuses on the amount of movement allowed by the joint. On this basis, there are **synar-throses** (sin″ar thro′sēz) or immovable joints **amphi-arthroses** (am″fe ar thro′sēz) or slightly movable joints, and **diarthroses** (di″ar thro′sēz) or freely movable joints. Freely movable joints predominate in the limbs, where mobility is important. Immovable and slightly movable joints are restricted mainly to the axial skeleton, where firm attachments and protection of internal organs are priorities.

Structurally, there are *fibrous, cartilaginous,* and *synovial joints* based on whether fibrous tissue, cartilage, or a joint cavity separates the bony regions at the joint. As a general rule, fibrous joints are immovable and synovial joints are freely movable. Although cartilaginous joints have both immovable and slightly movable examples, most are amphiarthrotic. Since the structural classification is more clear-cut, we will focus on that classification scheme here. Table 5.3 shows the functional categories of joints. Table 5.4 shows the structural categories of joints.

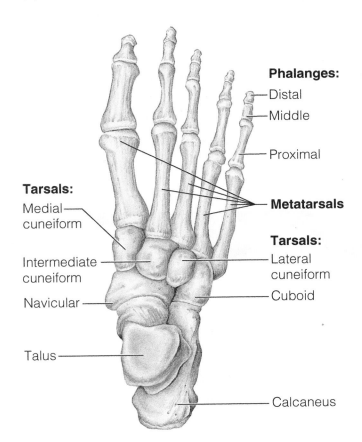

Phalanges:
— Distal
— Middle
— Proximal

Metatarsals

Tarsals:
Medial cuneiform
Intermediate cuneiform
Navicular
Talus

Tarsals:
Lateral cuneiform
Cuboid
Calcaneus

FIGURE 5.27   Bones of the right foot, superior view.

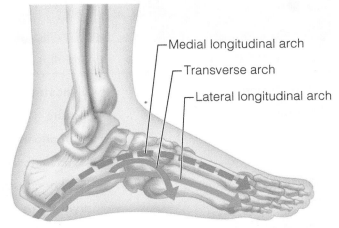

— Medial longitudinal arch
— Transverse arch
— Lateral longitudinal arch

FIGURE 5.28   Arches of the foot.

TABLE 5.3   A Functional Classification of Articulations

Functional Category	Structural Category and Type	Description	Example(s)
Synarthrosis (no movement)	*Fibrous* **Suture**	Fibrous connections plus interlocking projections	Between the bones of the skull
	Gomphosis	Fibrous connections plus insertion in alveolar process	Between the teeth and jaws
	Cartilaginous **Synchondrosis**	Interposition of cartilage plate	Epiphyseal cartilages
	Bony fusion **Synostosis**	Conversion of other articular form to a solid mass of bone	Portions of the skull, epiphyseal lines
Amphiarthrosis (little movement)	*Fibrous* **Syndesmosis**	Ligamentous connection	Between the tibia and fibula
	Cartilaginous **Symphysis**	Connection by a fibrocartilage pad	Between right and left pubic bones of pelvis; between adjacent vertebral bodies along vertebral column
Diarthrosis (free movement)	**Synovial**	Complex joint bounded by joint capsule and containing synovial fluid	Numerous; subdivided by range of movement
	Monaxial	Permits movement in one plane	Elbow, ankle
	Biaxial	Permits movement in two planes	Ribs, wrist
	Triaxial	Permits movement in all three planes	Shoulder, hip

TABLE 5.4   A Structural Classification of Articulations

Structural Category	Structural Type	Functional Category
Bony fusion	**Synostosis**	Synarthrosis
Fibrous joint	**Suture**	Synarthrosis
	Gomphosis	Synarthrosis
	Syndesmosis	Amphiarthrosis
Cartilaginous joint	**Synchondrosis**	Synarthrosis
	Symphysis	Amphiarthrosis
Synovial joint	**Monaxial** **Biaxial** **Triaxial**	Diarthroses

A Closer Look

Them Bones, Them Bones Goin' to Walk Around—Clinical Advances in Bone Repair

ALTHOUGH bones have remarkable self-regenerative powers, some conditions are just too severe for bones to effect repair. Examples include extensive shattering (as in automobile accidents), poor circulation in old bones, and certain birth defects. Here we address healing problems that bones cannot handle themselves. Let's take a look at some techniques currently used to expedite bone repair.

Electrical stimulation of fracture sites dramatically increases the speed and completeness of healing in slowly healing fractures. For years it has been known that bone tissue is deposited in regions of negative electrical charge (its stressed regions) and absorbed in regions of positive charge, but we are still not sure how electricity promotes healing. One theory is that negative fields prevent parathyroid hormone from stimulating the bone-absorbing osteoclast cells at the fracture site. Another theory is that the fields induce production of growth chemicals that stimulate the osteoblasts.

Ultrasound, introduced as the basis of an imaging technique in Chapter 1, can speed the repair of fresh fractures. Daily exposure to pulsed low-power ultrasound waves reduces the healing time of broken arm and shin bones by 35 to 45 percent. It apparently stimulates cartilage cells to make a fibrocartilage callus.

The most troublesome injuries to bones are non-union fractures, in which the two parts of a split bone fail to join. Such fractures traditionally have been treated with grafts, in which sections of bone are taken from the hip and inserted into the gap. However, this requires several painful grafting sessions, and one-third of the grafts fail to heal. A potential improvement is the **free vascular fibular graft technique,** which uses pieces of the fibula to replace missing bone. One reason that traditional grafts often fail is that a blood supply cannot reach their interior. This new technique grafts normal blood vessels along with the bone sections, and subsequent remodeling leads to a good replica of the preinjury bone.

Although bone implants have proved effective in adults, they have been less satisfactory for children with growing bones. This problem has been partly resolved, at least for knee replacement candidates, with **self-extendible endoprostheses.** The telescopic sleeve of these devices (see the figure) undergoes continual automatic elongation of the limb enforced by knee bending. Over-lengthening of the prosthesis is prevented by tension in the surrounding tissue which increases after each elongation and then gradually decreases as the soft tissues grow.

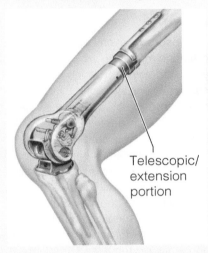

Telescopic/
extension
portion

The self-extending leg implant. Lengthening occurs at the telescopic/extension portion.

Much research has gone into developing **bone substitutes** (crushed cadaver bone or synthetic materials) to fill the gaps in non-union defects. Crushed bone from human cadavers is mixed with water to form a paste that can be molded into the desired shape or packed into small, difficult-to-reach spaces. However, cadaver bone is a foreign tissue that the immune system may reject, and the body sometimes fails to replace it with new bone, as it must for healing to occur. Furthermore, there is a slight but real risk that the cadaver bone contains disease organisms.

Presently several types of artificial bone materials, which can serve as a scaffolding on which new bone can grow, are available. ProOsteon, made from coral, avoids the rejection problems seen with cadaveric bone. The coral is heat-treated to kill its living cells and convert its calcium carbonate to hydroxyapatite, the mineral in bone. The coral graft is then carved to the desired shape, coated with a natural substance that induces bone formation (bone morphogenic protein), and implanted. Osteoblasts and blood vessels migrate from the adjacent natural bone into the coral implant, gradually replacing it with living bone. Research has also produced several types of ceramic bone substitutes. One is TCP, a biodegradable ceramic

substance soft enough to be shaped but, like the "coral bone," not very strong. TCP's biggest application has been to replace parts of non-weight-bearing bones, such as skull bones.

Norian SRS, a bone cement made of calcium phosphate, provides immediate structural support to fractured or osteoporotic sites. Mixed at the time of surgery, Norian SRS paste is injected into areas of damaged bone to create an internal "cast." The paste hardens in minutes and cures into a substance with greater compressive strength than spongy bone. Because its crystalline structure is the same as that of natural bone, it continues to provide support as it is gradually remodeled and replaced by host

bone. However, Norian SRS can be used only on bone ends because it cannot resist the strong compressive and bending stresses occurring at the central shaft.

Perhaps the most promising product being tested is Osteo-Medica's bioceramic called Megagraft 1000. Made from mildly heated, chemically synthesized hydroxyapatite, bioceramic is stronger than the bone substitutes just described above. Better still, it can be molded and carved into long pieces that are placed in gaps in the shafts of long bones. It essentially works as an artificial bone graft. Thus far in animal tests, it has been shown to bear weight well after several months of initial healing and natural remodeling.

Fibrous Joints

In **fibrous joints,** the bones are united by fibrous tissue. The best examples of this type of joint are the *sutures* of the skull (Figure 5.29a). In sutures, the irregular edges of the bones interlock and are bound tightly together by connective tissue fibers, allowing essentially no movement to occur. In **syndesmoses** (sin-dez-mo'sēz), the connecting fibers are longer than those of sutures; thus the joint has more "give."

The joint connecting the distal ends of the tibia and fibula is a syndesmosis (Figure 5.29b).

Cartilaginous Joints

In **cartilaginous joints,** the bone ends are connected by cartilage. Examples of this joint type that are slightly movable (amphiarthrotic) are the *pubic symphysis* of the pelvis (Figure 5.29e) and *intervertebral joints* of the spinal column

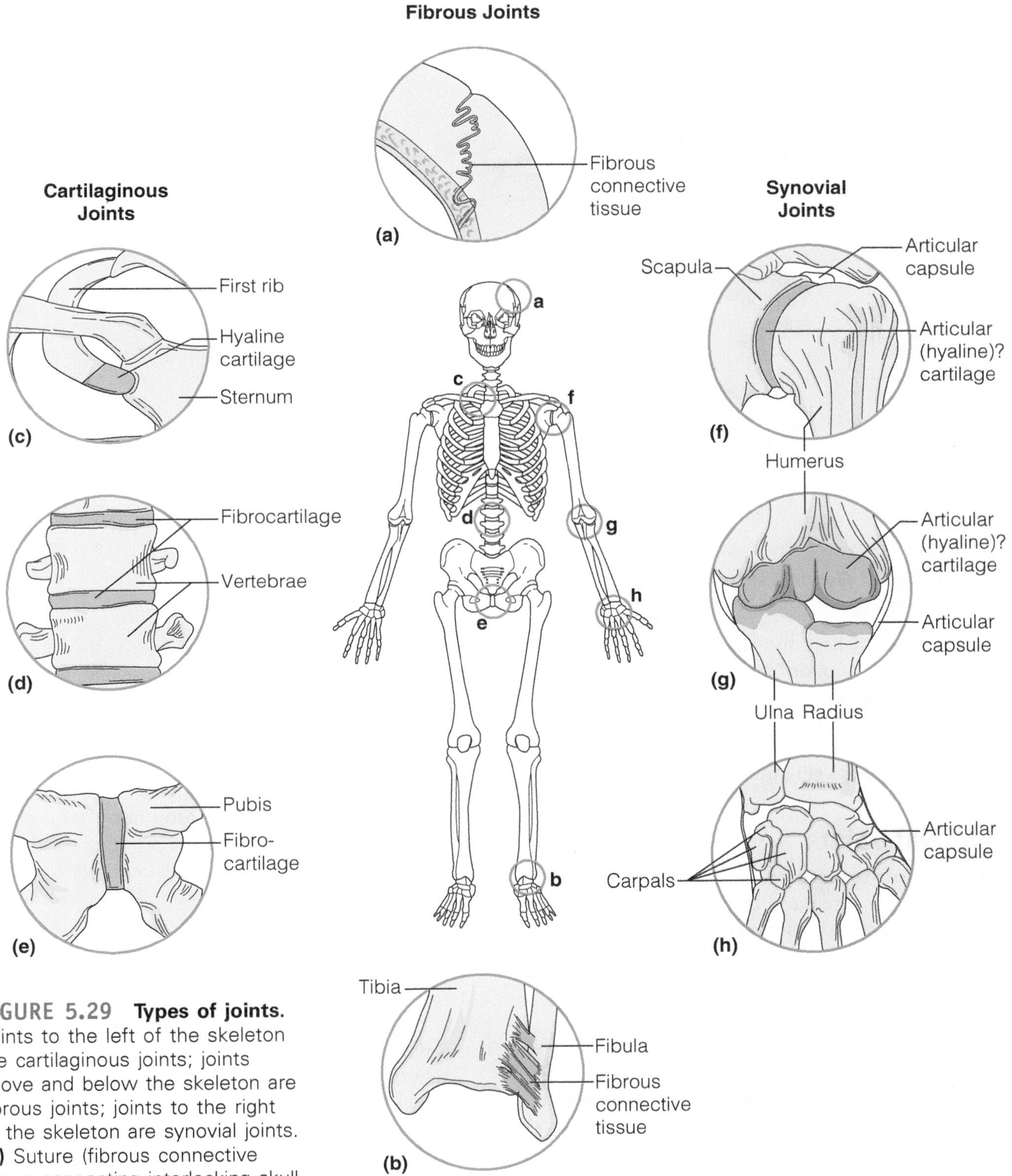

Fibrous Joints

Cartilaginous Joints

Synovial Joints

FIGURE 5.29 Types of joints. Joints to the left of the skeleton are cartilaginous joints; joints above and below the skeleton are fibrous joints; joints to the right of the skeleton are synovial joints. **(a)** Suture (fibrous connective tissue connecting interlocking skull bones). **(b)** Syndesmosis (fibrous connective tissue connecting the distal ends of the tibia and fibula). **(c)** Synchondrosis (joint between costal cartilage of rib 1 and the sternum). **(d)** Symphyses (intervertebral discs of fibrocartilage connecting adjacent vertebrae). **(e)** Symphysis (fibrocartilaginous pubic symphysis connecting the pubic bones anteriorly). **(f)** Synovial joint (multiaxial shoulder joint). **(g)** Synovial joint (uniaxial elbow joint). **(h)** Synovial joints (biaxial intercarpal joints of the hand).

Q   *How does this joint type differ structurally from cartilaginous and fibrous joints?*

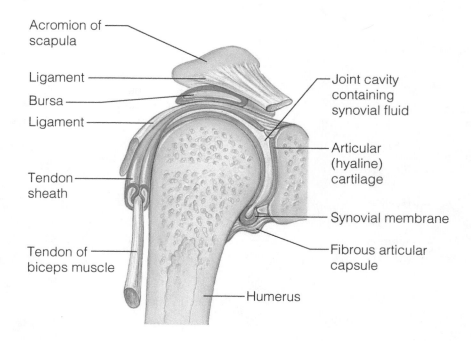

Acromion of scapula

Ligament

Bursa

Ligament

Tendon sheath

Tendon of biceps muscle

Joint cavity containing synovial fluid

Articular (hyaline) cartilage

Synovial membrane

Fibrous articular capsule

Humerus

FIGURE 5.30   General structure of a synovial joint.

(Figure 5.29d), where the articulating bone surfaces are connected by pads (discs) of fibrocartilage. The hyaline-cartilage epiphyseal plates of growing long bones and the cartilaginous joints between the first ribs and the sternum are immovable (synarthrotic) cartilaginous joints (Figure 5.29c).

Synovial Joints

Synovial joints are those in which the articulating bone ends are separated by a joint cavity containing synovial fluid (see Figure 5.29f–h). They account for all joints of the limbs.

All synovial joints have four distinguishing features (Figure 5.30):

- **Articular cartilage.** Articular (hyaline) cartilage covers the ends of the bones forming the joint.
- **Fibrous articular capsule.** The joint surfaces are enclosed by a sleeve or capsule of fibrous connective tissue, and the capsule is lined with a smooth *synovial membrane* (the reason these joints are called synovial joints).

- **Joint cavity.** The articular capsule encloses a cavity, called the joint cavity, which contains lubricating synovial fluid.
- **Reinforcing ligaments.** The fibrous capsule is usually reinforced with ligaments.

Bursae and tendon sheaths are not strictly part of synovial joints, but they are often found closely associated with them (Figure 5.30). Essentially bags of lubricant, they act like ball bearings to reduce friction between adjacent structures during joint activity. **Bursae** (ber'se; "purse") are flattened fibrous sacs lined with synovial membrane and containing a thin film of synovial fluid. They are common where ligaments, muscles, skin, tendons, or bones rub together. A **tendon sheath,** also shown in Figure 5.30, is essentially an elongated bursa that wraps completely around a tendon subjected to friction, like a bun around a hot dog.

Homeostatic Imbalance

A *dislocation* happens when a bone is forced out of its normal position in the joint cavity. The process of returning the bone to its proper position, called *reduction,* should be done only by a physician. Attempts by an untrained person to "snap the bone back into its socket" are usually more harmful than helpful. ▲

A   *It has a joint cavity instead of cartilage or fibrous tissue separating the articulating bones.*

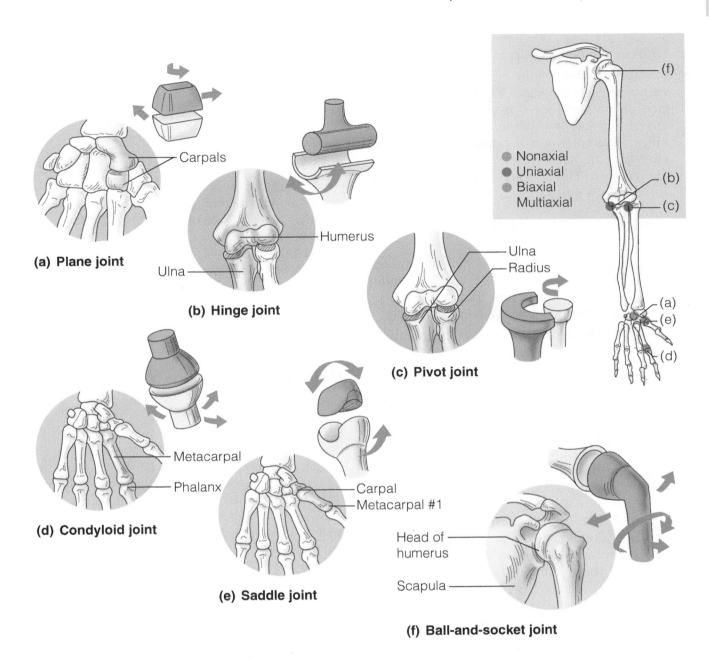

FIGURE 5.31 Types of synovial joints. (a) Plane joint (intercarpal and intertarsal joints). **(b)** Hinge joint (elbow and interphalangeal joints). **(c)** Pivot joint (proximal joint between the radius and the ulna). **(d)** Condyloid joint (knuckles). **(e)** Saddle joint (carpometacarpal joint of the thumb). **(f)** Ball-and-socket joint (shoulder and hip joints).

Types of Synovial Joints Based on Shape

The shapes of the articulating bone surfaces determine what movements are allowed at a joint. Based on such shapes, our synovial joints can be classified as *gliding, plane, hinge, pivot,* *condyloid, saddle,* and *ball-and-socket joints* (Figure 5.31).

- In a **plane joint** (Figure 5.31a), the articular surfaces are essentially flat, and only short slipping or gliding movements are allowed. The movements of plane joints are *nonaxial;* that is, gliding does not involve rotation around any axis. The intercarpal joints of the wrist are the best examples of plane joints.

- In a **hinge joint** (Figure 5.31b), the cylindrical end of one bone fits into a trough-shaped surface on another bone. Angular movement is allowed in just one plane, like a mechanical hinge. Examples are the elbow joint, ankle joint, and the joints between the phalanges of the fingers. Hinge joints are classified as *uniaxial* (u″ne-aks′e-al; "one axis"); they allow movement around one axis only, as indicated by the single magenta arrow in Figure 5.31b.

- **Gliding joints** (planar) have flattened faces. These relatively flat articular surfaces slide across one another with limited movement due to ligaments restricting movement.

- In a **pivot joint** (Figure 5.31c), the rounded end of one bone fits into a sleeve or ring of bone (and possibly ligaments). Because the rotating bone can turn only around its long axis, pivot joints are also uniaxial joints (see the single arrow in Figure 5.31c). The proximal radioulnar joint and the joint between the atlas and the dens of the axis are examples.

- In a **condyloid joint** (kon′dĭ-loid; "knuckle-like"), the egg-shaped articular surface of one bone fits into an oval concavity in another (Figure 5.31d). Both of these articular surfaces are oval. Condyloid joints allow the moving bone to travel (1) from side to side and (2) back and forth, but the bone cannot rotate around its long axis. Movement occurs around two axes, hence these joints are *biaxial* (*bi* = two), as in knuckle (metacarpophalangeal) joints.

- In **saddle joints,** each articular surface has both convex and concave areas, like a saddle (Figure 5.31e). These biaxial joints allow essentially the same movements as condyloid joints. The best examples of saddle joints are the carpometacarpal joints in the thumb, and the movements of these joints are clearly demonstrated by twiddling your thumbs.

- In a **ball-and-socket joint** (Figure 5.31f), the spherical head of one bone fits into a round socket in another. These *multiaxial* joints allow movement in all axes, including rotation (see the three arrows in Figure 5.31f), and are

the most freely moving synovial joints. The shoulder and hip are examples.

The various types of movements that occur at synovial joints are discussed in detail in the next section.

Function of Synovial Joints

To understand human movement, you must be aware of the relationship between structure and function at each articulation. To *describe* human movement, you need a frame of reference that enables accurate and precise communication. We can classify the synovial joints according to their anatomical and functional properties. To demonstrate the basis for that classification, we will use a simple model to describe the movements that occur at a typical synovial joint.

Describing Dynamic Motion

Take a pencil (or a pen) as your model, and stand it upright on the surface of a desk or table (Figure 5.32a). The pencil represents a bone, and the desktop represents an articular surface. A little imagination and a lot of twisting, pushing, and pulling will demonstrate that there are only three ways to move the model. Considering them one at a time will provide a frame of reference for us to analyze complex movements:

Possible Movement 1: The pencil point can move. If you hold the pencil upright, without securing the point, you can push the pencil point across the surface. This kind of motion, *gliding* (Figure 5.32b), is an example of **linear motion.** You could slide the point forward or backward, from side to side, or diagonally. However you move the pencil, the motion can be described by using two lines of reference (axes). One line represents forward–backward motion, the other left–right movement. For example, a simple movement along one axis could be described as "forward 1 cm" or "left 2 cm." A diagonal movement could be described with both axes, as in "backward 1 cm and to the right 2.5 cm."

Possible Movement 2: The pencil shaft can change its angle with the surface. With the tip held in position, you can move the free (eraser) end of the

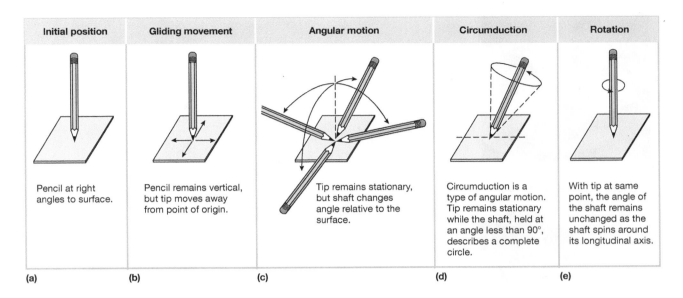

Initial position	Gliding movement	Angular motion	Circumduction	Rotation
Pencil at right angles to surface.	Pencil remains vertical, but tip moves away from point of origin.	Tip remains stationary, but shaft changes angle relative to the surface.	Circumduction is a type of angular motion. Tip remains stationary while the shaft, held at an angle less than 90°, describes a complete circle.	With tip at same point, the angle of the shaft remains unchanged as the shaft spins around its longitudinal axis.
(a)	(b)	(c)	(d)	(e)

FIGURE 5.32   A simple model of articular motion.

pencil forward and backward, from side to side, or at some intermediate angle. These movements, which change the angle between the shaft and the desktop, are examples of **angular motion** (Figure 5.32c). We can describe such motion by the angle the pencil shaft makes with the surface.

Any angular movement can be described with reference to the same two axes (forward–backward, left–right) and the angular change (in degrees). In one instance, however, a special term is used to describe a complex angular movement. Grasp the pencil eraser and move the pencil in any direction until it is no longer vertical. Now swing the eraser through a complete circle (Figure 5.32d). This movement, which corresponds to the path of your arm when you draw a large circle on a chalkboard, is very difficult to describe. Anatomists avoid the problem by using a special term, **circumduction** (sir-kum-DUK-shun; *circum,* around), for this type of angular motion.

Types of Movements at Synovial Joints

In descriptions of motion at synovial joints, phrases such as "bend the leg" or "raise the arm" are not sufficiently precise. Anatomists use descriptive terms that have specific meanings. We will consider these motions with reference to the basic categories of movement discussed previously: gliding, angular motion, and rotation.

Linear Motion (Gliding)

In **gliding,** two opposing surfaces slide past one another, as in possible movement 1. Gliding occurs between the surfaces of articulating carpal bones, between tarsal bones, and between the clavicles and the sternum. The movement can occur in almost any direction, but the amount of movement is slight, and rotation is generally prevented by the capsule and associated ligaments.

Angular Motion

Examples of angular motion include *flexion, extension, abduction, adduction,* and *circumduction* (Figure 5.33). Descriptions of these movements are based on reference to an individual in the anatomical position.

Flexion and Extension **Flexion** (FLEK-shun) is movement in the anterior–posterior plane that reduces the angle between the articulating elements. **Extension** occurs in the same plane, but it increases the angle between articulating elements (Figure 5.33a). These terms are usually applied to the movements of the long bones of the limbs, but they are also used to describe movements of the axial skeleton. For example, when you bring your head

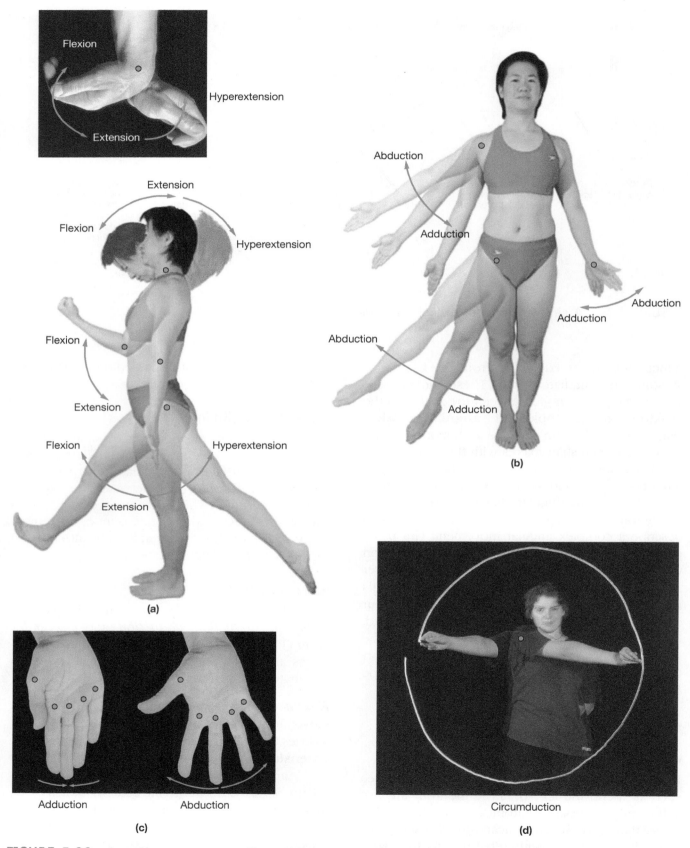

FIGURE 5.33 Angular movements. The red dots indicate the locations of the joints involved in the movements illustrated.

toward your chest, you flex the intervertebral joints of the neck. When you bend down to touch your toes, you flex the intervertebral joints of the spine. Extension reverses these movements, returning you to the anatomical position. When a person is in the anatomical position, all of the major joints of the axial and appendicular skeletons (except the ankle) are at full extension. (Special terms used to describe movements of the ankle joint are introduced shortly.)

Flexion of the shoulder joint or hip joint moves the limbs anteriorly, whereas extension moves them posteriorly. Flexion of the wrist joint moves the hand anteriorly, and extension moves it posteriorly. In each of these examples, extension can be continued past the anatomical position. Extension past the anatomical position is called **hyperextension** (see Figure 5.33b). When you hyperextend your neck, you can gaze at the ceiling. Hyperextension of many joints, such as the elbow or the knee, is prevented by ligaments, bony processes, or soft tissues.

Abduction and Adduction **Abduction** (*ab,* from) is movement *away from the longitudinal axis of the body* in the frontal plane (Figure 5.33b). For example, swinging the upper limb to the side is abduction of the limb. Moving it back to the anatomical position constitutes **adduction** (*ad,* to). Adduction of the wrist moves the heel of the hand and fingers *toward* the body, whereas abduction moves them farther away. Spreading the fingers or toes apart abducts them, because they move *away from* a central digit (Figure 5.33c). Bringing them together constitutes adduction. (Fingers move toward or away from the middle finger; toes move toward or away from the second toe.) Abduction and adduction always refer to movements of the appendicular skeleton, not to those of the axial skeleton.

Circumduction We introduced a special type of angular motion, circumduction, in our model. Moving your arm in a loop is circumduction (Figure 5.33d), as when you draw a large circle on a chalkboard. Your hand moves in a circle, but your arm does not rotate.

Rotation

Rotational movements are also described with reference to a figure in the anatomical position. Rotation of the head may involve **left rotation** or **right rotation** (Figure 5.34a). Limb rotation may be described by reference to the longitudinal axis

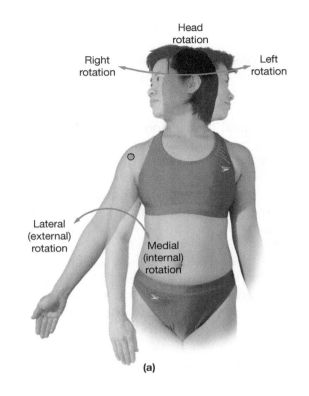

(a)

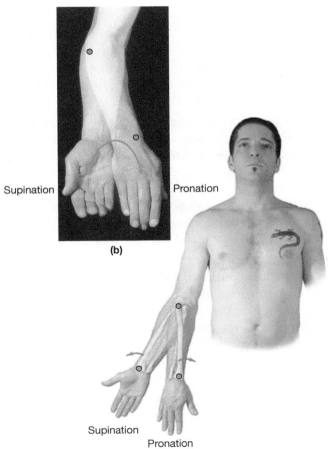

(b)

FIGURE 5.34 **Rotational movements.**

of the trunk. During **medial rotation,** also known as *internal rotation* or *inward rotation,* the anterior surface of a limb turns toward the long axis of the trunk (see Figure 5.34a). The reverse movement is called **lateral rotation,** *external rotation,* or *outward rotation.*

The proximal articulation between the radius and the ulna permits rotation of the radial head. As the shaft of the radius rotates, the distal epiphysis of the radius rolls across the anterior surface of the ulna. This movement, called **pronation** (prō-NĀ-shun), turns the wrist and hand from palm facing front to palm facing back (Figure 5.34b). The opposing movement, in which the palm is turned anteriorly, is **supination** (soo-pi-NĀ-shun). The forearm is supinated in the anatomical position. This view makes it easier to follow the path of the blood vessels, nerves, and tendons, which rotate with the radius during pronation.

Special Movements

Several special terms apply to specific articulations or unusual types of movement (Figure 5.35):

- **Inversion** (*in,* into + *vertere,* to turn) is a twisting motion of the foot that turns the sole inward, elevating the medial edge of the sole. The opposite movement is called **eversion** (ē-VER-zhun; *e,* out).

- **Dorsiflexion** is flexion at the ankle joint and elevation of the sole, as when you dig in your heel. **Plantar flexion** (*planta,* sole), the opposite movement, extends the ankle joint and elevates the heel, as when you stand on tiptoe. However, it is also acceptable (and simpler) to use "flexion and extension at the ankle," rather than "dorsiflexion and plantar flexion."

- **Opposition** is movement of the thumb toward the surface of the palm or the pads of other fingers. Opposition enables you to grasp and hold objects between your thumb and palm. It involves movement at the first carpometacarpal and metacarpophalangeal joints. Flexion at the fifth metacarpophalangeal joint can assist this movement.

- **Protraction** entails moving a part of the body anteriorly in the horizontal plane. **Retraction** is the reverse movement. You protract your jaw when you grasp your upper lip with your lower teeth, and you protract your clavicles when you cross your arms.

- **Elevation** and **depression** occur when a structure moves in a superior or an inferior direction, respectively. You depress your mandible when you open your mouth; you elevate your mandible as you close your mouth. Another familiar elevation occurs when you shrug your shoulders.

- **Lateral flexion** occurs when your vertebral column bends to the side. This movement is most pronounced in the cervical and thoracic regions.

Homeostatic Imbalance of Joints

Few of us pay attention to our joints unless something goes wrong with them. Joint pain and inflammation may be caused by many things. For example, falling on one's knee can cause a painful *bursitis,* called "water on the knee," due to inflammation of bursae or synovial membrane. Sprains and dislocations are other types of joint problems that result in swelling and pain. In a *sprain,* the ligaments or tendons reinforcing a joint are damaged by excessive stretching, or they are torn away from the bone. Since both tendons and ligaments are cords of dense fibrous connective tissue with a poor blood supply, sprains heal slowly and are extremely painful.

Few inflammatory joint disorders cause more pain and suffering than arthritis. The term **arthritis** (*arth* = joint; *itis* = inflammation) describes over 100 different inflammatory or degenerative diseases that damage the joints. In all its forms, arthritis is the most widespread, crippling disease in the United States. One out of seven Americans suffers its ravages. All forms of arthritis have the same initial symptoms: pain, stiffness, and swelling of the joint. Then, depending on the specific form, certain changes in the joint structure occur.

Acute forms of arthritis usually result from bacterial invasion and are treated with antibiotic drugs. The synovial membrane thickens and fluid production decreases, leading to increased friction and pain. Chronic forms of arthritis include osteoarthritis, rheumatoid arthritis, and gouty arthritis, which differ substantially in their later symptoms and consequences. We will focus on these forms here.

Osteoarthritis (OA), the most common form of arthritis, is a chronic degenerative condition that typically affects the aged. OA, also called "wear-and-tear arthritis," affects the articular cartilages. Over the years, there is a softening, fraying, and eventual breakdown of the cartilage. As the disease progresses, the exposed bone thickens and extra bone tissue, called

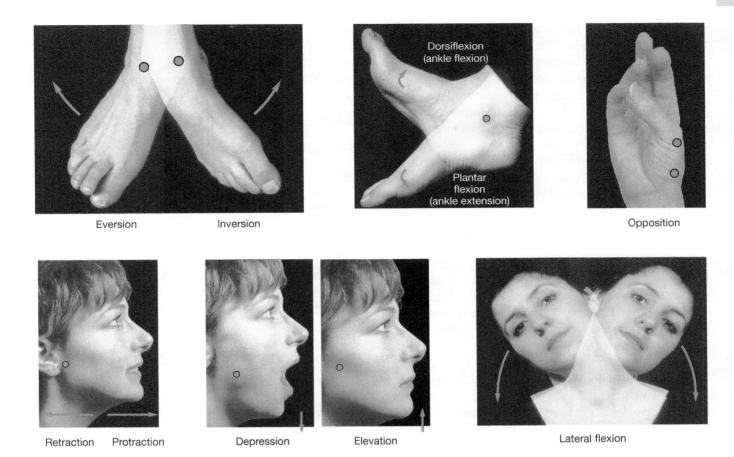

Eversion   Inversion

Dorsiflexion (ankle flexion)

Plantar flexion (ankle extension)

Opposition

Retraction   Protraction

Depression   Elevation

Lateral flexion

FIGURE 5.35   **Special movements.**

bone spurs, grows around the margins of the eroded cartilage and restricts joint movement. Patients complain of stiffness on arising that lessens with activity, and the affected joints may make a crunching noise (*crepitus*) when moved. The joints most commonly affected are those of the fingers, the cervical and lumbar joints of the spine, and the large, weight-bearing joints of the lower limbs (knees and hips).

The course of osteoarthritis is usually slow and irreversible, but it is rarely crippling. In most cases, its symptoms are controllable with a mild analgesic such as aspirin, moderate activity to maintain joint mobility, and rest when the joint becomes very painful. Some people with OA claim that rubbing capsaicin (a hot pepper extract) on the skin over painful joints provides relief. Others swear to the pain-reducing ability of glucosamine sulfate, a nutritional supplement.

Rheumatoid (roo'mah-toid) **arthritis (RA)** is a chronic inflammatory disorder. Its onset is insidious and usually occurs between the ages of 40 and 50, but it may occur at any age. It affects three times as many women as men. Many joints, particularly those of the fingers, wrists, ankles, and feet, are affected at the same time and usually in a symmetrical manner. For example, if the right elbow is affected, most likely the left elbow will be affected also. The course of RA varies and is marked by remissions and flare-ups (*rheumat* = susceptible to change or flux).

RA is an autoimmune disease—a disorder in which the body's immune system attempts to destroy its own tissues. The initial trigger for this reaction is unknown, but some suspect that it results from certain bacterial or viral infections.

RA begins with inflammation of the synovial membranes. The membranes thicken and the joints swell as synovial fluid accumulates. Inflammatory cells (white blood cells and others) enter the joint cavity from the blood and release a deluge of inflammatory chemicals that destroy body tissues when released inappropriately as in RA. In time the inflamed synovial membrane. Patients are advised to lose weight if obese, to avoid foods such as liver, kidneys, and sardines, which are high in nucleic acids, and to avoid alcohol, which inhibits excretion of uric acid by the kidneys thickens into a *pannus* ("rag"), an abnormal tissue that clings to and erodes articular cartilages. As the cartilage is destroyed, scar tissue forms and connects the bone ends. The scar tissue eventually ossifies, and the bone ends become firmly fused (*ankylosis*) and often deformed (see Figure 5.36). Not all cases of RA progress to the severely crippling ankylosis stage, but all cases involve restricted joint movement and extreme pain.

Current therapy for RA involves many different kinds of drugs. Some, like methotrexate and cyclosporin, are powerful drugs that can neutralize the inflammatory chemicals in the joint space and (hopefully) prevent joint deformity. However, drug therapy is usually begun with aspirin, which in large doses is an effective anti-inflammatory agent. Exercise is recommended to maintain as much joint mobility as possible. Cold packs are used to relieve the swelling and pain, and heat helps to relieve morning stiffness. Replacement joints or bone removal are the last resort for severely crippled RA patients.

Gouty (gow'te) **arthritis,** or **gout,** is a disease in which uric acid (a normal waste product of nucleic acid metabolism) accumulates in the blood and may be deposited as needle-shaped crystals in the soft tissues of joints. This leads to an agonizingly painful attack that typically affects a single joint, often in the great toe. Gout is most common in males and rarely appears before the age of thirty. It tends to run in families, so genetic factors are definitely implicated.

Untreated gout can be very destructive; the bone ends fuse and the joint becomes immobilized. Fortunately, several drugs (colchicine, ibuprofen, and others) are successful in preventing acute gout attacks. Patients are advised to lose weight if obese, to avoid foods such as liver, kidneys, and sardines, which are high in nucleic acids, and to avoid alcohol, which inhibits excretion of uric acid by the kidneys. ▲

Developmental Aspects of the Skeleton

As described earlier, the first "long bones" in the very young fetus are formed of hyaline cartilage, and the earliest "flat bones" of the skull are actually fibrous membranes. As the fetus develops and grows, both the flat and the long bone models are converted to bone (Figure 5.37). At birth, some fontanels still remain in the skull to allow for brain growth, but these areas are usually fully ossified by 2 years of age. By the end of adolescence, the epiphyseal plates of long bones that provide for longitudinal growth in childhood have become fully ossified, and long-bone growth ends.

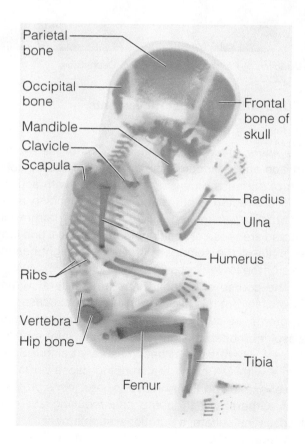

FIGURE 5.37 Ossification centers in the skeleton of a 12-week-old fetus are indicated by the darker areas. Lighter regions are still fibrous or cartilaginous.

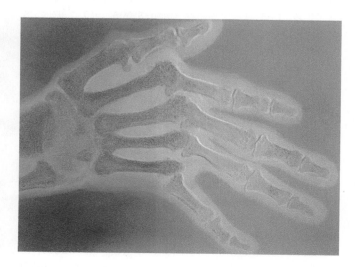

FIGURE 5.36 X-ray of a hand deformed by rheumatoid arthritis.

Systems in Sync

Homeostatic Relationships between the Skeletal System and Other Body Systems

Endocrine System
- Skeletal system provides some bony protection
- Hormones regulate uptake and release of calcium from bone; hormones promote long-bone growth and maturation

Lymphatic System/Immunity
- Skeletal system provides some protection to lymphatic organs; lymphocytes involved in immune response originate in bone marrow
- Lymphatic system drains leaked tissue fluids; immune cells protect against pathogens

Digestive System
- Skeletal system provides some bony protection to intestines, pelvic organs, and liver
- Digestive system provides nutrients needed for bone health and growth

Urinary System
- Skeletal system protects pelvic organs (bladder, etc.)
- Urinary system activates vitamin D; disposes of nitrogenous wastes

Muscular System
- Skeletal system provides levers plus calcium for muscle activity
- Muscle pull on bones increases bone strength and viability; helps determine bone shape

Nervous System
- Skeletal system protects brain and spinal cord; depot for calcium ions needed for neural function
- Nerves innervate bone and joint capsules, providing for pain and joint sense

Respiratory System
- Skeletal system (rib cage) protects lungs by enclosure
- Respiratory system provides oxygen; disposes of carbon dioxide

Cardiovascular System
- Bone marrow cavities provide site for blood cell formation; matrix stores calcium needed for cardiac muscle activity
- Cardiovascular system delivers nutrients and oxygen to bones; carries away wastes

Reproductive System
- Skeletal system protects some reproductive organs by enclosure
- Gonads produce hormones that influence form of skeleton and epiphyseal closure

Integumentary System
- Skeletal system provides support for body organs including the skin
- Skin provides vitamin D needed for proper calcium absorption and use

Skeletal System

6

The Muscular System

KEY TERMS

Because flexing muscles look like mice scurrying beneath the skin, some scientist long ago dubbed them *muscles,* from the Latin word *mus* meaning "little mouse." Indeed, the rippling muscles of professional boxers or weight lifters is often the first thing that comes to mind when one hears the word *muscle.* But muscle is also the dominant tissue in the heart and in the walls of other hollow organs of the body. In all its forms, it makes up nearly half the body's mass.

The essential function of muscle is *contraction,* or *shortening*—a unique characteristic that sets it apart from any other body tissue. As a result of this ability, muscles are responsible for essentially all body movement and can be viewed as the "machines" of the body.

Overview of Muscle Tissues

Muscle Types

There are three types of muscle tissue—skeletal, cardiac, and smooth. As summarized in Table 6.1, these differ in their cell structure, body location, and how they are stimulated to contract. But, before we explore their differences, let's look at some of the ways they are the same.

First, skeletal and smooth muscle cells are elongated. For this reason, these types of muscle cells (but not cardiac muscle cells) are called **muscle fibers.** Second, the ability of muscle to shorten, or contract, depends on two types of *myofilaments,* the muscle cell equivalents of the microfilaments of the cytoskeleton. A third similarity has to do with terminology. Whenever you see the prefixes *myo-* and *mys-* ("muscle") and *sarco-* ("flesh"), you will know that muscle is being referred to. For example, in muscle cells, the cytoplasm is called *sarcoplasm* (sar'ko-plaz"um).

Skeletal Muscle

Skeletal muscle fibers are packaged into the organs called *skeletal muscles* that attach to the body's skeleton. As the skeletal muscles cover our bony "underpinnings," they help form the much smoother contours of the body. Skeletal muscle fibers are cigar-shaped, multinucleate cells, and the largest of the muscle fiber types—some ranging up to 30 cm (nearly 1 foot) in

length. Indeed, the fibers of large, hardworking muscles, such as the antigravity muscles of the hip, are so big and coarse that they can be seen with the naked eye.

Skeletal muscle is also known as **striated muscle** (because its fibers appear to be striped) and as **voluntary muscle** (because it is the only muscle type subject to conscious control). However, it is important to recognize that skeletal muscles are often activated by reflexes (without our "willed command") as well. When you think of skeletal muscle tissue, the key words to keep in mind are **skeletal, striated,** and **voluntary.** Skeletal muscle tissue can contract rapidly and with great force, but it tires easily and must rest after short periods of activity.

Skeletal muscle fibers, like most living cells, are soft and surprisingly fragile. Yet skeletal muscles can exert tremendous power—indeed, the force they generate is often much greater than that required to lift the weight. How so? The reason they are not ripped apart as they exert force is that thousands of their fibers are bundled together by connective tissue, which provides strength and support to the muscle as a whole (Figure 6.1). Each muscle fiber is enclosed in a delicate connective tissue sheath called an **endomysium** (en"do-mis'e-um). Several sheathed muscle fibers are then wrapped by a coarser fibrous membrane called a **perimysium** to form a bundle of fibers called a **fascicle** (fas'ĭ-kul). Many fascicles are bound together by an even tougher "overcoat" of connective tissue called an **epimysium,** which covers the entire muscle. The epimysia blend into the strong, cordlike **tendons,** or into sheetlike **aponeuroses** (ap"o-nu-ro'sēz), which attach muscles indirectly to bones, cartilages, or connective tissue coverings of each other.

Besides simply acting to anchor muscles, tendons perform several functions. The most important are providing durability and conserving space. Tendons are mostly tough collagenic fibers, so they can cross rough bony projections, which would tear the more delicate muscle tissues. Because of their relatively small size, more tendons than fleshy muscles can pass over a joint.

Many people think of muscles as always having an enlarged "belly" that tapers down to a tendon at each end. However, muscles vary considerably in

TABLE 6.1   Comparison of Skeletal, Cardiac, and Smooth Muscles

Characteristic	Skeletal/Striated	Cardiac/Striated	Smooth/Nonstriated
Body location	Attached to bones or, for some facial muscles, to skin	Walls of the heart	Mostly in walls of hollow visceral organs (other than the heart)
Cell shape and appearance	Single, very long, cylindrical, multinucleate cells with very obvious striations	Branching chains of cells; uninucleate, striations; intercalated discs	Single, fusiform, uninucleate; no striations
Regulation of contraction	Voluntary; via nervous system controls	Involuntary; the heart has a pacemaker; also nervous system controls; hormones	Involuntary; nervous system controls; hormones, chemicals, stretch
Speed of contraction	Slow to fast	Slow	Very slow
Rhythmic contraction	No	Yes	Yes, in some

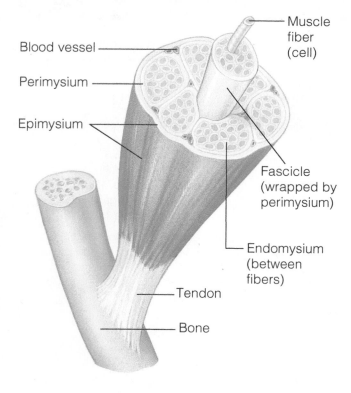

Blood vessel

Perimysium

Epimysium

Muscle fiber (cell)

Fascicle (wrapped by perimysium)

Endomysium (between fibers)

Tendon

Bone

FIGURE 6.1 Connective tissue wrappings of skeletal muscle.

the way their fibers are arranged. Many are spindle-shaped as just described, but in others, the fibers are arranged in a fan shape or a circle.

Smooth Muscle

Smooth muscle has no striations and is involuntary, which means that we cannot consciously control it. Found mainly in the walls of hollow visceral organs such as the stomach, urinary bladder, and respiratory passages, smooth muscle propels substances along a definite tract, or pathway, within the body. We can best describe smooth muscle using the terms **visceral, nonstriated,** and **voluntary.**

Smooth muscle cells are spindle-shaped and have a single nucleus (see also Table 6.1). They are arranged in sheets or layers. Most often there are two such layers, one running circularly and the

other longitudinally, as shown in Figure 6.2a. As the two layers alternately contract and relax, they change the size and shape of the organ. Movement of food through the digestive tract and emptying the bowels and bladder are examples of "housekeeping" activities normally handled by smooth muscles. Smooth muscle contraction is slow and sustained. If skeletal muscle is like a speedy wind-up car that quickly runs down, then smooth muscle is like a steady, heavy-duty engine that lumbers along tirelessly.

Cardiac Muscle

Cardiac muscle is found in only one place in the body—the heart. The heart serves as a pump, propelling blood into the blood vessels and to all tissues of the body. Cardiac muscle is like skeletal muscle in that it is striated and like smooth muscle in that it is involuntary and cannot be consciously controlled by most of us. Important key words to jog your memory for this muscle type are **cardiac, striated,** and **involuntary.**

The cardiac fibers are cushioned by small amounts of soft connective tissue and arranged in spiral or figure 8–shaped bundles, as shown in Figure 6.2b. When the heart contracts, its internal chambers become smaller, forcing the blood into the large arteries leaving the heart. Recall that cardiac muscle fibers are branching cells joined by special junctions called *intercalated discs* (see Figure 3.16). These two structural features and the spiral arrangement of the muscle bundles in the heart allow heart activity to be closely coordinated. Cardiac muscle usually contracts at a fairly steady rate set by the heart's "in-house" pacemaker, but the heart can also be stimulated by the nervous system to shift into "high gear" for short periods, as when you race to catch a bus.

Muscle Functions

Muscle plays four important roles in the body: it *produces movement, maintains posture, stabilizes joints,* and *generates heat.*

Producing Movement

Just about all movements of the human body are a result of muscle contraction. Mobility of the body as a whole reflects the activity of skeletal muscles, which are responsible for all locomotion (walking,

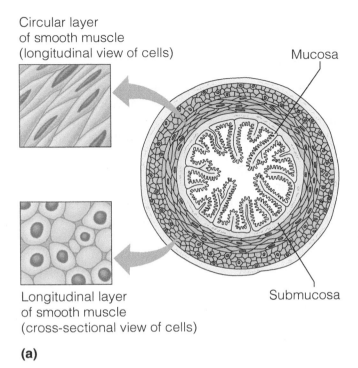

Circular layer
of smooth muscle
(longitudinal view of cells)

Mucosa

Submucosa

Longitudinal layer
of smooth muscle
(cross-sectional view of cells)

(a)

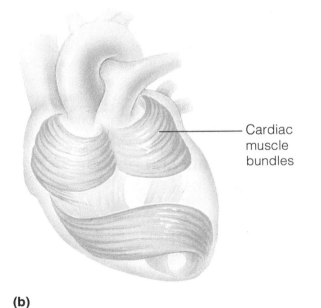

Cardiac
muscle
bundles

(b)

**FIGURE 6.2   Arrangement of smooth and
cardiac muscle cells. (a)** Diagrammatic view of a
cross section of the intestine. The longitudinal and
circular layers of muscles yield cross-sectional and
longitudinal views, respectively, of the smooth
muscle cells. **(b)** Longitudinal view of the heart,
showing the spiral arrangement of the cardiac
muscle cells in its walls.

swimming, and cross-country skiing, for example)
and manipulation. They enable us to respond
quickly to changes in the external environment. For
example, their speed and power enable us to jump
out of the way of a runaway car and then follow its
flight with our eyes. They also allow us to express
our emotions with the silent language of smiles and
frowns.

These are distinct from the smooth muscle of
blood vessel walls and cardiac muscle of the heart,
which work together to circulate blood and maintain blood pressure, and the smooth muscle of
other hollow organs, which forces fluids (urine,
bile) and other substances (food, a baby) through
internal body channels.

Maintaining Posture

We are rarely aware of the workings of the skeletal
muscles that maintain body posture. Yet, they function almost continuously, making one tiny adjustment after another so that we can maintain an erect
or seated posture despite the never-ending downward pull of gravity.

Stabilizing Joints

As the skeletal muscles pull on bones to cause
movements, they also stabilize the joints of the
skeleton. Indeed, muscle tendons are extremely
important in reinforcing and stabilizing joints that
have poorly fitting articulating surfaces (the shoulder joint, for example).

Generating Heat

The fourth function of muscle, generation of body
heat, is a by-product of muscle activity. As ATP is
used to power muscle contraction, nearly three-
quarters of its energy escapes as heat. This heat is
vital in maintaining normal body temperature.
Since skeletal muscle accounts for at least 40 percent of body mass, it is the muscle type most
responsible for heat generation.

As you can see, each of the three muscle types
has a structure and function well suited for its job
in the body. But since the term **muscular system**
applies specifically to skeletal muscle, we will be
concentrating on this muscle type in this chapter.
The most important structural and functional
aspects of the three muscle types are outlined in
Table 6.1.

Microscopic Anatomy of Skeletal Muscle

As mentioned above and illustrated in Figure 6.3a, skeletal muscle cells are multinucleate. Many oval nuclei can be seen just beneath the plasma membrane, which is called the **sarcolemma** (sar″ko-lem′ah; "muscle husk") in muscle cells. The nuclei are pushed aside by long ribbonlike organelles, the **myofibrils** (mi″o-fi′brilz), which nearly fill the cytoplasm. Alternating **light (I)** and **dark (A) bands** along the length of the perfectly aligned myofibrils give the muscle cell as a whole its striped appearance. (Think of the second letter of *light*, I, and the second letter of *dark*, A, to help you remember which band is which.) A closer look at the banding pattern reveals that the light I band has a midline interruption, a darker area called the *Z disc*, and the dark A band has a lighter central area called the *H zone* (Figure 6.3b). The *M line* in the center of the H zone contains tiny protein rods that hold adjacent thick filaments together.

So why are we bothering with all these terms—dark this and light that? Because the banding pattern reveals the working structure of the myofibrils. First, we find that the myofibrils are actually chains of tiny contractile units called **sarcomeres** (sar′ko-merz), which are aligned end-to-end like boxcars in a train along the length of the myofibrils. Second, it is the arrangement of even smaller structures (myofilaments) *within* sarcomeres that actually produces the banding pattern.

Let's examine how the arrangement of the myofilaments leads to the banding pattern. There are two types of threadlike protein **myofilaments** within each of our "boxcar" sarcomeres (Figure 6.3c). The larger **thick filaments,** also called *myosin filaments,* are made mostly of bundled molecules of the protein **myosin,** but they also contain ATPase enzymes, which split ATP to generate the power for muscle contraction. Notice that the thick filaments extend the entire length of the dark A band. Also, notice that the midparts of the thick filaments are smooth, but their ends are studded with small projections (Figure 6.3d). These projections, or myosin *heads,* are called **cross bridges** when they link the thick and thin filaments together during contraction. The **thin filaments** are composed of the contractile protein called **actin,** plus some regulatory proteins that play a role in allowing (or preventing) myosin head–binding to actin. The thin filaments, also called *actin filaments,* are anchored to the Z disc (a disclike membrane). Notice that the light I band includes parts of two adjacent sarcomeres and contains *only* the thin filaments. Although the thin filaments overlap the ends of the thick filaments, they do not extend into the middle of a relaxed sarcomere, and thus the central region (the H zone, which lacks actin filaments and looks a bit lighter) is sometimes called the *bare zone.* When contraction occurs, and the actin-containing filaments slide toward each other into the center of the sarcomeres, these light zones disappear because the actin and myosin filaments are completely overlapped. For now, however, just recognize that it is the precise arrangement of the myofilaments in the myofibrils that produces the banding pattern, or striations, in skeletal muscle cells.

Not shown in Figure 6.3 is another very important muscle fiber organelle—the **sarcoplasmic reticulum (SR),** a specialized smooth endoplasmic reticulum. The interconnecting tubules and sacs of the SR surround each and every myofibril just as the sleeve of a loosely crocheted sweater surrounds your arm. The major role of this elaborate system is to store calcium and to release it on demand when the muscle fiber is stimulated to contract. As you will see, calcium provides the final "go" signal for contraction.

Sliding Filaments and Muscle Contraction

When a skeletal muscle fiber contracts, (1) the H zones and I bands get smaller, (2) the zones of overlap get larger, (3) the Z lines move closer together, and (4) the width of the A band remains constant (Figure 6.4). These observations make sense only if the thin filaments are sliding toward the center of each sarcomere, alongside the thick filaments; this explanation is known as the **sliding filament theory.** The contraction weakens with the disappearance of the I bands, at which point the Z lines are in contact with the ends of the thick filaments.

During a contraction, sliding occurs in every sarcomere along the myofibril. As a result, the myofibril gets shorter. Because myofibrils are attached to the sarcolemma at each Z line and at

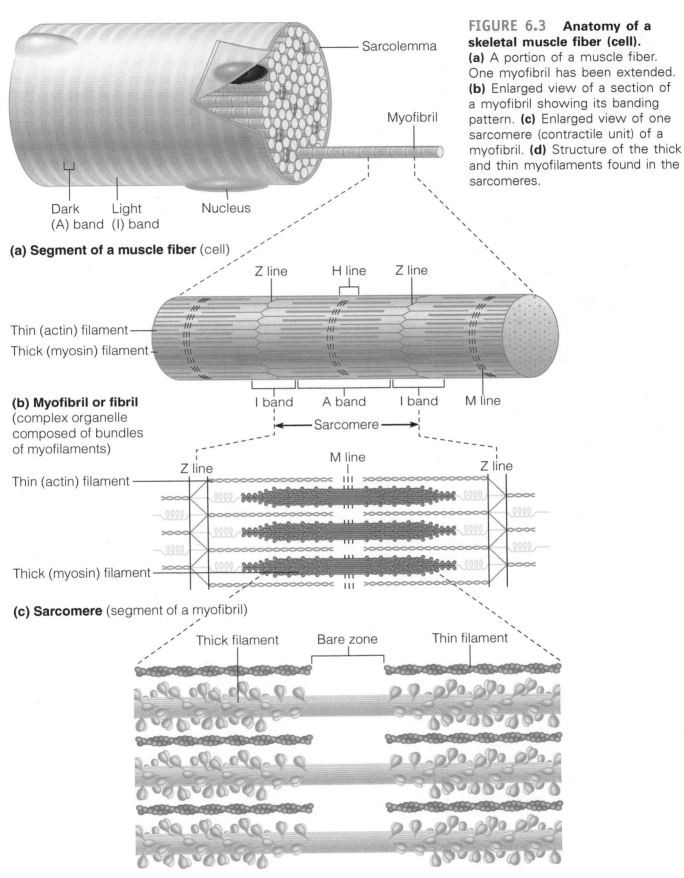

FIGURE 6.3   **Anatomy of a skeletal muscle fiber (cell).**
(a) A portion of a muscle fiber. One myofibril has been extended. **(b)** Enlarged view of a section of a myofibril showing its banding pattern. **(c)** Enlarged view of one sarcomere (contractile unit) of a myofibril. **(d)** Structure of the thick and thin myofilaments found in the sarcomeres.

Sarcolemma

Myofibril

Dark (A) band   Light (I) band   Nucleus

(a) Segment of a muscle fiber (cell)

Z line   H line   Z line

Thin (actin) filament

Thick (myosin) filament

I band   A band   I band   M line

Sarcomere

(b) Myofibril or fibril (complex organelle composed of bundles of myofilaments)

Z line   M line   Z line

Thin (actin) filament

Thick (myosin) filament

(c) Sarcomere (segment of a myofibril)

Thick filament   Bare zone   Thin filament

(d) Myofilament structure (within one sarcomere)

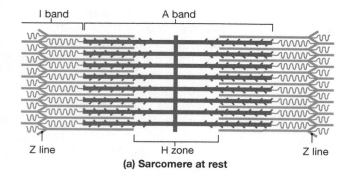

(a) Sarcomere at rest

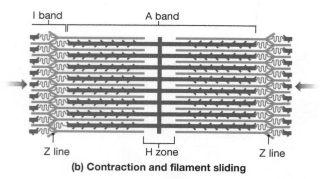

(b) Contraction and filament sliding

FIGURE 6.4   Changes in the appearance of a sarcomere during the contraction of a skeletal muscle fiber. (a) During a contraction, the A band stays the same width, but the Z lines move closer together and the I band gets smaller. **(b)** When the ends of a myofibril are free to move, the sarcomeres shorten simultaneously and the ends of the myofibril are pulled toward its center.

either end of the muscle fiber, when myofibrils get shorter, so does the muscle fiber.

You now know *how* the myofilaments in a sarcomere change position during a contraction, but not *why* these changes occur. To understand this process in detail, we must take a closer look at the contraction process and its regulation.

The Contraction of Skeletal Muscle

Most of the rest of this chapter describes how muscles contract and how those contractions are harnessed to do what you want them to do. First, you have to understand some basic physical principles that apply to muscle cells. When muscle cells contract, they pull on the attached tendon fibers the way a line of people might pull on a rope. The pull, called *tension,* is an active force:

Energy must be expended to produce it. Tension is applied *to* some object, whether a rope, a rubber band, or a book on a tabletop.

Muscle cells can use energy to shorten and generate tension, through interactions between thick and thin filaments, but not to lengthen and generate compression, or a push applied to an object. In other words, muscle cells can pull, but they cannot push.

With that background, we can investigate the mechanics of muscle contraction in some detail. Figure 6.5 provides an overview of the "big picture" we will be examining.

- Normal skeletal muscle is under neural control: Contraction occurs only when skeletal muscle fibers are activated by neurons whose cell bodies are in the central nervous system (brain and spinal cord). A neuron can activate a muscle fiber through stimulation of its sarcolemma. What follows is called **excitation–contraction coupling.**

- The first step in excitation–contraction coupling is the release of calcium ions from the cisternae of the sarcoplasmic reticulum.

- The calcium ions then trigger interactions between thick filaments and thin filaments, resulting in muscle fiber contraction and the consumption of energy in the form of ATP.

- These filament interactions produce active tension.

- The muscle will respond completely if the stimulus is above the threshold or not at all if the stimulus is below the threshold.

The Control of Skeletal Muscle Activity

Skeletal muscle fibers contract only under the control of the nervous system. Communication between the nervous system and a skeletal muscle fiber occurs at a specialized intercellular connection known as a **neuromuscular junction (NMJ),** or *myoneural junction* (Figure 6.6a).

Each skeletal muscle fiber is controlled by a neuron at a single neuromuscular junction midway along the fiber's length. A single axon branches within the perimysium to form a number of fine branches. Each branch ends at an expanded **synaptic terminal** (Figure 6.6b). The cytoplasm of the synaptic terminal contains mitochondria and

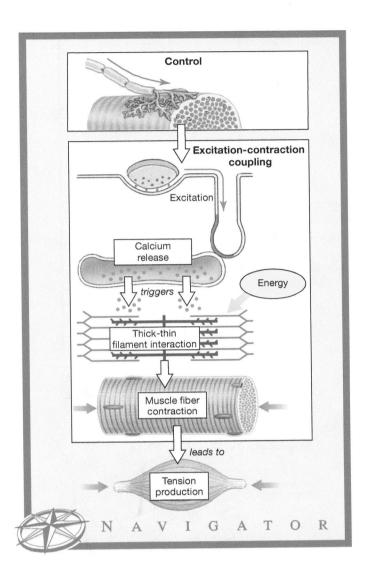

FIGURE 6.5 An overview of skeletal muscle contraction. The major factors are indicated here as a series of interrelated steps and processes. Each factor will be described further in a related section of the text. A simplified version of this figure will appear in later figures as a Navigator icon; its presence indicates that we are taking another step in the discussion.

vesicles filled with molecules of **acetylcholine** (as-ē-til-Kō-lēn), or **ACh.** Acetylcholine is a *neurotransmitter,* a chemical released by a neuron to change the permeability or other properties of another cell membrane. In this case, the release of ACh from the synaptic terminal can alter the permeability of the sarcolemma and trigger the contraction of the muscle fiber.

The **synaptic cleft,** a narrow space, separates the synaptic terminal of the neuron from the opposing sarcolemmal surface. This surface, which contains membrane receptors that bind ACh, is known as the **motor end plate.** The motor end plate has deep creases called *junctional folds,* which increase its surface area and thus the number of available ACh receptors. The synaptic cleft and the sarcolemma also contain molecules of the enzyme **acetylcholinesterase** (**AChE,** or *cholinesterase*), which breaks down ACh.

A neuron stimulates a muscle fiber through a series of steps (Figure 6.6c):

Step 1 **The Arrival of an Action Potential.** The stimulus for ACh release is the arrival of an electrical nerve impulse, or **action potential,** at the synaptic terminal. An action potential is a sudden change in the transmembrane potential that travels along the length of the axon.

Step 2 **The Release of ACh.** When the action potential reaches the synaptic terminal, permeability changes in the membrane trigger the exocytosis of ACh into the synaptic cleft. This is accomplished when vesicles in the synaptic terminal fuse with the cell membrane of the neuron.

Step 3 **ACh Binding at the Motor End Plate.** ACh molecules diffuse across the synaptic cleft and bind to ACh receptors on the surface of the sarcolemma at the motor end plate. ACh binding changes the permeability of the motor end plate to sodium ions. The extracellular fluid contains a high concentration of sodium ions, whereas sodium ion concentrations inside the cell are very low. When the membrane permeability to sodium increases, sodium ions rush into the sarcoplasm. This influx continues until AChE removes the ACh from the receptors.

Step 4 **Appearance of an Action Potential in the Sarcolemma.** The sudden inrush of sodium ions results in the generation of an action potential in the sarcolemma. This electrical impulse originates at the edges of the motor end plate, sweeps across the entire membrane surface, and travels inward along each T tubule. The arrival of an action potential at the synaptic terminal thus leads to the appearance of an action potential in the sarcolemma.

Step 5 **Return to Initial State.** Even before the action potential has spread across the entire sarcolemma, the ACh has been broken down by AChE. Some of the breakdown products will be absorbed by the synaptic terminal and used to resynthesize

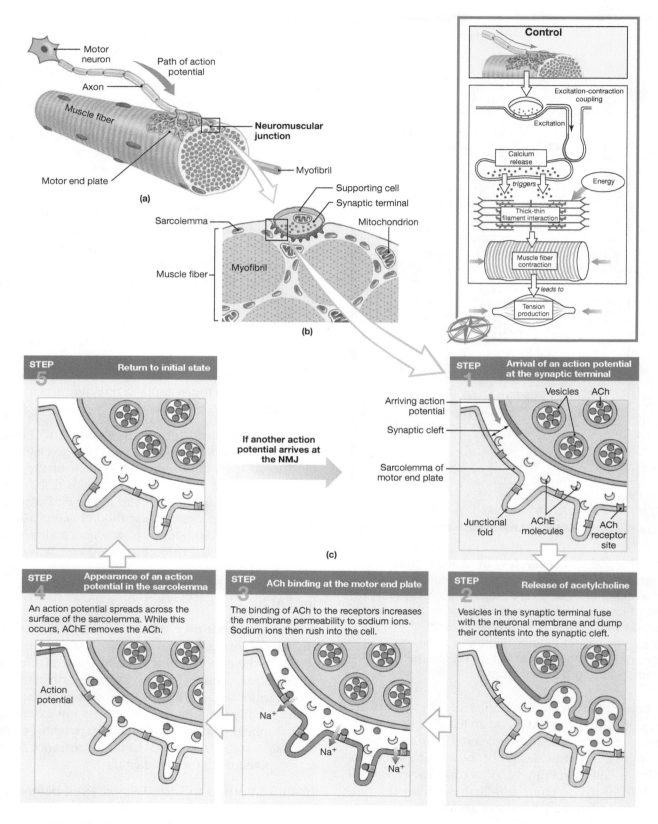

FIGURE 6.6 Skeletal muscle innervation. The Navigator in the shadow box highlights your location in the discussion. **(a)** A diagrammatic view of a neuromuscular junction. **(b)** Details of the neuromuscular junction. **(c)** Changes at the motor end plate that trigger an action potential in the sarcolemma.

ACh for subsequent release. This sequence of events can now be repeated should another action potential arrive at the synaptic terminal.

Excitation–Contraction Coupling

The link between the generation of an action potential in the sarcolemma and the start of a muscle contraction is called **excitation–contraction coupling.** This coupling occurs at the triads. On reaching a triad, an action potential triggers the release of Ca^{2+} from the cisternae of the sarcoplasmic reticulum. The change in the permeability of the SR to Ca^{2+} is temporary, lasting only about 0.03 seconds. Yet within a millisecond, the Ca^{2+} concentration in and around the sarcomere reaches 100 times resting levels. Because the terminal cisternae are situated at the zones of overlap, where the thick and thin filaments interact, the effect of calcium release on the sarcomere is almost instantaneous.

Troponin is the lock that keeps the active sites inaccessible. Calcium is the key to that lock. Troponin binds to actin and to tropomyosin, and the tropomyosin molecules cover the active sites and prevent interactions between thick filaments and thin filaments. Each troponin molecule also has a binding site for calcium; this site is empty when the muscle fiber is at rest. Calcium binding changes the shape of the troponin molecule and weakens the bond between tropinin and actin. The troponin molecule then changes position, rolling the tropomyosin strand away from the active sites (Figure 6.7). At this point, the **contraction cycle** begins.

The Contraction Cycle

Figure 6.8 details the molecular events that occur during the contraction cycle. In the resting sarcomere, each myosin head is already "energized"—charged with the energy that will be used

to power a contraction. The myosin head functions as ATPase, an enzyme that can break down ATP. At the start of the contraction cycle, each myosin head has already split a molecule of ATP and stored the energy released in the process. The breakdown products, ADP and phosphate (often represented as P), remain bound to the myosin head.

The contraction cycle involves five interlocking steps (see Figure 6.8):

Step 1 **Exposure of Active Sites.** The calcium ions entering the sarcoplasm bind to troponin. This binding weakens the bond between the troponin–tropomyosin complex and actin. The troponin molecule then changes position, pulling the tropomyosin molecule away from the active sites on actin and allowing interaction with the energized myosin heads.

Step 2 **Formation of Cross-Bridges.** When the active sites are exposed, the energized myosin heads bind to them, forming cross-bridges.

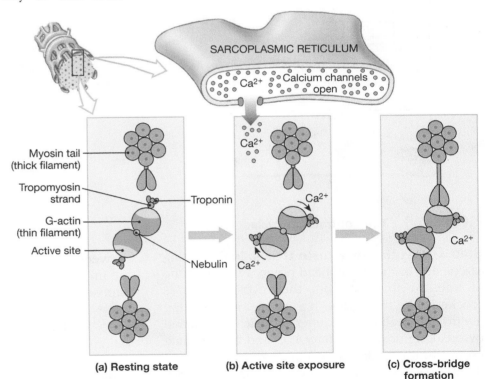

(a) **Resting state**   (b) **Active site exposure**   (c) **Cross-bridge formation**

FIGURE 6.7   The exposure of active sites. (a) In a resting sarcomere, the tropomyosin strands cover the active sites on the thin filaments, preventing cross-bridge formation. **(b)** When calcium ions enter the sarcomere, they bind to troponin, which rotates and swings the tropomyosin away from the active sites. **(c)** Cross-bridge formation then occurs, and the contraction cycle begins.

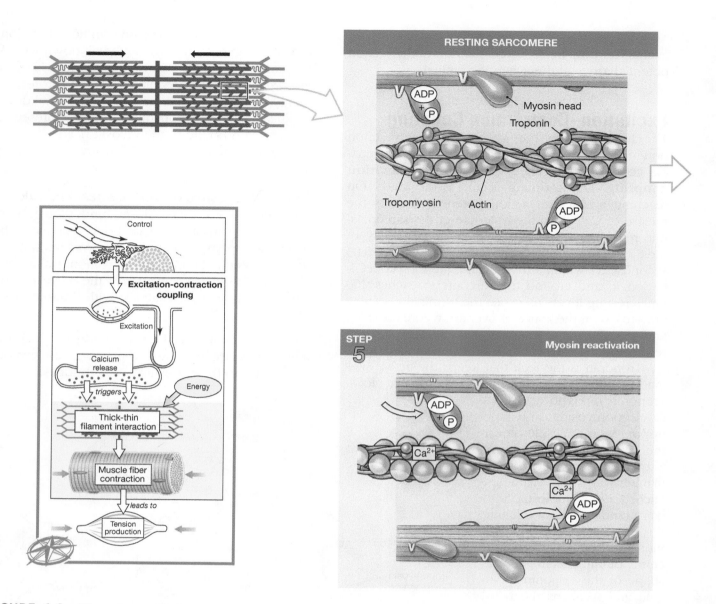

FIGURE 6.8   The contraction cycle.

Step 3   Pivoting of Myosin Heads. In the resting sarcomere, each myosin head points away from the M line. In this position, the myosin head is "cocked" like the spring in a mousetrap. Cocking the myosin head requires energy, which is obtained by breaking down ATP into ADP and a phosphate group. In the cocked position, both the ADP and the phosphate are still bound to the myosin head. After cross-bridge formation, the stored energy is released as the myosin head pivots toward the M line. This action is called the *power stroke;* when it occurs, the ADP and phosphate group are released.

Step 4   Detachment of Cross-Bridges. When another ATP binds to the myosin head, the link between the active site on the actin molecule and the myosin head is broken. The active site is now exposed and able to form another cross-bridge.

Step 5   Reactivation of Myosin. Myosin reactivation occurs when the free myosin head splits the ATP into ADP and a phosphate group. The energy released in this process is used to recock the myosin head. The entire cycle will now be repeated, several times each second, as long as calcium ion concentrations remain elevated and ATP reserves are sufficient. Each power stroke shortens the sarcomere by about 1 percent, because all the sarcomeres contract together, the entire muscle shortens at the same rate. The speed at which

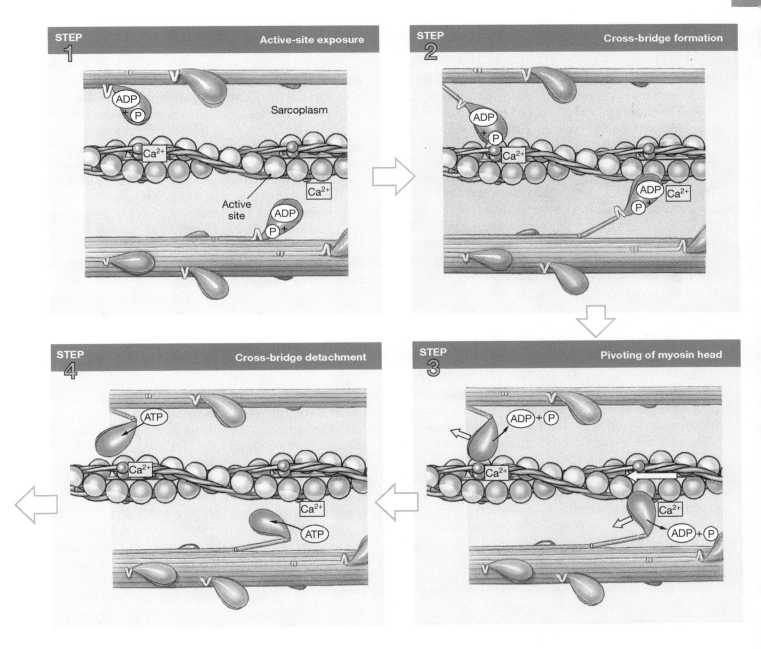

shortening occurs depends on the cycling rate (the number of power strokes per second): The higher the resistance, the slower the cycling rate.

To better understand how tension is produced in a muscle fiber, imagine that you are on a tug-of-war team. You reach forward, grab the rope with both hands, and pull it in. This action corresponds to cross-bridge attachment and pivoting. You then release the rope, reach forward and grab it, and pull once again. Your actions are not coordinated with the rest of your team; if everyone let go at the same time, your opponents would pull the rope away. So at any given time, some people are reaching and grabbing, some are pulling, and others are

letting go. The amount of tension produced is thus a function of how many people are pulling at any given moment. The situation is comparable in a muscle fiber; the myosin heads along a thick filament work together in a similar way to pull a thin filament toward the center of the sarcomere.

Each myofibril consists of a string of sarcomeres, and in a contraction all of the thin filaments are pulled toward the centers of the sarcomeres. If neither end of the myofibril is held in position, both ends move toward the middle, as illustrated in Figure 6.9a. This kind of contraction seldom occurs in an intact skeletal muscle, because one end of the muscle (the *origin*) is usually fixed in position during a contraction, while the other end (the *insertion*) moves. In that case, the free end moves toward the fixed end (see Figure 6.9b). If neither end of the myofibril can move, thick and thin filament interactions consume energy and generate tension, but sliding cannot occur. This kind of contraction, called *isometric,* will be the topic of a later section.

Relaxation

The duration of a contraction depends on (1) the duration of stimulation at the neuromuscular junction, (2) the presence of free calcium ions in the sarcoplasm, and (3) the availability of ATP. A single stimulus has only a brief effect on a muscle fiber because the ACh released after a single action potential arrives at the synaptic terminal does not remain intact for long. Whether it is bound to the sarcolemma or free in the synaptic cleft, the released ACh is rapidly broken down and inactivated by AChE. Inside the muscle fiber, the permeability changes in the SR are also very brief. Thus, a contraction will continue only if additional action potentials arrive at the synaptic terminal in rapid succession. When they do, the continual release of ACh into the synaptic cleft produces a series of action potentials in the sarcolemma that keeps Ca^{2+} levels elevated in the sarcoplasm. Under these conditions, the contraction cycle will be repeated over and over.

If just one action potential arrives at the neuromuscular junction, Ca^{2+} concentrations in the sarcoplasm will quickly return to normal resting levels. Two mechanisms are involved in this process: (1) active Ca^{2+} transport across the cell membrane into the extracellular fluid and (2) active Ca^{2+} transport into the SR. Of the two, transport into the SR is far more important. Virtually as soon as the calcium ions have been released, the SR returns to its normal permeability and begins actively absorbing Ca^{2+} from the surrounding sarcoplasm. As Ca^{2+} concentrations in the sarcoplasm fall, (1) calcium ions detach from troponin, (2) troponin returns to its original position, and (3) the active sites are re-covered by tropomyosin. The contraction has ended.

Once the contraction has ended, the sarcomere does not automatically return to its original length. Sarcomeres shorten actively, but there is no active mechanism for reversing the process. External forces must act on the contracted muscle fiber to stretch the myofibrils and sarcomeres to their original dimensions.

When death occurs, circulation ceases and the skeletal muscles are deprived of nutrients and oxygen. Within a few hours, the skeletal muscle fibers have run out of ATP and the sarcoplasmic reticulum becomes unable to pump Ca^{2+} out of the sarcoplasm. Calcium ions diffusing into the sarcoplasm from the extracellular fluid or leaking out of the sarcoplasmic reticulum then trigger a sustained contraction. Without ATP, the cross-bridges cannot detach from the active sites, so skeletal muscles throughout the body become locked in the contracted position. Because all the skeletal muscles are involved, the individual becomes "stiff as a board." This physical state—**rigor mortis**—lasts until the lysosomal enzymes released by autolysis break down the Z lines and titin filaments 15–25 hours later. The timing is dependent on environmental factors, such as temperature. Forensic pathologists can estimate the time of death on the basis of the degree of rigor mortis and environmental conditions.

Before you proceed, review the entire sequence of events from neural activation through excitation–contraction coupling to the completion of a contraction. Table 6.2 provides a review of the contraction process, from ACh release to the end of the contraction.

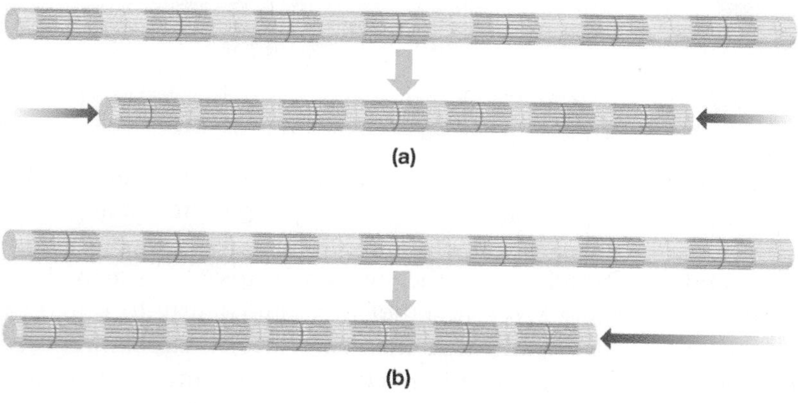

(a)

(b)

FIGURE 6.9   Shortening during a contraction. (a) When both ends are free to move, the ends of a contracting muscle fiber move toward the center of the muscle fiber. **(b)** When one end of a myofibril is fixed in position and the other end free to move, the free end is pulled toward the fixed end.

TABLE 6.2   Steps Involved in Skeletal Muscle Contraction

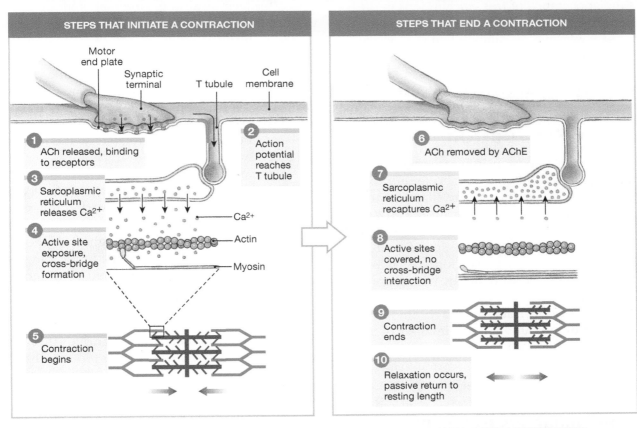

STEPS THAT INITIATE A CONTRACTION:

1. At the neuromuscular junction (NMJ), ACh released by the synaptic terminal binds to receptors on the sarcolemma.

2. The resulting change in the transmembrane potential of the muscle fiber leads to the production of an action potential that spreads across the entire surface of the muscle fiber and along the T tubules.

3. The sarcoplasmic reticulum (SR) releases stored calcium ions, increasing the calcium concentration of the sarcoplasm in and around the sarcomeres.

4. Calcium ions bind to troponin, producing a change in the orientation of the troponin–tropomyosin complex that exposes active sites on the thin (actin) filaments. Cross-bridges form when myosin heads bind to active sites on F actin.

5. The contraction begins as repeated cycles of cross-bridge binding, pivoting, and detachment occur, powered by the hydrolysis of ATP. These events produce filament sliding, and the muscle fiber shortens.*

STEPS THAT END A CONTRACTION:

6. Action potential generation ceases as ACh is broken down by acetylcholinesterase (AChE).

7. The SR reabsorbs calcium ions, and the concentration of calcium ions in the sarcoplasm declines.

8. When calcium ion concentrations approach normal resting levels, the troponin–tropomyosin complex returns to its normal position. This change re-covers the active sites and prevents further cross-bridge interaction.

9. Without cross-bridge interactions, further sliding cannot take place, and the contraction ends.

10. Muscle relaxation occurs, and the muscle returns passively to its resting length.

*There is a refractory period during which the muscle is incapable of repeating the action; this is the amount of time needed for the membrane to be ready for a second stimulus. The **absolute refractory period** is the internal during which a second action could not be initiated, no matter how strong the stimulus. The **relative refractory period** is the time during which a second action could take place but is inhibited with a lessened response.

100 Keys | Skeletal muscle fibers shorten as thin filaments interact with thick filaments and sliding occurs. The trigger for contraction is the appearance of free calcium ions in the sarcoplasm; the calcium ions are released by the sarcoplasmic reticulum when the muscle fiber is stimulated by the associated motor neuron. Contraction is an active process; the return to resting length is entirely passive.

Tension Production

When sarcomeres shorten in a contraction, they shorten the muscle fiber. This shortening exerts tension on the connective tissue fibers attached to the muscle fiber. The tension produced by an individual muscle fiber can vary, and in the next section we will consider the specific factors involved. In a subsequent section, we will see that the tension produced by an entire skeletal *muscle* can vary even more widely, because not only can tension production vary among the individual muscle fibers, but the number of stimulated muscle fibers can change from moment to moment.

Tension Production by Muscle Fibers

The amount of tension produced by an individual muscle fiber ultimately depends on the number of pivoting cross-bridges. There is no mechanism to regulate the amount of tension produced in that contraction by changing the number of contracting sarcomeres. When calcium ions are released, they are released from all triads in the muscle fiber. Thus, a muscle fiber is either "on" (producing tension) or "off" (relaxed). Tension production at the level of the individual muscle fiber *does* vary, depending on (1) the fiber's resting length at the time of stimulation, which determines the degree of overlap between thick and thin filaments, and (2) the frequency of stimulation, which affects the internal concentration of calcium ions and thus the amount bound to troponins.

Length–Tension Relationships

When many people pull on a rope, the amount of tension produced is proportional to the number of people pulling. Similarly, in a skeletal muscle fiber, the amount of tension generated during a contraction depends on the number of pivoting cross-bridges in all the sarcomeres along all the myofibrils. The number of cross-bridges that can form, in turn, depends on the degree of overlap between thick filaments and thin filaments within these sarcomeres. When the muscle fiber is stimulated to contract, only myosin heads in the zones of overlap can bind to active sites and produce tension. The tension produced by the entire muscle fiber can thus be related to the structure of individual sarcomeres.

A sarcomere works most efficiently within an optimal range of lengths (Figure 6.10a). When the resting sarcomere length is within this range, the maximum number of cross-bridges can form, and the tension produced is highest. If the resting sarcomere length falls outside the range—if the sarcomere is compressed and shortened, or stretched and lengthened—it cannot produce as much tension when stimulated. This is because the amount of tension produced is largely determined by the number of cross-bridges that form. An increase in sarcomere length reduces the tension produced by reducing the size of the zone of overlap and the number of potential cross-bridge interactions (Figure 6.10b). When the zone of overlap is reduced to zero, thin and thick filaments cannot interact at all. Under these conditions, the muscle fiber cannot produce any active tension, and a contraction cannot occur. Such extreme stretching of a muscle fiber is normally opposed by the titin filaments in the muscle fiber, which tie the thick filaments to the Z lines, and by the surrounding connective tissues, which limit the degree of muscle stretch.

A decrease in the resting sarcomere length reduces efficiency because the stimulated sarcomere cannot shorten very much before the thin filaments extend across the center of the sarcomere and collide with or overlap the thin filaments of the opposite side (Figure 6.10c). This disrupts the precise three-dimensional relationship between thick and thin filaments and interferes with the binding of myosin heads to active sites and the propagation of the action potential along the transverse tubules. Because the number of cross-bridges is reduced, tension declines in the stimulated muscle fiber. Tension production falls to zero

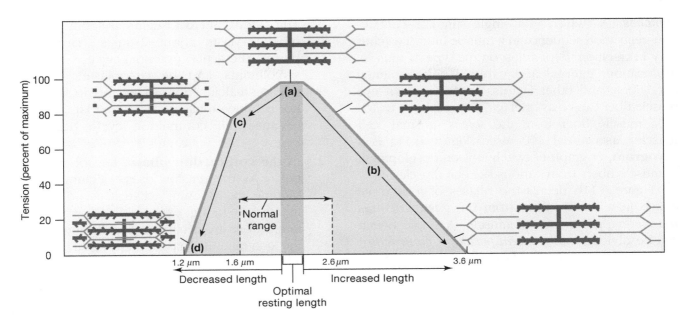

FIGURE 6.10 **The effect of sarcomere length on active tension. (a)** Maximum tension is produced when the zone of overlap is large but the thin filaments do not extend across the sarcomere's center. **(b)** If the sarcomeres are stretched too far, the zone of overlap is reduced or disappears, and cross-bridge interactions are reduced or cannot occur. **(c)** At short resting lengths, thin filaments extending across the center of the sarcomere interfere with the normal orientation of thick and thin filaments, reducing tension production. **(d)** When the thick filaments contact the Z lines, the sarcomere cannot shorten—the myosin heads cannot pivot and tension cannot be produced. The width of the light purple area represents the normal range of resting sarcomere lengths.

when the resting sarcomere is as short as it can be (Figure 6.10d). At this point, the thick filaments are jammed against the Z lines and the sarcomere cannot shorten further. Although cross-bridge binding can still occur, the myosin heads cannot pivot and generate tension, because the thin filaments cannot move.

In summary, skeletal muscle fibers contract most forcefully when stimulated over a narrow range of resting lengths. The normal range of resting sarcomere lengths in the body is 75 to 130 percent of the optimal length (see Figure 6.10). The arrangement of skeletal muscles, connective tissues, and bones normally prevents extreme compression or excessive stretching. For example, straightening your elbow stretches your *biceps brachii muscle,* but the bones and ligaments of the elbow stop this movement before the muscle fibers stretch too far. During an activity such as walking, in which muscles contract and relax cyclically, muscle fibers are stretched to a length very close to "ideal" before they are stimulated to contract. When muscles must contract over a larger range of resting lengths, they often "team up" to improve efficiency.

The Frequency of Stimulation

A single stimulation produces a single contraction, or *twitch*, that may last 7–100 milliseconds, depending on the muscle stimulated. Although muscle twitches can be produced by electrical stimulation in a laboratory and can generate heat when you are shivering, they are too brief to be part of any normal activity. The duration of a contraction can be extended by repeated stimulation, and a muscle fiber undergoing such a sustained contraction produces more tension than it does in a single twitch. To understand why, we need to take a closer look at tension production during a twitch and then follow the changes that occur as the rate of stimulation increases. This is a subject with real importance, as all consciously and subconsciously directed muscular activities—standing, walking, running, reaching, and so forth—involve sustained muscular contractions rather than twitches.

Twitches A **twitch** is a single stimulus–contraction–relaxation sequence in a muscle fiber. Twitches vary in duration, depending on the type of muscle, its location, internal and external environmental conditions, and other factors. Twitches in an eye muscle fiber can be as brief as 7.5 msec, but a twitch in a muscle fiber from the *soleus,* a small calf muscle, lasts about 100 msec. Figure 6.11a is a **myogram,** or graph of twitch tension development in muscle fibers from various skeletal muscles.

Figure 6.11b details the phases of a 40-msec twitch in a muscle fiber from the *gastrocnemius muscle,* a prominent calf muscle. A single twitch can be divided into a *latent period,* a *contraction phase,* and a *relaxation phase:*

1. The **latent period** begins at stimulation and typically lasts about 2 msec. During this period, the action potential sweeps across the sarcolemma, and the sarcoplasmic reticulum releases calcium ions. The muscle fiber does not produce tension during the latent period, because the contraction cycle has yet to begin.

2. In the **contraction phase,** tension rises to a peak. As the tension rises, calcium ions are binding to troponin, active sites on thin filaments are being exposed, and cross-bridge interactions are occurring. For this muscle fiber, the contraction phase ends roughly 15 msec after stimulation.

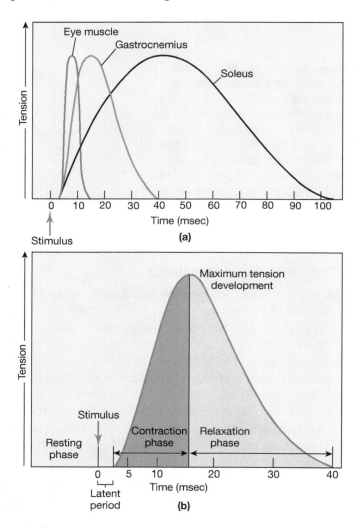

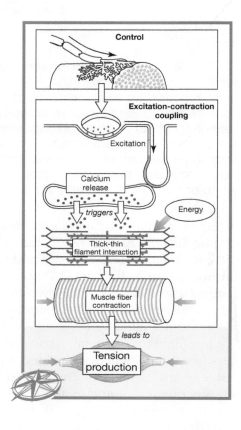

FIGURE 6.11 The development of tension in a twitch. (a) A myogram showing differences in tension over time for a twitch in different skeletal muscles. **(b)** The details of tension over time for a single twitch in the gastrocnemius muscle. Notice the presence of a latent period, which corresponds to the time needed for the conduction of an action potential and the subsequent release of calcium ions by the sarcoplasmic reticulum.

3. The **relaxation phase** lasts about 25 msec. During this period, calcium levels are falling, active sites are being covered by tropomyosin, and the number of active cross-bridges is declining. As a result, tension falls to resting levels.

Treppe If a skeletal muscle is stimulated a second time immediately after the relaxation phase has ended, the resulting contraction will develop a slightly higher maximum tension than did the contraction after the first stimulus. The increase in peak tension indicated in Figure 6.12a will continue over the first 30–50 stimulations. Thereafter, the amount of tension produced will remain constant. Because the tension rises in stages, like the steps in a staircase, this phenomenon is called **treppe** (TREP-eh), a German word meaning "stairs." The rise is thought to result from a gradual increase in the concentration of calcium ions in the sarcoplasm, in part because the ion pumps in the sarcoplasmic reticulum have too little time to recapture the ions between stimulations.

Wave Summation and Incomplete Tetanus If a second stimulus arrives before the relaxation phase has ended, a second, more powerful contraction occurs. The addition of one twitch to another in this way constitutes the **summation of twitches,** or **wave summation** (Figure 6.12b). The duration of a single twitch determines the maximum time available to produce wave summation. For example, if a twitch lasts 20 msec (1/50 sec), subsequent stimuli must be separated by less than 20 msec—a stimulation rate of more than 50 stimuli per second. This rate is usually expressed in terms of *stimulus frequency,* which is the number of stimuli per unit time. In this instance, a stimulus frequency of greater than 50 per second produces wave summation, whereas a stimulus frequency of less than 50 per second will produce individual twitches and treppe.

If the stimulation continues and the muscle is never allowed to relax completely, tension will rise until it reaches a peak value roughly four times the maximum produced by treppe (Figure 6.12c). A muscle producing almost peak tension during rapid cycles of contraction and relaxation is in **incomplete tetanus** (*tetanos,* convulsive tension).

Complete Tetanus Complete tetanus occurs when a higher stimulation frequency eliminates the relaxation phase (Figure 6.12d). During complete tetanus, action potentials arrive so rapidly that the sarcoplasmic reticulum does not have time to reclaim the calcium ions. The high Ca^{2+} concentration in the cytoplasm prolongs the contraction, making it continuous.

Tension Production by Skeletal Muscles

Now that you are familiar with the basic mechanisms of muscle contraction at the level of the individual muscle fiber, we can begin to examine the performance of skeletal muscles—the organs of the muscular system. In this section, we will consider the coordinated contractions of an entire population of skeletal muscle fibers. The amount of tension produced in the skeletal muscle *as a whole* is determined by (1) the tension produced by the stimulated muscle fibers and (2) the total number of muscle fibers stimulated.

As muscle fibers actively shorten, they pull on the attached tendons which become streched. The tension is transferred in turn to bones which are moved against an external load.

A myogram performed in the laboratory generally measures the tension in a tendon. A single twitch is so brief in duration that there isn't enough time to activate a significant percentage of the available cross-bridges. Twitches are therefore ineffective in terms of performing useful work.

However, if a second twitch occurs before the tension returns to zero, tension will peak at a higher level, because additional cross-bridges will form. Think of pushing a child on a swing: You push gently to start the swing moving; if you push harder the second time, the child swings higher because the energy of the second push is added to the energy remaining from the first. Each successive contraction begins before the tension has fallen to resting levels, so the tension continues to rise until it peaks. During a tetanic contraction, there is enough time for essentially all of the potential cross-bridges to form, and tension peaks. Muscles are rarely used this way in the body, but they can be made to contract tetanically in the laboratory.

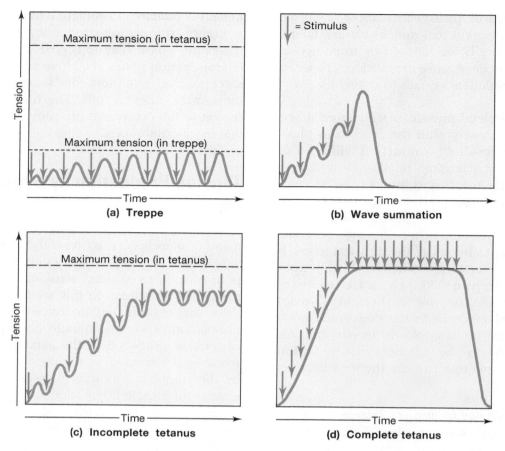

FIGURE 6.12 Effects of repeated stimulations. (a) Treppe is an increase in peak tension with each successive stimulus delivered shortly after the completion of the relaxation phase of the preceding twitch. **(b)** Wave summation occurs when successive stimuli arrive before the relaxation phase has been completed. **(c)** Incomplete tetanus occurs if the stimulus frequency increases further. Tension production rises to a peak, and the periods of relaxation are very brief. **(d)** During complete tetanus, the stimulus frequency is so high that the relaxation phase is eliminated; tension plateaus at maximal levels.

Motor Units and Tension Production

The amount of tension produced by the muscle as a whole is the sum of the tensions generated by the individual muscle fibers, since they are all pulling together. Thus, you can control the amount of tension produced by a skeletal muscle by controlling the number of stimulated muscle fibers.

A typical skeletal muscle contains thousands of muscle fibers. Although some motor neurons control a few muscle fibers, most control hundreds of them. All the muscle fibers controlled by a single motor neuron constitute a **motor unit.** All fibers respond a once in an "all-or-none" manner. The size of a motor unit is an indication of how fine the control of movement can be. In the muscles of the eye, where precise control is extremely important, a motor neuron may control 4–6 muscle fibers. We have much less precise control over our leg muscles, where a single motor neuron may control 1000–2000 muscle fibers.

The force of response can be increased according to the **graded strength principle:** The more frequent the stimuli or the larger area stimulated, the greater the response.

Muscle performance can be considered in terms of **force,** the maximum amount of tension produced by a particular muscle or muscle group, and **endurance,** the amount of time during which the individual can perform a particular activity. Two major factors determine the performance capabilities of any skeletal muscle: (1) the types of muscle fibers in the muscle and (2) physical conditioning or training.

Clinical Note

The Disease Called Tetanus

Children are often told to be careful around rusty nails. But it's not the rust or the nail, but instead an infection by the very common bacterium *Clostridium tetani* that causes the disease called **tetanus.** Although this disease and the normal muscle response to rapid neural stimulation share the same name, the mechanisms involved are very different.

Clostridium bacteria occur in soil and virtually everywhere else in the environment, but they can thrive only in tissues with low oxygen levels. For this reason, a deep puncture wound, such as that from a nail, is much more likely to result in tetanus than a shallow, open cut that bleeds freely. When active in body tissues, these bacteria release a powerful toxin that affects the central nervous system. Motor neurons, which control skeletal muscles throughout the body, are particularly sensitive to it. The toxin suppresses the mechanism that inhibits motor neuron activity. The result is a sustained, powerful contraction of skeletal muscles throughout the body.

The incubation period (the time between exposure and the development of symptoms) is generally less than 2 weeks. The most common early complaints are headache, muscle stiffness, and difficulty in swallowing. Because it soon becomes difficult to open the mouth, the disease is also called *lockjaw*. Widespread muscle spasms typically develop within 2 or 3 days of the initial symptoms and continue for a week before subsiding. After 2–4 weeks, patients who survive recover with no aftereffects.

Severe tetanus has a 40–60 percent mortality rate; that is, for every 100 people who develop severe tetanus, 40 to 60 die. Approximately 500,000 cases of tetanus occur worldwide each year, but only about 100 of them occur in the United States, thanks to an effective immunization program. (Recommended immunization involves a "tetanus shot" followed by a booster shot every 10 years.) In unimmunized patients, severe symptoms can be prevented by early administration of an antitoxin—in most cases, *human tetanus immune globulin*. However, this treatment does not reduce symptoms that have already appeared.

Types of Skeletal Muscle Fibers

The human body has three major types of skeletal muscle fibers: *fast fibers, slow fibers*, and *intermediate fibers* (Table 6.3).

Fast Fibers

Most of the skeletal muscle fibers in the body are called **fast fibers,** because they can contract in 0.01 sec or less after stimulation. Fast fibers are large in diameter and contain densely packed myofibrils, large glycogen reserves, and relatively few mitochondria. The tension produced by a muscle fiber is directly proportional to the number of myofibrils, so muscles dominated by fast fibers produce powerful contractions. However, fast fibers fatigue rapidly because their contractions use ATP in massive amounts, and there are relatively few mitochondria to generate ATP. As a result, prolonged activity is supported primarily by anaerobic metabolism. Other names used to refer to these muscle fibers include *white muscle fibers, fast-twitch glycolytic fibers*, and *Type II-B fibers*.

Slow Fibers

Slow fibers have only about half the diameter of fast fibers and take three times as long to reach peak tension after stimulation. These fibers are specialized to enable them to continue contracting for extended periods, long after a fast fiber would have become fatigued. The most important specializations improve mitochondrial performance.

One of the main characteristics of slow muscle fibers is that they are surrounded by a more extensive network of capillaries than is typical of fast muscle tissue; thus, they have a dramatically higher oxygen supply to support mitochondrial activity. Slow fibers also contain the red pigment **myoglobin** (MĪ-ō-glō-bin). This globular protein is structurally related to hemoglobin, the red oxygen-carrying pigment in blood. Both myoglobin and hemoglobin reversibly bind oxygen molecules. Although other muscle fiber types contain small amounts of myoglobin, it is most abundant in slow fibers. As a result, resting slow fibers contain substantial oxygen reserves that can be mobilized

TABLE 6.3   Properties of Skeletal Muscle Fiber Types

Property	Slow	Intermediate	Fast
Cross-sectional diameter	Small	Intermediate	Large
Tension	Low	Intermediate	High
Contraction speed	Slow	Fast	Fast
Fatigue resistance	High	Intermediate	Low
Color	Red	Pink	White
Myoglobin content	High	Low	Low
Capillary supply	Dense	Intermediate	Scarce
Mitochondria	Many	Intermediate	Few
Glycolytic enzyme concentration in sarcoplasm	Low	High	High
Substrates used for ATP generation during contraction	Lipids, carbohydrates, amino acids (aerobic)	Primarily carbohydrates (anaerobic)	Carbohydrates (anaerobic)
Alternative names	Type I, S (slow), red, SO (slow oxidizing), slow-twitch oxidative	Type II-A, FR (fast resistant), fast-twitch oxidative	Type II-B, FF (fast fatigue), white, fast-twitch glycolytic

during a contraction. Because slow fibers have both an extensive capillary supply and a high concentration of myoglobin, skeletal muscles dominated by slow fibers are dark red. Slow fibers are also known as *red muscle fibers, slow-twitch oxidative fibers,* and *Type I fibers.*

With oxygen reserves and a more efficient blood supply, the mitochondria of slow fibers can contribute more ATP during contraction. In addition, the cross-bridges in slow fibers cycle more slowly than those of fast fibers, and this reduces demand for ATP. Thus, slow fibers are less dependent on anaerobic metabolism than are fast fibers. Some of the mitochondrial energy production involves the breakdown of stored lipids rather than glycogen, so glycogen reserves of slow fibers are smaller than those of fast fibers. Slow fibers also contain more mitochondria than do fast fibers. Figure 6.13 compares the appearance of fast and slow fibers.

Intermediate Fibers

Most properties of **intermediate fibers** are intermediate between those of fast fibers and slow fibers. In appearance, intermediate fibers most closely resemble fast fibers, for they contain little myoglobin and are relatively pale. They have a more extensive capillary network around them, however, and are more resistant to fatigue than are fast fibers. Intermediate fibers are also known as *fast-twitch oxidative fibers* and *Type II-A fibers.*

Muscle Performance and the Distribution of Muscle Fibers

The percentages of fast, intermediate, and slow fibers in a skeletal muscle can be quite variable. In muscles that contain a mixture of fast and intermediate fibers, the proportion can change with physical conditioning. For example, if a muscle is

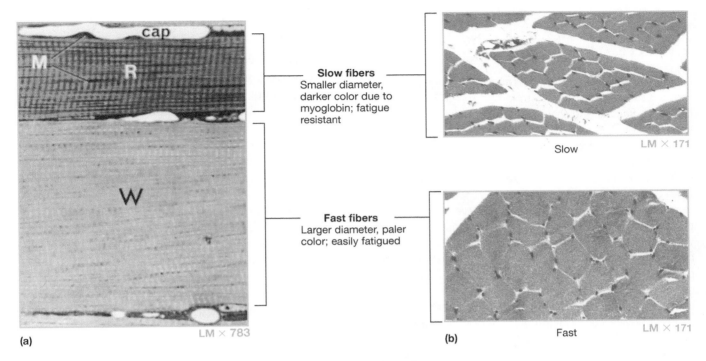

FIGURE 6.13 **Fast versus slow fibers.** **(a)** A longitudinal section, showing more mitochondria (M) and a more extensive capillary supply (cap) in a slow fiber (R, for red) than in a fast fiber (W, for white). **(b)** Cross sections of both types of fibers. Note the larger diameter of fast fibers.

used repeatedly for endurance events, some of the fast fibers will develop the appearance and functional capabilities of intermediate fibers. The muscle as a whole will thus become more resistant to fatigue.

Muscles dominated by fast fibers appear pale and are often called **white muscles.** Chicken breasts contain "white meat" because chickens use their wings only for brief intervals, as when fleeing from a predator, and the power for flight comes from the anaerobic process of glycolysis in the fast fibers of their breast muscles. As we saw earlier, the extensive blood vessels and myoglobin in slow fibers give these fibers a reddish color; muscles dominated by slow fibers are therefore known as **red muscles.** Chickens walk around all day, and these movements are powered by aerobic metabolism in the slow fibers of the "dark meat" of their legs.

Most human muscles contain a mixture of fiber types and so appear pink. However, there are no slow fibers in muscles of the eye or hand, where swift, but brief, contractions are required. Many back and calf muscles are dominated by slow fibers; these muscles contract almost continuously to maintain an upright posture. The percentage of fast versus slow fibers in each muscle is genetically determined. As noted earlier, the ratio of intermediate fibers to fast fibers can increase as a result of athletic training.

Muscle Hypertrophy and Atrophy

As a result of repeated, exhaustive stimulation, muscle fibers develop more mitochondria, a higher concentration of glycolytic enzymes, and larger glycogen reserves. Such muscle fibers have more myofibrils than do fibers that are less used, and each myofibril contains more thick and thin filaments. The net effect is **hypertrophy,** or an enlargement of the stimulated muscle. The number of muscle fibers does not change significantly, but the muscle as a whole enlarges because each muscle fiber increases in diameter.

Hypertrophy occurs in muscles that have been repeatedly stimulated to produce near-maximal tension. The intracellular changes that occur increase the amount of tension produced when these muscles contract. The muscles of a bodybuilder are excellent examples of muscular hypertrophy.

Clinical Note

A skeletal muscle that is not regularly stimulated by a motor neuron loses muscle tone and mass. The muscle becomes flaccid, and the muscle fibers become smaller and weaker. This reduction in muscle size, tone, and power is called **atrophy**. Individuals paralyzed by spinal injuries or other damage to the nervous system will gradually lose muscle tone and size in the areas affected. Even a temporary reduction in muscle use can lead to muscular atrophy; you can easily observe this effect by comparing "before and after" limb muscles in someone who has worn a cast. Muscle atrophy is initially reversible, but dying muscle fibers are not replaced. In extreme atrophy, the functional losses are permanent. That is why physical therapy is crucial for people who are temporarily unable to move normally. Electrical stimulation by an external device can substitute for nerve stimulation and prevent or reduce muscle atrophy.

Because skeletal muscles depend on motor neurons for stimulation, disorders that affect the nervous system can indirectly affect the muscular system. In *polio*, a virus attacks motor neurons in the spinal cord and brain, causing muscular paralysis and atrophy.

Providing Energy for Muscle Contraction

As a muscle contracts, the bonds of ATP molecules are hydrolyzed to release the needed energy. Surprisingly, muscles store very limited supplies of ATP—only 4 to 6 seconds' worth, just enough to get you going. Since ATP is the *only* energy source that can be used directly to power muscle activity, ATP must be regenerated continuously if contraction is to continue.

Essentially, working muscles use three pathways for ATP regeneration:

1. **Direct phosphorylation of ADP by creatine phosphate** (Figure 6.14a). The unique high-energy molecule **creatine phosphate (CP)** is found in muscle fibers but not other cell types. As ATP is being depleted, interactions between CP and ADP result in transfers of a high-energy phosphate group from CP to ADP, thus regenerating more ATP in a fraction of a second. Although muscle cells store perhaps five times as much CP as ATP, the CP supplies are also soon exhausted (in about 20 seconds).

2. **Aerobic respiration** (Figure 6.14b). At rest and during light to moderate exercise, some 95 percent of the ATP used for muscle activity comes from aerobic respiration. **Aerobic respiration** occurs in the mitochondria and involves a series of metabolic pathways that use oxygen. These pathways are collectively referred to as *oxidative phosphorylation*. During aerobic respiration, glucose is broken down completely to carbon dioxide and water, and some of the energy released as the bonds are broken is captured in the bonds of ATP molecules. Although aerobic respiration provides a rich ATP harvest (36 ATP per 1 glucose), it is fairly slow and requires continuous delivery of oxygen and nutrient fuels to the muscle to keep it going.

3. **Anaerobic glycolysis and lactic acid formation** (Figure 6.14c). The initial steps of glucose breakdown occur via a pathway called *glycolysis*, which does not use oxygen and hence is an *anaerobic* (literally "without oxygen") part of the metabolic pathway. During glycolysis, which occurs in the cytosol, glucose is broken down to pyruvic acid, and small amounts of energy are captured in ATP bonds (2 ATP per 1 glucose molecule). As long as enough oxygen is present, the pyruvic acid then enters the oxygen-requiring aerobic pathways that occur within the mitochondria to produce more ATP as described above. However, when muscle activity is intense, or oxygen and glucose delivery is temporarily inadequate to meet the needs of the working muscles, the sluggish aerobic mechanisms cannot keep up with the demands for ATP. Under these conditions, the pyruvic acid generated during glycolysis is converted to **lactic acid,** and the overall process is referred to as **anaerobic glycolysis.**

Anaerobic glycolysis produces only about 5 percent as much ATP from each glucose molecule as aerobic respiration. However, it is some 2½ times faster, and it can provide most of the ATP needed for 30 to 60 seconds of strenuous muscle activity. The main shortcomings of anaerobic glycolysis are that it uses

Q *Which of these methods of ATP generation is commonly used by the leg muscles of a long-distance cyclist?*

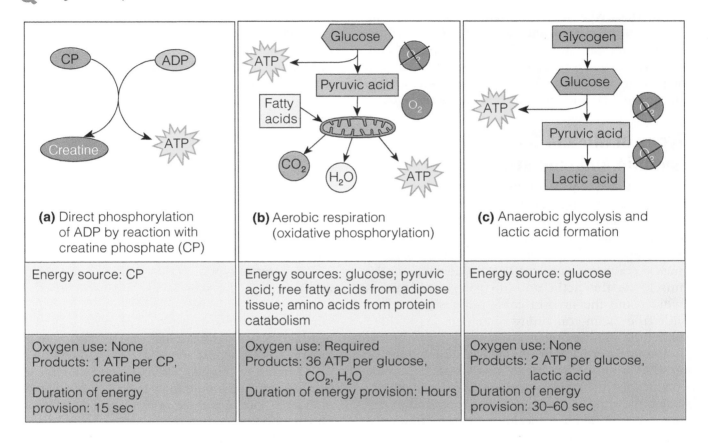

(a) Direct phosphorylation of ADP by reaction with creatine phosphate (CP)	(b) Aerobic respiration (oxidative phosphorylation)	(c) Anaerobic glycolysis and lactic acid formation
Energy source: CP	Energy sources: glucose; pyruvic acid; free fatty acids from adipose tissue; amino acids from protein catabolism	Energy source: glucose
Oxygen use: None Products: 1 ATP per CP, creatine Duration of energy provision: 15 sec	Oxygen use: Required Products: 36 ATP per glucose, CO_2, H_2O Duration of energy provision: Hours	Oxygen use: None Products: 2 ATP per glucose, lactic acid Duration of energy provision: 30–60 sec

FIGURE 6.14 Methods of regenerating ATP during muscle activity. The fastest mechanism is **(a)** direct phosphorylation; the slowest is **(b)** aerobic respiration.

huge amounts of glucose for a small ATP harvest, and accumulating lactic acid promotes muscle fatigue and muscle soreness.

Muscle Fatigue and Oxygen Debt

If we exercise our muscles strenuously for a long time, **muscle fatigue** occurs. A muscle is fatigued when it is unable to contract even though it is still being stimulated. Without rest, an active or working muscle begins to tire and contracts more weakly until it finally ceases reacting and stops contracting. Muscle fatigue is believed to result from the **oxygen debt** that occurs during prolonged muscle activity: A person is not able to take in oxygen fast enough to

keep the muscles supplied with all the oxygen they need when they are working vigorously. Obviously, then, the work that a muscle can do and how long it can work without becoming fatigued depend on how good its blood supply is. When muscles lack oxygen, lactic acid begins to accumulate in the muscle via the anaerobic mechanism described above. In addition, the muscle's ATP supply starts to run low. The increasing acidity in the muscle and the lack of ATP cause the muscle to contract less and less effectively and finally to stop contracting altogether.

True muscle fatigue, in which the muscle quits entirely, rarely occurs in most of us because we feel fatigued long before it happens and we simply slow down or stop our activity. It *does* happen commonly in marathon runners. Many of them have literally collapsed when their muscles became fatigued and could no longer work.

A   *The aerobic mechanism (b).*

Oxygen debt, which always occurs to some extent during vigorous muscle activity, must be "paid back" whether or not fatigue occurs. During the recovery period after activity, the individual breathes rapidly and deeply. This continues until the muscles have received the amount of oxygen needed to get rid of the accumulated lactic acid and make ATP and creatine phosphate reserves.

Types of Muscle Contractions— Isotonic and Isometric

Until now, we have been discussing contraction in terms of shortening behavior, but muscles do not always shorten when they contract. (I can hear you saying, "What kind of double-talk is that?"—but pay attention.) The event that is common to all muscle contractions is that *tension* develops in the muscle as the actin and myosin myofilaments interact and the myosin cross bridges attempt to slide the actin-containing filaments past them within the muscle fibers.

Isotonic contractions (literally, "same tone" or tension) are more familiar to most of us. In isotonic contractions, the myofilaments are successful in their sliding movements, the muscle shortens, and movement occurs. Bending the knee, rotating the arms, and smiling are all examples of isotonic contractions.

Contractions in which the muscles do not shorten are called **isometric contractions** (literally, "same measurement" or length). In isometric contractions, the myosin myofilaments are "skidding their wheels," and the tension in the muscle keeps increasing. They are trying to slide, but the muscle is pitted against some more or less immovable object. For example, muscles are contracting isometrically when you try to lift a 400-pound dresser alone. When you straighten a bent elbow, the triceps muscle is contracting isotonically. But when you push against a wall with bent elbows, the wall doesn't move, and the triceps muscles, which cannot shorten to straighten the elbows, are contracting isometrically.

Muscle Tone

One aspect of skeletal muscle activity cannot be consciously controlled. Even when a muscle is voluntarily relaxed, some of its fibers remain contracted—first one group and then another.

Their contraction is not visible, but, as a result of it, the muscle remains firm, healthy, and constantly ready for action. This state of continuous partial contractions is called **muscle tone** or **tonus.** Muscle tone is the result of different motor units, which are scattered through the muscle, being stimulated by the nervous system in a systematic way.

Homeostatic Imbalance

If the nerve supply to a muscle is destroyed (as in an accident), the muscle is no longer stimulated in this manner, and it loses tone and becomes paralyzed. Soon after, it becomes *flaccid* (flak'sid), or soft and flabby, and begins to *atrophy* (waste away). ▲

Effect of Exercise on Muscles

The amount of work done by a muscle is reflected in changes in the muscle itself. Muscle inactivity (due to a loss of nerve supply, immobilization, or whatever the cause) always leads to muscle weakness and wasting. Muscles are no exception to the saying, "Use it or lose it!"

Conversely, regular exercise increases muscle size, strength, and endurance. However, not all types of exercise produce these effects—in fact, there are important differences in the benefits of exercise.

Aerobic, or **endurance,** types of exercise such as participating in an aerobics class, jogging, or biking (Figure 6.15a), result in stronger, more flexible muscles with greater resistance to fatigue. These changes come about, at least partly, because the blood supply to the muscles increases, and the individual muscle cells form more mitochondria and store more oxygen. However, aerobic exercise benefits much more than the skeletal muscles. It makes overall body metabolism more efficient, improves digestion (and elimination), enhances neuromuscular coordination, and makes the skeleton stronger. The heart enlarges (*hypertrophies*) so that more blood is pumped out with each beat, fat deposits are cleared from the blood vessel walls, and the lungs become more efficient in gas exchange. These benefits may be permanent or temporary, depending on how often and how vigorously one exercises.

Aerobic exercise does *not* cause the muscles to increase much in size, even though the exercise may go on for hours. The bulging muscles of a bodybuilder or professional weight lifter result

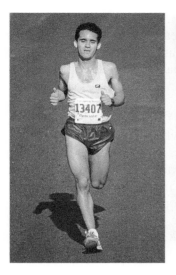 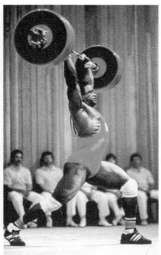

(a)   **(b)**

FIGURE 6.15 **The effects of aerobic training versus strength training. (a)** A marathon runner. **(b)** A weight lifter.

mainly from **resistance,** or **isometric, exercises** (Figure 6.15b) in which the muscles are pitted against some immovable object (or nearly so). Resistance exercises require very little time and little or no special equipment. A few minutes every other day is usually sufficient. A wall can be pushed against, and buttock muscles can be strongly contracted even while standing in line at the grocery store. The key is forcing the muscles to contract with as much force as possible. The increased muscle size and strength that results is due mainly to enlargement of individual muscle cells (they make more contractile filaments), rather than an increase in their number. The amount of connective tissue that reinforces the muscle also increases.

Because endurance and resistance exercises produce different patterns of muscle response, it is important to know what your exercise goals are. Lifting weights will not improve your endurance for a marathon. By the same token, jogging will do little to improve your muscle definition for competing in the Mr. or Ms. Muscle contest, nor will it make you stronger for moving furniture. Obviously, the best exercise program for most people is one that includes both types of exercise.

Muscle Movements, Types, and Names

This section is a bit of a hodge-podge. It includes some topics that don't really fit together, but they don't fit anywhere else any better. For example, there are five very basic understandings about gross muscle activity. I call these the *Five Golden Rules* of skeletal muscle activity because until you understand them, comprehending muscle movements and appreciating muscle interactions is nearly impossible. These golden rules are summarized for your quick review in Table 6.4.

Levers

Skeletal muscles do not work in isolation. For muscles attached to the skeleton, the nature and site of the connection determine the force, speed, and range of the movement produced. These characteristics are interdependent, and the relationships can explain a great deal about the general organization of the muscular and skeletal systems.

The force, speed, or direction of movement produced by contraction of a muscle can be modified by attaching the muscle to a lever. A **lever** is a rigid structure—such as a board, a crowbar, or a bone—that moves on a fixed point called the **fulcrum.** A lever moves when an applied force (AF) is sufficient to overcome any resistance (R) that would otherwise oppose or prevent such movement. In the body, each bone is a lever and each joint is a fulcrum, and muscles provide the applied force. The resistance

TABLE 6.4	The Five Golden Rules of Skeletal Muscle Activity

1. With a few exceptions, all muscles cross at least one joint.
2. Typically, the bulk of the muscle lies proximal to the joint crossed.
3. All muscles have at least two attachments: the origin and the insertion.
4. Muscles can only pull; they never push.
5. During contraction, the muscle insertion moves toward the origin.

can vary from the weight of an object held in the hand to the weight of a limb or the weight of the entire body, depending on the situation. The important thing about levers is that they can change (1) the direction of an applied force, (2) the distance and speed of movement produced by an applied force, and (3) the effective strength of an applied force.

Classes of Levers

There are three classes of levers, and examples of each are found in the human body (Figure 6.16). The seesaw or teeter-totter is an example of a **first-class lever.** In such a lever, the fulcrum (F) lies between the applied force (AF) and the resistance (R). The body has few first-class levers. One, involved with extension of the neck, is shown in Figure 6.16a.

In a **second-class lever** (Figure 6.16b), the resistance is located between the applied force and the fulcrum. A familiar example is a loaded wheelbarrow. The weight of the load is the resistance, and the upward lift on the handle is the applied force. Because in this arrangement the force is always farther from the fulcrum than the resistance is, a small force can move a larger weight. That is, the effective force is increased. Notice, however, that when a force moves the handle, the load moves more slowly and covers a shorter distance. Thus the effective force is increased at the expense of speed and distance. The body has few second-class levers. Ankle extension (plantar flexion) by the calf muscles involves a second-class lever (Figure 6.16b).

Third-class levers are the most common levers in the body. In this lever system, a force is applied between the resistance and the fulcrum (Figure 6.16c). The effect is the reverse of that for a second-class lever: Speed and distance traveled are increased at the expense of effective force. In the example shown (the biceps brachii muscle, which flexes the elbow), the resistance is six times farther from the fulcrum than is the applied force. The effective force is reduced to the same degree. The muscle must generate 180 kg of tension at its attachment to the forearm to support 30 kg held in the hand. However, the distance traveled and the speed of movement are increased by that same 6:1 ratio: The load will travel 45 cm when the point of attachment moves 7.5 cm.

Although not every muscle operates as part of a lever system, the presence of levers provides speed and versatility far in excess of what we would predict on the basis of muscle physiology alone. Skeletal muscle fibers resemble one another closely, and their abilities to contract and generate tension are quite similar. Consider a skeletal muscle that can shorten 1 cm while it exerts a 10-kg pull. Without using a lever, this muscle would be performing efficiently only when moving a 10-kg weight a distance of 1 cm. By using a lever, however, the same muscle operating at the same efficiency could move 20 kg a distance of 0.5 cm, 5 kg a distance of 2 cm, or 1 kg a distance of 10 cm.

100 Keys | Most skeletal muscles can shorten to roughly 70 percent of their "ideal" resting length. The versatility in terms of power, speed, and range of body movements results from differences in the positions of muscle attachments relative to the joints involved.

This chapter focuses on the functional anatomy of skeletal muscles and muscle groups. You must learn a number of new terms, and this section attempts to help you understand them. It may also help you to create a vocabulary list from the terms introduced. Once you are familiar with the basic terminology, the names and actions of skeletal muscles are easily understood.

Origins and Insertions

Earlier in this chapter we noted that when both ends of a myofibril are free to move, the ends move toward the center during a contraction. In the body, however, the ends of a skeletal muscle are always attached to other structures that limit their movement. In most cases, one end is fixed in position, and during a contraction, the other end moves toward the fixed end. The place where the fixed end attaches to a bone, cartilage, or connective tissue is called the **origin** of the muscle. The site where the movable end attaches to another structure is called the **insertion** of the muscle. The origin is typically proximal to the insertion. When a muscle contracts, it produces a specific **action,** or movement. Actions are described using the terms introduced (flexion, extension, adduction, and so forth).

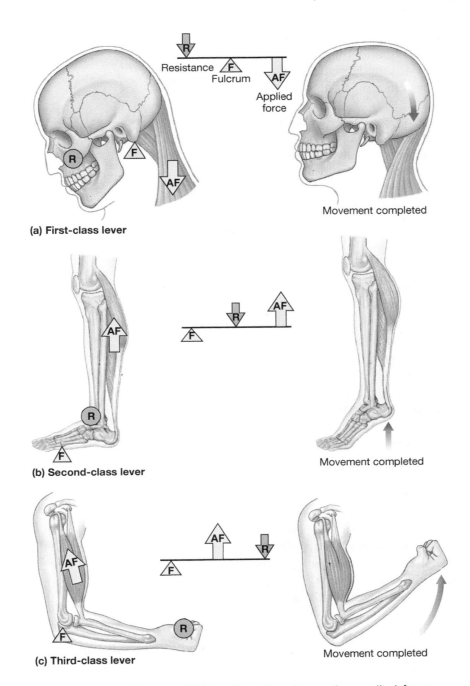

Resistance
Fulcrum
Applied force
Movement completed

(a) First-class lever

Movement completed

(b) Second-class lever

Movement completed

(c) Third-class lever

FIGURE 6.16 **The three classes of levers. (a)** In a first-class lever, the applied force and the resistance are on opposite sides of the fulcrum. **(b)** In a second-class lever, the resistance lies between the applied force and the fulcrum. **(c)** In a third-class lever, the force is applied between the resistance and the fulcrum.

As an example, consider the *gastrocnemius muscle*, a calf muscle that extends from the distal portion of the femur to the calcaneus. As Figure 6.16b shows, when the gastrocnemius muscle contracts, it pulls the calcaneus toward the knee. As a result, we say that the gastrocnemius muscle has its origin at the femur and its insertion at the calcaneus; its action can be described as "extension at the ankle" or "plantar flexion."

The decision as to which end is the origin and which is the insertion is usually based on movement from the anatomical position. Part of the fun of studying the muscular system is that you can actually do the movements and think about the muscles involved. As a result, laboratory discussions of the muscular system tend to resemble disorganized aerobics classes.

Generally speaking, body movement occurs when muscles contract across joints. The type of movement depends on the mobility of the joint and on where the muscle is located in relation to the joint. The most obvious examples of the action of muscles on bones are the movements that occur at the joints of the limbs. However, less freely movable bones are also tugged into motion by the muscles, such as the vertebrae's movements when the torso is bent to the side.

The most common types of body movements are described next and shown in Figure 6.17. Try to demonstrate each movement as you read the following descriptions:

- **Flexion.** A movement, generally in the sagittal plane, that decreases the angle of the joint and brings two bones closer together (Figure 6.17a and b). Flexion is typical of hinge joints (bending the knee or elbow), but it is also common at ball-and-socket joints (bending forward at the hip).

- **Extension.** Extension is the opposite of flexion, so it is a movement that increases the angle, or the distance, between two bones or parts of the body (straightening the knee or elbow). If extension is greater than 180° (as when you tip your head or your torso posteriorly so that your chin points toward the ceiling), it is hyperextension (Figure 6.17a and b).

- **Rotation.** Rotation is movement of a bone around its longitudinal axis (Figure 6.17c). Rotation is a common movement of ball-and-socket joints and describes the movement of the atlas around the dens of the axis (as in shaking your head "no").

- **Abduction.** Abduction is moving a limb away (generally on the frontal plane) from the midline, or median plane, of the body (Figure 6.17d). The terminology also applies to the fanning movement of the fingers or toes when they are spread apart.

- **Adduction.** Adduction is the opposite of abduction, so it is the movement of a limb toward the body midline (Figure 6.17d).

Q The other movement that the biceps brachii muscle (shown in this illustration) can bring about is to move the torso toward the bar when you chin yourself. Would the forearm still be the insertion for that movement?

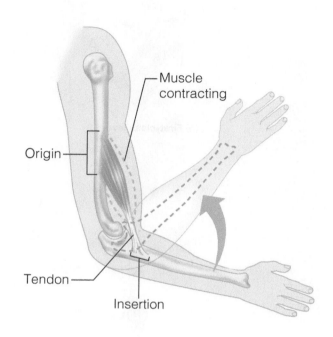

- **Circumduction.** Circumduction is a combination of flexion, extension, abduction, and adduction commonly seen in ball-and-socket joints such as the shoulder. The proximal end of the limb is stationary, and its distal end moves in a circle. The limb as a whole outlines a cone (Figure 6.17d).

Special Movements

Certain movements do not fit into any of the previous categories and occur at only a few joints. Some of these special movements are shown in Figure 6.17.

- **Dorsiflexion and plantar flexion.** Up and down movements of the foot at the ankle are given special names. Lifting the foot so that its superior surface approaches the shin (standing on your heels) is called dorsiflexion, whereas depressing the foot (pointing the toes) is called plantar flexion (Figure 6.17e).

A No, the insertion in this case would be its attachment to the humerus, and the attachment on the forearm (which is held steady during this movement) is the insertion.

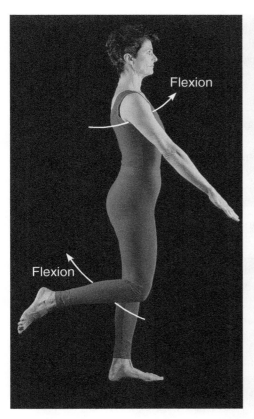
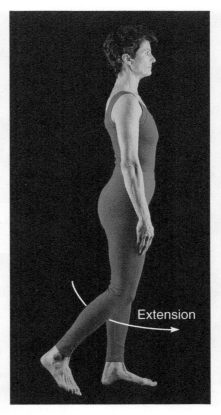
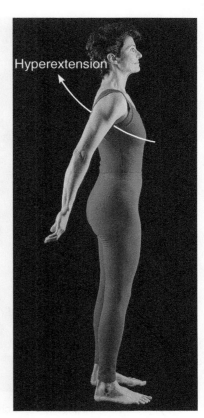

(a) Flexion and extension of the shoulder and knee

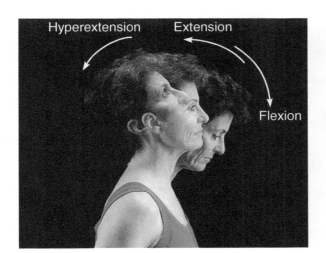

(b) Flexion, extension, and hyperextension

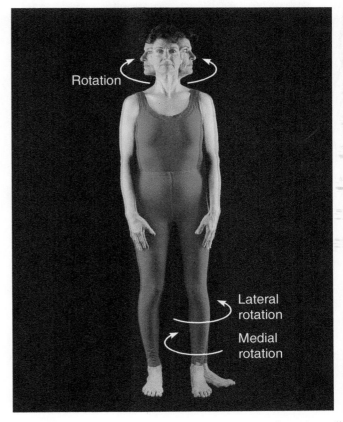

(c) Rotation

FIGURE 6.17   **Body movements.**

(continued)

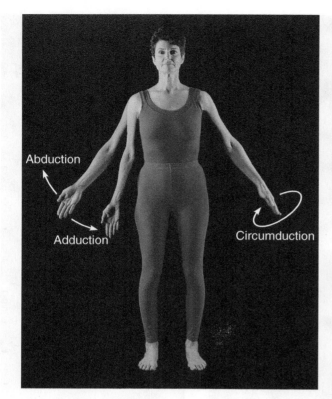

(d) Abduction, adduction, and circumduction

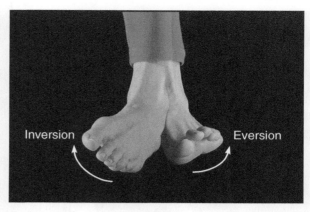

(f) Inversion and eversion

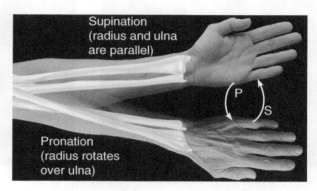

(g) Supination (S) and pronation (P)

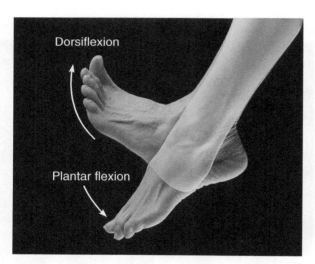

(e) Dorsiflexion and plantar flexion

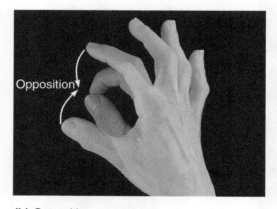

(h) Opposition

FIGURE 6.17 *(continued)*

Dorsiflexion of the foot corresponds to extension of the hand at the wrist, whereas plantar flexion of the foot corresponds to flexion of the hand.

- **Inversion and eversion.** Inversion and eversion are also special movements of the foot (Figure 6.17f). To invert the foot, turn the sole medially. To evert the foot, turn the sole laterally.

- **Supination and pronation.** The terms supination (soo″pĭ-na′shun; "turning backward") and pronation (pro-na′shun; "turning forward") refer to movements of the radius around the ulna (Figure 6.17g). Supination occurs when the forearm rotates laterally so that the palm faces anteriorly, and the radius and ulna are parallel. Pronation occurs when the forearm rotates medially so that the palm faces posteriorly. Pronation brings the radius across the ulna so that the two bones form an X. A helpful memory trick: If you lift a cup of soup up to your mouth *on your palm,* you are supinating ("soup"-inating).

- **Opposition.** In the palm of the hand, the saddle joint between metacarpal 1 and the carpals allows opposition of the thumb (Figure 6.17h). This is the action by which you move your thumb to touch the tips of the other fingers on the same hand. It is this unique action that makes the human hand such a fine tool for grasping and manipulating things.

Interactions of Skeletal Muscles in the Body

Muscles can't push—they can only pull as they contract—so most often body movements are the result of the activity of two or more muscles acting together or against each other. Muscles are arranged in such a way that whatever one muscle (or group of muscles) can do, other muscles can reverse. Because of this, muscles are able to bring about an immense variety of movements.

The muscle that has the major responsibility for causing a particular movement is called the **prime mover.** (This physiological term has been borrowed by the business world to label a person who gets things done.) Muscles that oppose or reverse a movement are **antagonists** (an-tag′o-nists). When

a prime mover is active, its antagonist is stretched and relaxed. Antagonists can be prime movers in their own right. For example, the biceps of the arm (prime mover of elbow flexion) is antagonized by the triceps (a prime mover of elbow extension).

Synergists (sin′er-jists; *syn* = together, *erg* = work) help prime movers by producing the same movement or by reducing undesirable movements. When a muscle crosses two or more joints, its contraction will cause movement in all the joints crossed unless synergists are there to stabilize them. For example, the finger-flexor muscles cross both the wrist and the finger joints. You can make a fist without bending your wrist because synergist muscles stabilize the wrist joints and allow the prime mover to act on the finger joints.

Fixators are specialized synergists. They hold a bone still or stabilize the origin of a prime mover so all the tension can be used to move the insertion bone. The postural muscles that stabilize the vertebral column are fixators, as are the muscles that anchor the scapulae to the thorax.

In summary, although prime movers seem to get all the credit for causing certain movements, the actions of antagonistic and synergistic muscles are also important in effecting smooth, coordinated, and precise movements.

Naming Skeletal Muscles

Like bones, muscles come in many shapes and sizes to suit their particular tasks in the body. Muscles are named on the basis of several criteria, each of which focuses on a particular structural or functional characteristic. Paying close attention to these cues can greatly simplify your task of learning muscle names and actions:

- **Direction of the muscle fibers.** Some muscles are named in reference to some imaginary line, usually the midline of the body or the long axis of a limb bone. When a muscle's name includes the term *rectus* (straight), its fibers run parallel to that imaginary line. For example, the rectus femoris is the straight muscle of the thigh, or femur. Similarly, the term *oblique* as part of a muscle's name tells you that the muscle fibers run obliquely (at a slant) to the imaginary line.

A Closer Look

Are Athletes Looking Good and Doing Better with Anabolic Steroids?

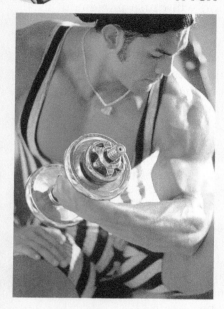

EVERYONE loves a winner, and top athletes are popular and make lots of money. It is not surprising that some will grasp at anything to increase their performance—including anabolic steroids. These hormones, engineered by pharmaceutical companies, were introduced in the 1950s to treat victims of certain muscle-wasting diseases and anemia and to prevent muscle atrophy in patients immobilized after surgery. Testosterone, a natural anabolic steroid hormone made by the body, triggers the increase in muscle and bone mass and other physical changes that occur during puberty and convert boys into men. Convinced that huge doses of the anabolic steroids could enhance masculinizing effects in grown men, many athletes were using the steroids by the early 1960s, and the practice is still going strong today. Indeed, it is estimated that one out of every ten young men has tried steroids, so use is no longer confined to athletes looking for the edge.

The use of these drugs has been banned by most international athletic competitions, and users (and prescribing physicians or drug dealers) are naturally reluctant to talk about it. Nonetheless, there is little question that many professional bodybuilders and athletes competing in events that require great muscle strength (such as discus throwing and weight lifting) are heavy users. Sports figures such as football players have also admitted to using steroids to help them prepare for games. Advantages of anabolic steroids cited by athletes include increased muscle mass and strength, increased oxygen-carrying capacity of the blood (because of greater red blood cell volume), and an increase in aggressive behavior (the urge to "steamroller the other guy").

But do the drugs do all that is claimed for them? Research studies have reported increases in isometric strength and body weight in steroid users. Although these are results weightlifters dream about, there is a hot dispute over whether the drugs also enhance the fine muscle coordination and endurance needed by runners and others.

Do the claimed slight advantages conferred by steroid use outweigh the risks? Absolutely not! Physicians say they cause bloated faces (a sign of steroid excess), shriveled testes, and infertility; damage the liver and promote liver cancer; and cause changes in blood-cholesterol levels (which may place long-term users at risk for coronary heart disease). Additionally, about one-third of anabolic steroid users develop serious psychiatric problems. Manic behavior in which the users undergo Jekyll–Hyde personality swings and become extremely violent (the so-called 'roid rage) is common; so, too, are depression and delusions.

A recent arrival on the scene, sold over the counter as a "nutritional performance enhancer," is androstenedione, which is converted to testosterone in the body. It is taken orally and much of it is destroyed by the liver soon after ingestion, but the few milligrams that survive temporarily boost testosterone levels. "Wannabe" athletes from the fifth grade up are said to be sweeping the supplement off the drugstore shelves.

This is troubling; androstenedione is not regulated by the U.S. Food and Drug Administration (FDA) and its long-term effects are unpredictable. Ongoing studies have found that males who took the supplement developed elevated levels of the female hormone estrogen as well as testosterone (raising their risk of feminizing effects such as enlarged breasts), early puberty, and stunted bone growth.

The question of why athletes use these drugs is easy to answer. Some say they are willing to do almost anything to win, short of killing themselves. Are they unwittingly doing this as well?

- **Relative size of the muscle.** Such terms as *maximus* (largest), *minimus* (smallest), and *longus* (long) are often used in the names of muscles—for example, the gluteus maximus is the largest muscle of the gluteus muscle group.

- **Location of the muscle.** Some muscles are named for the bone with which they are associated. For example, the temporalis and frontalis muscles overlie the temporal and frontal bones of the skull, respectively.

- **Number of origins.** When the term *biceps, triceps,* or *quadriceps* forms part of a muscle name, one can assume that the muscle has two, three, or four origins, respectively. For example, the biceps muscle of the arm has two heads, or origins, and the triceps muscle has three.

- **Location of the muscle's origin and insertion.** Occasionally, muscles are named for their attachment sites. For example, the sternocleidomastoid muscle has its origin on the sternum (*sterno*) and clavicle (*cleido*) and inserts on the *mastoid* process of the temporal bone.

- **Shape of the muscle.** Some muscles have a distinctive shape that helps to identify them. For example, the deltoid muscle is roughly triangular (*deltoid* means "triangular").

- **Action of the muscle.** When muscles are named for their actions, terms such as *flexor, extensor,* and *adductor* appear in their names. For example, the adductor muscles of the thigh all bring about its adduction, and the extensor muscles of the wrist all extend the wrist.

Arrangement of Fascicles

Skeletal muscles consist of fascicles, but fascicle arrangements vary, producing muscles with different

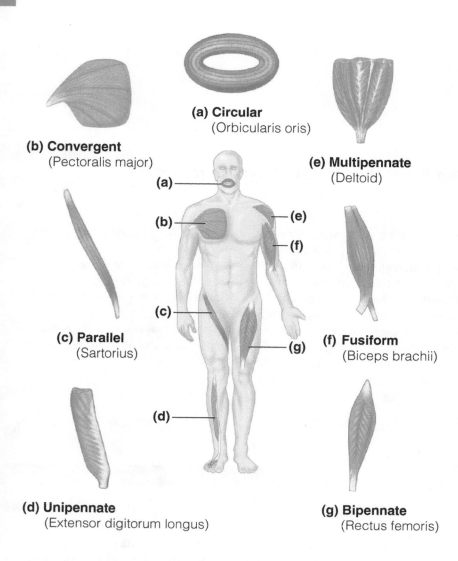

(a) **Circular**
(Orbicularis oris)

(b) **Convergent**
(Pectoralis major)

(a) ——

(b) ——

(c) ——

(d) ——

(e) ——

(f) ——

(g) ——

(e) **Multipennate**
(Deltoid)

(f) **Fusiform**
(Biceps brachii)

(c) **Parallel**
(Sartorius)

(d) **Unipennate**
(Extensor digitorum longus)

(g) **Bipennate**
(Rectus femoris)

FIGURE 6.18 **Relationship of fascicle arrangement to muscle structure.**

structures and functional properties. The most common patterns of fascicle arrangement are described next.

The pattern is **circular** when the fascicles are arranged in concentric rings (Figure 6.18a). Circular muscles are typically found surrounding external body openings which they close by contracting. A general term for such muscles is *sphincters* ("squeezers"). Examples are the orbicularis muscles surrounding the eyes and mouth.

In a **convergent** muscle, the fascicles converge toward a single insertion tendon. Such a muscle is triangular or fan-shaped like the pectoralis major muscle of the anterior thorax (Figure 6.18b).

In a **parallel** arrangement, the length of the fascicles run parallel to the long axis of the muscle. These muscles are straplike (Figure 6.18c). A modification of the parallel arrangement, called

fusiform, results in a spindle-shaped muscle with an expanded belly (midsection) like the biceps brachii muscle of the arm (Figure 6.18f).

In a **pennate** (pen′āt; "feather") pattern, short fascicles attach obliquely to a central tendon. In the extensor digitorum muscle of the leg, the fascicles insert into only one side of the tendon and the muscle is *unipennate* (Figure 6.18d). If the fascicles insert into opposite sides of the tendon or from several different sides, the muscle is *bipennate* (Figure 6.18g) or *multipennate* (Figure 6.18e), respectively.

A muscle's fascicle arrangement determines its range of motion and power. The longer and the more nearly parallel the fascicles are to a muscle's long axis, the more the muscle can shorten, but such muscles are not usually very powerful. Muscle power depends more on the total number of muscle

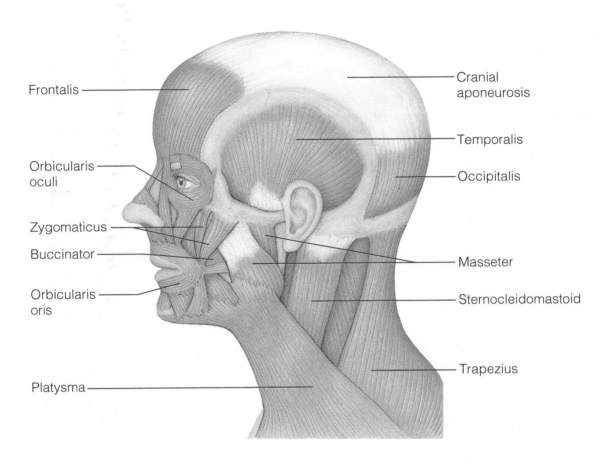

Frontalis

Cranial aponeurosis

Temporalis

Occipitalis

Orbicularis oculi

Zygomaticus

Buccinator

Masseter

Orbicularis oris

Sternocleidomastoid

Trapezius

Platysma

FIGURE 6.19   Superficial muscles of the face and neck.

cells in the muscle. The stocky bipennate and multipennate muscles, which pack in the most fibers, shorten very little but are very powerful.

Gross Anatomy of Skeletal Muscles

It is beyond the scope of this book to describe the hundreds of skeletal muscles of the human body. Only the most important muscles are described here. In addition, all the superficial muscles considered are summarized in Tables 6.5 and 6.6 and are illustrated in overall body views in Figures 6.25 and 6.26, which accompany the tables.

Head and Neck Muscles

The head muscles (Figure 6.19) are an interesting group. They have many specific functions but are usually grouped into two large categories—facial muscles and chewing muscles. Facial muscles are unique because they are inserted into soft tissues such as other muscles or skin. When they pull on the skin of the face, they permit us to smile faintly, grin widely, frown, pout, deliver a kiss, and so forth. The chewing muscles begin the breakdown of food for the body.

Facial Muscles

Frontalis   The frontalis covers the frontal bone as it runs from the cranial aponeurosis to the skin of the eyebrows, where it inserts. This muscle allows you to raise your eyebrows, as in surprise, and to wrinkle your forehead. At the posterior end of the cranial aponeurosis is the small **occipitalis** muscle, which covers the posterior aspect of the skull and pulls the scalp posteriorly.*

---

*Although the current references on anatomic terminology refer to the frontalis and occipitalis as the *frontal* and *occipital bellies* of the *epicranius* ("over the cranium") muscle, we will continue to use the terms frontalis and occipitalis here.

Orbicularis Oculi   The orbicularis oculi (or-bik"u-la'ris ok'u-li) has fibers that run in circles around the eyes. It allows you to close your eyes, squint, blink, and wink.

Orbicularis Oris   The orbicularis oris is the circular muscle of the lips. Because it closes the mouth and protrudes the lips, it is often called the "kissing" muscle.

Buccinator   The fleshy buccinator (bu'sĭ-na"tor) muscle runs horizontally across the cheek and inserts into the orbicularis oris. It flattens the cheek (as in whistling or blowing a trumpet). It is also listed as a chewing muscle because it compresses the cheek to hold the food between the teeth during chewing.

Zygomaticus   The zygomaticus (zi"go-mat'i-kus) extends from the corner of the mouth to the cheekbone. It is often referred to as the "smiling" muscle because it raises the corners of the mouth upward.

Chewing Muscles

The buccinator muscle, which is a member of this group, is described with the facial muscles.

Masseter   The masseter (mă-se'ter) covers the angle of the lower jaw as it runs from the zygomatic process of the temporal bone to the mandible. This muscle closes the jaw by elevating the mandible.

Temporalis   The temporalis is a fan-shaped muscle overlying the temporal bone. It inserts into the mandible and acts as a synergist of the masseter in closing the jaw.

Neck Muscles

For the most part, the neck muscles, which move the head and shoulder girdle, are small and straplike. Only two neck muscles are considered here.

Platysma   The platysma is a single sheetlike muscle that covers the anterolateral neck (see Figure 6.19). It originates from the connective tissue covering of the chest muscles and inserts into the area around the mouth. Its action is to pull the corners of the mouth inferiorly, producing a downward sag of the mouth.

Sternocleidomastoid   The paired sternocleidomastoid (ster"no-kli"do-mas'toid) muscles are two-headed muscles, one found on each side of the neck. Of the two heads of each muscle, one arises from the sternum and the other arises from the clavicle. The heads fuse before inserting into the mastoid process of the temporal bone. When both sternocleidomastoid muscles contract together, they flex your neck. (It is this action of bowing the head that has led some people to call these muscles the "prayer" muscles.) If just one muscle contracts, the head is rotated toward the opposite side.

⚖ Homeostatic Imbalance

In some difficult births, one of these muscles may be injured and develop spasms. A baby injured in this way has *torticollis* (tor"ti-kol'is), or wryneck. ▲

Trunk Muscles

The trunk muscles include (1) those that move the vertebral column (most of which are posterior anti-gravity muscles); (2) anterior thorax muscles, which move the ribs, head, and arms; and (3) muscles of the abdominal wall, which help to move the vertebral column and, most importantly, form the muscular "natural girdle" of the abdominal body wall.

Anterior Muscles   (Figure 6.20)

Pectoralis Major   The pectoralis (pek"to-ra'lis) major is a large fan-shaped muscle covering the upper part of the chest. Its origin is from the sternum, shoulder girdle, and the first six ribs. It inserts on the proximal end of the humerus. This muscle forms the anterior wall of the axilla and acts to adduct and flex the arm.

Intercostal Muscles   The intercostal muscles are deep muscles found between the ribs. (Although they are not shown in Figure 6.20, which only shows superficial muscles, they are illustrated in Figure 6.25.) The external intercostals are important in breathing because they help to raise the rib cage for breathing air in. The internal intercostals, which lie deep to the external intercostals, depress the rib cage, which helps to move air out of the lungs when you exhale forcibly.

Muscles of the Abdominal Girdle   The anterior abdominal muscles (rectus abdominis, external and internal obliques, and transversus abdominis) form a natural "girdle" that reinforces the body trunk. Taken together, they resemble the structure of plywood because the fibers of each muscle or muscle pair run in a different direction. Just as

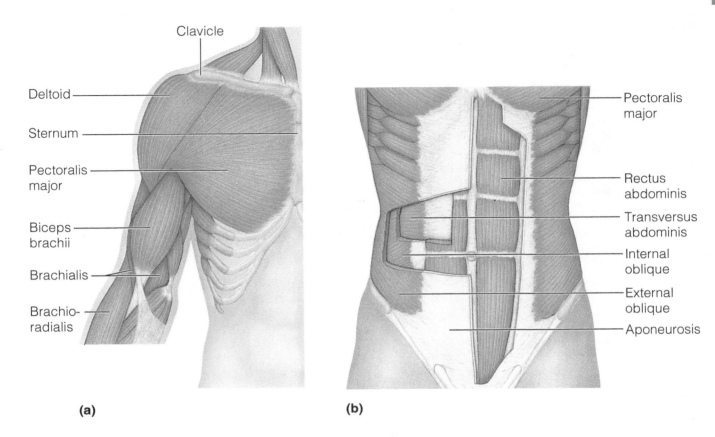

Clavicle

Deltoid

Sternum

Pectoralis major

Biceps brachii

Brachialis

Brachio-radialis

Pectoralis major

Rectus abdominis

Transversus abdominis

Internal oblique

External oblique

Aponeurosis

(a)

(b)

FIGURE 6.20 Muscles of the anterior trunk, shoulder, and arm.
(a) Muscles crossing the shoulder joint, causing movements of the arm.
The platysma of the neck is removed. **(b)** Muscles of the abdominal wall.
Portions of the superficial muscles of the right side of the abdomen are
cut away to reveal the deeper muscles.

plywood is exceptionally strong for its thickness, the abdominal muscles form a muscular wall that is well suited for its job of containing and protecting the abdominal contents.

- **Rectus abdominis.** The paired straplike rectus abdominis muscles are the most superficial muscles of the abdomen. They run from the pubis to the rib cage, enclosed in an aponeurosis. Their main function is to flex the vertebral column. They also compress the abdominal contents during defecation and childbirth and are involved in forced breathing.

- **External oblique.** The external oblique muscles are paired superficial muscles that make up the lateral walls of the abdomen. Their fibers run downward and medially from the last eight ribs and insert into the ilium. Like the rectus abdominis, they flex the vertebral column, but they also rotate the trunk and bend it laterally.

- **Internal oblique.** The internal oblique muscles are paired muscles deep to the external obliques. Their fibers run at right angles to those of the external obliques. They arise from the iliac crest and insert into the last three ribs. Their functions are the same as those of the external obliques.

- **Transversus abdominis.** The transversus abdominis is the deepest muscle of the abdominal wall and has fibers that run horizontally across the abdomen. It arises from the lower ribs and iliac crest and inserts into the pubis. This muscle compresses the abdominal contents.

Posterior Muscles (Figure 6.21)

Trapezius The trapezius (trah-pe′ze-us) muscles are the most superficial muscles of the posterior

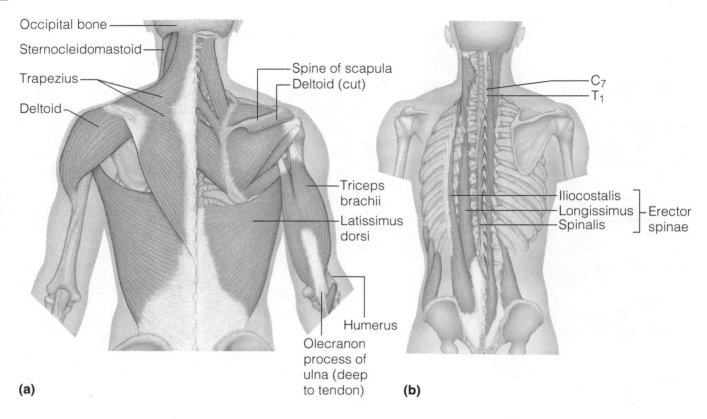

Occipital bone
Sternocleidomastoid
Trapezius
Deltoid

Spine of scapula
Deltoid (cut)
Triceps brachii
Latissimus dorsi
Humerus
Olecranon process of ulna (deep to tendon)

(a)

C₇
T₁
Iliocostalis
Longissimus
Spinalis
Erector spinae

(b)

FIGURE 6.21   Muscles of the posterior neck, trunk, and arm.
(a) Superficial muscles. **(b)** The erector spinae muscles (longissimus, iliocostalis, and spinalis), deep muscles of the back.

neck and upper trunk. When seen together, they form a diamond- or kite-shaped muscle mass. Their origin is very broad. Each muscle runs from the occipital bone of the skull down the vertebral column to the end of the thoracic vertebrae. They then flare laterally to insert on the scapular spine and clavicle. The trapezius muscles extend the head (thus they are antagonists of the sternocleidomastoids). They also can elevate, depress, adduct, and stabilize the scapula.

Latissimus Dorsi   The latissimus (lah-tis′ĭ-mus) dorsi is the large, flat muscle pair that covers the lower back. It originates on the lower spine and ilium and then sweeps superiorly to insert into the proximal end of the humerus. The latissimus dorsi extends and adducts the humerus. These are very important muscles when the arm must be brought down in a power stroke, as when swimming or striking a blow.

Erector Spinae   The erector spinae (e-rek′tor spi′ne) group is a prime mover of back extension. These

paired muscles are deep muscles of the back; they are shown in Figure 6.21b. Each erector spinae is a composite muscle consisting of three muscle columns (longissimus, iliocostalis, and spinalis) that collectively span the entire length of the vertebral column. These muscles not only act as powerful back extensors ("erectors"), but also provide resistance that helps control the action of bending over at the waist. Following injury to back structures, these muscles go into spasms, a common source of lower back pain.

Deltoid   The deltoids are fleshy, triangle-shaped muscles that form the rounded shape of your shoulders (see Figure 6.21a). Because they are so bulky, they are a favorite injection site (Figure 6.22) when relatively small amounts of medication (less than 5 ml) must be given intramuscularly (into muscle). The origin of each deltoid winds across the shoulder girdle from the spine of the scapula to the clavicle. It inserts into the proximal humerus. The deltoids are the prime movers of arm abduction.

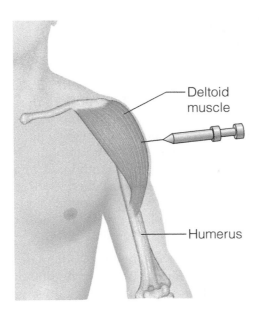

Deltoid
muscle

Humerus

FIGURE 6.22   The fleshy deltoid muscle is a favored site for administering intramuscular injections.

Muscles of the Upper Limb

The upper limb muscles fall into three groups. The first group includes muscles that arise from the shoulder girdle and cross the shoulder joint to insert into the humerus (see Figures 6.20 and 6.21a). These muscles, which move the arm, have already been considered—the pectoralis major, latissimus dorsi, and deltoid.

The second group causes movement at the elbow joint. These muscles enclose the humerus and insert on the forearm bones. Only the muscles of this second group will be described in this section. The third group includes the muscles of the forearm, which insert on the hand bones and cause their movement. The muscles of this last group are thin and spindle-shaped, and there are many of them. They will not be considered here except to mention their general naming and function. As a rule, the forearm muscles have names that reflect their activities. For example, the flexor carpi and flexor digitorum muscles, found on the anterior aspect of the forearm, cause flexion of the wrist and fingers, respectively. The extensor carpi and extensor digitorum muscles, found on the lateral and posterior aspect of the forearm, extend the same structures. (Some of these muscles are described briefly in Table 6.6 and illustrated in Figure 6.26.)

Muscles of the Humerus That Act on the Forearm

All *anterior* arm muscles cause elbow flexion. In order of decreasing strength, these are the bra-chialis, biceps brachii, and brachioradialis (Figures 6.20a and 6.25).

Biceps Brachii   The biceps brachii (bra′ke-i) is the most familiar muscle of the forearm because it bulges when the elbow is flexed (see Figure 6.20a). It originates by two heads from the shoulder girdle and inserts into the radial tuberosity. This muscle is the powerful prime mover for flexion of the forearm and acts to supinate the forearm. The best way to remember its action is that "it turns the corkscrew *and* pulls the cork."

Brachialis   The brachialis lies deep to the biceps muscle and is as important as the biceps in elbow flexion.

Brachioradialis   The brachioradialis is a fairly weak muscle that arises on the humerus and inserts into the distal forearm (see Figures 6.20a and 6.25). Hence, it resides mainly in the forearm.

Triceps Brachii   The triceps muscle is the only muscle fleshing out the posterior humerus (see Figure 6.21a). Its three heads arise from the shoulder girdle and proximal humerus, and it inserts into the olecranon process of the ulna. Being the powerful prime mover of elbow extension, it is the antagonist of the biceps brachii. This muscle is often called the "boxer's" muscle because it can deliver a straight-arm knockout punch.

Muscles of the Lower Limb

Muscles that act on the lower limb cause movement at the hip, knee, and foot joints. They are among the largest, strongest muscles in the body and are specialized for walking and balancing the body. Because the pelvic girdle is composed of heavy, fused bones that allow little movement, no special group of muscles is necessary to stabilize it. This is very different from the shoulder girdle, which requires several fixator muscles.

Many muscles of the lower limb span two joints and can cause movement at both of them. Therefore, the terms *origin* and *insertion* are often interchangeable in referring to these muscles.

Muscles acting on the thigh are massive muscles that help hold the body upright against the pull of gravity and cause various movements at the hip joint. Muscles acting on the leg form the flesh of the thigh. (Recall that in common usage, the term *leg* refers to the whole lower limb, but anatomically, the term refers only to that part between the knee and the ankle.) The thigh muscles cross the knee and cause its flexion or extension. Because many of the thigh muscles also have attachments on the pelvic girdle, they can cause movement at the hip joint as well.

Muscles originating on the leg cause assorted movements of the ankle and foot. Only three muscles of this group will be considered, but there are many others that act to extend and flex the ankle and toe joints.

Muscles Causing Movement at the Hip Joint   (Figure 6.23)

Gluteus Maximus   The gluteus maximus (gloo′te- us max′ĭ-mus) is a superficial muscle of the hip that forms most of the flesh of the buttock (Figure 6.23a). It is a powerful hip extensor that acts to bring the thigh in a straight line with the pelvis. Although it is not very important in walking, it is probably the most important muscle for extending the hip when power is needed, as when climbing stairs and when jumping. It originates from the sacrum and iliac bones and inserts on the gluteal tuberosity of the femur.

Gluteus Medius   The gluteus medius runs from the ilium to the femur, beneath the gluteus maximus for most of its length. The gluteus medius is

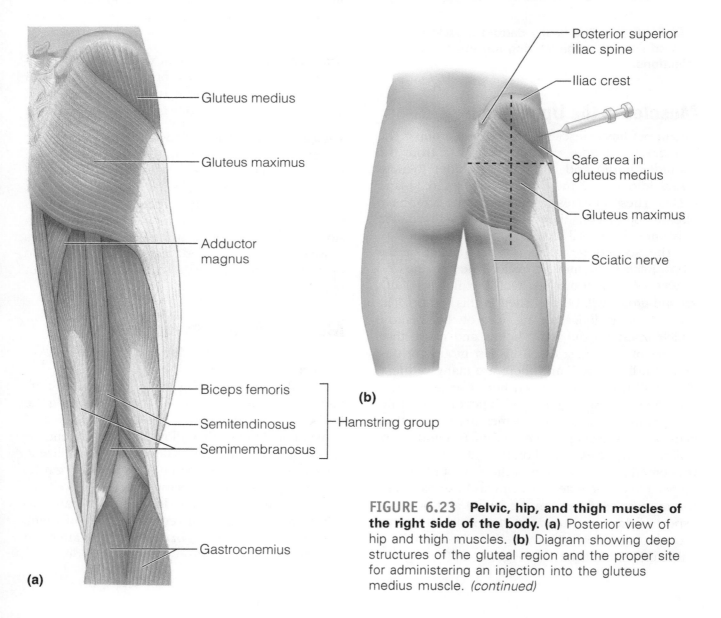

FIGURE 6.23 Pelvic, hip, and thigh muscles of the right side of the body. (a) Posterior view of hip and thigh muscles. **(b)** Diagram showing deep structures of the gluteal region and the proper site for administering an injection into the gluteus medius muscle. *(continued)*

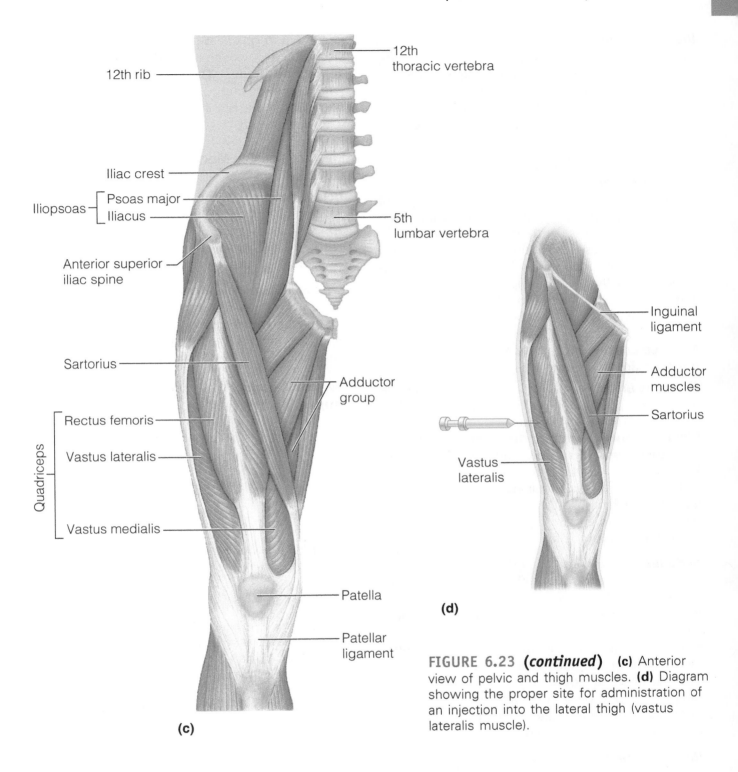

(c)

(d)

FIGURE 6.23 (continued) **(c)** Anterior view of pelvic and thigh muscles. **(d)** Diagram showing the proper site for administration of an injection into the lateral thigh (vastus lateralis muscle).

a hip abductor and is important in steadying the pelvis during walking. The gluteus medius is an important site for giving intramuscular injections, particularly when more than 5 ml is administered (see Figure 6.23b). Although it might appear that the large, fleshy gluteus maximus that forms the bulk of the buttock mass would be a better choice, notice that the medial part of each buttock overlies the large *sciatic nerve;* hence this area must be carefully avoided. This can be accomplished by *mentally* dividing the buttock into four equal quadrants (shown by the division lines on Figure 6.23b). The upper outer quadrant then overlies the gluteus medius muscle, which is usually a very safe site for an intramuscular injection.

Iliopsoas   The iliopsoas (il″e-o-so′as; the *p* is silent) is a fused muscle composed of two muscles, the *iliacus* and the *psoas major* (Figure 6.23c). It runs from the iliac bone and lower vertebrae deep inside the pelvis to insert on the lesser trochanter of the femur. It is a prime mover of hip flexion. It also acts to keep the upper body from falling backward when we are standing erect.

Adductor Muscles   The muscles of the adductor group form the muscle mass at the medial side of each thigh (Figure 6.23c). As their name indicates, they adduct or press the thighs together. However, since gravity does most of the work for them, they tend to become flabby very easily. Special exercises are usually needed to keep them toned. The adductors have their origin on the pelvis and insert on the proximal aspect of the femur.

Muscles Causing Movement at the Knee Joint   (Figure 6.23)

Hamstring Group   The muscles forming the muscle mass of the posterior thigh are the hamstrings (Figure 6.23a). The group consists of three muscles, the **biceps femoris, semimembranosus,** and **semitendinosus,** which originate on the ischial tuberosity and run down the thigh to insert on both sides of the proximal tibia. Their name comes from the fact that butchers use their tendons to hang hams (consisting of thigh and hip muscles) for smoking. These tendons can be felt at the back of the knee.

Sartorius   Compared to other thigh muscles described here, the thin, straplike sartorius (sarto′re-us) muscle is not too important. However, it is the most superficial muscle of the thigh so it is rather hard to miss (Figure 6.23c). It runs obliquely across the thigh from the anterior iliac crest to the medial side of the tibia. It is a weak thigh flexor. The sartorius is commonly referred to as the "tailor's" muscle because it acts as a synergist to bring about the cross-legged position in which old-time tailors are often shown.

Quadriceps Group   The quadriceps (kwod′rĭ-seps) group consists of four muscles—the **rectus femoris** and three **vastus muscles**—that flesh out the anterior thigh. The vastus muscles originate from the femur; the rectus femoris originates on the pelvis. All four muscles insert into the tibial tuberosity via the patellar ligament. The group as a whole acts to extend the knee powerfully, as when kicking a football. Because the rectus femoris crosses two joints, the hip and the knee, it can also help to flex the hip. The vastus lateralis and rectus femoris are sometimes used as intramuscular injection sites (Figure 6.23d), particularly in infants, who have poorly developed gluteus muscles.

Muscles Causing Movement at the Ankle and Foot   (Figure 6.24)

Tibialis Anterior   The tibialis anterior is a superficial muscle on the anterior leg. It arises from the upper tibia and then parallels the anterior crest as it runs to the tarsal bones, where it inserts by a long tendon. It acts to dorsiflex and invert the foot.

Extensor Digitorum Longus   Lateral to the tibialis anterior, this muscle arises from the lateral tibial condyle and proximal radius and inserts into the phalanges of toes 2 to 5. It is a prime mover of toe extension and a dorsiflexor of the foot.

Fibularis Muscles   The three fibularis muscles— **longus, brevis,** and **tertius**—are found on the lateral part of the leg. They arise from the fibula and insert into the metatarsal bones of the foot.

Prove It Yourself

Palpate Muscles as They Contract

The following demonstrations will help you locate and identify specific muscles discussed in this chapter:

- Go into a deep bend. Now palpate your *gluteus maximus* muscle as you extend your hip to stand up again.
- Sit down and have a friend hold on to your leg. Demonstrate the contraction of the anterior *rectus femoris* by trying to extend your knee against resistance. Note how the patellar tendon reacts. The *biceps femoris* of the posterior thigh comes into play when you flex your knee against your friend's applied resistance.
- Now stand on your toes. Have a friend palpate the lateral and medial heads of your *gastrocnemius* and follow it to its insertion in the calcaneal tendon.
- Dorsiflex and invert your foot while palpating your *tibialis anterior* muscle, which parallels the sharp anterior crest of the tibia laterally.

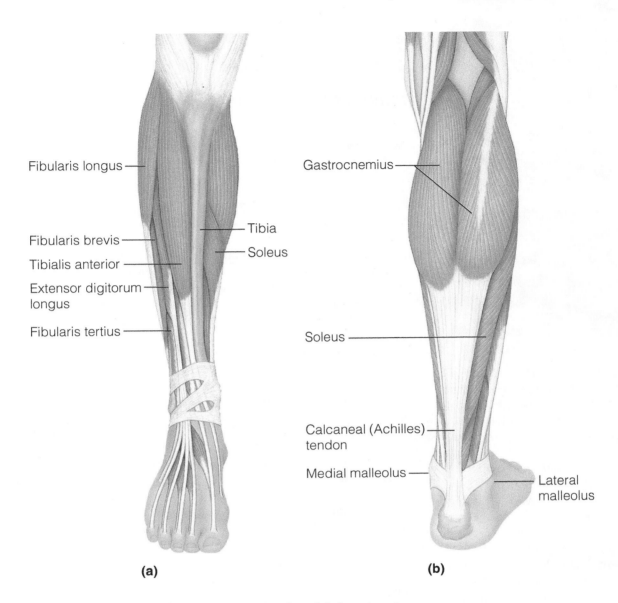

FIGURE 6.24 **Superficial muscles of the right leg. (a)** Anterior view;
(b) posterior view.

The group as a whole plantar flexes and everts the foot.

Gastrocnemius The gastrocnemius (gas"trok-ne′ me-us) muscle is a two-bellied muscle that forms the curved calf of the posterior leg. It arises by two heads, one from each side of the distal femur, and inserts through the large *calcaneal (Achilles) tendon* into the heel of the foot. It is a prime mover for plantar flexion of the foot; for this reason, it is often called the "toe dancer's" muscle. If its insertion tendon is cut, walking is very

difficult. The foot drags because the heel cannot be lifted.

Soleus Deep to the gastrocnemius is the fleshy soleus muscle. Because it arises on the tibia and fibula (rather than the femur), it does not affect knee movement, but like the gastrocnemius, it is a strong plantar flexor of the foot.

Remember that most of the superficial muscles previously described are shown in anterior and posterior views of the body as a whole in Figures 6.25 and 6.26 and are summarized in Tables 6.5 and 6.6.

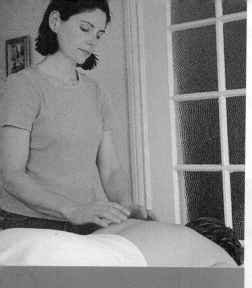

Focus on Careers
Massage Therapist

To be effective, a massage therapist needs a thorough understanding of anatomy and physiology.

> "Anatomy and physiology classes are fascinating because you're really learning how your own body works."

MANY of us think of massage simply as something that feels good. While this is certainly true, there's a lot of skill involved in massaging the body correctly.

Diana Syverud, part-owner of the Berkeley Massage and Self-Healing Center in Berkeley, California, doesn't just make her clients feel good; she helps them recover from injuries and prevent further problems. Many of them suffer from pain due to overusing certain muscles. "Most often, I see people who spend hours at the computer," she explains. "This can lead to trouble with the flexor carpi ulnaris, trapezius, and other muscles in the neck and back. But you don't need to have a desk job to experience muscle and tendon problems. I treat musicians who are sore from spending hours playing the violin and waitresses who have painful wrists from carrying heavy trays."

Training for massage therapists varies widely. State requirements for hours of training vary from 200 to 500 hours or more. Some states also require therapists to be licensed, while others do not. Syverud studied in Washington, where she completed an 850-hour program plus an optional internship. Regardless of their length, all effective massage programs require an understanding of anatomy and physiology; Syverud estimates it made up more than one-third of her course work.

"When I was studying anatomy and physiology, sometimes I wondered why I had to learn all that," she admits. "But today, I'm glad I did. It's important for me to know where muscles are located in the body and where they attach. For instance, sometimes a muscle may contract and pinch the sciatic nerve, causing excruciating pain. I check to determine which muscle is contracted and use various massage techniques to release it. I also help clients who have no specific muscular problems stretch and strengthen their muscles, increasing their range of motion." She notes another reason she's glad she took those classes: some parts of the body are better left untouched. "It's important to know the areas of the body where massage is contraindicated, such as in the area of the esophagus or hyoid bone."

"Anatomy and physiology classes are fascinating because you're really learning how your own body works," she comments. "This knowledge is valuable, for your clients' sake and for your own welfare."

Syverud's favorite aspect of her work is the one-on-one contact. "Typically I meet with a client for at least an hour at a time, often over a period of several months," she says. "Many initially come for a specific reason, then stay with me for years, long after we've resolved their original problem. We might meet weekly while they're in pain, then switch to monthly appointments to help prevent future problems." Some customers are referred to her by chiropractors, but most come on their own. If she feels their problems require more than massage, she refers them to appropriate health-care practitioners such as chiropractors, psychiatrists, or internists.

While Syverud is in private practice, many massage therapists work in spas, health clubs, or chiropractic offices. Often employers prefer to hire graduates of programs accredited by the American Massage Therapy Association (AMTA). Please note that accreditation procedures vary from state to state. For more information about the field, contact AMTA

820 Davis Street, Suite 100
Evanston, IL 60201
(847) 864-0123
http://www.amtamassage.org

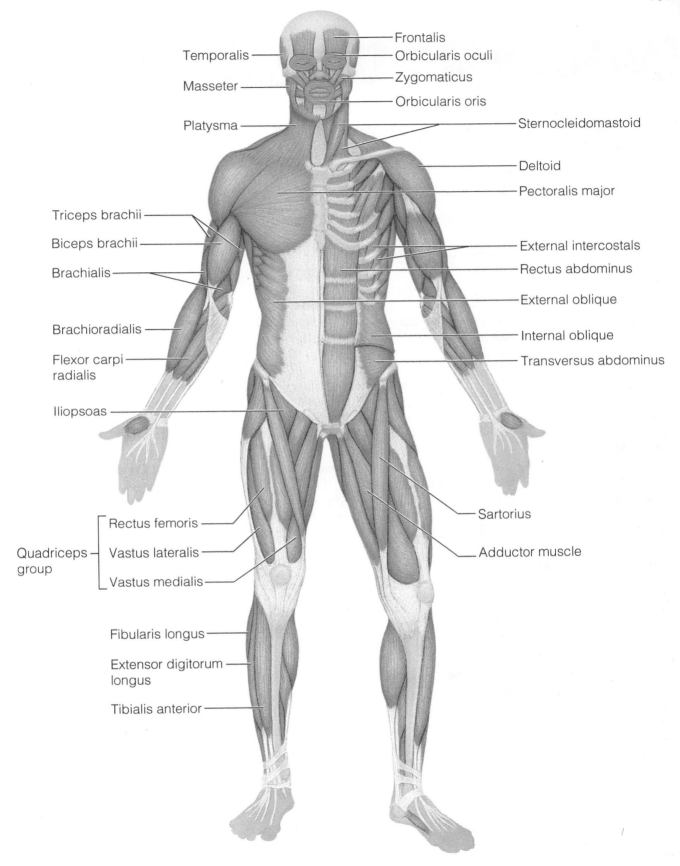

Frontalis
Temporalis
Orbicularis oculi
Zygomaticus
Masseter
Orbicularis oris
Platysma
Sternocleidomastoid
Deltoid
Pectoralis major
Triceps brachii
Biceps brachii
External intercostals
Rectus abdominus
Brachialis
External oblique
Brachioradialis
Internal oblique
Flexor carpi
radialis
Transversus abdominus
Iliopsoas
Sartorius
Rectus femoris
Quadriceps
group
Vastus lateralis
Adductor muscle
Vastus medialis
Fibularis longus
Extensor digitorum
longus
Tibialis anterior

FIGURE 6.25 **Major superficial muscles of the anterior surface of the body.**

TABLE 6.5   Superficial Anterior Muscles of the Body   (See Figure 6.25)

Name	Origin	Insertion	Primary Action(s)
Head/Neck Muscles			
Frontalis	Cranial aponeurosis	Skin of eyebrows	Raises eyebrows
Orbicularis oculi	Frontal bone and maxilla	Tissue around eyes	Blinks and closes eyes
Orbicularis oris	Mandible and maxilla	Skin and muscle around mouth	Closes and protrudes lips
Temporalis	Temporal bone	Mandible	Closes jaw
Zygomaticus	Zygomatic bone	Skin and muscle at corner of lips	Raises corner of mouth
Masseter	Temporal bone	Mandible	Closes jaw
Buccinator	Maxilla and mandible near molars	Orbicularis oris	Compresses cheek as in whistling and sucking; holds food between teeth during chewing
Sternocleidomastoid	Sternum and clavicle	Temporal bone (mastoid process)	Flexes neck; rotates head
Platysma	Connective tissue covering of superior chest muscles	Tissue around mouth	Pulls corners of mouth inferiorly
Trunk Muscles			
Pectoralis major	Sternum, clavicle, and first to sixth ribs	Proximal humerus	Adducts and flexes humerus
Rectus abdominis	Pubis	Sternum and fifth to seventh ribs	Flexes vertebral column
External oblique	Lower eight ribs	Iliac crest	Flexes and rotates vertebral column
Arm/Shoulder Muscles			
Biceps brachii	Scapula of shoulder girdle	Proximal radius	Flexes elbow and supinates forearm
Brachialis	Distal humerus	Proximal ulna	Flexes elbow
Deltoid	See Table 6.4		Abducts arm
Hip/Thigh/Leg Muscles			
Iliopsoas	Ilium and lumbar vertebrae	Femur (lesser trochanter)	Flexes hip
Adductor muscles	Pelvis	Proximal femur	Adduct thigh
Sartorius	Ilium	Proximal tibia	Flexes thigh on hip
Quadriceps group (vastus medialis, intermedius, and lateralis; and the rectus femoris)	Vasti: Femur Rectus femoris: Pelvis	Tibial tuberosity via patellar ligament Tibial tuberosity via patellar ligament	All extend knee; rectus femoris also flexes hip on thigh
Tibialis anterior	Proximal tibia	First cuneiform (tarsal) and first metatarsal of foot	Dorsiflexes and inverts foot
Extensor digitorum longus	Proximal tibia and radius	Distal toes 2–5	Extends toes and dorsiflexes foot
Fibularis muscles	Fibula	Metatarsals of foot	Plantar flex and evert foot

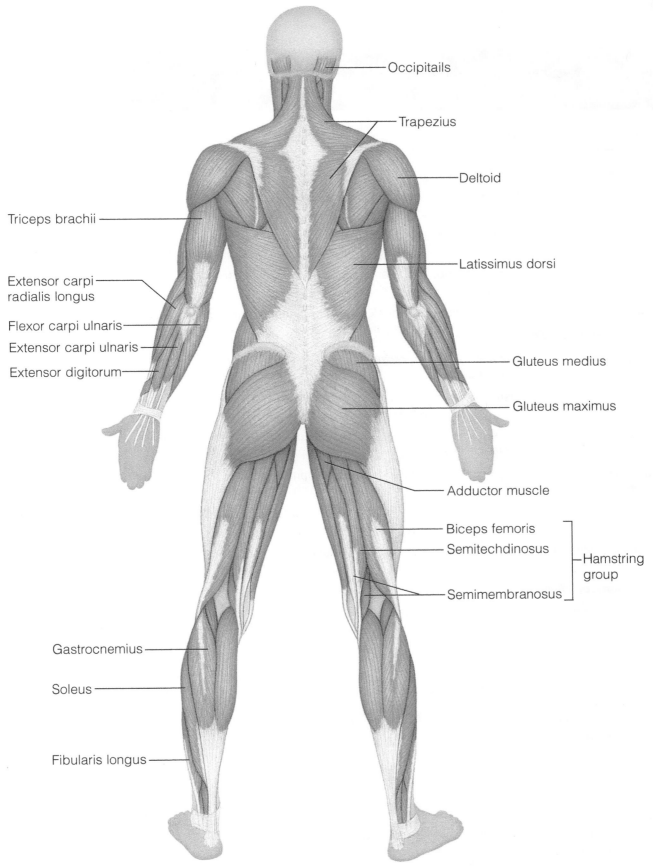

Occipitails

Trapezius

Deltoid

Triceps brachii

Latissimus dorsi

Extensor carpi
radialis longus

Flexor carpi ulnaris

Extensor carpi ulnaris

Extensor digitorum

Gluteus medius

Gluteus maximus

Adductor muscle

Biceps femoris

Semitechdinosus

Semimembranosus

Hamstring
group

Gastrocnemius

Soleus

Fibularis longus

FIGURE 6.26 **Major superficial muscles of the posterior surface of
the body.**

TABLE 6.6	Superficial Posterior Muscles of the Body (Some Forearm Muscles Also Shown) (See Figure 6.26)

Name	Origin	Insertion	Primary Action(s)
Neck/Trunk/Shoulder Muscles			
Trapezius	Occipital bone and all cervical and thoracic vertebrae	Scapular spine and clavicle	Extends neck and adducts scapula
Latissimus dorsi	Lower spine and iliac crest	Proximal humerus	Extends and adducts humerus
Erector spinae*	Iliac crests, ribs 3–12, and vertebrae	Ribs, thoracic and cervical vertebrae	Extends back
Deltoid	Scapular spine and clavicle	Humerus (deltoid tuberosity)	Abducts humerus
Arm/Forearm Muscles			
Triceps brachii	Shoulder girdle and proximal humerus	Olecranon process of ulna	Extends elbow
Flexor carpi radialis	Distal humerus	Second and third metacarpals	Flexes wrist and abducts hand (see Figure 6.25)
Flexor carpi ulnaris	Distal humerus and posterior ulna	Carpals of wrist and fifth metacarpal	Flexes wrist and adducts hand
Flexor digitorum superficialis†	Distal humerus, ulna and radius	Middle phalanges of second to fifth fingers	Flexes wrist and fingers
Extensor carpi radialis	Humerus	Base of second and third metacarpals	Extends wrist and abducts hand
Extensor digitorum	Distal humerus	Distal phalanges of second to fifth fingers	Extends fingers and wrist
Hip/Thigh/Leg Muscles			
Gluteus maximus	Sacrum and ilium	Proximal femur (gluteal tuberosity)	Extends hip (when forceful extension is required)
Gluteus medius	Ilium	Proximal femur	Abducts thigh; steadies pelvis during walking
Hamstring muscles (semitendinosus, semimembranosus, biceps femoris)	Ischial tuberosity	Proximal tibia (head of fibula in the case of biceps femoris)	Flex knee and extend hip
Gastrocnemius	Distal femur	Calcaneus (heel via calcaneal tendon)	Plantar flexes foot and flexes knee
Soleus	Proximal tibia and fibula	Calcaneus	Plantar flexes foot

*Erector spinae is a deep muscle group and not shown in Figure 6.26.

†Although its name indicates that it is a superficial muscle, the flexor digitorum superficialis lies deep to the flexor carpi radialis and is not visible in a superficial view.

Developmental Aspects of the Muscular System

In the developing embryo, the muscular system is laid down in segments (much like the structural plan of an earthworm), and then each segment is invaded by nerves. The muscles of the thoracic and lumbar regions become very extensive since they must cover and move the bones of the limbs. Development of the muscles and their control by the nervous system occur rather early in pregnancy. The expectant mother is often astonished by the first movements (called the *quickening*) of the fetus, which usually occur by the sixteenth week of pregnancy.

Homeostatic Imbalance

Very few congenital muscular problems occur. The exception to this is *muscular dystrophy*—a group of inherited muscle-destroying diseases that affect specific muscle groups. The muscles enlarge due to fat and connective tissue deposit, but the muscle fibers degenerate and atrophy.

The most common and serious form is *Duchenne's muscular dystrophy*, which is expressed almost exclusively in males. This tragic disease is usually diagnosed between the ages of 2 and 6 years. Active, normal-appearing children become clumsy and begin to fall frequently as their muscles weaken. The disease progresses relentlessly from the extremities upward, finally affecting the head and chest muscles. Most victims must use wheelchairs by the age of 12 and generally do not live beyond young adulthood. Although the cause of muscular dystrophy has been pinned down (the diseased muscle fibers lack a protein [called dystrophin] that helps maintain the sarcolemma), a cure is still elusive.

Initially after birth, a baby's movements are all gross reflex types of movements. Because the nervous system must mature before the baby can control muscles, we can trace the increasing efficiency of the nervous system by observing a baby's development of muscle control. This development proceeds in a cephalic/caudal direction, and gross muscular movements precede fine ones. Babies can raise their heads before they can sit up and can sit up before they can walk. Muscular control also proceeds in a proximal/distal direction; that is, babies can wave "bye-bye" and pull objects to themselves before using the pincher grasp to pick up a pin. All through childhood, the control of the skeletal muscles by the nervous system becomes more and more precise. By midadolescence, we have reached the peak level of development of this natural control and can simply accept it or bring it to a fine edge by athletic training.

Because of its rich blood supply, skeletal muscle is amazingly resistant to infection throughout life, and given good nutrition, relatively few problems afflict skeletal muscles. It should be repeated, however, that muscles, like bones, *will* atrophy, even with normal tone, if they are not used continually. On the other hand, a lifelong program of regular exercise keeps the whole body operating at its best possible level.

Homeostatic Imbalance

One rare disease that can affect muscles during adulthood is *myasthenia gravis* (mi"as-the'ne-ah gra'vis; *asthen* = weakness; *gravi* = heavy), a disease characterized by drooping of the upper eyelids, difficulty in swallowing and talking, and generalized muscle weakness and fatigability. The disease involves a shortage of acetylcholine receptors at the neuromuscular junction. The blood of many of these patients contains antibodies to acetylcholine receptors, which suggests that myasthenia gravis is an autoimmune disease. Although the receptors may initially be present in normal numbers, they appear to be destroyed as the disease progresses. Whatever the case, the muscle cells are not stimulated properly and get progressively weaker. Death usually occurs as a result of the inability of the respiratory muscles to function. This is called *respiratory failure*.

As we age, the amount of connective tissue in the muscles increases and the amount of muscle tissue decreases; thus the muscles become stringier, or more sinewy. Since the skeletal muscles represent so much of the body weight, body weight begins to decline in the elderly person as this natural loss in muscle mass occurs. Another result of the loss in muscle mass is a decrease in muscle strength; strength decreases by about 50 percent by the age of 80. Regular exercise can help offset the effects of aging on the muscular system, and frail elders who begin to "pump iron" (use leg and hand weights) can rebuild muscle mass and dramatically increase their strength.

Systems in Sync

Homeostatic Relationships between the Muscular System and Other Body Systems

Nervous System
- Facial muscle activity allows emotions to be expressed
- Nervous system stimulates and regulates muscle activity

Endocrine System
- Growth hormone and androgens influence skeletal muscle strength and mass

Respiratory System
- Muscular exercise increases respiratory capacity
- Respiratory system provides oxygen and disposes of carbon dioxide

Lymphatic System/Immunity
- Physical exercise may enhance or depress immunity depending on its intensity
- Lymphatic vessels drain leaked tissue fluids; immune system protects muscles from disease

Cardiovascular System
- Skeletal muscle activity increases efficiency of cardiovascular functioning; helps prevent atherosclerosis and causes cardiac hypertrophy
- Cardiovascular system delivers oxygen and nutrients to muscles; carries away wastes

Digestive System
- Physical activity increases gastrointestinal mobility when at rest
- Digestive system provides nutrients needed for muscle health; liver metabolizes lactic acid

Reproductive System
- Skeletal muscle helps support pelvic organs (e.g., uterus in females); assists erection of penis and clitoris
- Testicular androgen promotes increased skeletal muscle size

Urinary System
- Physical activity promotes normal voiding behavior; skeletal muscle forms the voluntary sphincter of the urethra
- Urinary system disposes of nitrogenous wastes

Integumentary System
- Muscular exercise enhances circulation to skin and improves skin health; exercise also increases body heat, which the skin helps dissipate
- Skin protects the muscles by external enclosure

Muscular System

Skeletal System
- Skeletal muscle activity maintains bone health and strength
- Bones provide levers for muscle activity

Unit 4

Integration and Regulatory Mechanisms

7

The Nervous System

KEY TERMS

You are driving down the freeway, and a horn blares on your right. You swerve to your left. Charlie leaves a note on the kitchen table: "See you later—have the stuff ready at 6." You know that the "stuff" is chili with taco chips. You are dozing, and your infant son makes a soft cry. Instantly, you awaken. What do all these events have in common? They are all everyday examples of the functioning of your nervous system, which has your body cells humming with activity nearly all the time.

The **nervous system** is the master controlling and communicating system of the body. Every thought, action, and emotion reflects its activity. Its signaling device, or means of communicating with body cells, is electrical impulses, which are rapid and specific and cause almost immediate responses.

To carry out its normal role, the nervous system has three overlapping functions (Figure 7.1): (1) Much like a sentry, it uses its millions of sensory receptors to *monitor changes* occurring both inside and outside the body. These changes are called **stimuli,** and the gathered information is called **sensory input.** (2) It *processes and interprets* the sensory input and makes decisions about what should be done at each moment—a process called **integration.** (3) It then *effects a response* by activating muscles or glands (effectors) via **motor output.** An example will illustrate how these functions work together. When you are driving and see a red light just ahead (sensory input), your nervous system integrates this information (red light means "stop") and sends motor output to the muscles of your right leg and foot, and your foot goes for the brake pedal (the response).

The nervous system does not work alone to regulate and maintain body homeostasis; the endocrine system is a second important regulating system. While the nervous system controls with rapid electrical nerve impulses, the endocrine system organs produce hormones that are released into the blood. Thus, the endocrine system typically brings about its effects in a more leisurely way.

Organization of the Nervous System

We have only one nervous system, but, because of its complexity, it is difficult to consider all its parts at the same time. So, to simplify its study, we divide it in terms of its structures (structural classification)

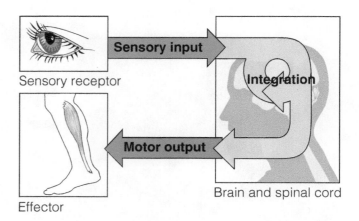

FIGURE 7.1   The nervous system's functions.

or in terms of its activities (functional classification). Each of these classification schemes is described briefly below, and their relationships are illustrated in Figure 7.2. It is not necessary to memorize this whole scheme now, but as you are reading the descriptions, try to get a "feel" for the major parts and how they fit together. This will make your learning task easier as you make your way through this chapter. Later you will meet all these terms and concepts again and in more detail.

Structural Classification

The structural classification, which includes all nervous system organs, has two subdivisions—the central nervous system and the peripheral nervous system (see Figure 7.2).

The **central nervous system (CNS)** consists of the brain and spinal cord, which occupy the dorsal body cavity and act as the integrating and command centers of the nervous system. They interpret incoming sensory information and issue instructions based on past experience and current conditions.

The **peripheral** (pĕ-rif′er-al) **nervous system (PNS),** the part of the nervous system outside the CNS, consists mainly of the nerves that extend from the brain and spinal cord. **Spinal nerves** carry impulses to and from the spinal cord. **Cranial** (kra′ne-al) **nerves** carry impulses to and from the brain. These nerves serve as communication lines. They link all parts of the body by carrying impulses from the sensory receptors to the CNS and from the CNS to the appropriate glands or muscles.

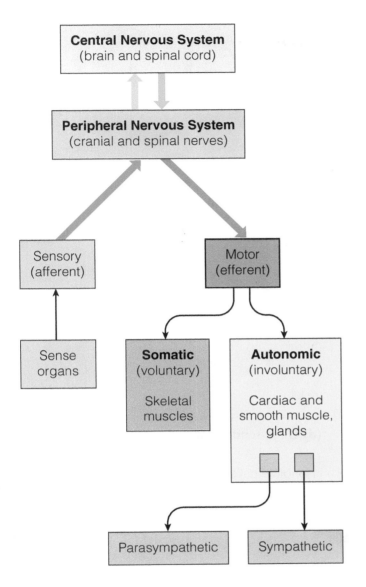

central nervous system from sensory receptors located in various parts of the body. Sensory fibers delivering impulses from the skin, skeletal muscles, and joints are called *somatic* (*soma* = body) *sensory* (afferent) *fibers,* whereas those transmitting impulses from the visceral organs are called *visceral sensory fibers,* or *visceral afferents.* The sensory division keeps the CNS constantly informed of events going on both inside and outside the body.

The **motor,** or **efferent** (ef'er-rent), **division** carries impulses *from* the CNS to effector organs, the muscles and glands. These impulses activate muscles and glands; that is, they *effect* (bring about) a motor response.

The motor division in turn has two subdivisions (see Figure 7.2):

1. The **somatic** (so-mat'ik) **nervous system** allows us to consciously, or voluntarily, control our skeletal muscles. Hence, this subdivision is often referred to as the **voluntary nervous system.** However, not all skeletal muscle activity controlled by this motor division is voluntary. Skeletal muscle reflexes, like the stretch reflex for example, are initiated involuntarily by these same fibers.

2. The **autonomic** (aw"to-nom'ik) **nervous system (ANS)** regulates events that are automatic, or involuntary, such as the activity of smooth and cardiac muscles and glands. This subdivision, commonly called the **involuntary nervous system,** itself has two parts, the *sympathetic* and *parasympathetic,* which typically bring about opposite effects. What one stimulates, the other inhibits. These will be described later.

Although it is simpler to study the nervous system in terms of its subdivisions, you should recognize that these subdivisions are made for the sake of convenience only. Remember that the nervous system acts as a coordinated unit, both structurally and functionally.

FIGURE 7.2   Organization of the nervous system. Organizational flowchart showing that the central nervous system receives input via sensory fibers and issues commands via motor fibers. The sensory and motor fibers together form the nerves that constitute the peripheral nervous system.

The organs making up the CNS and PNS are discussed at length later in this chapter.

Functional Classification

The functional classification scheme is concerned only with PNS structures. It divides them into two principal subdivisions (see Figure 7.2).

The **sensory,** or **afferent** (af'er-ent), **division** consists of nerve fibers that convey impulses *to* the

Nervous Tissue: Structure and Function

Even though it is complex, nervous tissue is made up of just two principal types of cells—*supporting cells* and *neurons.*

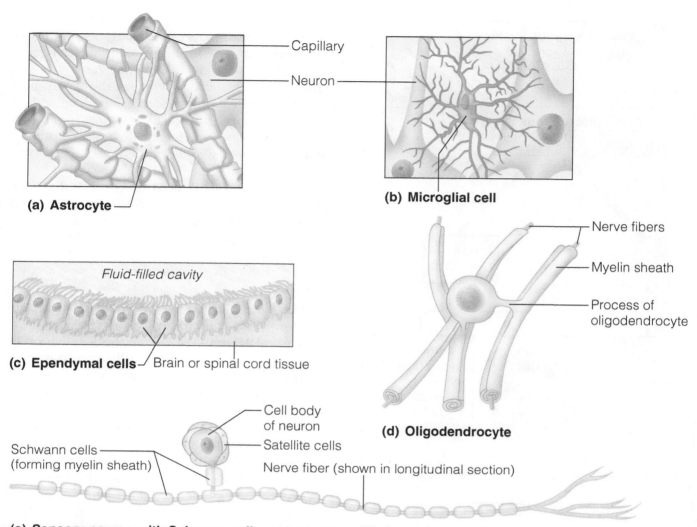

(a) Astrocyte

(b) Microglial cell

Capillary

Neuron

Nerve fibers

Myelin sheath

Process of
oligodendrocyte

Fluid-filled cavity

(c) Ependymal cells / Brain or spinal cord tissue

(d) Oligodendrocyte

Cell body
of neuron

Satellite cells

Schwann cells
(forming myelin sheath)

Nerve fiber (shown in longitudinal section)

(e) Sensory neuron with Schwann cells and satellite cells

FIGURE 7.3   Supporting (glial) cells of nervous tissues. Astrocytes
(a) form a living barrier between neurons and capillaries in the CNS.
Microglia **(b)** are phagocytes, whereas ependymal cells **(c)** line the fluid-
filled cavities of the CNS. The oligodendrocytes **(d)** form myelin sheaths
around nerve fibers in the CNS. **(e)** The relationship of Schwann cells
(myelinating cells) and satellite cells to a neuron in the peripheral
nervous system.

Supporting Cells

Supporting cells in the CNS are "lumped together" as
neuroglia (nu-rog′le-ah), literally, "nerve glue."
Neuroglia includes many types of cells that generally
support, insulate, and protect the delicate neurons
(Figure 7.3). In addition, each of the different types
of neuroglia, also simply called **glia** (gle′ah) or glial
cells, has special functions. The CNS glia include:

- **Astrocytes:** abundant star-shaped cells that
  account for nearly half of the neural tissue. Their

numerous projections have swollen ends that
cling to neurons, bracing them and anchoring
them to their nutrient supply lines, the blood
capillaries (Figure 7.3a). Astrocytes form a living
barrier between capillaries and neurons and
play a role in making exchanges between the
two. In this way, they help protect the neurons
from harmful substances that might be in the
blood. Astrocytes also help control the chemical
environment in the brain by picking up excess
ions and recapturing released neurotransmitters.

- **Microglia** (mi-krog′le-ah): spiderlike phago-cytes that dispose of debris, including dead brain cells and bacteria (Figure 7.3b).

- **Ependymal** (ĕ-pen′dĭ-mal) **cells:** these glial cells line the cavities of the brain and the spinal cord (Figure 7.3c). The beating of their cilia helps to circulate the cerebrospinal fluid that fills those cavities and forms a protective cushion around the CNS.

- **Oligodendrocytes** (ol″ĭ-go-den′dro-sītz): glia that wrap their flat extensions tightly around the nerve fibers, producing fatty insulating coverings called *myelin sheaths* (Figure 7.3d).

Although they somewhat resemble neurons structurally (both cell types have cell extensions), glia are not able to transmit nerve impulses, a function that is highly developed in neurons. Another important difference is that glia never lose their ability to divide, whereas most neurons do. Consequently, most brain tumors are *gliomas,* or tumors formed by glial cells (neuroglia).

Supporting cells in the PNS come in two major varieties—Schwann cells and satellite cells (Figure 7.3e). **Schwann cells** form the myelin sheaths around nerve fibers that are found in the PNS. **Satellite cells** act as protective, cushioning cells.

Neurons

Anatomy

Neurons, also called **nerve cells,** are highly specialized to transmit messages (nerve impulses) from one part of the body to another. Although neurons differ structurally, they have many common features (Figure 7.4). All have a cell body, which contains the nucleus and is the metabolic center of the cell, and one or more slender processes extending from the cell body.

The **cell body** is the metabolic center of the neuron. It contains the usual organelles except for centrioles (which confirms the amitotic nature of most neurons). The rough ER, called **Nissl** (nis′l) **substance,** and **neurofibrils,** intermediate filaments that are important in maintaining cell shape, are particularly abundant in the cell body.

The armlike **processes,** or **fibers,** vary in length from microscopic to 3 to 4 feet. The longest ones in humans reach from the lumbar region of the spine to the great toe. Neuron processes that convey incoming messages (electrical signals)

toward the cell body are **dendrites** (den′drītz), whereas those that generate nerve impulses and typically conduct them *away* from the cell body are **axons** (ak′sonz). Neurons may have hundreds of the branching dendrites (*dendr* = tree), depending on the neuron type, but each neuron has only one axon, which arises from a conelike region of the cell body called the **axon hillock.**

An occasional axon gives off a *collateral branch* along its length, but all axons branch profusely at their terminal end, forming hundreds to thousands of **axon terminals.** These terminals contain hundreds of tiny vesicles, or membranous sacs, that contain chemicals called **neurotransmitters.** As we said, axons transmit nerve impulses away from the cell body. When these impulses reach the axon terminals, they stimulate the release of neurotransmitters into the extracellular space.

Each axon terminal is separated from the next neuron by a tiny gap called the **synaptic** (sĭ-nap′tik) **cleft.** Such a functional junction is called a **synapse** (*syn* = to clasp or join). Although they are close, neurons never actually touch other neurons. We will learn more about synapses and the events that occur there a bit later.

Most long nerve fibers are covered with a whitish, fatty material, called **myelin** (mi′ĕ-lin), which has a waxy appearance. Myelin protects and insulates the fibers and increases the transmission rate of nerve impulses. Axons outside the CNS are myelinated by Schwann cells, specialized supporting cells that wrap themselves tightly around the axon in jelly-roll fashion (Figure 7.5). When the wrapping process is done, a tight coil of wrapped membranes, the **myelin sheath,** encloses the axon. Most of the Schwann cell cytoplasm ends up just beneath the outermost part of its plasma membrane. This part of the Schwann cell, external to the myelin sheath, is called the **neurilemma** (nu″rĭ-lem′mah, "neuron husk"). Since the myelin sheath is formed by many individual Schwann cells, it has gaps or indentations, called **nodes of Ranvier** (rahn-vēr), at regular intervals (see Figure 7.4).

Myelinated fibers are also found in the central nervous system. However, there it is oligodendrocytes that form CNS myelin sheaths (see Figure 7.3d). In contrast to Schwann cells, each of which deposits myelin around a small segment of

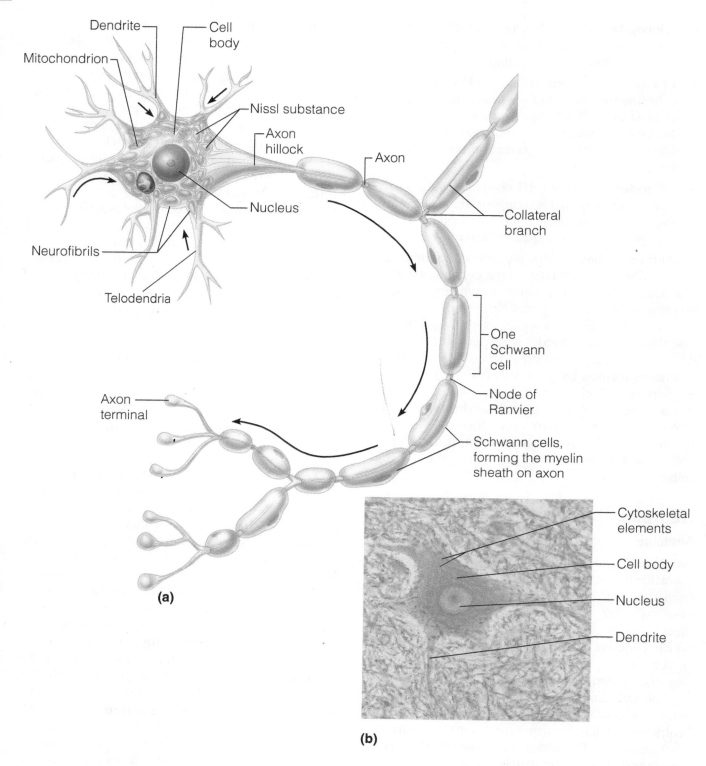

Dendrite

Cell body

Mitochondrion

Nissl substance

Axon hillock

Axon

Nucleus

Collateral branch

Neurofibrils

Telodendria

One Schwann cell

Node of Ranvier

Schwann cells, forming the myelin sheath on axon

Axon terminal

Cytoskeletal elements

Cell body

Nucleus

Dendrite

(a)

(b)

FIGURE 7.4 Structure of a typical motor neuron. (a) Diagrammatic view.
(b) Photomicrograph (265×).

Q Why does the myelin sheath that is produced by Schwann cells have gaps in it?

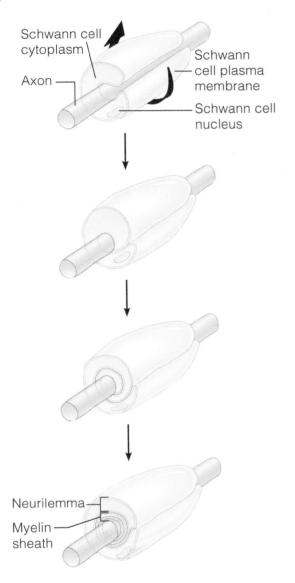

Schwann cell cytoplasm

Axon

Schwann cell plasma membrane

Schwann cell nucleus

Neurilemma

Myelin sheath

FIGURE 7.5 Relationship of Schwann cells to axons in the peripheral nervous system. As illustrated (top to bottom), a Schwann cell envelops part of an axon in a trough and then rotates around the axon. Most of the Schwann cell cytoplasm comes to lie just beneath the exposed part of its plasma membrane. The tight coil of plasma membrane material surrounding the axon is the myelin sheath. The Schwann cell cytoplasm and exposed membrane are referred to as the *neurilemma*.

A Because the sheath is produced by several Schwann cells that arrange themselves end to end along the nerve fiber, each Schwann cell forming only one tiny segment of the sheath.

one nerve fiber, the oligodendrocytes with their many flat extensions can coil around as many as 60 different fibers at the same time. Although the myelin sheaths formed by oligodendrocytes and those formed by Schwann cells are quite similar, the CNS sheaths lack a neurilemma. Because the neurilemma remains intact (for the most part) when a peripheral nerve fiber is damaged, it plays an important role in fiber regeneration, an ability that is largely lacking in the central nervous system.

Homeostatic Imbalance

The importance of the myelin insulation to nerve transmission is best illustrated by observing what happens when it is not there. In people with *multiple sclerosis (MS)*, the myelin sheaths around the fibers are gradually destroyed, converted to hardened sheaths called *scleroses*. As this happens, the current is short-circuited, and the affected person loses the ability to control his or her muscles and becomes increasingly disabled. Multiple sclerosis is an autoimmune disease in which a protein component of the sheath is attacked. As yet there is no cure, but injections of interferon (a hormonelike substance released by some immune cells) and oral doses of bovine myelin appear to provide some relief. ▲

Clusters of neuron cell bodies and collections of nerve fibers are named differently when they are in the CNS than when they are part of the PNS. For the most part, cell bodies are found in the CNS in clusters called **nuclei.** This well-protected location within the bony skull or vertebral column is essential to the well-being of the nervous system—remember that neurons do not routinely undergo cell division after birth. The cell body carries out most of the metabolic functions of a neuron, so if it is damaged the cell dies and is not replaced. Small collections of cell bodies called **ganglia** (gang'le-ah; **ganglion,** singular) are found in a few sites outside the CNS in the PNS. Bundles of nerve fibers (neuron processes) running through the CNS are called **tracts,** whereas in the PNS they are called **nerves.** The terms *white matter* and *gray matter* refer respectively to myelinated versus unmyelinated regions of the CNS. As a general rule, the **white matter** consists of dense collections of myelinated fibers (tracts), and **gray matter** contains mostly unmyelinated fibers and cell bodies.

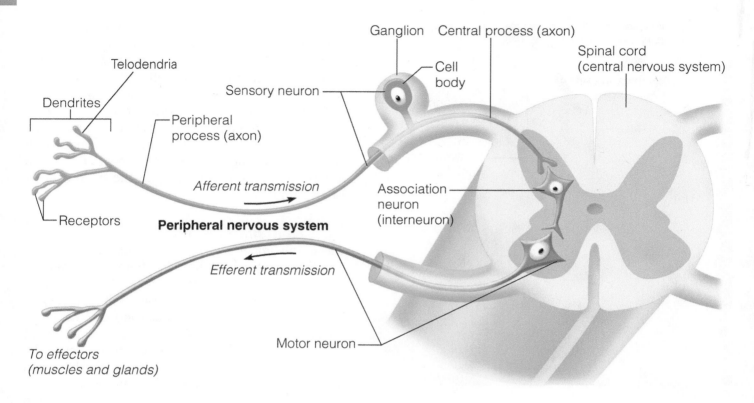

FIGURE 7.6 Neurons classified by function. Sensory (afferent) neurons conduct impulses from sensory receptors (in the skin, viscera, muscles) to the central nervous system; most cell bodies are in ganglia in the PNS. Motor (efferent) neurons transmit impulses from the CNS (brain or spinal cord) to effectors in the body periphery. Association neurons (interneurons) complete the communication pathway between sensory and motor neurons; their cell bodies reside in the CNS.

Classification

Neurons may be classified either according to how they function or according to their structure.

Functional Classification Functional classification groups neurons according to the direction the nerve impulse is traveling relative to the CNS. On this basis, there are sensory, motor, and association neurons (Figure 7.6). Neurons carrying impulses from sensory receptors (in the internal organs or the skin) to the CNS are **sensory,** or **afferent, neurons.** (*Afferent* literally means "to go toward.") The *cell bodies* of sensory neurons are always found in a *ganglion* outside the CNS. Sensory neurons keep us informed about what is happening both inside and outside the body.

The *dendrite* and finely branched **telodendria** endings of the sensory neurons are usually associated with specialized **receptors** that are activated

by specific changes occurring nearby. The very complex receptors of the special sense organs (vision, hearing, equilibrium, taste, and smell) are covered separately in Chapter 8. The simpler types of sensory receptors seen in the skin (**cutaneous sense organs**) and in the muscles and tendons (**proprioceptors** [pro"pre-o-sep'torz]) are shown in Figure 7.7. The pain receptors (actually bare dendrite endings) are the least specialized of the cutaneous receptors. They are also the most numerous, because pain warns us that some type of body damage is occurring or is about to occur. However, strong stimulation of any of the cutaneous receptors (for example, by searing heat, extreme cold, or excessive pressure) is also interpreted as pain.

The proprioceptors detect the amount of stretch, or tension, in skeletal muscles, their tendons, and joints. They send this information to the brain so that the proper adjustments can be made

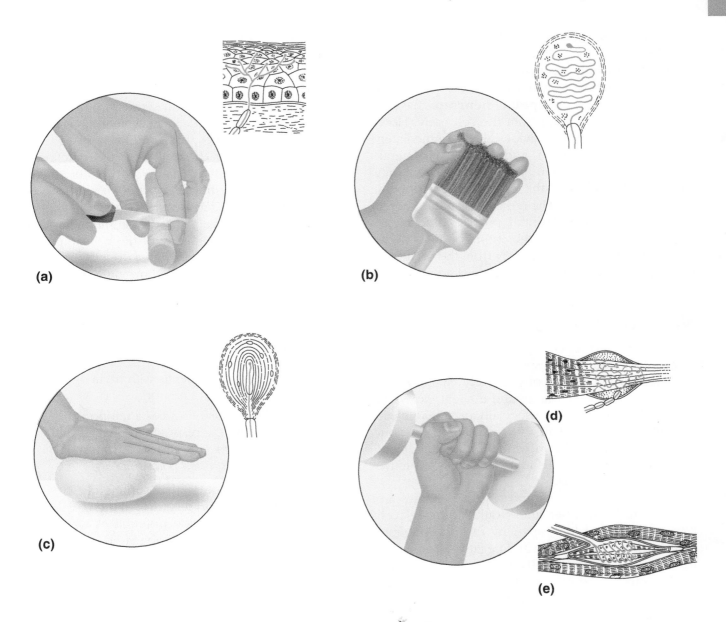

FIGURE 7.7 **Types of sensory receptors.** **(a)** Naked nerve endings (pain and temperature receptors). **(b)** Meissner's corpuscle (touch receptor). **(c)** Pacinian corpuscle (deep pressure receptor). **(d)** Golgi tendon organ (proprioceptor). **(e)** Muscle spindle (proprioceptor).

to maintain balance and normal posture. *Propria* comes from the Latin word meaning "one's own," and the proprioceptors constantly advise our brain of our own movements.

Neurons carrying impulses from the CNS to the viscera and/or muscles and glands are **motor,** or **efferent, neurons** (see Figure 7.6). The cell bodies of motor neurons are always located in the CNS.

The third category of neurons is the **association neurons,** or **interneurons.** They connect the motor and sensory neurons in neural pathways. Like the motor neurons, their cell bodies are always located in the CNS.

Structural Classification Structural classification is based on the number of processes extending from the cell body. If there are several, the neuron is a **multipolar neuron.** Since all motor and association neurons are multipolar, this is the most common structural type. Neurons with two processes—an axon and a dendrite—are called **bipolar neurons.** Bipolar neurons are rare in adults, found only in some special sense organs (eye, nose), where they act in sensory processing as receptor cells. **Unipolar neurons** have a single process emerging from the cell body. However, it is very short and divides almost immediately into proximal (central) and distal (peripheral) processes. Unipolar neurons are unique in that only the small branches at the end of the peripheral process are dendrites. The remainder of the peripheral process and the central process function as axons; thus, in this case, the axon conducts nerve impulses both toward *and* away from the cell body. Sensory neurons found in PNS ganglia are unipolar.

Neurons: Electrical Signals

The inside of the cell membrane has a slight negative charge with respect to the outside. The cause is a slight excess of positively charged ions outside the cell membrane, and a slight excess of negatively charged ions (especially proteins) inside the cell membrane. This unequal charge distribution is created by differences in the permeability of the membrane to various ions, as well as by active transport mechanisms.

Although the positive and negative charges are attracted to each other and would normally rush together, they are kept apart by the phospholipid membrane. When positive and negative charges are held apart, a **potential difference** is said to exist between them. We refer to the potential difference across a cell membrane as the **transmembrane potential.**

The unit of measurement of potential difference is the *volt* (V). Most cars, for example, have 12-V batteries. The transmembrane potentials of cells are much smaller, typically in the vicinity of 0.07 V. Such a value is usually expressed as 70 mV, or 70 *millivolts* (thousandths of a volt). The transmembrane potential in an undisturbed cell is called the **resting potential.** Each type of cell has a characteristic resting potential between −10 mV (−0.01 V) and −100 mV (−0.1 V), with the minus sign signifying that the inside of the cell membrane contains an excess of negative charges compared with the outside. Examples include fat cells (−40 mV), thyroid cells (−50 mV), neurons (−70 mV), skeletal muscle cells (−85 mV), and cardiac muscle cells (−90 mV).

If the lipid barrier were removed, the positive and negative charges would rush together and the potential difference would be eliminated. The cell membrane thus acts like a dam across a stream. Just as a dam resists the water pressure that builds up on the upstream side, a cell membrane resists electrochemical forces that would otherwise drive ions into or out of the cell. The water retained behind a dam and the ions held on either side of the cell membrane have *potential energy*—stored energy that can be released to do work.

In this section, we will focus on the membrane properties of neurons; many of the principles discussed also apply to other types of cells.

Figure 7.8 introduces the important membrane processes we will be examining.

- All living cells have a transmembrane potential that varies from moment to moment depending on the activities of the cell. The *resting potential* is the transmembrane potential of a resting cell. All neural activities begin with a change in the resting potential of a neuron.

- A typical stimulus produces a temporary, localized change in the resting potential. The effect, which decreases with distance from the stimulus, is called a *graded potential*.

- If the graded potential is sufficiently large, it produces an *action potential* in the membrane of the axon. An action potential is an electrical impulse that is propagated across the surface of an axon and does not diminish as it moves away from its source. This impulse travels along the axon to one or more synapses.

- *Synaptic activity* then produces graded potentials in the cell membrane of the postsynaptic cell. The process typically involves the release of neurotransmitters, such as ACh, by the presynaptic cell. These compounds bind to receptors on the postsynaptic cell membrane, changing its permeability. The mechanism is comparable to that of the neuromuscular junction.

- The response of the postsynaptic cell ultimately depends on what the stimulated receptors do and what other stimuli are influencing the cell at the same time. The integration of stimuli at the level of the individual cell is the simplest form of *information processing* in the nervous system.

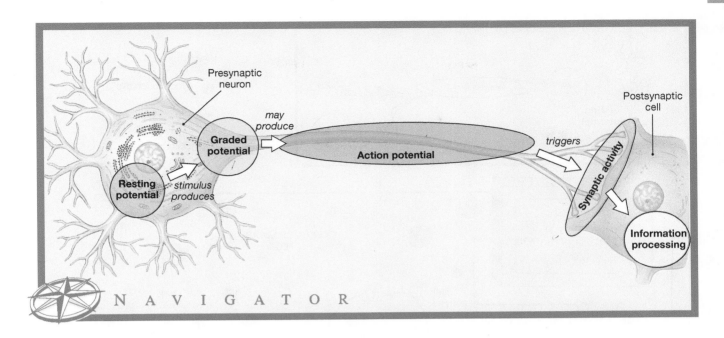

FIGURE 7.8 **An overview of neural activities.** The important membrane processes are shown in order of their presentation in the text. This figure will be repeated, in simplified form, as a Navigator icon in other figures whenever we are changing topics.

When you understand each of the foregoing processes, you will know how neurons process information and communicate with one another and with peripheral effectors.

The Transmembrane Potential

There are three important concepts regarding the transmembrane potential:

1. The intracellular fluid (cytosol) and extracellular fluid differ markedly in ionic composition. The extracellular fluid (ECF) contains high concentrations of sodium ions (Na^+) and chloride ions (Cl^-), whereas the cytosol contains high concentrations of potassium ions (K^+) and negatively charged proteins.

2. If the cell membrane were freely permeable, diffusion would continue until all the ions were evenly distributed across the membrane and a state of equilibrium existed. But an even distribution does not occur, because cells have selectively permeable membranes. Ions cannot freely cross the lipid portions of the cell membrane; they can enter or leave the cell only through membrane channels.

Many kinds of membrane channels exist, each with its own properties. At the resting potential, or transmembrane potential of an undisturbed cell, ion movement occurs through *leak channels*—membrane channels that are always open. Active transport mechanisms also move specific ions into or out of the cell.

3. The cell's passive and active transport mechanisms do not ensure an equal distribution of charges across its membrane, because membrane permeability varies by ion. For example, negatively charged proteins inside the cell cannot cross the membrane, and it is easier for K^+ to diffuse out of the cell through a potassium channel than it is for Na^+ to enter the cell through a sodium channel. As a result, the inner surface has an excess of negative charges with respect to the outer surface.

Both passive and active forces act across the cell membrane to determine the transmembrane potential at any moment. Figure 7.9 provides a brief overview of the state of the membrane at the normal resting potential.

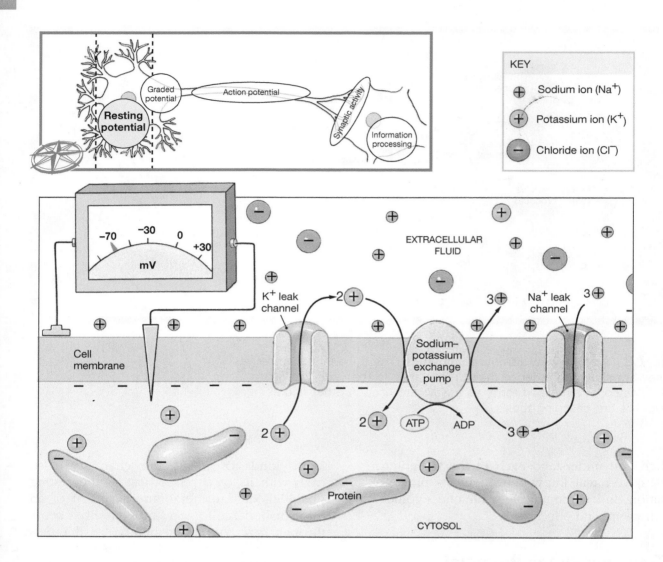

FIGURE 7.9   An Introduction to the resting potential. The resting potential is the transmembrane potential of an undisturbed cell. The phospholipid bilayer of the cell membrane is represented by a simple blue band. The Navigator icon highlights the resting potential to indicate "You are here!"

Passive Forces Acting across the Membrane

The passive forces acting across the membrane are both chemical and electrical in nature.

Chemical Gradients   Because the intracellular concentration of potassium ions is relatively high, these ions tend to move out of the cell through open potassium channels. The movement is driven by a concentration gradient, or *chemical gradient*. Similarly, a chemical gradient for sodium ions tends to drive those ions into the cell.

Electrical Gradients   Because the cell membrane is much more permeable to potassium than to sodium, potassium ions leave the cytoplasm more rapidly than sodium ions enter. As a result, the cytosol along the interior of the membrane exhibits a net loss of positive charges, leaving an excess of negatively charged proteins. At the same time, the extracellular fluid near the outer surface of the cell membrane displays a net gain of positive charges. The positive and negative charges are separated by the cell membrane, which restricts the free movement of ions. Whenever positive and negative ions are held apart, a *potential difference* arises.

The size of a potential difference is measured in volts (V) or millivolts (mV; thousandths of a volt). The resting potential varies widely, depending on the type of cell, but averages about 0.07 V for many cells, including most neurons. We will use this value in our discussion, usually expressing it as −70 mV (see Figure 7.9). The minus sign signifies that the inner surface of the cell membrane is negatively charged with respect to the exterior.

Positive and negative charges attract one another. If nothing separates them, oppositely charged ions will move together and eliminate the potential difference between them. A movement of charges to eliminate a potential difference is called a **current.** If a barrier (such as a cell membrane) separates the oppositely charged ions, the amount of current depends on how easily the ions can cross the membrane. The **resistance** of the membrane is a measure of how much the membrane restricts ion movement. If the resistance is high, the current is very small, because few ions can cross the membrane. If the resistance is low, the current is very large, because ions flood across the membrane. The resistance of a cell membrane can be changed by the opening or closing of ion channels. The ensuing changes result in currents that bring ions into or out of the cytoplasm.

The Electrochemical Gradient Electrical gradients can either reinforce or oppose the chemical gradient for each ion. The **electrochemical gradient** for a specific ion is the sum of the chemical and electrical forces acting on that ion across the cell membrane. The electrochemical gradients for K^+ and Na^+ are the primary factors affecting the resting potential of most cells, including neurons. We will consider the forces acting on each ion independently.

The intracellular concentration of potassium ions is relatively high, whereas the extracellular concentration is very low. Therefore, the chemical gradient for potassium ions tends to drive them out of the cell, as indicated by the black arrow in Figure 7.10a. However, the electrical gradient opposes this movement, because K^+ inside and outside of the cell are attracted to the negative charges on the inside of the cell membrane, and repelled by the positive charges on the outside of the cell membrane. The size and direction of the

electrical gradient is indicated by the white arrow in Figure 7.10a. The chemical gradient is strong enough to overpower the electrical gradient, but this weakens the force driving K^+ out of the cell; the net driving force is represented by the gray arrow.

If the cell membrane were freely permeable to K^+ but impermeable to other positively charged ions, potassium ions would continue to leave the cell until the electrical gradient (opposing the exit of K^+ from the cell) was as strong as the chemical gradient (driving K^+ out of the cell). The transmembrane potential at which there is no net movement of a particular ion across the cell membrane is called the *equilibrium potential* for that ion. For potassium ions, this equilibrium occurs at a transmembrane potential of about −90 mV, as illustrated in Figure 7.10b. The resting membrane potential is typically −70 mV, a value very close to the equilibrium potential for K^+; the difference is due primarily to the continuous leakage of Na^+ into the cell.

The sodium ion concentration in the extracellular fluid is relatively high, whereas that inside the cell is extremely low. As a result, there is a strong chemical gradient driving Na^+ into the cell (the black arrow in Figure 7.10c). In addition, the extracellular sodium ions are attracted by the excess of negative charges on the inner surface of the cell membrane, and the relative size and direction of this electrical gradient is indicated by the white arrow in Figure 7.11c. This means that electrical forces and chemical forces drive Na^+ into the cell, and the net driving force is represented by the gray arrow.

If the cell membrane were freely permeable to Na^+, these ions would continue to enter the cell until the interior of the cell membrane contained enough excess positive charges to reverse the electrical gradient. In other words, ion movement would continue until the interior developed such a strongly positive charge that repulsion between the positive charges would prevent any further net movement of Na^+ into the cell. The equilibrium potential for Na^+ is approximately +66mV, as illustrated in Figure 7.11d. The resting potential is nowhere near that value, because the resting membrane permeability to Na^+ is very low, and because ion pumps in the cell membrane are able to eject sodium ions as fast as they cross the membrane.

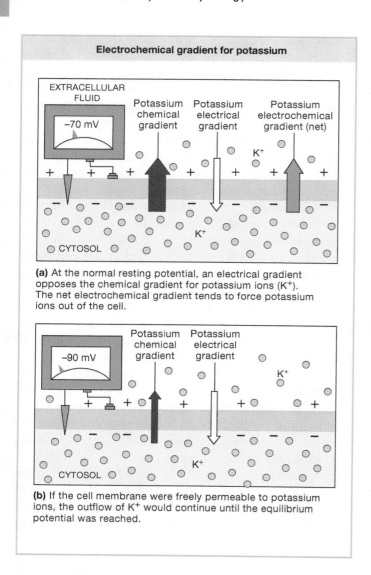

(a) At the normal resting potential, an electrical gradient opposes the chemical gradient for potassium ions (K^+). The net electrochemical gradient tends to force potassium ions out of the cell.

(b) If the cell membrane were freely permeable to potassium ions, the outflow of K^+ would continue until the equilibrium potential was reached.

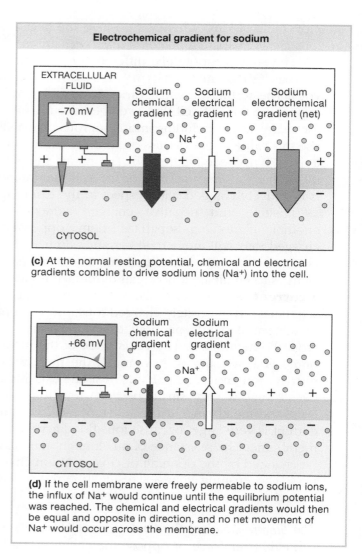

(c) At the normal resting potential, chemical and electrical gradients combine to drive sodium ions (Na^+) into the cell.

(d) If the cell membrane were freely permeable to sodium ions, the influx of Na^+ would continue until the equilibrium potential was reached. The chemical and electrical gradients would then be equal and opposite in direction, and no net movement of Na^+ would occur across the membrane.

FIGURE 7.10   Electrochemical gradients for potassium and sodium ions.

An electrochemical gradient is a form of *potential energy*. Potential energy is stored energy—the energy of position, as exists in a stretched spring, a charged battery, or water behind a dam. Without a cell membrane, diffusion would eliminate all electrochemical gradients. In effect, the cell membrane acts like a dam across a river. Without the dam, water would simply respond to gravity and flow downstream, gradually losing energy. With the dam in place, even a small opening will release water under tremendous pressure. Similarly, any stimulus that increases the permeability of the cell membrane to sodium or potassium ions will produce sudden and dramatic ion movement. For example, a stimulus that opens sodium ion channels will trigger an immediate rush of Na^+ into the cell. The nature of the stimulus does not determine the amount of ion movement; if the stimulus opens the door, the electrochemical gradient will do the rest.

Active Forces across the Membrane: The Sodium–Potassium Exchange Pump

We can compare a cell to a leaky fishing boat loaded with tiny fish. The hull represents the cell membrane; the fish, K^+; and the ocean water, Na^+. As the boat rumbles and rolls, water comes in through the cracks, and fish swim out. If the boat is to stay afloat and the catch kept, the water must be pumped out, and the lost fish recaptured.

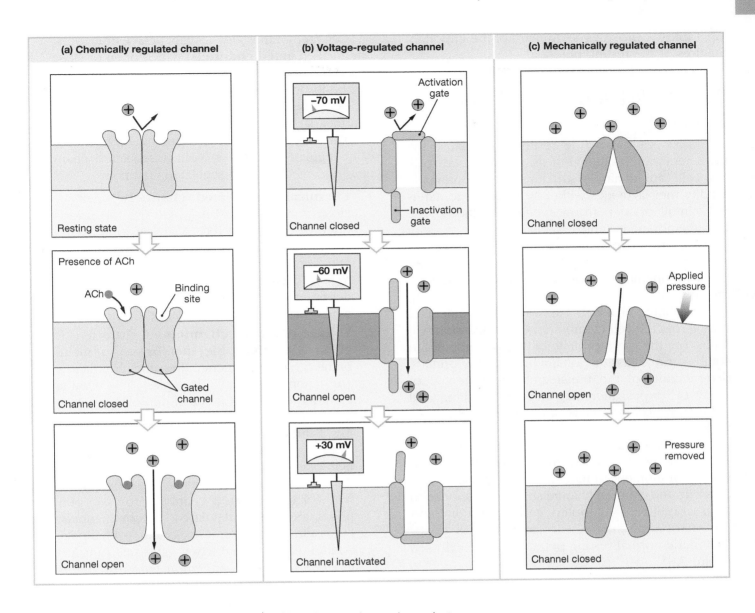

FIGURE 7.11   Gated channels. Na$^+$ channels are shown here, but comparable gated channels regulate the movements of other cations and anions. **(a)** A chemically regulated Na$^+$ channel that opens in response to the presence of ACh at a binding site. **(b)** A voltage-regulated Na$^+$ channel that responds to changes in the transmembrane potential. At the normal resting potential, the channel is closed; at a membrane potential of −60 mV, the channel opens; at +30 mV, the channel is inactivated. **(c)** A mechanically regulated channel, which opens in response to distortion of the membrane.

Similarly, at the normal resting potential, the cell must bail out sodium ions that leak in and recapture potassium ions that leak out. The "bailing" occurs through the activity of an exchange pump powered by ATP. The ion pump involved is the carrier protein *sodium–potassium ATPase.* This pump exchanges three intracellular sodium ions for two extracellular potassium ions. At the normal resting potential, this pump's primary significance is that it ejects sodium ions as quickly as they enter the cell. Thus, the activity of the exchange pump exactly balances the passive forces of diffusion, and the resting potential remains stable.

Table 7.1 provides a summary of the important features of the resting potential.

Changes in the Transmembrane Potential

As noted previously, the resting potential is the transmembrane potential of an "undisturbed" cell. Yet cells are dynamic structures that continually modify their activities, either in response to external stimuli or to perform specific functions. The transmembrane potential is equally dynamic, rising or falling in response to temporary changes in membrane permeability. Those changes result from the opening or closing of specific membrane channels.

Membrane channels control the movement of ions across the cell membrane. Our discussion will focus on the permeability of the membrane to sodium and potassium ions, which are the primary determinants of the transmembrane potential of many cell types, including neurons. Sodium and potassium ion channels are either passive or active.

Passive channels, or **leak channels,** are always open. However, their permeability can vary from moment to moment as the proteins that make up the channel change shape in response to local conditions. As noted earlier, sodium and potassium leak channels are important in establishing the normal resting potential of the cell (see Figure 7.8).

Cell membranes also contain **active channels,** often called **gated channels,** which open or close in response to specific stimuli. Each gated channel can be in one of three states: (1) closed but capable of opening, (2) open (**activated**), or (3) closed and incapable of opening (**inactivated**).

Three classes of gated channels exist: chemically regulated channels, voltage-regulated channels, and mechanically regulated channels.

1. **Chemically regulated channels** open or close when they bind specific chemicals (Figure 7.11a). The receptors that bind acetylcholine (ACh) at the neuromuscular junction are chemically regulated channels. Chemically regulated channels are most abundant on the dendrites and cell body of a neuron, the areas where most synaptic communication occurs.

2. **Voltage-regulated channels** are characteristic of areas of **excitable membrane,** a membrane capable of generating and conducting an action potential. Examples of excitable membranes are the axons of unipolar and multipolar neurons, and the sarcolemma (including T tubules) of skeletal muscle fibers and cardiac muscle cells. Voltage-regulated channels open or close in response to changes in the transmembrane potential. The most important voltage-regulated channels, for our purposes, are voltage-regulated sodium channels, potassium channels, and calcium channels. Sodium channels have two gates that function independently: an *activation gate* that opens

---

TABLE 7.1   The Resting Potential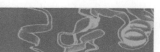

- Because the cell membrane is highly permeable to potassium ions, the resting potential is fairly close to -90 mV, the equilibrium potential for K^+.

- Although the electrochemical gradient for sodium ions is very large, the membrane's permeability to these ions is very low. Consequently, Na^+ has only a small effect on the normal resting potential, making it just slightly less negative than it would otherwise be.

- The sodium–potassium exchange pump ejects 3 Na^+ ions for every 2 K^+ ions that it brings into the cell. It thus serves to stabilize the resting potential when the ratio of Na^+ entry to K^+ loss through passive channels is 3:2

- At the normal resting potential, these passive and active mechanisms are in balance. The resting potential varies widely with the type of cell. A typical neuron has a resting potential of approximately -70 mV.

on stimulation, letting sodium ions into the cell, and an *inactivation gate* that closes to stop the entry of sodium ions (Figure 7.11b).

3. **Mechanically regulated channels** open or close in response to physical distortion of the membrane surface (Figure 7.11c). Such channels are important in sensory receptors that respond to touch, pressure, or vibration.

At the resting potential, most gated channels are closed. The opening of gated channels alters the rate of ion movement across the cell membrane and thus changes the transmembrane potential. The distribution of membrane channels can vary from one region of the cell membrane to another, affecting how and where a cell responds to specific stimuli. For example, whereas chemically regulated sodium channels are widespread on the surfaces of a neuron, voltage-regulated sodium channels are most abundant on the axon, its branches, and the synaptic terminals, and mechanically regulated channels are typically located only on the dendrites of sensory neurons.

100 Keys | A transmembrane potential exists across the cell membrane. It is there because (1) the cytosol differs from extracellular fluid in chemical and ionic composition and (2) the cell membrane is selectively permeable. The transmembrane potential can change from moment to moment, as the cell membrane changes its permeability in response to chemical or physical stimuli.

Physiology

Nerve Impulses Stimulus carried by membrane excitation: on *irritability*, the ability to respond to a stimulus and convert it into a nerve impulse, and *conductivity*, the ability to transmit the impulse to other neurons, muscles, or glands. We will consider these functional abilities next.

The plasma membrane of a resting, or inactive, neuron is **polarized**, which means that there are fewer positive ions sitting on the inner face of the neuron's plasma membrane than there are on its outer face in the tissue fluid that surrounds it (Figure 7.12). The major positive ions inside the cell are potassium (K^+), whereas the major positive ions outside the cell are sodium (Na^+). As long as the inside remains more negative as compared to the outside, the neuron will stay inactive.

Many different types of stimuli excite neurons to become active and generate an impulse. For example, light excites the eye receptors, sound excites some of the ear receptors, and pressure excites some cutaneous receptors of the skin. However, *most* neurons in the body are excited by neurotransmitters released by other neurons, as will be described shortly. Regardless of what the stimulus is, the result is always the same—the permeability properties of the cell's plasma membrane change for a very brief period. *Normally*, sodium ions cannot diffuse through the plasma membrane to any great extent; but when the neuron is adequately stimulated, the "gates" of sodium channels in the membrane open. Because sodium is in much higher concentration outside the cell, it will then diffuse quickly into the neuron. (Remember the laws of diffusion?) This inward rush of sodium ions changes the polarity of the neuron's membrane at that site, an event called **depolarization.** Locally, the inside is now more positive, and the outside is less positive, a situation called a **graded potential.** However, if the stimulus is strong enough and the sodium influx is great enough, the local depolarization (graded potential) activates the neuron to initiate and transmit a long distance signal called an **action potential,** also called a **nerve impulse** in neurons. The nerve impulse is an **all-or-none response** like firing a gun. It is either propagated (conducted) over the entire axon, or it doesn't happen at all. The nerve impulse never goes partway along an axon's length, nor does it die out with distance as do graded potentials.

Almost immediately after the sodium ions rush into the neuron, the membrane permeability changes again, becoming impermeable to sodium ions but permeable to potassium ions. So potassium ions are allowed to diffuse out of the neuron into the tissue fluid, and they do so very rapidly. This outflow of positive ions from the cell restores the electrical conditions at the membrane to the polarized, or resting, state, an event called **repolarization.** *Until repolarization occurs, a neuron cannot conduct another impulse.* After repolarization occurs, the initial concentrations of the sodium and potassium ions inside and outside the neuron are restored by activation of the sodium-potassium pump. This pump uses ATP (cellular energy) to pump excess sodium ions out of the cell and to bring potassium ions back into it. Once

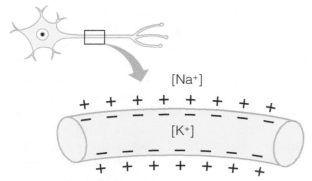

(a) Resting membrane

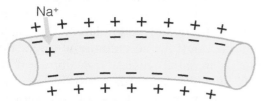

(b) Stimulus initiates local depolarization

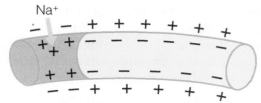

(c) Depolarization and generation of the action potential

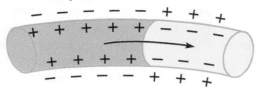

(d) Propagation of the action potential

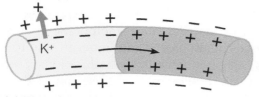

(e) Repolarization

(f) Restoration of ionic concentrations via sodium-potassium pump

FIGURE 7.12 The nerve impulse. (a) Resting membrane electrical conditions. The external face of the membrane is slightly positive; its internal face is slightly negative. The chief extracellular ion is sodium (Na^+), whereas the chief intracellular ion is potassium (K^+). The membrane is relatively impermeable to both ions. **(b)** Stimulus initiates local depolarization. A stimulus changes the permeability of a "patch" of the membrane, and sodium ions diffuse rapidly into the cell through voltage regulated channels. This changes the polarity of the membrane (the inside becomes more positive; the outside becomes more negative). **(c)** Depolarization and generation of an action potential. If the stimulus is strong enough, depolarization causes membrane polarity to be completely reversed and an action potential is initiated. **(d)** Propagation of the action potential. Depolarization of the first membrane patch causes permeability changes in the adjacent membrane, and the events described in (b) are repeated. Thus, the action potential propagates rapidly along the entire length of the membrane. **(e)** Repolarization. Potassium ions diffuse out of the cell as membrane permeability changes again, restoring the negative charge on the inside of the membrane and the positive charge on the outside surface. Repolarization occurs in the same direction as depolarization. **(f)** The ionic conditions of the resting state are restored later by the activity of the sodium-potassium pump.

100 Keys | The stronger the stimulus, the greater the area that is affected, thus more neurons carry the impulse in an all-or-none manner.

begun, these sequential events spread along the entire neuronal membrane.

The events just described explain propagation of a nerve impulse along unmyelinated fibers. Fibers that have myelin sheaths conduct impulses much faster because the nerve impulse literally jumps, or leaps, from node to node along the length of the fiber. This occurs because no current can flow across the axon membrane where there is fatty myelin insulation. This faster type of impulse propagation is called **saltatory** (sal'tah-to"re) **conduction** (*saltare* = to dance or leap). Figure 7.13 demonstrates saltatory propagation along a myelinated axon.

So far we have explained only the irritability aspect of neuronal functioning. What about conductivity—how does the electrical impulse traveling along one neuron get across the synapse

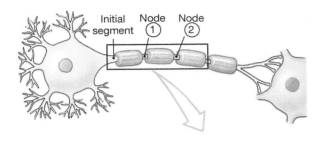

FIGURE 7.13 Saltatory propagation along a myelinated axon. This process will continue along the entire length of the axon.

to the next neuron (or effector cell) to influence its activity? The answer is that *it* doesn't! When the action potential reaches the axon terminal, the tiny vesicles containing the neurotransmitter chemical fuse with the axonal membrane, causing a pore-like opening to form and releasing the neurotransmitter. The neurotransmitter molecules diffuse across the synapse* and bind to receptors on the membrane of the next neuron (Figure 7.14). If enough neurotransmitter is released, the whole series of events described above (sodium entry, depolarization, etc.) will occur, leading to generation of a nerve impulse in the neuron beyond the synapse. The electrical changes prompted by neurotransmitter binding are very brief because the neurotransmitter is quickly removed from the synapse, either by re-uptake into the axonal terminal or by enzymatic breakdown. This limits the effect of each nerve impulse to a period shorter than the blink of an eye.

Notice that the transmission of an **impulse** is an *electrochemical event.* Transmission down the length of the neuron's membrane is basically *electrical,* but the next neuron is stimulated by a neurotransmitter, which is a *chemical.* Since each neuron both receives signals from and sends signals to scores of other neurons, it carries on "conversations" with many different neurons at the same time.

*Although most neurons communicate via the *chemical* type of synapse described above, there are some examples of *electrical* synapses in which the neurons are physically joined by gap junctions and electrical currents actually flow from one neuron to the next.

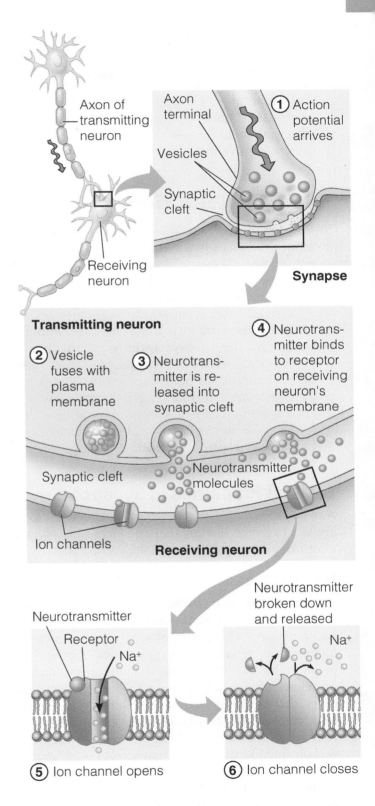

FIGURE 7.14 How neurons communicate at chemical synapses. The events occurring at the synapse are numbered in order.

100 Keys | "Information" travels within the nervous system primarily in the form of propagated electrical signals known as **action potentials.** The most important information—including vision and balance sensations, and the motor commands to skeletal muscles—is carried by large-diameter myelinated axons.

Synaptic Function

In the nervous system, messages move from one location to another in the form of action potentials along axons. These electrical events are also known as **nerve impulses.** To be effective, a message must be not only propagated along an axon, but also transferred in some way to another cell. At a synapse between two neurons, the impulse passes from the **presynaptic neuron** to the **postsynaptic neuron**. A synapse may also involve other types of postsynaptic cells. For example, the neuromuscular junction is a synapse where the postsynaptic cell is a skeletal muscle fiber. We will now take a closer look at the mechanisms involved in **synaptic function.**

General Properties of Synapses

A synapse may be *electrical,* with direct physical contact between the cells, or *chemical,* involving a neurotransmitter.

Electrical Synapses

At **electrical synapses,** the presynaptic and postsynaptic membranes are locked together at gap junctions. The lipid portions of the opposing membranes, separated by only 2 nm, are held in position by binding between integral membrane proteins called *connexons.* These proteins contain pores that permit the passage of ions between the cells. Because the two cells are linked in this way, changes in the transmembrane potential of one cell will produce local currents that affect the other cell as if the two shared a common membrane. As a result, an electrical synapse propagates action potentials quickly and efficiently from one cell to the next.

Electrical synapses are located in both the CNS and PNS, but they are extremely rare. They are present in some areas of the brain, including the

vestibular nuclei, in the eye, and in at least one pair of PNS ganglia (the *ciliary ganglia*).

Chemical Synapses

The situation at a **chemical synapse** is far more dynamic than that at an electrical synapse, because the cells are not directly coupled. For example, an action potential that reaches an electrical synapse will *always* be propagated to the next cell. But at a chemical synapse, an arriving action potential *may or may not* release enough neurotransmitter to bring the postsynaptic neuron to threshold. In addition, other factors may intervene and make the postsynaptic cell more or less sensitive to arriving stimuli. In essence, the postsynaptic cell at a chemical synapse is not a slave to the presynaptic neuron; its activity can be adjusted, or "tuned," by a variety of factors.

Chemical synapses are by far the most abundant type of synapse. Most synapses between neurons, and all communications between neurons and other types of cells, involve chemical synapses. Normally, communication across a chemical synapse can occur in only one direction: from the presynaptic membrane to the postsynaptic membrane.

Although acetylcholine is the neurotransmitter that has received the most attention, there are other important chemical transmitters. Based on their effects on postsynaptic membranes, neurotransmitters are often classified as excitatory or inhibitory. **Excitatory neurotransmitters** cause depolarization and promote the generation of action potentials, whereas **inhibitory neurotransmitters** cause hyperpolarization and suppress the generation of action potentials.

This classification is useful, but not always precise. For example, acetylcholine typically produces a depolarization in the postsynaptic membrane, but acetylcholine released at neuromuscular junctions in the heart has an inhibitory effect, producing a transient hyperpolarization of the postsynaptic membrane. This situation highlights an important aspect of neurotransmitter function: *The effect of a neurotransmitter on the postsynaptic membrane depends on the properties of the receptor, not on the nature of the neurotransmitter.*

We will continue our discussion of chemical synapses with a closer look at a synapse that releases the neurotransmitter **acetylcholine (ACh).** We will then briefly examine the activities of other important neurotransmitters.

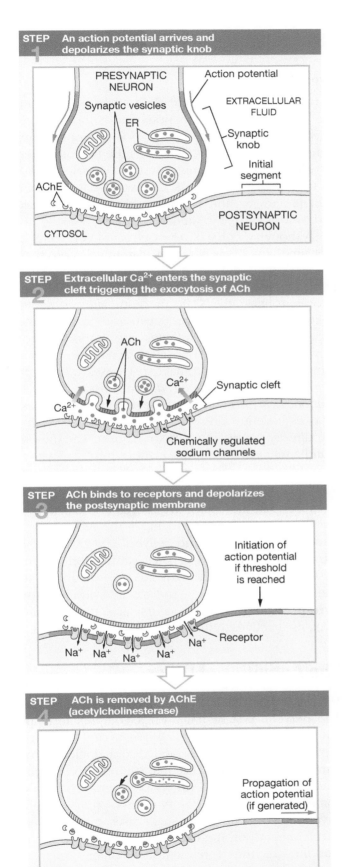

STEP 1 An action potential arrives and depolarizes the synaptic knob

PRESYNAPTIC NEURON

Synaptic vesicles

ER

AChE

CYTOSOL

Action potential

EXTRACELLULAR FLUID

Synaptic knob

Initial segment

POSTSYNAPTIC NEURON

STEP 2 Extracellular Ca^{2+} enters the synaptic cleft triggering the exocytosis of ACh

ACh

Ca^{2+}

Ca^{2+}

Synaptic cleft

Chemically regulated sodium channels

STEP 3 ACh binds to receptors and depolarizes the postsynaptic membrane

Initiation of action potential if threshold is reached

Na$^+$ Na$^+$ Na$^+$ Na$^+$

Na$^+$ Receptor

STEP 4 ACh is removed by AChE (acetylcholinesterase)

Propagation of action potential (if generated)

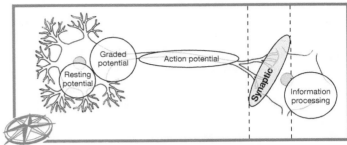

FIGURE 7.15   Events in the functioning of a cholinergic synapse.

Cholinergic Synapses

Synapses that release ACh are known as **cholinergic synapses.** The neuromuscular junction is an example of a cholinergic synapse. ACh, the most widespread (and best-studied) neurotransmitter, is released (1) at all neuromuscular junctions involving skeletal muscle fibers, (2) at many synapses in the CNS, (3) at all neuron-to-neuron synapses in the PNS, and (4) at all neuromuscular and neuroglandular junctions within the parasympathetic division of the ANS.

At a cholinergic synapse between two neurons, the presynaptic and postsynaptic membranes are separated by a synaptic cleft that averages 20 nm (0.02 μm) in width. Most of the ACh in the synaptic knob is packaged in synaptic vesicles, each containing several thousand molecules of the neurotransmitter. A single synaptic knob may contain a million such vesicles.

Events at a Cholinergic Synapse

Figure 7.15 diagrams the events that occur at a cholinergic synapse after an action potential arrives at a synaptic knob. For convenience, we will assume that this synapse is adjacent to the initial segment of the axon, a common arrangement that is relatively easy to illustrate.

Step 1 **An Action Potential Arrives and Depolarizes the Synaptic Knob** (see Figure 7.15). The normal stimulus for neurotransmitter release is the depolarization of the synaptic knob by the arrival of an action potential.

Step 2 **Calcium modulation: Extracellular Calcium Ions Enter the Synaptic Knob, Triggering the Exocytosis of ACh.** The depolarization of the synaptic knob opens voltage-regulated calcium channels. In the brief period during which these channels remain open, calcium ions rush into the knob. Their arrival triggers exocytosis and the release of ACh into the synaptic cleft. The ACh is released in packets of roughly 3000 molecules, the average number of ACh molecules in a single vesicle. The release of ACh stops very soon, because the calcium ions that triggered exocytosis are rapidly removed from the cytoplasm by active transport mechanisms; they are either pumped out of the cell or transferred into mitochondria, vesicles, or the endoplasmic reticulum.

Step 3 ACh Binds to Receptors and Depolarizes the Postsynaptic Membrane. The ACh released through exocytosis diffuses across the synaptic cleft toward receptors on the postsynaptic membrane. These receptors are chemically regulated ion channels. The primary response is an increased permeability to Na^+, producing a depolarization that lasts about 20 msec.*

This depolarization is a graded potential: The greater the amount of ACh released at the presynaptic membrane, the larger the depolarization. If the depolarization brings the adjacent area of excitable membrane to threshold, an action potential will appear in the postsynaptic neuron.

Step 4   ACh Is Removed by AChE. The effects on the postsynaptic membrane are temporary, because the synaptic cleft and the postsynaptic membrane contain the enzyme *acetylcholinesterase (AChE, or cholinesterase)*. Roughly half of the ACh released at the presynaptic membrane is broken down before it reaches receptors on the postsynaptic membrane. ACh molecules that succeed in binding to receptor sites are generally broken down within 20 msec of their arrival.

AChE breaks down molecules of ACh into **acetate** and **choline.** The choline is actively absorbed by the synaptic knob and is used to synthesize more ACh, using acetate provided by *coenzyme A (CoA)*. Coenzymes derived from vitamins are required in many enzymatic reactions. Acetate diffusing away from the synapse can be absorbed and metabolized by the postsynaptic cell or by other cells and tissues.

---

*These channels also let potassium ions out of the cell, but because sodium ions are driven by a much stronger electrochemical gradient, the net effect is a slight depolarization of the postsynaptic membrane.

Table 7.2 summarizes the events that occur at a cholinergic synapse.

Synaptic Delay

A 0.2–0.5-msec **synaptic delay** occurs between the arrival of the action potential at the synaptic knob and the effect on the postsynaptic membrane. Most of that delay reflects the time involved in calcium influx and neurotransmitter release, not in the neurotransmitter's diffusion—the synaptic cleft is narrow, and neurotransmitters can diffuse across it in very little time.

Although a delay of 0.5 msec is not very long, in that time, an action potential may travel more than 7 cm (about 3 in.) along a myelinated axon. When information is being passed along a chain of interneurons in the CNS, the cumulative synaptic delay may exceed the propagation time along the axons. This is why reflexes are important for survival—they involve only a few synapses and thus provide rapid and automatic responses to stimuli. *The fewer synapses involved, the shorter the total synaptic delay and the faster the response.* The fastest reflexes have just one synapse, with a sensory neuron directly controlling a motor neuron. The muscle spindle reflexes are an important example.

Synaptic Fatigue

Because ACh molecules are recycled, the synaptic knob is not totally dependent on the ACh synthesized in the cell body and delivered by axoplasmic transport. But under intensive stimulation, resynthesis and transport mechanisms may be unable to keep pace with the demand for neurotransmitter. **Synaptic fatigue** then occurs, and the synapse remains inactive until ACh has been replenished.

The Activities of Other Neurotransmitters

The nervous system relies on a complex form of chemical communication. Whereas it was once thought that neurons responded to a single neurotransmitter, we now realize that each neuron is continuously exposed to a variety of neurotransmitters. Some usually have excitatory effects, others usually have inhibitory effects. Yet in all cases, the observed effects depend on the nature of the receptor rather than the structure of the neurotransmitter.

Major categories of neurotransmitters include *biogenic amines, amino acids, neuropeptides,*

TABLE 7.2   Synaptic Activity

THE SEQUENCE OF EVENTS AT A TYPICAL CHOLINERGIC SYNAPSE:

STEP 1:

- An arriving action potential depolarizes the synaptic knob.

STEP 2:

- Calcium ions enter the cytoplasm of the synaptic knob.
- ACh is released through exocytosis of neurotransmitter vesicles.

STEP 3:

- ACh diffuses across the synaptic cleft and binds to receptors on the postsynaptic membrane.
- Chemically regulated sodium channels on the postsynaptic surface are activated, producing a graded depolarization.
- ACh release ceases because calcium ions are removed from the cytoplasm of the synaptic knob.

STEP 4:

- The depolarization ends as ACh is broken down into acetate and choline by AChE.
- The synaptic knob reabsorbs choline from the synaptic cleft and uses it to resynthesize ACh.

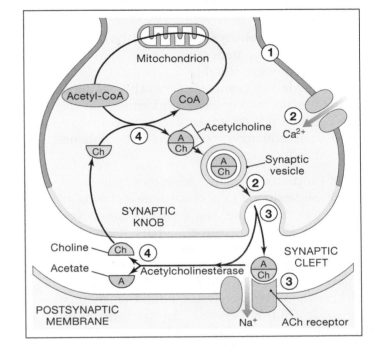

dissolved gases, and a variety of other compounds. Here we will consider only a few of the most important neurotransmitters.

- **Norepinephrine** (nor-ep-i-NEF-rin), or **NE,** is a neurotransmitter that is widely distributed in the brain and in portions of the ANS. Norepinephrine is also called *noradrenaline,* and synapses that release NE are known as **adrenergic synapses.** Norepinephrine typically has an excitatory, depolarizing effect on the postsynaptic membrane, but the mechanism is quite distinct from that of ACh. Its effects last longer than ACh, up to several minutes.

- **Dopamine** (DŌ-puh-mēn), a CNS neurotransmitter released in many areas of the brain, may have either inhibitory or excitatory effects. Inhibitory effects play an important role in our precise control of movements. For example, dopamine release in one portion of the brain prevents the overstimulation of neurons that control

skeletal muscle tone. If the neurons that produce dopamine are damaged or destroyed, the result can be the characteristic rigidity and stiffness of *Parkinson's disease.* At other sites, dopamine release has excitatory effects. Cocaine inhibits the removal of dopamine from synapses in specific areas of the brain. The resulting rise in dopamine concentrations at these synapses is responsible for the "high" experienced by cocaine users.

- **Serotonin** (ser-o-TŌ-nin) is another important CNS neurotransmitter. Inadequate serotonin production can have widespread effects on a person's attention and emotional states and may be responsible for many cases of severe chronic depression. *Fluoxetine (Prozac), Paxil, Zoloft,* and related antidepressant drugs inhibit the reabsorption of serotonin by synaptic knobs (hence their classification as *selective serotonin reuptake inhibitors,* or *SSRIs*). This inhibition leads to increased serotonin concentrations at synapses; over time, the increase may relieve the symptoms of depression. Interactions among serotonin, norepinephrine, and other neurotransmitters are thought to be involved in the regulation of sleep and wake cycles.

- **Gamma aminobutyric** (a-MĒ-nō-bū-TĒR-ik) **acid,** or **GABA,** generally has an inhibitory effect. Although roughly 20 percent of the synapses in the brain release GABA, its functions remain incompletely understood. In the CNS, GABA release appears to reduce anxiety, and some antianxiety drugs work by enhancing this effect.

The functions of many neurotransmitters are not well understood. In a clear demonstration of the principle "the more you look, the more you see," at least 50 neurotransmitters have been identified, including certain amino acids, peptides, polypeptides, prostaglandins, and ATP. In addition, two gases, nitric oxide and carbon monoxide, are now known to be important neurotransmitters. Nitric oxide (NO) is generated by synaptic terminals that innervate smooth muscle in the walls of blood vessels in the PNS, and at synapses in several regions of the brain. Carbon monoxide (CO), best known as a component of automobile exhaust, is also generated by specialized synaptic knobs in the brain, where it functions as a neurotransmitter. Our knowledge of the significance of these compounds and the mechanisms involved in their synthesis and release remains incomplete.

Enzymes are a common target for recreational drugs. Monoamine oxidase (MAO) is an enzyme that breaks down both natural and ingested neurotransmitters. Several antidepressants block MAO, which inhibits its natural function of breaking down dopamine, seratonin, and norepinephrine.

100 Keys | At a chemical synapse, a synaptic terminal releases a neurotransmitter that binds to the postsynaptic cell membrane. The result is a temporary, localized change in the permeability or function of the postsynaptic cell. This change may have broader effects on the cell, depending on the nature and number of stimulated receptors. Many drugs affect the nervous system by stimulating receptors that otherwise respond only to neurotransmitters. These drugs can have complex effects on perception, motor control, and emotional states.

Neuromodulators

Although it is convenient to discuss each synapse as if it were releasing only one chemical, synaptic knobs may release a mixture of active compounds, either through diffusion across the membrane or via exocytosis, in the company of neurotransmitter molecules. These compounds may have a variety of functions. Those that alter the rate of neurotransmitter release by the presynaptic neuron or change the postsynaptic cell's response to neurotransmitters are called **neuromodulators** (noo-rō-MOD-ū-lā-torz). These substances are typically **neuropeptides,** small peptide chains synthesized and released by the synaptic knob. Most neuromodulators act by binding to receptors in the presynaptic or postsynaptic membranes and activating cytoplasmic enzymes.

Neuromodulators called **opioids** (Ō-pē-oydz) have effects similar to those of the drugs *opium* and *morphine,* because they bind to the same group of postsynaptic receptors. Four classes of opioids are identified in the CNS: (1) **endorphins** (en-DOR-finz), (2) **enkephalins** (en-KEF-a-linz), (3) **endomorphins,** and (4) **dynorphins** (dī-NOR-finz). The primary function of opioids is probably the relief of pain—they inhibit the release of the neurotransmitter *substance P* at synapses that relay pain sensations. Dynorphins have far more powerful analgesic (pain-relieving) effects than morphine or the other opioids.

In general, neuromodulators (1) have long-term effects that are relatively slow to appear, (2) trigger responses that involve a number of steps and intermediary compounds, (3) may affect the presynaptic membrane, the postsynaptic membrane, or both, and (4) can be released alone or in the company of a neurotransmitter. Table 7.3 lists major neurotransmitters and neuromodulators of the brain and spinal cord, and their primary effects (if known). In practice, it can be very difficult to distinguish neurotransmitters from neuromodulators on either biochemical or functional grounds: A neuropeptide may function in one site as a neuromodulator and in another as a neurotransmitter. For this reason, Table 7.3 does not distinguish between neurotransmitters and neuromodulators.

How Neurotransmitters and Neuromodulators Work

Functionally, neurotransmitters and neuromodulators fall into one of three groups: (1) *compounds*

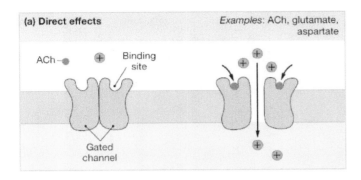

(a) **Direct effects**   *Examples*: ACh, glutamate, aspartate

ACh
Binding site
Gated channel

(b) **Indirect effects via G proteins**   *Examples*: E, NE, dopamine, histamine, GABA

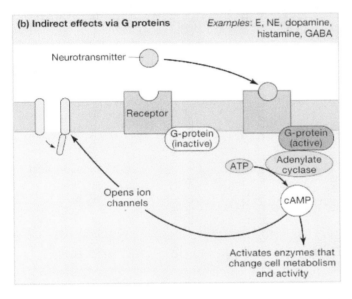

Neurotransmitter
Receptor
G-protein (inactive)
G-protein (active)
ATP
Adenylate cyclase
Opens ion channels
cAMP
Activates enzymes that change cell metabolism and activity

(c) **Indirect effects via intracellular enzymes**   *Examples*: Nitric oxide, carbon monoxide

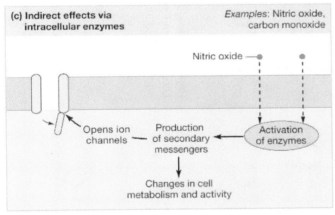

Nitric oxide
Opens ion channels
Production of secondary messengers
Activation of enzymes
Changes in cell metabolism and activity

that have a direct effect on membrane potential, (2) compounds that have an indirect effect on membrane potential, or (3) lipid-soluble gases that exert their effects inside the cell.

Information Processing by Individual Neurons

A single neuron may receive information across thousands of synapses, and, as we have seen, some of the neurotransmitters arriving at the postsynaptic cell at any moment may be excitatory, whereas others may be inhibitory. The net effect on the transmembrane potential of the cell body—specifically, in the area of the axon hillock—determines how the neuron responds from moment to moment. If the net effect is a depolarization at the axon hillock, that depolarization will affect the transmembrane potential at the initial segment. If threshold is reached at the initial segment, an action potential will be generated and propagated along the axon.

Thus it is really the axon hillock that integrates the excitatory and inhibitory stimuli affecting the cell body and dendrites at any given moment. This integration process, which determines the rate of action potential generation at the initial segment, is the simplest level of **information processing** in the nervous system. The excitatory and inhibitory stimuli are integrated through interactions between *postsynaptic potentials,* which we discuss next. Higher levels of information processing involve interactions among neurons and interactions among groups of neurons.

Postsynaptic Potentials

Postsynaptic potentials are graded potentials that develop in the postsynaptic membrane in response to a neurotransmitter. Two major types of postsynaptic potentials develop at neuron-to-neuron synapses: excitatory postsynaptic potentials and inhibitory postsynaptic potentials.

An **excitatory postsynaptic potential,** or **EPSP,** is a graded depolarization caused by the arrival of a neurotransmitter at the postsynaptic membrane. An EPSP results from the opening of chemically regulated membrane channels that lead to depolarization of the cell membrane. For example, the graded depolarization produced by the binding of ACh is an EPSP. Because it is a graded potential, an EPSP affects only the area immediately surrounding the synapse.

We have already noted that not all neurotransmitters have an excitatory (depolarizing) effect. An **inhibitory postsynaptic potential,** or **IPSP,** is a graded hyperpolarization of the postsynaptic membrane. For example, an IPSP may result from the opening of chemically regulated potassium channels. While the hyperpolarization continues, the neuron is said to be **inhibited,** because a larger-than-usual depolarizing stimulus must be provided to bring the membrane potential to threshold. A stimulus sufficient to shift the transmembrane

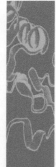

TABLE 7.3 Representative Neurotransmitters and Neuromodulators

Class and Neurotransmitter	Chemical Structure	Mechanism of Action	Location(s)	Comments
Acetylcholine	$CH_3-N^+-CH_2-CH_2-O-C-CH_3$ (with O double bond)	Primarily direct, through binding to chemically regulated channels	CNS: Synapses throughout brain and spinal cord PNS: Neuromuscular junctions; preganglionic synapses of ANS; neuroglandular junctions of parasympathetic division and (rarely) sympathetic division of ANS; amacrine cells of retina	Widespread in CNS and PNS; best known and most studied of the neurotransmitters
BIOGENIC AMINES				
Norepinephrine	$NH_2-CH_2-CH_2-$ (catechol ring with OH)	Indirect: G proteins and second messengers	CNS: Cerebral cortex, hypothalamus, brain stem, cerebellum, spinal cord PNS: Most neuromuscular and neuroglandular junctions of sympathetic division of ANS	Involved in attention and consciousness, control of body temperature, and regulation of pituitary gland secretion
Epinephrine	$CH_2-NH-CH_2-CH-$ (catechol ring with OH)	Indirect: G proteins and second messengers	CNS: Thalamus, hypothalamus, midbrain, spinal cord	Uncertain functions
Dopamine	$NH_2-CH_2-CH_2-$ (catechol ring)	Indirect: G proteins and second messengers	CNS: Hypothalamus, midbrain, limbic system, cerebral cortex, retina	Regulation of subconscious motor function; receptor abnormalities have been linked to development of schizophrenia
Serotonin	$NH_2-CH_2-CH_2-$ (indole ring with OH)	Primarily indirect: G proteins and second messengers	CNS: Hypothalamus, limbic system, cerebellum, spinal cord, retina	Important in emotional states, moods, and body temperature; several illicit hallucinogenic drugs, such as *Ecstasy*, target serotonin receptors
Histamine	$NH_2-CH_2-CH_2-$ (imidazole ring)	Indirect: G proteins and second messengers	CNS: Neurons in hypothalamus, with axons projecting throughout the brain	Receptors are primarily on presynaptic membranes; functions in sexual arousal, pain threshold, pituitary hormone secretion, thirst, and blood pressure control

AMINO ACIDS

Neurotransmitter	Structure	Mechanism	Site	Effects
Excitatory: **Glutamate**	O=C(HO)—CH—CH₂—CH₂—C(O)—OH with NH₂	Indirect: G proteins and second messengers Direct: opens calcium channels on pre- and postsynaptic membranes	CNS: Cerebral cortex and brain stem	Important in memory and learning; most important excitatory neurotransmitter in the brain
Aspartate	O=C(HO)—CH—CH₂—C(O)—OH with NH₂	Direct or indirect (G proteins), depending on type of receptor	CNS: Cerebral cortex, retina, and spinal cord	Used by pyramidal cells that provide voluntary motor control over skeletal muscles
Inhibitory: **Gamma γ aminobutyric acid (GABA)**	NH₂—CH₂—CH₂—CH₂—C(O)—OH	Direct or indirect (G proteins), depending on type of receptor	CNS: Cerebral cortex, cerebellum, interneurons throughout brain and spinal cord	Direct effects: open Cl^- channels; indirect effects: open K^+ channels and block entry of Ca^{2+}
Glycine	NH₂—CH₂—C(O)—OH	Direct: Opens Cl^- channels	CNS: Interneurons in brain stem, spinal cord, and retina	Produces postsynaptic inhibition; the poison *strychnine* produces fatal convulsions by blocking glycine receptors

NEUROPEPTIDES

Neurotransmitter	Structure	Mechanism	Site	Effects
Substance P	Arg–Pro–Lys–Pro–Glu–Gln–Phe–Gly–Leu–Met	Indirect: G proteins and second messengers	CNS: Synapses of pain receptors within spinal cord, hypothalamus, and other areas of the brain PNS: Entericnervous system (network of neurons along the digestive tract)	Important in pain pathway, regulation of pituitary gland function, control of digestive tract reflexes
Neuropeptide Y	36-amino-acid peptide	As above	CNS: hypothalamus PNS: sympathetic neurons	Stimulates appetite and food intake
Opioids Endorphins	31-amino-acid peptide	Indirect: G proteins and second messengers	CNS: Thalamus, hypothalamus, brain stem, retina	Pain control; emotional and behavioral effects poorly understood
Enkephalins	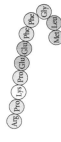 Tyr–Gly–Gly–Phe–Met	As above	CNS: Basal nuclei, hypothalamus, midbrain, pons, medulla oblongata, spinal cord	As above

(continued)

TABLE 7.3 (continued)

Class and Neurotransmitter	Chemical Structure	Mechanism of Action	Location(s)	Comments
Endomorphin	9-or 10-amino-acid peptide	As above	CNS: Thalamus, hypothalamus, basal nuclei	As above
Dynorphin	[peptide structure: Tyr–Gly–Gly–Phe–Leu–Arg–Arg–Ile–Arg–Pro–Lys–Leu–Lys–Trp–Asp–Asn–Gln]	As above	CNS: hypothalamus, midbrain, medulla oblongata	As above
PURINES				
ATP, GTP		Direct or indirect (G proteins), depending on type of receptor	CNS: Spinal cord PNS: Autonomic ganglia	
Adenosine		Indirect: G proteins and second messengers	CNS: Cerebral cortex, hippocampus, cerebellum	Produces drowsiness; stimulatory effect of caffeine is due to inhibition of adenosine activity
HORMONES				
ADH, oxytocin, insulin,glucagon, secretin, CCK, GIP, VIP, inhibins, ANP, BNP, and many others	Peptide containing fewer than 200 amino acids	Typically indirect: G proteins and second messengers	CNS: Brain (widespread)	Numerous, complex, and incompletely understood
GASES				
Carbon monoxide (CO)	$C = O$	Indirect: By diffusion to enzymes activating second messengers	CNS: Brain PNS: Some neuromuscular and neuroglandular junctions	Localization and function poorly understood
Nitric oxide (NO)	$N = O$	As above	CNS: Brain, especially at blood vessels PNS: Some sympathetic neuromuscular and neuroglandular junctions	
LIPIDS				
Anandamide	[lipid structure]	Indirect: G proteins and second messengers	CNS: cerebral cortex, hippocampus, cerebellum in marijuana	Euphoria, drowsiness; receptors are targeted by the active ingredient

potential by 10 mV (from −70 mV to −60 mV) would normally produce an action potential, but if the transmembrane potential were reset at −85 mV by an IPSP, the same stimulus would depolarize it to only −75 mV, which is below threshold.

Summation

An individual EPSP has a small effect on the transmembrane potential, typically producing a depolarization of about 0.5 mV at the postsynaptic

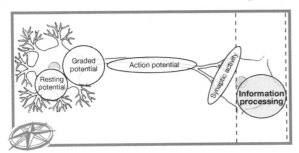

membrane. Before an action potential will arise in the initial segment, local currents must depolarize that region by at least 10 mV. Therefore, a single EPSP will not result in an action potential, even if the synapse is on the axon hillock. But individual EPSPs combine through the process of **summation,** which integrates the effects of all the graded potentials that affect one portion of the cell membrane. The graded potentials may be EPSPs, IPSPs, or both. We will consider EPSPs in our discussion.

Two forms of summation exist: temporal summation and spatial summation (Figure 7.16).

Temporal summation (*tempus,* time) is the addition of stimuli occurring in rapid succession at a *single synapse* that is active *repeatedly*. This form of summation can be likened to using a bucket to fill up a bathtub; you can't fill the tub with a single bucket of water, but you will fill it eventually if you keep repeating the process. In the case of temporal summation, the water in a bucket corresponds to the sodium ions that enter the cytoplasm during an EPSP. A typical EPSP lasts about 20 msec, but under maximum stimulation an action potential can reach the synaptic knob each millisecond. Figure 7.16a shows what happens when a second EPSP arrives before the effects of the first EPSP have disappeared. Every time an action potential arrives, a group of vesicles discharges ACh into the synaptic cleft; every time more ACh molecules arrive at the postsynaptic membrane, more chemically regulated channels open, and the degree of depolarization increases. In this way, a series

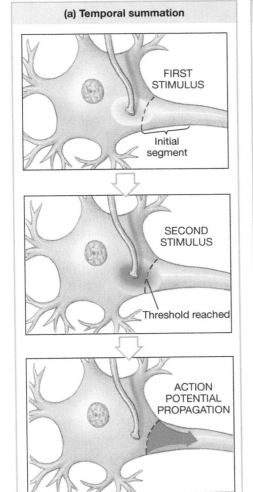

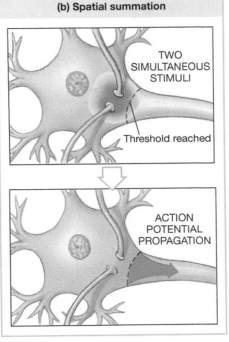

FIGURE 7.16 Temporal and spatial summation. (a) Temporal summation occurs on a membrane that receives two depolarizing stimuli from the same source in rapid succession. The effects of the second stimulus are added to those of the first. **(b)** Spatial summation occurs when sources of stimulation arrive simultaneously, but at different locations. Local currents spread the depolarizing effects, and areas of overlap experience the combined effects.

of small steps can eventually bring the initial segment to threshold.

Spatial summation occurs when simultaneous stimuli applied at different locations have a cumulative effect on the transmembrane potential. In other words, spatial summation involves *multiple synapses* that are active *simultaneously*. In terms of our bucket analogy, you could fill the bathtub immediately if 50 friends emptied their buckets into it all at the same time.

In spatial summation, more than one synapse is active at the same time (Figure 7.16b), and each "pours" sodium ions across the postsynaptic membrane, producing a graded potential with localized effects. At each active synapse, the sodium ions that produce the EPSPs spread out along the inner surface of the membrane and mingle with those entering at other synapses. As a result, the effects on the initial segment are cumulative. The degree of depolarization depends on how many synapses are active at any moment, and on their distance from the initial segment. As in temporal summation, an action potential results when the transmembrane potential at the initial segment reaches threshold.

Facilitation

Consider a situation in which summation of EPSPs is underway, but the initial segment has not been depolarized to threshold. The closer the initial segment is to threshold, the easier it will be for the *next* depolarizing stimulus to trigger an action potential. A neuron whose transmembrane potential shifts closer to threshold is said to be **facilitated.** The larger the degree of facilitation, the smaller is the additional stimulus needed to trigger an action potential. In a highly facilitated neuron, even a small depolarizing stimulus produces an action potential.

Facilitation can result from the summation of EPSPs or from the exposure of a neuron to certain drugs in the extracellular fluid. For example, the nicotine in cigarettes stimulates postsynaptic ACh receptors, producing prolonged EPSPs that facilitate CNS neurons.

Summation of EPSPs and IPSPs

Like EPSPs, IPSPs summate spatially and temporally. EPSPs and IPSPs reflect the activation of different types of chemically regulated channels, producing opposing effects on the transmembrane potential. The antagonism between IPSPs and EPSPs is an important mechanism in cellular information processing. In terms of our bucket analogy, EPSPs put water into the bathtub, and IPSPs take water out. If more buckets add water than remove water, the water level in the tub will rise. If more buckets remove water, the level will fall. If a bucket of water is removed every time another bucket is dumped in, the level will remain stable. Comparable interactions between EPSPs and IPSPs (Figure 7.17) determine the transmembrane potential at the boundary between the axon hillock and the initial segment.

Neuromodulators, hormones, or both can change the postsynaptic membrane's sensitivity to excitatory or inhibitory neurotransmitters. By shifting the balance between EPSPs and IPSPs, these compounds promote facilitation or inhibition of CNS and PNS neurons.

Principles of Functional Organization

The human body has about 10 million sensory neurons, one-half million motor neurons, and 20 *billion* interneurons. The sensory neurons deliver information to the CNS; the motor neurons distribute commands to peripheral effectors, such as skeletal muscles; and the interneurons interpret, plan, and coordinate the incoming and outgoing signals.

Neuronal Pools

The billions of interneurons of the CNS are organized into a much smaller number of **neuronal pools**—functional groups of interconnected neurons. A neuronal pool may be diffuse, involving neurons in several regions of the brain, or localized, with neurons restricted to one specific location in the brain or spinal cord. Estimates of the actual number of neuronal pools range between a few hundred and a few thousand. Each has a limited number of input sources and output destinations, and each may contain both excitatory and inhibitory neurons. The output of the entire neuronal pool may stimulate or depress activity in other parts of the brain or spinal cord, affecting the interpretation of sensory information or the coordination of motor commands.

The pattern of interaction among neurons provides clues to the functional characteristics of a neuronal pool. It is customary to refer to the "wiring diagrams" in Figure 7.18 as *neural circuits,* just as we refer to electrical circuits in the wiring of a house. We can distinguish five circuit patterns:

1. **Divergence** is the spread of information from one neuron to several neurons (see Figure 7.18a), or from one pool to multiple pools. Divergence permits the broad distribution of a specific input. Considerable divergence occurs when sensory neurons bring information into the CNS, for the information is distributed to neuronal pools throughout the spinal cord and brain. Visual information arriving from the eyes, for example, reaches your consciousness at the same time it is distributed to areas of the brain that control posture and balance at the subconscious level.

2. In **convergence,** several neurons synapse on a single postsynaptic neuron (see Figure 7.18b). Several patterns of activity in the presynaptic neurons can therefore have the same effect on the postsynaptic neuron. Through convergence, the same motor neurons can be subject to both conscious and subconscious control. For example, the movements of your diaphragm and ribs are now being controlled by your brain at the subconscious level. But the same motor neurons can also be controlled consciously, as when you take a deep breath and hold it. Two neuronal pools are involved, both synapsing on the same motor neurons.

3. In **serial processing,** information is relayed in a stepwise fashion, from one neuron to another or from one neuronal pool to the next (see Figure 7.18c). This pattern occurs as sensory information is relayed from one part of the brain to another. For example, pain sensations en route to your consciousness make two stops along the way, at neuronal pools along the pain pathway.

4. **Parallel processing** occurs when several neurons or neuronal pools process the same information simultaneously (see Figure 7.18d). Divergence must take place before parallel processing can occur. Thanks to parallel processing, many responses can occur simultaneously. For example, stepping on a sharp object stimulates sensory neurons that distribute the information to several neuronal pools. As a result of parallel processing, you might withdraw your foot, shift your weight, move your arms, feel the pain, and shout "Ouch!" all at the same time.

5. In **reverberation,** collateral branches of axons somewhere along the circuit extend back toward the source of an impulse and further stimulate the presynaptic neurons (see Figure 7.18e). Reverberation is like a positive feedback loop involving neurons: Once a reverberating circuit has been activated, it will continue to function until synaptic fatigue or inhibitory stimuli break the cycle. Reverberation can occur within a single neuronal pool,

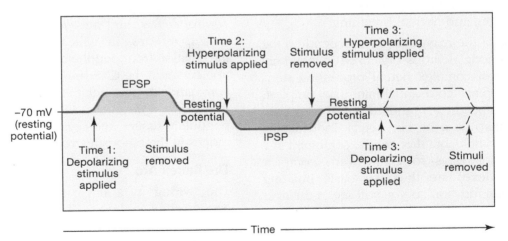

FIGURE 7.17 **Interactions between EPSPs and IPSPs.** At time 1, a small depolarizing stimulus produces an EPSP. At time 2, a small hyperpolarizing stimulus produces an IPSP of comparable magnitude. If the two stimuli are applied simultaneously, as they are at time 3, summation occurs. Because the two are equal in size but have opposite effects, the membrane potential remains at the resting level. If the EPSP were larger, a net depolarization would result; if the IPSP were larger, a net hyperpolarization would result instead.

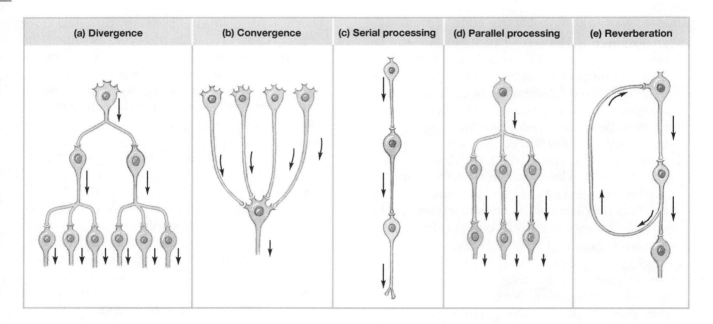

FIGURE 7.18   Neural circuits: the organization of neuronal pools.
(a) Divergence, a mechanism for spreading stimulation to multiple neurons or neuronal pools in the CNS. **(b)** Convergence, a mechanism providing input to a single neuron from multiple sources. **(c)** Serial processing, in which neurons or pools work sequentially. **(d)** Parallel processing, in which neurons or pools process information simultaneously. **(e)** Reverberation, a positive feedback mechanism.

or it may involve a series of interconnected pools. Highly complicated examples of reverberation among neuronal pools in the brain may help maintain consciousness, muscular coordination, and normal breathing.

The functions of the nervous system depend on the interactions among neurons organized in neuronal pools. The most complex neural processing steps occur in the spinal cord and brain. The simplest, which occur within the PNS and the spinal cord, control reflexes that are a bit like Legos: Individually, they are quite simple, but they can be combined in a great variety of ways to create very complex responses. Reflexes are thus the basic building blocks of neural function, as you will see in the next section.

An Introduction to Reflexes

Conditions inside or outside the body can change rapidly and unexpectedly. **Reflexes** are rapid, automatic responses to specific stimuli. Reflexes preserve homeostasis by making rapid adjustments in the function of organs or organ systems. The response shows little variability: Each time a particular reflex is activated, it usually produces the same motor response. Chapter 1 introduced the basic functional components involved in all types of homeostatic regulation: a *receptor,* an *integration control center,* and an *effector.* Here we consider *neural reflexes,* in which sensory fibers deliver information from peripheral receptors to an integration center in the CNS, and motor fibers carry motor commands to peripheral effectors. We will examine *endocrine reflexes,* in which the commands to peripheral tissues and organs are delivered by hormones in the bloodstream, in Chapter 9.

The Reflex Arc

The "wiring" of a single reflex is called a **reflex arc.** A reflex arc begins at a receptor and ends at a peripheral effector, such as a muscle fiber or a gland cell. Figure 7.19 diagrams the five steps in a simple neural reflex known as a *stretch reflex:*

Step 1   **The Arrival of a Stimulus and Activation of a Receptor.** A *receptor* is either a specialized cell or the dendrites of a sensory neuron. Receptors are sensitive to physical or chemical changes in the body and to changes in the external environment. If you lean on a tack, for

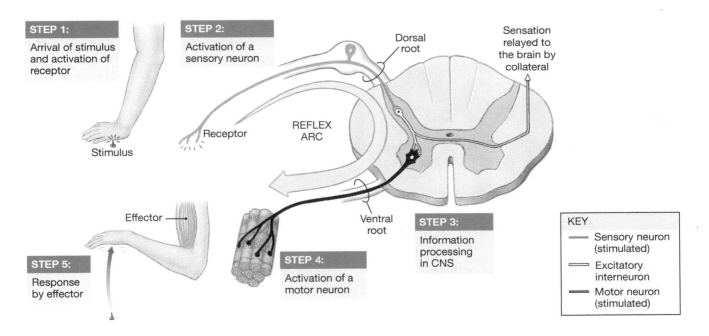

STEP 1: Arrival of stimulus and activation of receptor

STEP 2: Activation of a sensory neuron

Dorsal root

Sensation relayed to the brain by collateral

Stimulus

Receptor

REFLEX ARC

Effector

Ventral root

STEP 3: Information processing in CNS

STEP 5: Response by effector

STEP 4: Activation of a motor neuron

KEY
— Sensory neuron (stimulated)
═ Excitatory interneuron
▬ Motor neuron (stimulated)

FIGURE 7.19   Events in a neural reflex. A simple reflex arc, such as the withdrawal reflex, consists of a sensory neuron, an interneuron, and a motor neuron.

example, pain receptors in the palm of your hand are activated. These receptors, the dendrites of sensory neurons, respond to stimuli that cause or accompany tissue damage.

Step 2   The Activation of a Sensory Neuron. When the dendrites are stretched, there is a graded depolarization that leads to the formation and propagation of action potentials along the axons of the sensory neurons. This information reaches the spinal cord by way of a dorsal root. In our example, STEP 1 and STEP 2 involve the same cell. However, the two steps may involve different cells. For example, reflexes triggered by loud sounds begin when receptor cells in the inner ear release neurotransmitters that stimulate sensory neurons.

Step 3   Information Processing. In our example, information processing begins when excitatory neurotransmitter molecules, released by the synaptic knob of a sensory neuron, arrive at the postsynaptic membrane of an interneuron. The neurotransmitter produces an excitatory postsynaptic potential (EPSP), which is integrated with other stimuli arriving at the postsynaptic cell at that moment. The information processing is thus performed by the interneuron. In the simplest reflexes, such as the *stretch reflex*, considered in a later

section, the sensory neuron innervates a motor neuron directly. In that case, it is the motor neuron that performs the information processing. By contrast, complex reflexes introduced later in the chapter involve several interneurons, some releasing excitatory neurotransmitters (*excitatory interneurons*) and others inhibitory neurotransmitters (*inhibitory interneurons*).

Step 4   The Activation of a Motor Neuron. The axons of the stimulated motor neurons carry action potentials into the periphery—in this example, through the ventral root of a spinal nerve.

Step 5   The Response of a Peripheral Effector. The release of neurotransmitters by the motor neurons at synaptic knobs then leads to a response by a peripheral effector—in this case, a skeletal muscle whose contraction pulls your hand away from the tack.

A reflex response generally removes or opposes the original stimulus; in this case, the contracting muscle pulls your hand away from a painful stimulus. This reflex arc is therefore an example of *negative feedback*. By opposing potentially harmful changes in the internal or external environment, reflexes play an important role in homeostatic maintenance. The immediate reflex response is typically not the only response to a stimulus. The other responses, which are directed by your brain, involve multiple synapses and take longer to organize and coordinate.

Classification of Reflexes

Reflexes are classified on the basis of (1) their development, (2) the nature of the resulting motor response, (3) the complexity of the neural circuit involved, or (4) the site of information processing. These categories are not mutually exclusive—they represent different ways of describing a single reflex.

Development of Reflexes   **Innate reflexes** result from the connections that form between neurons during development. Such reflexes generally appear in a predictable sequence, from the simplest reflex responses (withdrawal from pain) to more complex motor patterns (chewing, suckling, or tracking objects with the eyes). The neural connections responsible for the basic motor patterns of an innate reflex are genetically or developmentally programmed. Examples include the reflexive removal of your hand from a hot stove top and blinking when your eyelashes are touched.

More complex, learned motor patterns are called **acquired reflexes.** An experienced driver steps on the brake when trouble appears ahead; a professional skier must make equally quick adjustments in body position while racing. These motor responses are rapid and automatic, but they were learned rather than preestablished. Such reflexes are enhanced by repetition. The distinction between innate and acquired reflexes is not absolute: Some people can learn motor patterns more quickly than others, and the differences probably have a genetic basis.

Most reflexes, whether innate or acquired, can be modified over time or suppressed through conscious effort. For example, while walking a tightrope over the Grand Canyon, you might ignore a bee sting on your hand, although under other circumstances you would probably withdraw your hand immediately, shouting and thrashing as well.

Nature of the Response   **Somatic reflexes** provide a mechanism for the involuntary control of the muscular system. *Superficial reflexes* are triggered by stimuli at the skin or mucous membranes. *Stretch reflexes* are triggered by the sudden elongation of a tendon;

a familiar example is the *patellar,* or **"knee-jerk,"** **reflex** that is usually tested during physical exams. These reflexes are also known as *deep tendon reflexes,* or *myotactic reflexes.* **Visceral reflexes,** or *autonomic reflexes,* control the activities of other systems.

The movements directed by somatic reflexes are neither delicate nor precise. You might therefore wonder why they exist at all, because we have voluntary control over the same muscles. In fact, somatic reflexes are absolutely vital, primarily because they are *immediate.* Making decisions and coordinating voluntary responses take time, and in an emergency—when you slip while descending a flight of stairs, or lean your hand against a knife edge—any delay increases the likelihood of severe injury. Thus, somatic reflexes provide a rapid response that can be modified later, if necessary, by voluntary motor commands.

Complexity of the Circuit   In the simplest reflex arc, a sensory neuron synapses directly on a motor neuron, which serves as the processing center. Such a reflex is a **monosynaptic reflex.** Transmission across a chemical synapse always involves a synaptic delay, but with only one synapse, the delay between the stimulus and the response is minimized. Most other types of reflexes have at least one interneuron between the sensory neuron and the motor neuron. The reflex diagrammed in Figure 7.19 is an example of this type of reflex. Such **polysynaptic reflexes** have a longer delay between stimulus and response. The length of the delay is proportional to the number of synapses involved. Polysynaptic reflexes can produce far more complicated responses than monosynaptic reflexes, because the interneurons can control motor neurons that activate several muscle groups simultaneously.

Processing Sites   In **spinal reflexes,** the important interconnections and processing events occur in the spinal cord. We will discuss these reflexes further in the next section. Reflexes processed in the brain, called **cranial reflexes,** will be considered later in this chapter.

Spinal Reflexes

Spinal reflexes range in complexity from simple monosynaptic reflexes involving a single segment of the spinal cord to polysynaptic reflexes that involve many segments. In the most complicated spinal reflexes, called **intersegmental reflex arcs,** many segments interact to produce a coordinated, highly variable motor response.

Monosynaptic Reflexes

In monosynaptic reflexes, there is little delay between sensory input and motor output. These reflexes control the most-rapid, stereotyped motor responses of the nervous system to specific stimuli.

The Stretch Reflex

The best-known monosynaptic reflex is the **stretch reflex,** which provides automatic regulation of skeletal muscle length. The **patellar reflex** is an example. When a physician taps your patellar tendon with a reflex hammer, receptors in the quadriceps muscle are stretched (Figure 7.20). The distortion of the receptors in turn stimulates sensory neurons that extend into the spinal cord and synapse on motor neurons that control the motor units in the stretched muscle. This leads to a reflexive contraction of the stretched muscle that extends the knee in a brief kick. To summarize: The stimulus (increasing muscle length) activates a sensory neuron, which triggers an immediate motor response (contraction of the stretched muscle) that counteracts the stimulus. Because the action potentials traveling toward and away from the spinal cord are conducted along large, myelinated Type A fibers, the entire reflex is completed within 20–40 msec.

The receptors in stretch reflexes are called *muscle spindles.* The stretching of muscle spindles produces a sudden burst of activity in the sensory neurons that monitor them. This in turn leads to stimulation of motor neurons that control the motor units in the stretched muscle. The result is a rapid increase in muscle tone, and this returns the muscle spindles to their resting length. The rate of action potential generation in the sensory neurons then declines, causing a drop in muscle tone to resting levels.

An Introduction to the Organization of the Brain

The adult human brain contains almost 98 percent of the body's neural tissue. A "typical" brain weighs 1.4 kg (3 lb) and has a volume of 1200 cc (71 in.^{3}). Brain size varies considerably among

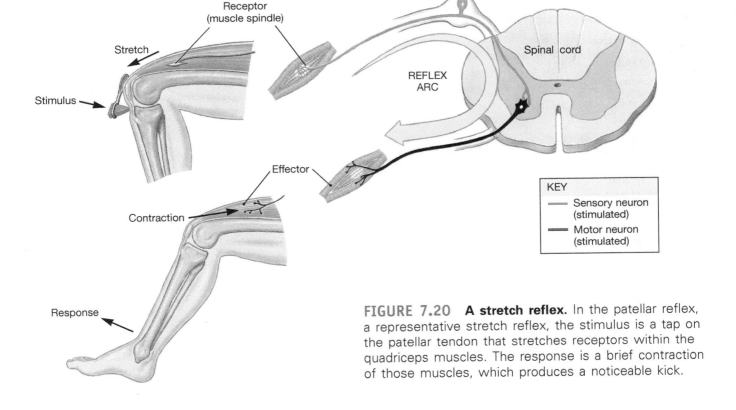

FIGURE 7.20 A stretch reflex. In the patellar reflex, a representative stretch reflex, the stimulus is a tap on the patellar tendon that stretches receptors within the quadriceps muscles. The response is a brief contraction of those muscles, which produces a noticeable kick.

individuals. The brains of males are, on average, about 10 percent larger than those of females, owing to differences in average body size. No correlation exists between brain size and intelligence. Individuals with the smallest brains (750 cc) and the largest brains (2100 cc) are functionally normal.

A Preview of Major Regions and Landmarks

The adult brain is dominated in size by the cerebrum (Figure 7.21). Viewed from the anterior and superior surfaces, the **cerebrum** (SER-e-brum, or se-RĒ-brum) of the adult brain can be divided into large, paired **cerebral hemispheres**. The surfaces of the cerebral hemispheres are highly folded and covered by **neural cortex (cortex,** rind or bark), a superficial layer of gray matter. This **cerebral cortex** forms a series of elevated ridges, or **gyri** (JĪ-rī; singular, **gyrus**) that serve to increase its surface area. The gyri are separated by shallow depressions called **sulci** (SUL-sī) or by deeper grooves called **fissures.** The cerebrum is the seat of most higher mental functions. Conscious thoughts, sensations, intellect, memory,

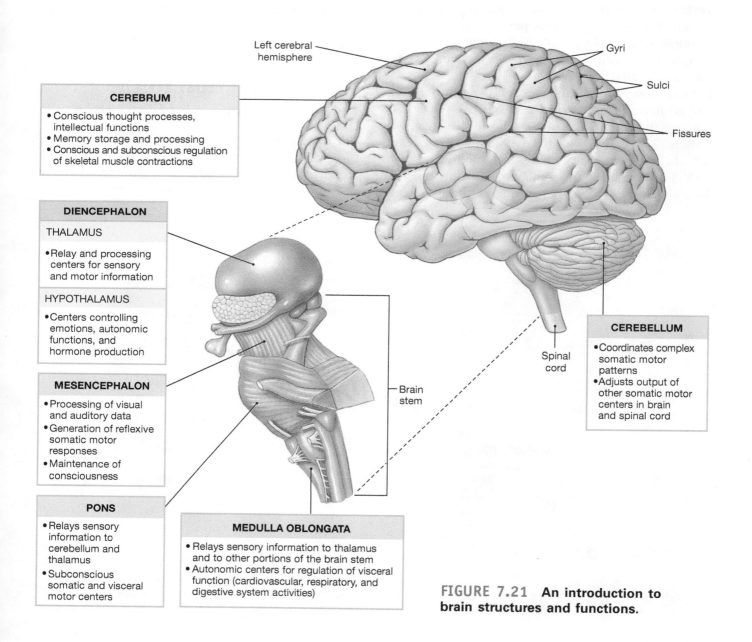

Left cerebral hemisphere

Gyri

Sulci

Fissures

CEREBRUM
- Conscious thought processes, intellectual functions
- Memory storage and processing
- Conscious and subconscious regulation of skeletal muscle contractions

DIENCEPHALON

THALAMUS
- Relay and processing centers for sensory and motor information

HYPOTHALAMUS
- Centers controlling emotions, autonomic functions, and hormone production

MESENCEPHALON
- Processing of visual and auditory data
- Generation of reflexive somatic motor responses
- Maintenance of consciousness

PONS
- Relays sensory information to cerebellum and thalamus
- Subconscious somatic and visceral motor centers

MEDULLA OBLONGATA
- Relays sensory information to thalamus and to other portions of the brain stem
- Autonomic centers for regulation of visceral function (cardiovascular, respiratory, and digestive system activities)

Brain stem

Spinal cord

CEREBELLUM
- Coordinates complex somatic motor patterns
- Adjusts output of other somatic motor centers in brain and spinal cord

FIGURE 7.21 An introduction to brain structures and functions.

and complex movements all originate in the cerebrum.[1]

The **cerebellum** (ser-e-BEL-um) is partially hidden by the cerebral hemispheres, but it is the second-largest part of the brain. Like the cerebrum, the cerebellum has hemispheres that are covered by a layer of gray matter, the *cerebellar cortex*. The cerebellum adjusts ongoing movements by comparing arriving sensations with previously experienced sensations, allowing you to perform the same movements over and over.

The other major anatomical regions of the brain can best be examined after the cerebral and cerebellar hemispheres have been removed (see Figure 7.21). The walls of the **diencephalon** (dī-en-SEF-a-lon; *dia,* through + *cephalon,* head) are composed of the **left thalamus** and **right thalamus** (THAL-a-mus; plural, *thalami*). Each thalamus contains relay and processing centers for sensory information. The **hypothalamus** (*hypo-,* below), or floor of the diencephalon, contains centers involved with emotions, autonomic function, and hormone production. The *infundibulum,* a narrow stalk, connects the hypothalamus to the **pituitary gland,** a component of the endocrine system. The hypothalamus and the pituitary gland are responsible for the integration of the nervous and endocrine systems.

The diencephalon is a structural and functional link between the cerebral hemispheres and the components of the brain stem. The **brain stem** contains a variety of important processing centers and nuclei that relay information headed to or from the cerebrum or cerebellum. The brain stem includes the *mesencephalon, pons,* and *medulla oblongata.*[1]

- The **mesencephalon** (**mesos,** middle), or midbrain, contains nuclei that process visual and auditory information and control reflexes triggered by these stimuli. For example, your immediate, reflexive responses to a loud, unexpected noise (eye movements and head turning) are directed by nuclei in the midbrain. This region also contains centers that help maintain consciousness.

- The **pons** of the brain connects the cerebellum to the brain stem (**pons** is Latin for "bridge").

In addition to tracts and relay centers, the pons also contains nuclei involved with somatic and visceral motor control.

- The spinal cord connects to the brain at the **medulla oblongata.** Near the pons, the posterior wall of the medulla oblongata is thin and membranous. The inferior portion of the medulla oblongata resembles the spinal cord in that it has a narrow central canal. The medulla oblongata relays sensory information to the thalamus and to centers in other portions of the brain stem. The medulla oblongata also contains major centers that regulate autonomic function, such as heart rate, blood pressure, and digestion.

The boundaries and general functions of the diencephalon and brain stem are indicated in Figure 7.21. In considering the individual components of the brain, we will begin at the inferior portion of the medulla oblongata. This region has the simplest organization found anywhere in the brain, and in many respects, it resembles the spinal cord. We will then ascend to regions of increasing structural and functional complexity until we reach the cerebral cortex, whose functions and capabilities are as yet poorly understood.

Embryology of the Brain

To understand the internal organization of the adult brain, we must consider its embryological origins. The central nervous system (CNS) begins as a hollow cylinder known as the **neural tube.** This tube has a fluid-filled internal cavity, the **neurocoel.** In the cephalic portion of the neural tube, three areas enlarge rapidly through expansion of the neurocoel. This enlargement creates three prominent divisions called **primary brain vesicles.** The primary brain vesicles are named for their relative positions: the *prosencephalon* (proz-en-SEF-a-lon; **proso,** forward + **enkephalos,** brain), or "forebrain"; the **mesencephalon,** or "midbrain"; and the *rhombencephalon* (rom-ben-SEF-a-lon), or "hindbrain."

The fates of the three primary divisions of the brain are summarized in Table 7.4. The prosencephalon and rhombencephalon are subdivided further, forming **secondary brain vesicles.** The prosencephalon forms the **telencephalon** (tel-en-SEF-a-lon; **telos,** end) and the diencephalon. The

---

[1]Some sources consider the brain stem to include the diencephalon. We will use the more restrictive definition here.

telencephalon will ultimately form the cerebrum of the adult brain. The walls of the mesencephalon thicken, and the neurocoel becomes a relatively narrow passageway, comparable to the central canal of the spinal cord. The portion of the rhombencephalon adjacent to the mesencephalon forms the **metencephalon** (met-en-SEF-a-lon; **meta,** after). The dorsal portion of the metencephalon will become the cerebellum, and the ventral portion will develop into the pons. The portion of the rhombencephalon closer to the spinal cord forms the **myelencephalon** (mī-el-en-SEF-a-lon; **myelon,** spinal cord), which will become the medulla oblongata.

Ventricles of the Brain

During development, the neurocoel within the cerebral hemispheres, diencephalon, metencephalon, and medulla oblongata expands to form chambers called **ventricles** (VEN-tri-kls). The ventricles are lined by cells of the *ependyma*.

Each cerebral hemisphere contains a large **lateral ventricle** (Figure 7.22). The **septum pellucidum**, a thin medial partition, separates the two lateral ventricles. Because there are *two* lateral ventricles, the ventricle in the diencephalon is called the **third ventricle**. Although the two lateral ventricles are not directly connected, each communicates with the third ventricle of the diencephalon through an **interventricular foramen** (*foramen of Monro*).

The mesencephalon has a slender canal known as the **mesencephalic aqueduct** (or *the aqueduct of the midbrain, aqueduct of Sylvius, or cerebral aqueduct*). This passageway connects the third ventricle with the **fourth ventricle.** The superior portion of the fourth ventricle lies between the posterior surface of the pons and the anterior surface of the cerebellum. The fourth ventricle extends into the superior portion of the medulla oblongata. This ventricle then narrows and becomes continuous with the central canal of the spinal cord.

The ventricles are filled with cerebrospinal fluid (CSF). The CSF continuously circulates from the ventricles and central canal into the *subarachnoid space* of the surrounding cranial meninges. The CSF passes between the interior and exterior of the CNS through three foramina in the roof of the fourth ventricle.

TABLE 7.4	Development of the Brain	
Primary Brain Vesicles (3 weeks)	**Secondary Brain Vesicles (6 weeks)**	**Brain Regions at Birth**
	Telencephalon	Cerebrum
Prosencephalon	Diencephalon	Diencephalon
Mesencephalon	Mesencephalon	Mesencephalon
	Metencephalon	Cerebellum and Pons
Rhombencephalon	Myelencephalon	Medulla oblongata

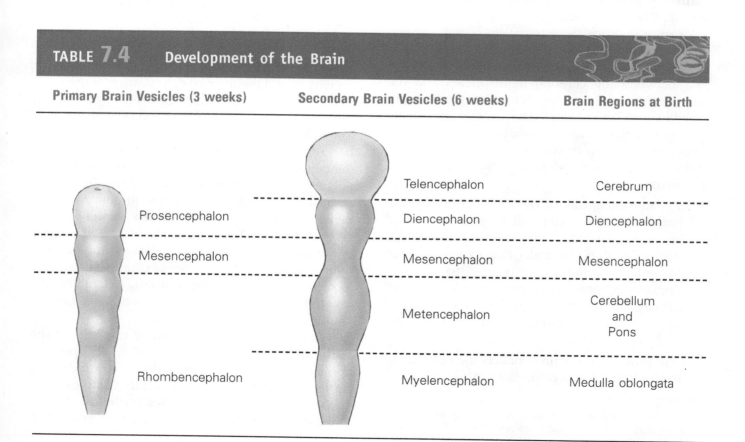

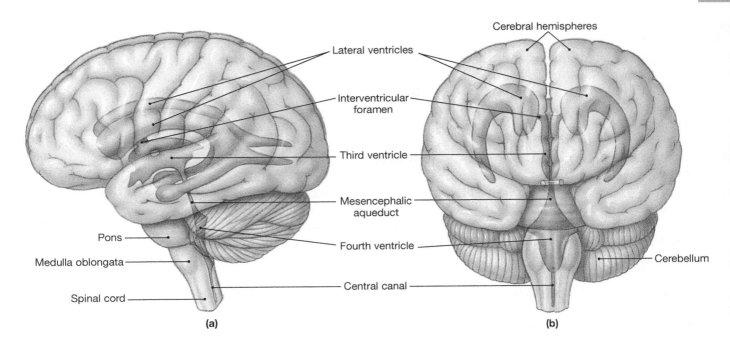

FIGURE 7.22   Ventricles of the brain. The orientation and extent of the ventricles as they would appear if the brain were transparent. **(a)** A lateral view. **(b)** An anterior view. ATLAS: Plates 10; 12a–c; 13a–e

100 Keys | The brain is a large, delicate mass of neural tissue containing internal passageways and chambers filled with cerebrospinal fluid. Each of the five major regions of the brain has specific functions. As you ascend from the medulla oblongata (which connects to the spinal cord) to the cerebrum, those functions become more complex and variable. Conscious thought and intelligence are provided by the neural cortex of the cerebral hemispheres.

Cerebrospinal Fluid

Cerebrospinal fluid (CSF) completely surrounds and bathes the exposed surfaces of the CNS. The CSF has several important functions, including the following:

- **Cushioning Delicate Neural Structures.**
- **Supporting the Brain.** In essence, the brain is suspended inside the cranium and floats in the CSF. A human brain weighs about 1400 g in air, but only about 50 g when supported by CSF.
- **Transporting Nutrients, Chemical Messengers, and Waste Products.** Except at the choroid plexus, where CSF is produced,

the ependymal lining is freely permeable and the CSF is in constant chemical communication with the interstitial fluid that surrounds the neurons and neuroglia of the CNS.

Functional Anatomy of the Adult Brain

The adult brain's unimpressive appearance gives few hints of its remarkable abilities. It is about two good fistfuls of pinkish gray tissue, wrinkled like a walnut, and with the texture of cold oatmeal. It weighs a little over three pounds. Because the brain is the largest and most complex mass of nervous tissue in the body, it is commonly discussed in terms of its four major regions—*cerebral hemispheres, diencephalon* (di"en-sef'ah-lon), *brain stem,* and *cerebellum* (Figure 7.23).

Cerebral Hemispheres

The paired **cerebral** (ser'e-bral) **hemispheres,** collectively called the **cerebrum,** are the most superior part of the brain and together are a good deal larger than the other three brain regions combined. In fact, as the cerebral hemispheres develop and grow, they enclose and obscure most of the brain stem, so many brain stem structures cannot normally be seen unless a sagittal section is made. Picture how a mushroom cap covers the top of its stalk, and you have a fairly good idea of how the cerebral hemispheres cover the diencephalon and the superior part of the brain stem (see Figure 7.23).

The entire surface of the cerebral hemispheres exhibits elevated ridges of tissue called **gyri** (ji're; **gyrus,** singular; "twisters"), separated by shallow grooves called **sulci** (sul'ki; **sulcus,** singular; "furrows"). Less numerous are the deeper grooves called **fissures** (Figure 7.24a), which separate large regions of the brain. Many of the fissures and gyri are important anatomical landmarks. The cerebral hemispheres are separated by a single deep fissure, the *longitudinal fissure.* Other fissures or sulci divide each cerebral hemisphere into a number of **lobes,** named for the cranial bones that lie over them (see Figure 7.24a and b).

Speech, memory, logical and emotional response, as well as consciousness, interpretation of sensation, and voluntary movement, are all functions of neurons of the cerebral cortex, and many of the functional areas of the cerebral hemispheres have been identified (Figure 7.24c). The **somatic sensory area** is located in the **parietal lobe** posterior to the **central sulcus.** Impulses

traveling from the body's sensory receptors (except for the special senses) are localized and interpreted in this area of the brain. The somatic sensory area allows you to recognize pain, coldness, or a light touch. As illustrated in Figure 7.25, the body is represented in an upside-down manner in the sensory area. This spatial map is called the **sensory** homunculus (ho-mung'ku-lus; "little man"). Body regions with the most sensory receptors—the lips and fingertips—send impulses to neurons that make up a large part of the sensory cortex. Furthermore, the sensory pathways are crossed pathways—meaning that the left side of the sensory cortex receives impulses from the right side of the body, and vice versa.

Impulses from the special sense organs are interpreted in other cortical areas (see Figure 7.24b and c). For example, the visual area is located in the posterior part of the **occipital lobe,** the auditory area is in the **temporal lobe** bordering the *lateral sulcus,* and the olfactory area is found deep inside the temporal lobe.

The **primary motor area** that allows us to consciously move our skeletal muscles is anterior to the central sulcus in the **frontal lobe.** The axons of these motor neurons form the major voluntary motor tract—the **corticospinal** (kor"tĭ-ko-spi'nal), or **pyramidal tract,** which descends

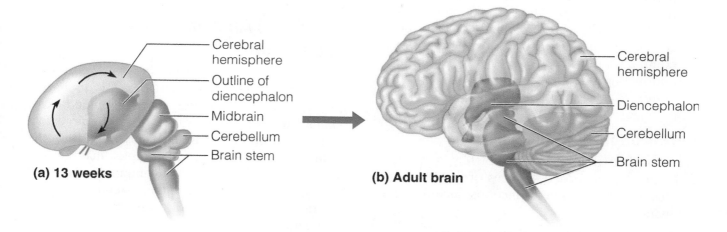

(a) 13 weeks

Cerebral hemisphere
Outline of diencephalon
Midbrain
Cerebellum
Brain stem

(b) Adult brain

Cerebral hemisphere
Diencephalon
Cerebellum
Brain stem

FIGURE 7.23   Development and regions of the human brain. The brain can be considered in terms of four main parts: cerebral hemispheres, diencephalon, brain stem, and cerebellum. In the developing brain **(a),** the cerebral hemispheres are forced to grow posteriorly and laterally over the other brain regions by the bones of the skull. In the adult brain **(b),** the cerebral hemispheres hide the diencephalon and the upper part of the brain stem. The left cerebral hemisphere is drawn so that it looks transparent, to reveal the location of the deeply situated diencephalon and superior part of the brain stem.

Q What sense(s) would be affected by temporal lobe damage? By occipital lobe damage?

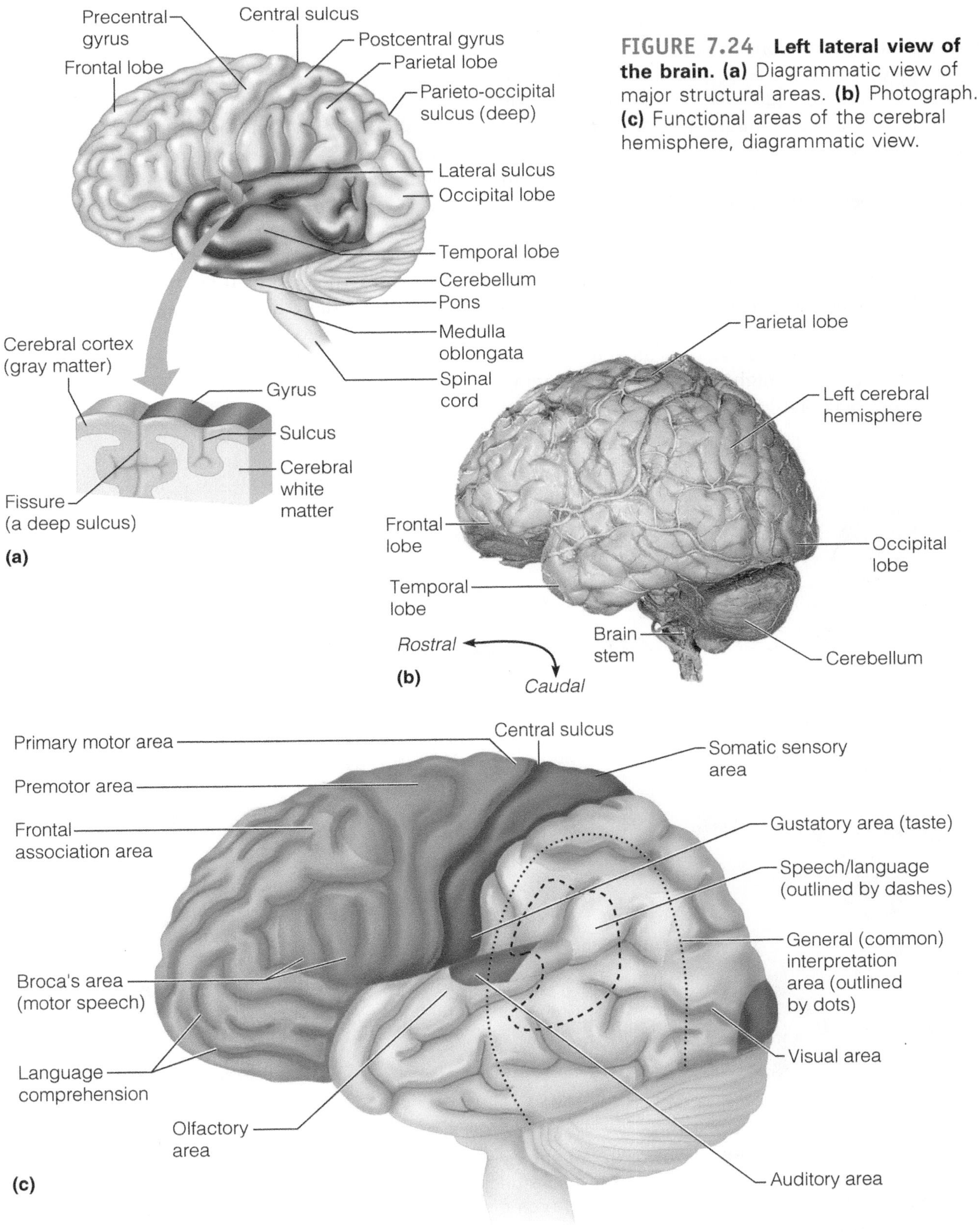

Precentral gyrus
Frontal lobe
Central sulcus
Postcentral gyrus
Parietal lobe
Parieto-occipital sulcus (deep)
Lateral sulcus
Occipital lobe
Temporal lobe
Cerebellum
Pons
Medulla oblongata
Spinal cord

Cerebral cortex (gray matter)
Gyrus
Sulcus
Cerebral white matter
Fissure (a deep sulcus)

(a)

FIGURE 7.24 Left lateral view of the brain. (a) Diagrammatic view of major structural areas. **(b)** Photograph. **(c)** Functional areas of the cerebral hemisphere, diagrammatic view.

Parietal lobe
Left cerebral hemisphere
Frontal lobe
Occipital lobe
Temporal lobe
Brain stem
Cerebellum

Rostral
Caudal

(b)

Primary motor area
Premotor area
Frontal association area
Central sulcus
Somatic sensory area
Gustatory area (taste)
Speech/language (outlined by dashes)
General (common) interpretation area (outlined by dots)
Broca's area (motor speech)
Language comprehension
Olfactory area
Visual area
Auditory area

(c)

A Damage to the temporal lobe (depending on its site) might affect hearing and/or the sense of smell. Occipital lobe damage would cause visual problems.

to the cord. As in the somatic sensory cortex, the body is represented upside-down and the pathways are crossed. Most of the neurons in this primary motor area control body areas having the finest motor control; that is, the face, mouth, and hands (see Figure 7.25). The body map on the motor cortex, as you might guess, is called the **motor** homunculus.

A specialized area that is very involved in our ability to speak, **Broca's** (bro'kahz) **area** (see Figure 7.24c), is found at the base of the precentral gyrus (the gyrus anterior to the central sulcus). Damage to this area, which is located in only one cerebral hemisphere (usually the left), causes inability to say words properly. You know what you want to say, but you can't vocalize the words.

Areas involved in higher intellectual reasoning and socially acceptable behavior are believed to

be in the anterior part of the frontal lobes. Complex memories appear to be stored in the temporal and frontal lobes. The **speech area** is located at the junction of the temporal, parietal, and occipital lobes. The speech area allows one to sound out words. This area (like Broca's area) is usually in only one cerebral hemisphere. The frontal lobes house areas involved with language comprehension (word meanings).

The cell bodies of neurons involved in the cerebral hemisphere functions named above are found only in the outermost **gray matter** of the cerebrum, the **cerebral cortex** (see Figure 7.24a). As noted earlier, the cortical region is highly ridged and convoluted, providing more room for the thousands of neurons found there.

Most of the remaining cerebral hemisphere tissue—the deeper **cerebral white matter** (see

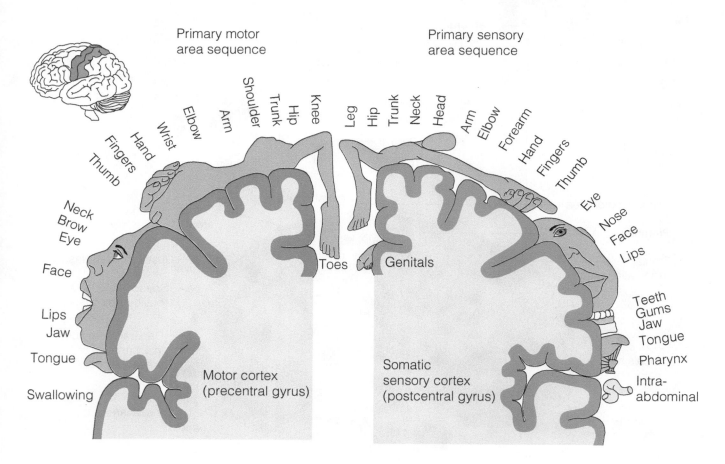

FIGURE 7.25 Sensory and motor areas of the cerebral cortex. The relative amount of cortical tissue devoted to each function is indicated by the amount of the gyrus occupied by the body area diagrams (homunculi). The primary motor cortex is shown on the right, the somatic sensory cortex is on the left.

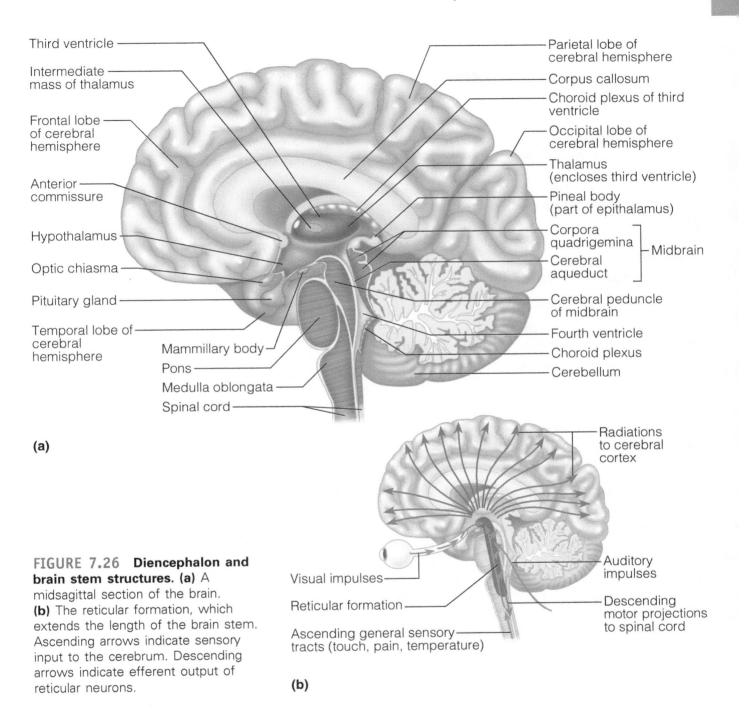

FIGURE 7.26 Diencephalon and brain stem structures. (a) A midsagittal section of the brain. **(b)** The reticular formation, which extends the length of the brain stem. Ascending arrows indicate sensory input to the cerebrum. Descending arrows indicate efferent output of reticular neurons.

Figure 7.24a)—is composed of fiber *tracts* (bundles of nerve fibers) carrying impulses to or from the cortex. One very large fiber tract, the **corpus callosum** (kah-lo′sum), connects the cerebral hemispheres (Figure 7.26). The corpus callosum arches above the structures of the brain stem and allows the cerebral hemispheres to communicate with one another. This is important because, as already noted, some of the cortical functional areas are in only one hemisphere.

Although most of the gray matter is in the cerebral cortex, there are several "islands" of gray matter, called the **basal nuclei,** or **basal ganglia,** buried deep within the white matter of the

*The term *basal ganglia* is a historical misnomer. Ganglia are peripheral nervous system structures but the basal ganglia are collections of nerve cell bodies *in the CNS.* Hence, *basal nuclei* is a more accurate term.

cerebral hemispheres. The basal nuclei help regulate voluntary motor activities by modifying instructions sent to the skeletal muscles by the primary motor cortex.

Homeostatic Imbalance

Individuals who have problems with their basal nuclei are often unable to walk normally or carry out other voluntary movements in the usual normal way. *Huntington's disease* (or *Huntington's chorea*) and *Parkinson's disease* are two examples of such syndromes. ▲

Diencephalon

The **diencephalon,** or **interbrain,** sits atop the brain stem and is enclosed by the cerebral hemispheres (see Figure 7.23). The major structures of the diencephalon are the *thalamus, hypothalamus,* and *epithalamus* (see Figure 7.26). The **thalamus,** which encloses the shallow *third ventricle* of the brain, is a relay station for sensory impulses passing upward to the sensory cortex. As impulses surge through the thalamus, we have a crude recognition of whether the sensation we are about to have is pleasant or unpleasant. The actual localization and interpretation of the sensation is done by the neurons of the sensory cortex.

The **hypothalamus** (literally, "under the thalamus") makes up the floor of the diencephalon. It is an important autonomic nervous system center because it plays a role in the regulation of body temperature, water balance, and metabolism. The hypothalamus is also the center for many drives and emotions, and as such, it is an important part of the so-called **limbic system,** or "emotional-visceral brain." For example, thirst, appetite, sex, pain, and pleasure centers are in the hypothalamus. Additionally, the hypothalamus regulates the pituitary gland (an endocrine organ) and produces two hormones of its own. The **pituitary gland** hangs from the anterior floor of the hypothalamus by a slender stalk. (Its function is discussed in Chapter 9.) The **mammillary bodies,** reflex centers involved in olfaction (the sense of smell), bulge from the floor of the hypothalamus posterior to the pituitary gland.

The **epithalamus** (ep"ĭ-thal'ah-mus) forms the roof of the third ventricle. Important parts of the epithalamus are the **pineal body** (part of the endocrine system) and the **choroid** (ko'roid) **plexus** of the third ventricle. The choroid plexuses, knots of capillaries within each ventricle, form the cerebrospinal fluid.

Brain Stem

The **brain stem** is about the size of a thumb in diameter and approximately 3 inches (approximately 7.5 cm) long. Its structures are the *midbrain, pons,* and *medulla oblongata*. In addition to providing a pathway for ascending and descending tracts, the brain stem has many small gray matter areas. These nuclei are part of the cranial nerves and control vital activities such as breathing and blood pressure. Identify the brain stem areas in Figure 7.26 as you read their descriptions that follow.

Midbrain   The **midbrain** is a relatively small part of the brain stem. It extends from the mammillary bodies to the pons inferiorly. The **cerebral aqueduct** is a tiny canal that travels through the midbrain and connects the third ventricle of the diencephalon to the fourth ventricle below. Anteriorly, the midbrain is composed primarily of two bulging fiber tracts, the **cerebral peduncles** (literally, "little feet of the cerebrum"), which convey ascending and descending impulses. Dorsally located are four rounded protrusions called the **corpora quadrigemina** (kor'por-ah kwah'''' drĭ-jem'ĭ-nah) because they reminded some anatomist of two pairs of twins (*gemini*). These bulging nuclei are reflex centers involved with vision and hearing.

Pons   The **pons** (ponz) is the rounded structure that protrudes just below the midbrain. *Pons* means "bridge," and this area of the brain stem is mostly fiber tracts. However, it does have important nuclei involved in the control of breathing.

Medulla Oblongata   The **medulla oblongata** (mĕ-dul'ah ob"long-gă'tah) is the most inferior part of the brain stem. It merges into the spinal cord below without any obvious change in structure. Like the pons, the medulla is an important fiber tract area. The medulla also contains many nuclei that regulate vital visceral activities. It contains centers that control heart rate, blood pressure, breathing, swallowing, and vomiting, among others. The **fourth ventricle** lies posterior to the pons and medulla and anterior to the cerebellum.

Reticular Formation   Extending the entire length of the brain stem is a diffuse mass of gray matter, the **reticular formation.** The neurons of the reticular formation are involved in motor control of the visceral organs. A special group of reticular formation neurons, the **reticular activating system (RAS),** plays a role in consciousness and the awake/sleep cycles (Figure 7.26b). Damage to this area can result in permanent unconsciousness (coma).

Cerebellum

The large, cauliflowerlike **cerebellum** (ser"e-bel'um) projects dorsally from under the occipital lobe of the cerebrum. Like the cerebrum, it has two hemispheres and a convoluted surface. The cerebellum also has an outer cortex made up of gray matter and an inner region of white matter.

The cerebellum provides the precise timing for skeletal muscle activity and controls our balance and equilibrium. Because of its activity, body movements are smooth and coordinated. Fibers reach the cerebellum from the equilibrium apparatus of the inner ear, the eye, the proprioceptors of the skeletal muscles and tendons, and many other areas. The cerebellum can be compared to an automatic pilot, continuously comparing the brain's "intentions" with actual body performance by monitoring body position and amount of tension in various body parts. When needed, it sends messages to initiate the appropriate corrective measures.

◢ Homeostatic Imbalance

If the cerebellum is damaged (for example, by a blow to the head, a tumor, or a stroke), movements become clumsy and disorganized—a condition called *ataxia*. Victims cannot keep their balance and may appear to be drunk because of the loss of muscle coordination. They are no longer able to touch their finger to their nose with eyes closed—a feat that normal individuals accomplish easily. ◢

Protection of the Central Nervous System

Nervous tissue is very soft and delicate, and the irreplaceable neurons are injured by even the slightest pressure. Nature has tried to protect the brain and spinal cord by enclosing them within bone (the skull and vertebral column), membranes (the meninges), and a watery cushion (cerebrospinal fluid). Protection from harmful substances in the blood is provided by the so-called blood-brain barrier.

Meninges

The three connective tissue membranes covering and protecting the CNS structures are **meninges** (mĕ-nin'jēz) (Figure 7.27). The outermost layer, the leathery **dura mater** (du'rah ma'ter), meaning "tough or hard mother," is a double-layered membrane where it surrounds the brain. One of its layers is attached to the inner surface of the skull, forming the periosteum (*periosteal layer*). The other, called the *meningeal layer,* forms the outermost covering of the brain and continues as the dura mater of the spinal cord. The dural layers are fused together except in three areas where they separate to enclose *dural sinuses* that collect venous blood.

In several places, the inner dural membrane extends inward to form a fold that attaches the brain to the cranial cavity. One of these folds, the **falx** (falks) **cerebri,** is shown in Figure 7.27a. Another such fold, the **tentorium cerebelli** separating the cerebellum from the cerebrum, is shown in Figures 7.27b and 7.28c.

The middle meningeal layer is the weblike **arachnoid** (ah-rak'noid) **mater** (see Fig. 7.27). *Arachnida* means "spider," and some think the arachnoid membrane looks like a cobweb. Its threadlike extensions span the **subarachnoid space** to attach it to the innermost membrane, the **pia** (pi'ah) **mater** ("gentle mother"). The delicate pia mater clings tightly to the surface of the brain and spinal cord, following every fold.

The subarachnoid space is filled with cerebrospinal fluid. Specialized projections of the arachnoid membrane, **arachnoid villi** (vih'li), protrude through the dura mater. The cerebrospinal fluid is absorbed into the venous blood in the dural sinuses through the arachnoid villi.

◢ Homeostatic Imbalance

Meningitis, an inflammation of the meninges, is a serious threat to the brain because bacterial or viral meningitis may spread into the nervous tissue of the CNS. This condition of brain inflammation is called *encephalitis* (en-sef-ah-li'tis). Meningitis is usually diagnosed by taking a sample of cerebrospinal fluid from the subarachnoid space. ◢

Cerebrospinal Fluid

Cerebrospinal (ser"e-bro-spi'nal) **fluid (CSF)** is a watery "broth" similar in its makeup to blood

Q *What would be the consequence of blocked arachnoid villi?*

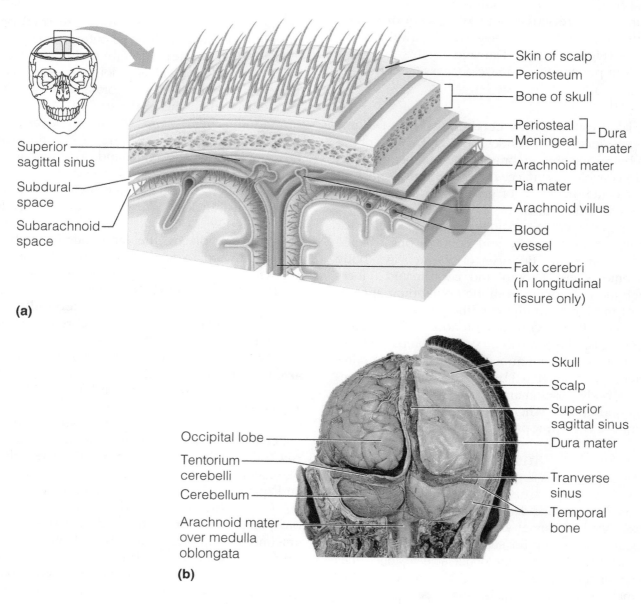

Skin of scalp
Periosteum
Bone of skull
Periosteal ⎫ Dura
Meningeal ⎭ mater
Arachnoid mater
Pia mater
Arachnoid villus
Blood vessel
Falx cerebri (in longitudinal fissure only)

Superior sagittal sinus
Subdural space
Subarachnoid space

(a)

Skull
Scalp
Superior sagittal sinus
Dura mater
Tranverse sinus
Temporal bone

Occipital lobe
Tentorium cerebelli
Cerebellum
Arachnoid mater over medulla oblongata

(b)

FIGURE 7.27 Meninges of the brain. (a) Three-dimensional frontal section showing the meninges—the dura mater, arachnoid mater, and pia mater—that surround and protect the brain. The relationship of the dura mater to the falx cerebri and the superior sagittal (dural) sinus is also shown. **(b)** Posterior view of the brain in place surrounded by the dura mater.

A *Hydrocephalus ("water on the brain"). The ventricles would expand as cerebrospinal fluid (unable to drain into the dural sinus) accumulated.*

Q Why are the lateral ventricles horn-shaped rather than oriented vertically like the third and fourth ventricles?

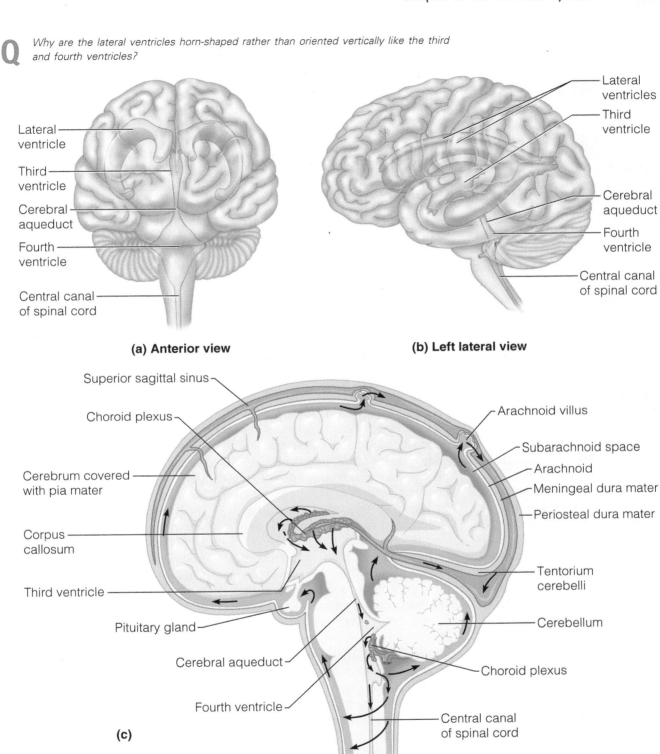

Lateral ventricle

Third ventricle

Cerebral aqueduct

Fourth ventricle

Central canal of spinal cord

(a) Anterior view

Lateral ventricles

Third ventricle

Cerebral aqueduct

Fourth ventricle

Central canal of spinal cord

(b) Left lateral view

Superior sagittal sinus

Choroid plexus

Cerebrum covered with pia mater

Corpus callosum

Third ventricle

Pituitary gland

Cerebral aqueduct

Fourth ventricle

(c)

Arachnoid villus

Subarachnoid space

Arachnoid

Meningeal dura mater

Periosteal dura mater

Tentorium cerebelli

Cerebellum

Choroid plexus

Central canal of spinal cord

FIGURE 7.28 Ventricles and location of the cerebrospinal fluid. (a) and **(b)** Three-dimensional views of the ventricles of the brain. **(c)** Circulatory pathway of the cerebrospinal fluid (indicated by arrows) within the central nervous system and the subarachnoid space. (The relative position of the right lateral ventricle is indicated by the pale blue area deep to the corpus callosum.)

A The bones of the skull restrict superior growth of the cerebral hemispheres (and their ventricles) during development, forcing them to grow posterolaterally, and the ventricles within them are bent into the arching horn-shape during that process.

A Closer Look

Alzheimer's, Parkinson's, and Huntington's— The Terrible Three

WHAT do former President Reagan and actor Michael J. Fox have in common? Not much, other than the fact that each was or is a victim of one of the terrible three CNS degenerative diseases.

Alzheimer's (altz'hi-merz) **disease (AD)** is a progressive degenerative disease of the brain that ultimately results in dementia (mental deterioration). Alzheimer's patients represent nearly half of all people in nursing homes. Between 5 and 15 percent of people over 65 develop this condition, and up to half of those over 85 die of it.

Its victims, which include the recently deceased President Reagan, exhibit memory loss (particularly for recent events), a short attention span and disorientation, and eventual language loss. Over a period of several years, formerly good-natured people become irritable, moody, confused, and sometimes violent. Ultimately, hallucinations occur.

AD is associated with a shortage of acetylcholine (ACh) and with structural changes in the brain, particularly in areas involved with cognition and memory. The gyri shrink, and the brain atrophies. Its precise cause is unknown, but some cases of AD appear to run in families.

Microscopic examinations of brain tissue reveal abnormal protein deposits (masses of cells and degenerated fibers around a *beta amyloid peptide* core) littering the brain like shrapnel between the neurons. They also show *neurofibrillary tangles* (twisted fibers within neuron cell bodies). It has been frustratingly difficult for researchers to uncover how beta amyloid peptide acts as a neurotoxin, particularly since it is also present in healthy brain cells (but in lower amounts). Just what tips things off balance to favor production of more beta amyloid is not understood, but it is known that this tiny peptide does its damage by enhancing calcium entry into certain brain neurons.

Another line of research has implicated a protein called *tau,* which appears to function like railroad ties to bind microtubule "tracks" together. In the brains of AD victims, tau abandons its microtubule stabilizing role and grabs onto other tau molecules, forming the spaghetti-like neurofibrillary tangles. These degenerative changes develop over a period of several years, during which time the family members watch the person they love "disappear." It is a long and painful process. It is hoped that the lines of investigation, particularly stem cell research, will eventually merge and point to a treatment, but at present, only drugs that ease symptoms by inhibiting ACh breakdown are useful.

Parkinson's disease, an example of basal nuclei problems, typically strikes people in their 50s and 60s (Michael J. Fox is an exception). It results from a degeneration of the dopamine-releasing neurons of the substantia nigra, and as those neurons deteriorate, the dopamine-deprived basal nuclei they target become overactive, causing the well-known symptoms of the disease. Afflicted individuals, including Michael J. Fox, have a persistent tremor at rest (exhibited by head nodding and a "pill-rolling" movement of the fingers), a forward-bent walking posture and shuffling gait, a stiff facial expression, and they have trouble initiating movement or getting their muscles going.

The cause of Parkinson's disease is still unknown. The drug L-dopa helps to alleviate some of the symptoms; however, L-dopa is not a cure, and as more and more neurons die off, it becomes ineffective. It also has undesirable side effects: severe nausea, dizziness, and in some, liver damage. A newer treatment drug is deprenyl. When given early on in the disease, deprenyl slows the neurological deterioration to some extent and delays the need to administer L-dopa for up to 18 months.

Alzheimer's, Parkinson's, and Huntington's—The Terrible Three *(continued)*

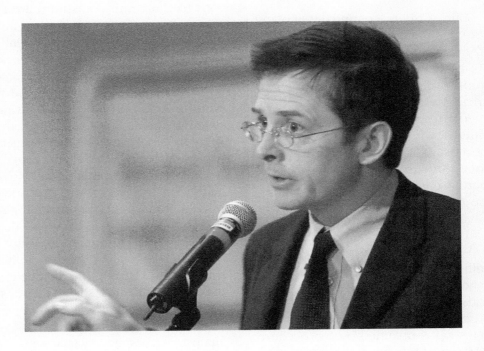

Deep-brain (thalamic) stimulation via implanted electrodes has proved helpful in alleviating tremors but does little else. More promising for long-term results are the intrabrain transplants of embryonic substantia nigra tissue, genetically engineered adult nigral cells, or dopamine-producing cells from fetal pigs; all these have produced some regression of disease symptoms. However, the use of fetal tissue is controversial and riddled with ethical and legal roadblocks.

Huntington's disease is a genetic disease that strikes during middle age and leads to massive degeneration of the basal nuclei and later of the cerebral cortex. Its initial symptoms in many are wild, jerky, and almost continuous flapping movements called *chorea* (Greek for "dance"). Although the movements appear to be voluntary, they are not. Late in the disease, marked mental deterioration occurs. Huntington's disease is progressive and usually fatal within 15 years of onset of symptoms.

The signs and symptoms of Huntington's disease are essentially the opposite of those of Parkinson's disease (overstimulation rather than inhibition of the motor drive), and Huntington's is usually treated with drugs that block, rather than enhance, dopamine's effects. As you can see, neurotransmitters, which are the "vocabulary" of neurons, can cause garbled neural language when things go wrong. As with Parkinson's disease, fetal tissue implants may provide promise for its treatment in the future.

plasma, from which it forms. However, it contains less protein, more vitamin C, and its ion composition is different.

CSF is continually formed from blood by the choroid plexuses. Choroid plexuses are clusters of capillaries hanging from the "roof" in each of the brain's ventricles. The CSF in and around the brain and cord forms a watery cushion that protects the fragile nervous tissue from blows and other trauma.

Inside the brain, CSF is continually moving (see Figure 7.28c). It circulates from the two lateral ventricles (in the cerebral hemispheres) into the third ventricle (in the diencephalon), and then through the cerebral aqueduct of the midbrain into the fourth ventricle dorsal to the pons and medulla oblongata. Some of the fluid reaching the fourth ventricle continues down the **central canal** of the spinal cord, but most of it circulates into the **subarachnoid space** through three openings in the walls of the fourth ventricle. The fluid returns to the blood in the dural sinuses through the arachnoid villi. Ordinarily, CSF forms and drains at a constant rate so that its normal pressure and volume (150 ml—about half a cup) are maintained. Any significant changes in CSF composition (or the appearance of blood cells in it) may be a sign of meningitis or certain other brain pathologies (such as tumors and multiple sclerosis). The CSF sample for testing is obtained by a procedure called a *lumbar (spinal) tap.* Since the withdrawal of fluid for testing decreases CSF fluid pressure, the patient must remain in a horizontal position (lying down) for 6 to 12 hours after the procedure to prevent an agonizingly painful "spinal headache."

Homeostatic Imbalance

If something obstructs its drainage (for example, a tumor), CSF begins to accumulate and exert pressure on the brain. This condition is *hydrocephalus* (hi-dro-sef'ah-lus), literally, "water on the brain." Hydrocephalus in a newborn baby causes the head to enlarge as the brain increases in size. This is possible in an infant because the skull bones have not yet fused. However, in an adult, this condition is likely to result in brain damage because the skull is hard, and the accumulating fluid crushes soft nervous tissue. Today hydrocephalus is treated surgically by inserting a shunt (a plastic tube) to direct the excess fluid into a vein in the neck. ▲

The Blood-Brain Barrier

No other body organ is so absolutely dependent on a constant internal environment as is the brain. Other body tissues can withstand the rather small fluctuations in the concentrations of hormones, ions, and nutrients that continually occur, particularly after eating or exercising. If the brain were exposed to such chemical changes, uncontrolled neural activity might result—remember that certain ions (sodium and potassium) are involved in initiating nerve impulses, and some amino acids serve as neurotransmitters. Consequently, neurons are kept separated from bloodborne substances by a so-called **blood-brain barrier,** composed of the *least* permeable capillaries in the whole body. Of water-soluble substances, only water, glucose, and essential amino acids pass easily through the walls of these capillaries. Metabolic wastes, such as urea, toxins, proteins, and most drugs are prevented from entering the brain tissue. Nonessential amino acids and potassium ions are not only prevented from entering the brain, but also are actively pumped from the brain into the blood across capillary walls. Although the bulbous "feet" of the astrocytes that cling to the capillaries may contribute to the barrier, the relative impermeability of the brain capillaries is most responsible for providing this protection.

The blood-brain barrier is virtually useless against fats, respiratory gases, and other fat-soluble molecules that diffuse easily through all plasma membranes. This explains why bloodborne alcohol, nicotine, and anesthetics can affect the brain.

Cerebrovascular Accident Commonly called *strokes,* **cerebrovascular** (ser"e-bro-vas'ku-lar) **accidents (CVAs)** are the third leading cause of death in the United States. CVAs occur when blood circulation to a brain area is blocked, as by a blood clot or a ruptured blood vessel, and vital brain tissue dies. After a CVA, it is often possible to determine the area of brain damage by observing the patient's symptoms. For example, if the patient has left-sided paralysis, the right motor cortex of the frontal lobe is most likely involved. *Aphasias* (ah-fa'ze-ahz) are a common result of damage to the left cerebral hemisphere, where the language areas are located. There are many types of aphasias, but the most common are *motor aphasia,* which involves damage to Broca's area and a loss of ability to speak, and *sensory aphasia,* in which a person loses the ability to understand written or spoken language. Aphasias are maddening to the victims because, as a rule, their intellect is unimpaired. Brain lesions can also cause marked changes in a person's disposition (for example, a change from a sunny to a foul personality). In such cases, a tumor as well as a CVA might be suspected.

Fewer than a third of those surviving a CVA are alive three years later. Even so, the picture is not hopeless. Some patients recover at least part of their lost faculties because undamaged neurons spread into areas where neurons have died and take over some lost functions. Indeed, most of the recovery seen after brain injury is due to this phenomenon.

Not all strokes are "completed." Temporary brain ischemia, or restriction of blood flow, is called a *transient ischemic attack (TIA)*. TIAs last from 5 to 50 minutes and are characterized by symptoms such as numbness, temporary paralysis, and impaired speech. Although these defects are not permanent, they do constitute "red flags" that warn of impending, more serious CVAs.

Spinal Cord

The cylindrical **spinal cord,** which is approximately 17 inches (42 cm) long, is a glistening white continuation of the brain stem. The spinal cord provides a two-way conduction pathway to and from the brain, and it is a major reflex center (the spinal reflexes are completed at this level). Enclosed within the vertebral column, the spinal cord extends from the foramen magnum of the skull to the first or second lumbar vertebra, where it ends just below the ribs (Figure 7.29). Like the brain, the spinal cord is cushioned and protected by meninges. Meningeal coverings do not end at the second lumbar vertebra (L$_2$), but instead extend well beyond the end of the spinal cord in the vertebral canal. Because there is no possibility of damaging the cord beyond L$_3$, the meningeal sac inferior to that point provides a nearly ideal spot for removing CSF for testing.

In humans, 31 pairs of spinal nerves arise from the cord and exit from the vertebral column to serve the body area close by. The spinal cord is about the size of a thumb for most of its length, but it is obviously enlarged in the cervical and lumbar regions where the nerves serving the upper and lower limbs arise and leave the cord. Because the

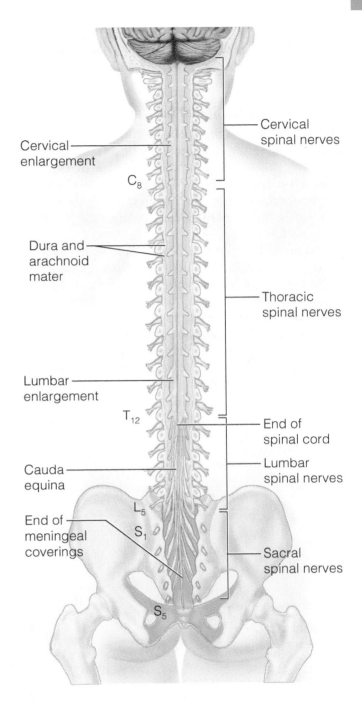

FIGURE 7.29 Anatomy of the spinal cord, posterior view.

vertebral column grows faster than the spinal cord, the spinal cord does not reach the end of the vertebral column and the spinal nerves leaving its inferior end must travel through the vertebral canal for some distance before exiting. This collection of spinal nerves at the inferior end of the vertebral canal is called the **cauda equina** (kaw'da e-kwi'nah) because it looks so much like a horse's tail (the literal translation of *cauda equina*).

Gray Matter of the Spinal Cord and Spinal Roots

The gray matter of the spinal cord looks like a butterfly or the letter H in cross section (Figure 7.30). The two posterior projections are the **dorsal,** or **posterior, horns;** the two anterior projections are the **ventral,** or **anterior, horns.** The gray matter surrounds the **central canal** of the cord, which contains CSF.

Neurons with specific functions can be located in the gray matter. The dorsal horns contain association neurons, or interneurons. The cell bodies of the sensory neurons, whose fibers enter the cord by the **dorsal root,** are found in an enlarged area called the **dorsal root ganglion.** If the dorsal root or its ganglion is damaged, sensation from the body area served will be lost. The ventral horns of the gray matter contain cell bodies of motor neurons of the somatic (voluntary) nervous system, which send their axons out the **ventral root** of the cord. The dorsal and ventral roots fuse to form the **spinal nerves.**

Homeostatic Imbalance

Damage to the ventral root results in a *flaccid paralysis* of the muscles served. In flaccid paralysis, nerve impulses do not reach the muscles affected; thus, no voluntary movement of those muscles is possible. The muscles begin to atrophy because they are no longer stimulated. ▲

White Matter of the Spinal Cord

White matter of the spinal cord is composed of myelinated fiber tracts—some running to higher centers, some traveling from the brain to the cord, and some conducting impulses from one side of the spinal cord to the other.

Because of the irregular shape of gray matter, the white matter on each side of the cord is divided into three regions—the **posterior, lateral,** and **anterior columns.** Each of the columns contains a number of fiber tracts made up of axons with the same destination and function. Tracts conducting sensory impulses to the brain are *sensory,* or *afferent, tracts.* Those carrying impulses from the brain to skeletal muscles are *motor,* or *efferent, tracts.* All tracts in the posterior columns are **ascending tracts** that carry sensory input to the

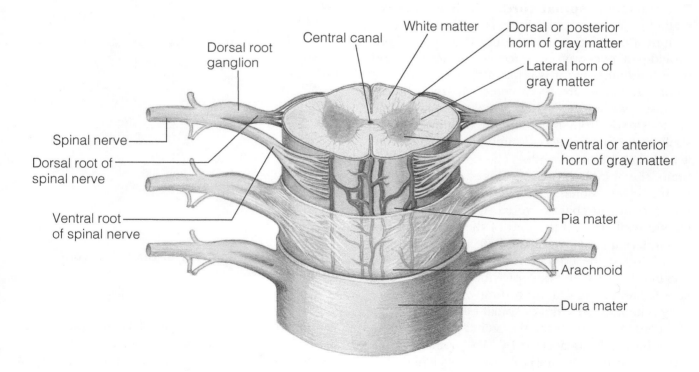

FIGURE 7.30 Spinal cord with meninges (three-dimensional view).

Labels: Dorsal root ganglion · Central canal · White matter · Dorsal or posterior horn of gray matter · Lateral horn of gray matter · Spinal nerve · Dorsal root of spinal nerve · Ventral root of spinal nerve · Ventral or anterior horn of gray matter · Pia mater · Arachnoid · Dura mater

brain. The lateral and anterior tracts contain both ascending and **descending (motor) tracts.**

The next section discusses the organization of sensory pathways in detail.

Homeostatic Imbalance

If the spinal cord is transected (cut crosswise) or crushed, *spastic paralysis* results. The affected muscles stay healthy because they are still stimulated by spinal reflex arcs, and movement of those muscles does occur. However, movements are involuntary and not controllable, and this can be as much of a problem as complete lack of mobility. In addition, because the spinal cord carries both sensory and motor impulses, a loss of feeling or sensory input occurs in the body areas below the point of cord destruction. Physicians often use a pin to see if a person can feel pain after spinal cord injury—to find out if regeneration is occurring. Pain is a hopeful sign in such cases. If the spinal cord injury occurs high in the cord, so that all four limbs are affected, the individual is a *quadriplegic* (kwod″ rĭ-ple′jik). If only the legs are paralyzed, the individual is a *paraplegic* (par″ă-ple′jik). ▲

The Organization of Sensory Pathways

A sensory neuron that delivers sensations to the CNS is often called a **first-order neuron.** The cell body of a first-order general sensory neuron is located in a dorsal root ganglion or cranial nerve ganglion. In the CNS, the axon of that sensory neuron synapses on an interneuron known as a **second-order neuron,** which may be located in the spinal cord or brain stem. If the sensation is to reach our awareness, the second-order neuron synapses on a **third-order neuron** in the thalamus. Somewhere along its length, the axon of the second-order neuron crosses over to the opposite side of the CNS. As a result, the right side of the thalamus receives sensory information from the left side of the body, and vice versa.

The axons of the third-order neurons ascend without crossing over and synapse on neurons of the primary sensory cortex of the cerebral hemisphere. As a result, the right cerebral hemisphere receives sensory information from the left side of the body, and the left cerebral hemisphere receives sensations from the right side. The reason for this

crossover is unknown. Although it has no apparent functional benefit, crossover occurs along sensory and motor pathways in all vertebrates.

Somatic Sensory Pathways

Somatic sensory pathways carry sensory information from the skin and musculature of the body wall, head, neck, and limbs. We will consider three major somatic sensory pathways: (1) the *posterior column pathway,* (2) the *anterolateral pathway,* and (3) the *spinocerebellar pathway.* These pathways utilize pairs of spinal tracts, symmetrically arranged on opposite sides of the spinal cord. All the axons within a tract share a common origin and destination.

Figure 7.31 indicates the relative positions of the spinal tracts involved. Note that tract names often give clues to their function. For example, if the name of a tract begins with *spino-,* the tract must *start* in the spinal cord and *end* in the brain. It must therefore be an ascending tract that carries sensory information. The rest of the name indicates the tract's destination. Thus, a *spinothalamic tract* begins in the spinal cord and carries sensory information to the thalamus.

If, on the other hand, the name of a tract ends in *-spinal,* the tract *ends* in the spinal cord and *starts* in a higher center of the brain. It must therefore be a descending tract that carries motor commands. The first part of the name indicates the nucleus or cortical area of the brain where the tract originates. For example, a *corticospinal tract* carries motor commands from the cerebral cortex to the spinal cord. Such tracts will be considered later in the chapter.

The Posterior Column Pathway

The **posterior column pathway** carries sensations of highly localized ("fine") touch, pressure, vibration, and proprioception (Figure 7.32a). This pathway, also known as the *dorsal column/medial lemniscus,* begins at a peripheral receptor and ends at the primary sensory cortex of the cerebral hemispheres. The spinal tracts involved are the left and right **fasciculus gracilis** (*gracilis,* delicate) and the left and right **fasciculus cuneatus** (*cuneus,* wedge-shaped). On each side of the posterior median sulcus, the fasciculus gracilis is medial to the fasciculus cuneatus.

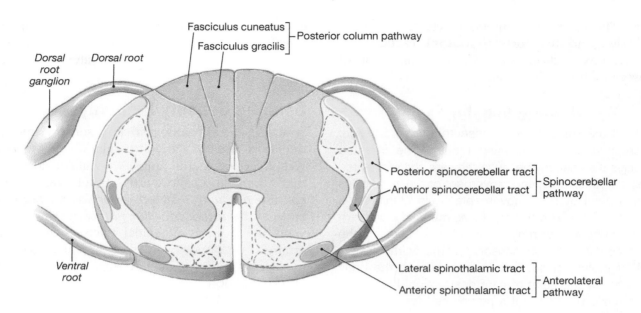

FIGURE 7.31   Sensory pathways and ascending tracts in the spinal cord.
A cross-sectional view of the spinal cord indicating the locations of the major ascending (sensory) tracts. For information about these tracts, see Table 7.5 Descending (motor) tracts (identified in Figure 7.5) are shown in dashed outline.

The axons of the first-order neurons reach the CNS within the dorsal roots of spinal nerves and the sensory roots of cranial nerves. The axons ascending within the posterior column are organized according to the region innervated. Axons carrying sensations from the inferior half of the body ascend within the fasciculus gracilis and synapse in the nucleus gracilis of the medulla oblongata. Axons carrying sensations from the superior half of the trunk, upper limbs, and neck ascend in the fasciculus cuneatus and synapse in the nucleus cuneatus.

Axons of the second-order neurons of the nucleus gracilis and nucleus cuneatus ascend to the thalamus. As they ascend, these axons cross over to the opposite side of the brain stem. The crossing of an axon from the left side to the right side, or vice versa, is called **decussation.** Once on the opposite side of the brain, the axons enter a tract called the **medial lemniscus** (*lemniskos,* ribbon). As it ascends, the medial lemniscus runs alongside a smaller tract that carries sensory information from the face, relayed from the sensory nuclei of the trigeminal nerve (V).

The axons in these tracts synapse on third-order neurons in one of the ventral nuclei of the

thalamus. These nuclei sort the arriving information according to (1) the nature of the stimulus and (2) the region of the body involved. Processing in the thalamus determines whether you perceive a given sensation as fine touch, or as pressure or vibration.

Our ability to localize the sensation—to determine precisely where on the body a specific stimulus originated—depends on the projection of information from the thalamus to the primary sensory cortex. Sensory information from the toes arrives at one end of the primary sensory cortex, and information from the head arrives at the other. When neurons in one portion of your primary sensory cortex are stimulated, you become aware of sensations originating at a specific location. If your primary sensory cortex were damaged or the projection fibers were cut, you could detect a light touch but would be unable to determine its source.

The same sensations are reported whether the cortical neurons are activated by axons ascending from the thalamus or by direct electrical stimulation. Researchers have electrically stimulated the primary sensory cortex in awake individuals during brain surgery and asked the subjects where they thought the stimulus originated. The results were used to create a functional map of the primary sensory cortex. Such a map, three of which are shown in Figure 7.32, is called a **sensory homunculus** ("little man").

The proportions of the sensory homunculus are very different from those of any individual. For example, the face is huge and distorted, with enormous lips and tongue, whereas the back is relatively tiny. These distortions occur because the area of sensory cortex devoted to a particular body region is proportional not to the region's absolute size, but to the *number of sensory receptors* it contains. In other words, many more cortical neurons are required to process sensory information arriving from the tongue, which has tens of thousands of taste and touch receptors, than to analyze sensations originating on the back, where touch receptors are few and far between.

The Anterolateral Pathway

The **anterolateral pathway** provides conscious sensations of poorly localized ("crude") touch, pressure, pain, and temperature. In this pathway, the axons of first-order sensory neurons enter the spinal cord and synapse on second-order neurons within the posterior gray horns. The axons of these interneurons cross to the opposite side of the spinal cord before ascending. This pathway includes relatively small tracts that deliver sensations to reflex centers in the brain stem as well as larger tracts that carry sensations destined for the cerebral cortex. We will ignore the smaller tracts in this discussion.

Sensations bound for the cerebral cortex ascend within the anterior or lateral spinothalamic tracts. The **anterior spinothalamic tracts** carry crude touch and pressure sensations (Figure 7.32b), whereas the **lateral spinothalamic tracts** carry pain and temperature sensations (Figure 7.32c). These tracts end at third-order neurons in the ventral nucleus group of the thalamus. After the sensations have been sorted and processed, they are relayed to the primary sensory cortex.

The perception that an arriving stimulus is painful rather than cold, hot, or vibrating depends on which second-order and third-order neurons are stimulated. The ability to localize that stimulus to a specific location in the body depends on the stimulation of an appropriate area of the primary sensory cortex. Any abnormality along the pathway can result in inappropriate sensations or inaccurate localization of the source. Consider these examples:

- An individual can experience painful sensations that are not real. For example, a person may continue to experience pain in an amputated limb. This *phantom limb pain* is caused by activity in the sensory neurons or interneurons along the anterolateral pathway. The neurons involved were once part of the labeled line that monitored conditions in the intact limb. These labeled lines and pathways are developmentally programmed, even individuals born without limbs can have phantom limb pain.

- An individual can feel pain in an uninjured part of the body when the pain actually originates at another location. For example, strong visceral pain sensations arriving at a segment of the spinal cord can stimulate interneurons that are part of the anterolateral pathway. Activity in these interneurons leads to the stimulation of the primary sensory cortex, so the individual feels pain in a specific part of the body surface. This phenomenon is called **referred pain.** Two familiar examples are (1) the pain of a heart attack, which is frequently felt in the left arm, and (2) the pain of appendicitis, which is generally felt first in the area around the navel and then in the right lower quadrant. These and additional examples are shown in Figure 7.33.

The Spinocerebellar Pathway

The cerebellum receives proprioceptive information about the position of skeletal muscles, tendons, and joints along the **spinocerebellar pathway** (Figure 7.34). This information does not reach our awareness. The axons of first-order sensory neurons synapse on interneurons in the dorsal gray horns of the spinal cord. The axons of these second-order neurons ascend in one of the spinocerebellar tracts:

- The **posterior spinocerebellar tracts** contain axons that do not cross over to the opposite side of the spinal cord. These axons reach the cerebellar cortex via the inferior cerebellar peduncle of that side.

- The **anterior spinocerebellar tracts** are dominated by axons that have crossed over to

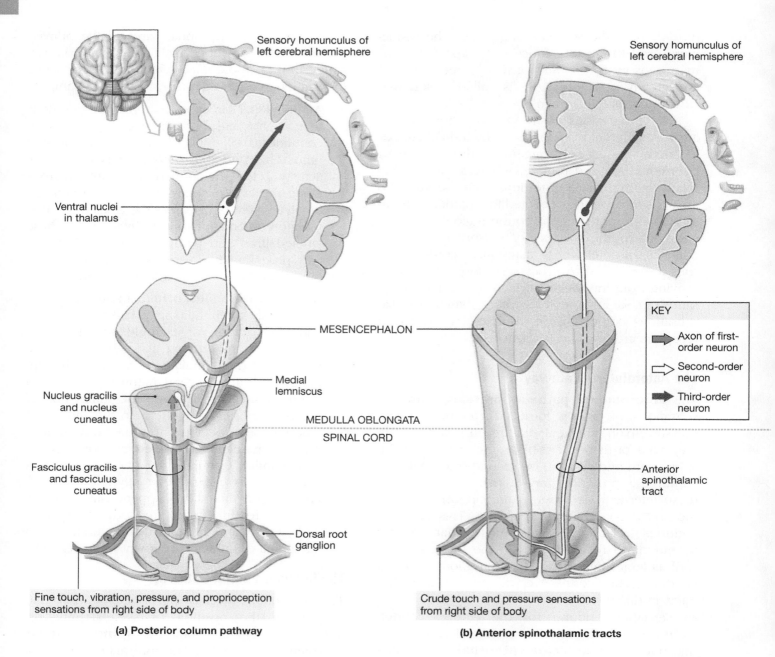

Sensory homunculus of
left cerebral hemisphere

Sensory homunculus of
left cerebral hemisphere

Ventral nuclei
in thalamus

MESENCEPHALON

KEY

Axon of first-
order neuron

Second-order
neuron

Third-order
neuron

Medial
lemniscus

Nucleus gracilis
and nucleus
cuneatus

MEDULLA OBLONGATA

SPINAL CORD

Fasciculus gracilis
and fasciculus
cuneatus

Anterior
spinothalamic
tract

Dorsal root
ganglion

Fine touch, vibration, pressure, and proprioception
sensations from right side of body

Crude touch and pressure sensations
from right side of body

(a) Posterior column pathway

(b) Anterior spinothalamic tracts

FIGURE 7.32   **The posterior column pathway, and the spinothalamic
tracts of the anterolateral pathway.** For clarity, only the pathways for
sensations originating on the right side of the body are shown. **(a)** The
posterior column pathway delivers fine touch, vibration, and proprioception
information to the primary sensory cortex on the opposite side of the body.
(b) The anterior spinothalamic tracts carry sensations of crude touch and
pressure to the primary sensory cortex on the opposite side of the body.
(c) The lateral spinothalamic tracts carry sensations of pain and temperature
to the primary sensory cortex on the opposite side of the body.

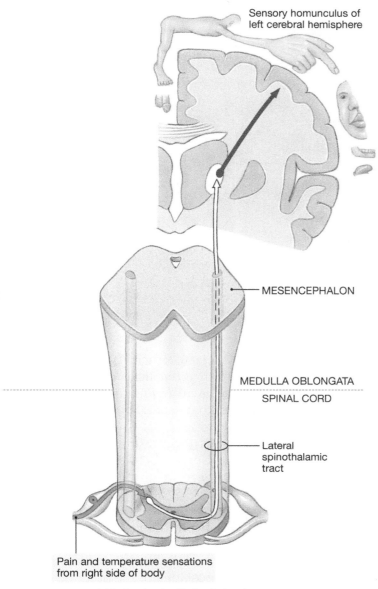

Sensory homunculus of
left cerebral hemisphere

MESENCEPHALON

MEDULLA OBLONGATA

SPINAL CORD

Lateral
spinothalamic
tract

Pain and temperature sensations
from right side of body

(c) Lateral spinothalamic tract

the opposite side of the spinal cord, although they do contain a significant number of un-crossed axons as well. The sensations carried by the anterior spinocerebellar tracts reach the cerebellar cortex via the superior cerebellar peduncle. Interestingly, many of the axons that cross over and ascend to the cerebellum then cross over again within the cerebellum, synapsing on the same side as the original stimulus. The functional significance of this "double cross" is unknown.

The information carried by the spinocerebellar pathway ultimately arrives at the *Purkinje cells* of the cerebellar cortex. Proprioceptive information from each part of the body is relayed to a specific portion of the cerebellar cortex. We will consider the integration of proprioceptive information and the role of the cerebellum in somatic motor control in a later section.

Table 7.5 reviews the somatic sensory pathways discussed in this section.

100 Keys | Most somatic sensory information is relayed to the thalamus for processing. A small fraction of the arriving information is projected to the cerebral cortex and reaches our awareness.

Visceral Sensory Pathways

Visceral sensory information is collected by interoceptors monitoring visceral tissues and organs, primarily within the thoracic and abdominopelvic cavities. These interoceptors include nociceptors, thermoreceptors, tactile receptors, baroreceptors, and chemoreceptors, although none of them are as numerous as they are in somatic tissues. The axons of the first-order neurons usually travel in company with autonomic motor fibers innervating the same visceral structures.

Cranial nerves V, VII, IX, and X carry visceral sensory information from the mouth, palate, pharynx, larynx, trachea, esophagus, and associated vessels and glands. This information is delivered to the **solitary nucleus,** a large nucleus in the medulla oblongata. The solitary nucleus is a major processing and sorting center for visceral sensory information; it has extensive connections with the various cardiovascular and respiratory centers as well as with the reticular formation.

The dorsal roots of spinal nerves $T_1–L_2$ carry visceral sensory information provided by receptors in organs located between the diaphragm and the pelvic cavity. The dorsal roots of spinal nerves $S_2–S_4$ carry visceral sensory information from organs in the inferior portion of the pelvic cavity, including the last portion of the large intestine, the urethra and base of the urinary bladder, and the prostate gland (males) or the cervix of the uterus and adjacent portions of the vagina (females).

The first-order neurons deliver the visceral sensory information to interneurons whose axons ascend within the anterolateral pathway. Most of the sensory information is delivered to the soli-

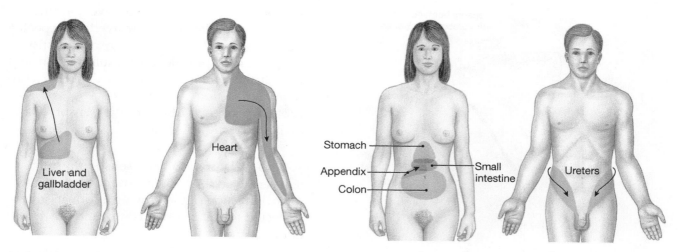

FIGURE 7.33   Referred pain. Pain sensations from visceral organs are often perceived as involving specific regions of the body surface innervated by the same spinal segments. Each region of perceived pain is labeled according to the organ at which the pain originates.

tary nucleus, and because it never reaches the primary sensory cortex we remain unaware of these sensations.

The Somatic Nervous System

Motor commands issued by the CNS are distributed by the somatic nervous system (SNS) and the autonomic nervous system (ANS). The somatic nervous system, also called the *somatic motor system,* controls the contractions of skeletal muscles. The output of the SNS is under voluntary control. The autonomic nervous system, or *visceral motor system,* controls visceral effectors, such as smooth muscle, cardiac muscle, and glands. Our interest here is the structure of the SNS. Throughout this discussion we will use the terms *motor neuron* and *motor control* to refer specifically to somatic motor neurons and pathways that control skeletal muscles.

Somatic motor pathways always involve at least two motor neurons: an **upper motor neuron,** whose cell body lies in a CNS processing center, and a **lower motor neuron,** whose cell body lies in a nucleus of the brain stem or spinal cord. The upper motor neuron synapses on the lower motor neuron, which in turn innervates a

single motor unit in a skeletal muscle. Activity in the upper motor neuron may facilitate or inhibit the lower motor neuron. Activation of the lower motor neuron triggers a contraction in the innervated muscle. Only the axon of the lower motor neuron extends outside the CNS. Destruction of or damage to a lower motor neuron eliminates voluntary and reflex control over the innervated motor unit.

Conscious and subconscious motor commands control skeletal muscles by traveling over three integrated motor pathways: the *corticospinal pathway,* the *medial pathway,* and the *lateral pathway.* Figure 7.35 indicates the positions of the associated motor (descending) tracts in the spinal cord. Activity within these motor pathways is monitored and adjusted by the basal nuclei and cerebellum. Their output stimulates or inhibits the activity of either (1) motor nuclei or (2) the primary motor cortex.

The Corticospinal Pathway

The **corticospinal pathway** (Figure 7.36), sometimes called the *pyramidal system,* provides voluntary control over skeletal muscles. This system begins at the *pyramidal cells* of the primary motor cortex. The axons of these upper motor neurons descend into the brain stem and spinal cord to synapse on lower motor neurons that control

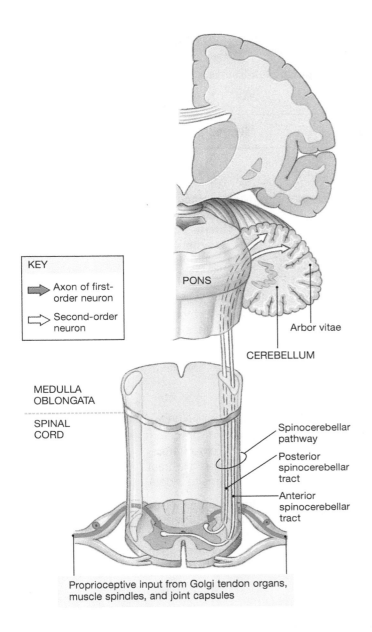

KEY

→ Axon of first-order neuron

⇨ Second-order neuron

PONS

Arbor vitae

CEREBELLUM

MEDULLA OBLONGATA

SPINAL CORD

Spinocerebellar pathway

Posterior spinocerebellar tract

Anterior spinocerebellar tract

Proprioceptive input from Golgi tendon organs, muscle spindles, and joint capsules

FIGURE 7.34 The spinocerebellar pathway.

the brain stem, and emerge on either side of the mesencephalon as the *cerebral peduncles*.

The Corticobulbar Tracts

Axons in the **corticobulbar** (kor-ti-kō-BUL-bar) **tracts** (*bulbar,* brain stem) synapse on lower motor neurons in the motor nuclei of cranial nerves III, IV, V, VI, VII, IX, XI, and XII. The corticobulbar tracts provide conscious control over skeletal muscles that move the eye, jaw, and face, and some muscles of the neck and pharynx. The corticobulbar tracts also innervate the motor centers of the medial and lateral pathways.

The Corticospinal Tracts

Axons in the **corticospinal tracts** synapse on lower motor neurons in the anterior gray horns of the spinal cord. As they descend, the corticospinal tracts are visible along the ventral surface of the medulla oblongata as a pair of thick bands, the **pyramids.** Along the length of the pyramids, roughly 85 percent of the axons cross the midline (decussate) to enter the descending **lateral corticospinal tracts** on the opposite side of the spinal cord. The other 15 percent continue uncrossed along the spinal cord as the **anterior corticospinal tracts.** At the spinal segment it targets, an axon in the anterior corticospinal tract crosses over to the opposite side of the spinal cord in the anterior white commissure before synapsing on lower motor neurons in the anterior gray horns.

The Motor Homunculus

The activity of pyramidal cells in a specific portion of the primary motor cortex will result in the contraction of specific peripheral muscles. The identities of the stimulated muscles depend on the region of motor cortex that is active. As in the primary sensory cortex, the primary motor cortex corresponds point by point with specific regions of the body. The cortical areas have been mapped out in diagrammatic form, creating a **motor homunculus.** Figure 7.36 shows the motor homunculus of the left cerebral hemisphere and the corticospinal pathway controlling skeletal muscles on the right side of the body.

The proportions of the motor homunculus are quite different from those of the actual body, because the motor area devoted to a specific region of the cortex is proportional to the number

skeletal muscles. In general, the corticospinal pathway is direct: The upper motor neurons synapse directly on the lower motor neurons. However, the corticospinal pathway also works indirectly, as it innervates centers of the medial and lateral pathways.

The corticospinal pathway contains three pairs of descending tracts: (1) the *corticobulbar tracts,* (2) the *lateral corticospinal tracts,* and (3) the *anterior corticospinal tracts.* These tracts enter the white matter of the internal capsule, descend into

TABLE 7.5   Principal Ascending (Sensory) Pathways

Pathway/Tract	Sensation(s)	Location of Neuron Cell Bodies		
		First-Order	Second-Order	Third-Order
POSTERIOR COLUMN PATHWAY				
Fasciculus gracilis	Proprioception and fine touch, pressure, and vibration from inferior half of body	Dorsal root ganglia of inferior half of body; axons enter CNS in dorsal roots and join fasciculus gracilis	Nucleus gracilis of meduila oblongata; axons cross over before entering medial lemniscus	Ventral nuclei of thalmus
Fasciculus cuneatus	Proprioception and fine touch, and ventral pressure, and vibration from superior half of body	Dorsal root ganglia of superior half of body; axons enter CNS in dorsal roots and join fasciculus cuneatus	Nucleus cuneatus of medulla oblongata; axons cross over before entering medial lemniscus	As above
SPINOTHALAMIC PATHWAY	Pain and temperature			
Lateral spinothalamic tracts		Dorsal root ganglia; axons enter CNS in dorsal roots	Interneurons in posterior gray horn; axons enter lateral spinothalamic tract on opposite side	Ventral nuclei of thalamus
Anterior spinothalamic tracts	Crude touch and pressure	As above	Interneurons in posterior gray horn; axons enter anterior spinothalamic tract on opposite side	As above
SPINOCEREBELLAR PATHWAY	Proprioception			
Posterior spinocerebellar tracts		Dorsal root ganglia; axons enter CNS in dorsal roots	Interneurons in posterior gray horn; axons enter posterior spinothalamic tract on same side	Not present
Anterior spinocerebellar tracts	Proprioception	As above	Interneurons in same spinal section; axons enter anterior spinocerebellar tract on the same or opposite side	Not present

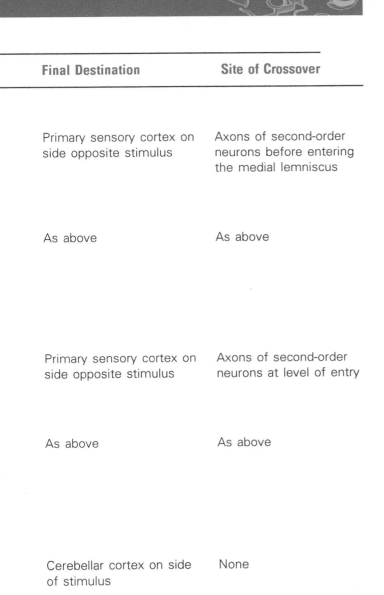

Final Destination	Site of Crossover
Primary sensory cortex on side opposite stimulus	Axons of second-order neurons before entering the medial lemniscus
As above	As above
Primary sensory cortex on side opposite stimulus	Axons of second-order neurons at level of entry
As above	As above
Cerebellar cortex on side of stimulus	None
Cerebellar cortex on side opposite (and side of) stimulus	Axons of most second-order neurons cross over before entering tract; many re-cross at cerebellum

of motor units involved in the region's control, not to its actual size. As a result, the homunculus provides an indication of the degree of fine motor control available. For example, the hands, face, and tongue, all of which are capable of varied and complex movements, appear very large, whereas the trunk is relatively small. These proportions are similar to those of the sensory homunculus (see Figure 7.32). The sensory and motor homunculi differ in other respects because some highly sensitive regions, such as the sole of the foot, contain few motor units, and some areas with an abundance of motor units, such as the eye muscles, are not particularly sensitive.

The Medial and Lateral Pathways

Several centers in the cerebrum, diencephalon, and brain stem may issue somatic motor commands as a result of processing performed at a subconscious level. These centers and their associated tracts were long known as the *extrapyramidal system (EPS),* because it was thought that they operated independently of, and in parallel with, the *pyramidal system* (corticospinal pathway). This classification scheme is both inaccurate and misleading, because motor control is integrated at all levels through extensive feedback loops and interconnections. It is more appropriate to group these nuclei and tracts in terms of their primary functions: The components of the **medial pathway** help control gross movements of the trunk and proximal limb muscles, whereas those of the **lateral pathway** help control the distal limb muscles that perform more precise movements.

The medial and lateral pathways can modify or direct skeletal muscle contractions by stimulating, facilitating, or inhibiting lower motor neurons. It is important to note that the axons of upper motor neurons in the medial and lateral pathways synapse on the same lower motor neurons innervated by the corticospinal pathway. This means that the various motor pathways interact not only within the brain, through interconnections between the primary motor cortex and motor centers in the brain stem, but also through excitatory

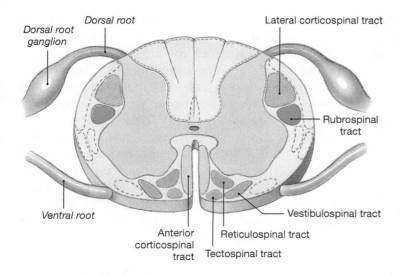

FIGURE 7.35 Descending (motor) tracts in the spinal cord. A cross-sectional view indicating the locations of the major descending (motor) tracts that contain the axons of upper motor neurons. The origins and destinations of these tracts are listed in *Table 7.6* Sensory tracts (shown in *Figure 7.32*) appear in dashed outline.

or inhibitory interactions at the level of the lower motor neuron.

The Medial Pathway

The medial pathway is primarily concerned with the control of muscle tone and gross movements of the neck, trunk, and proximal limb muscles. The upper motor neurons of the medial pathway are located in the *vestibular nuclei,* the *superior* and *inferior colliculi,* and the *reticular formation.*

The vestibular nuclei receive information, over the vestibulocochlear nerve (VIII), from receptors in the inner ear that monitor the position and movement of the head. These nuclei respond to changes in the orientation of the head, sending motor commands that alter the muscle tone, extension, and position of the neck, eyes, head, and limbs. The primary goal is to maintain posture and balance. The descending fibers in the spinal cord constitute the **vestibulospinal tracts.**

The superior and inferior colliculi are located in the *tectum,* or roof of the mesencephalon. The colliculi receive visual (superior) and auditory

(inferior) sensations. Axons of upper motor neurons in the colliculi descend in the **tectospinal tracts.** These axons cross to the opposite side immediately, before descending to synapse on lower motor neurons in the brain stem or spinal cord. Axons in the tectospinal tracts direct reflexive changes in the position of the head, neck, and upper limbs in response to bright lights, sudden movements, or loud noises.

The reticular formation is a loosely organized network of neurons that extends throughout the brain stem. The reticular formation receives input from almost every ascending and descending pathway. It also has extensive interconnections with the cerebrum, the cerebellum, and brain stem nuclei. Axons of upper motor neurons in the reticular formation descend into the **reticulospinal tracts** without crossing to the opposite side. The effects of reticular formation stimulation are determined by the region stimulated. For example, the stimulation of upper motor neurons in one portion of the reticular formation produces eye movements, whereas the stimulation of another portion activates respiratory muscles.

The Lateral Pathway

The lateral pathway is primarily concerned with the control of muscle tone and the more precise movements of the distal parts of the limbs. The upper motor neurons of the lateral pathway lie within the red nuclei of the mesencephalon. Axons of upper motor neurons in the red nuclei cross to the opposite side of the brain and descend into the spinal cord in the **rubrospinal tracts** (*ruber,* red). In humans, the rubrospinal tracts are small and extend only to the cervical spinal cord. There they provide motor control over distal muscles of the upper limbs; normally, their role is insignificant as compared with that of the lateral corticospinal tracts. However, the rubrospinal tracts can be important in maintaining motor control and muscle tone in the upper limbs if the lateral corticospinal tracts are damaged.

Table 7.6 reviews the major descending (motor) tracts discussed in this section.

The Basal Nuclei

The basal nuclei provide the background patterns of movement involved in voluntary motor activities. For example, they may control muscles that determine the background position of the trunk or limbs, or they may direct rhythmic cycles of movement, as in walking or running. These nuclei do not exert direct control over lower motor neurons. Instead, they adjust the activities of upper motor neurons in the various motor pathways based on input from all portions of the cerebral cortex, as well as from the substantia nigra.

The basal nuclei adjust or establish patterns of movement via two major pathways:

1. One group of axons synapses on thalamic neurons, whose axons extend to the premotor cortex, the motor association area that directs activities of the primary motor cortex. This arrangement creates a feedback loop that changes the sensitivity of the pyramidal cells and alters the pattern of instructions carried by the corticospinal tracts.

2. A second group of axons synapses in the reticular formation, altering the excitatory or inhibitory output of the reticulospinal tracts.

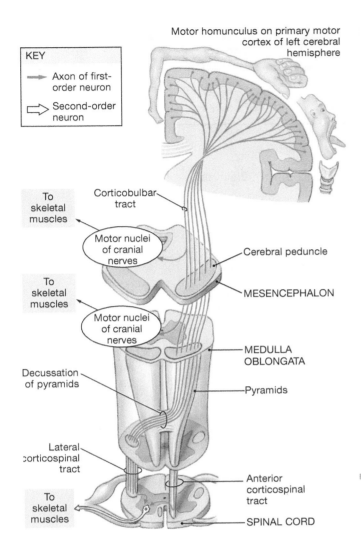

KEY

→ Axon of first-order neuron

⇨ Second-order neuron

Motor homunculus on primary motor cortex of left cerebral hemisphere

To skeletal muscles

Corticobulbar tract

Motor nuclei of cranial nerves

Cerebral peduncle

MESENCEPHALON

To skeletal muscles

Motor nuclei of cranial nerves

MEDULLA OBLONGATA

Decussation of pyramids

Pyramids

Lateral corticospinal tract

To skeletal muscles

Anterior corticospinal tract

SPINAL CORD

FIGURE 7.36   The corticospinal pathway. The corticospinal pathway originates at the primary motor cortex. The corticobulbar tracts end at the motor nuclei of cranial nerves on the opposite side of the brain. Most fibers in this pathway cross over in the medulla and enter the lateral corticospinal tracts; the rest descend in the anterior corticospinal tracts and cross over after reaching target segments in the spinal cord.

The Basal Nuclei and Cerebellum

The basal nuclei and cerebellum are responsible for coordination and feedback control over muscle contractions, whether those contractions are consciously or subconsciously directed.

Clinical Note

The term **cerebral palsy** refers to a number of disorders that affect voluntary motor performance; they appear during infancy or childhood and persist throughout the life of the affected individual. The cause may be trauma associated with premature or unusually stressful birth, maternal exposure to drugs (including alcohol), or a genetic defect that causes the improper development of motor pathways. Problems during labor and delivery may produce compression or interruption of placental circulation or oxygen supplies. If the oxygen concentration in fetal blood declines significantly for as little as 5–10 minutes, CNS function can be permanently impaired. The cerebral cortex, cerebellum, basal nuclei, hippocampus, and thalamus are likely targets, producing abnormalities in motor skills, posture and balance, memory, speech, and learning abilities.

TABLE 7.6   Principal Descending (Motor) Pathways

Tract	Location of Upper Motor Neurons	Site of Destination	Crossover	Action
CORTICOSPINAL PATHWAY				
Corticobulbar tracts	Primary motor cortex (cerebral hemisphere)	Lower motor neurons of cranial nerve nuclei in brain stem	Brain stem	Conscious motor control of skeletal muscles
Lateral corticospinal tracts	As above	Lower motor neurons of anterior gray horns of spinal cord	Pyramids of medulla oblongata	As above
Anterior corticospinal tracts	As above	As above	Level of lower motor neuron	As above
MEDIAL PATHWAY				
Vestibulospinal tracts	Vestibular nuclei (at border of pons and medulla oblongata)	As above	None (uncrossed)	Subconscious regulation of balance and muscle tone
Tectospinal tracts	Tectum (mesencephalon: superior and inferior colliculi)	Lower motor neurons of anterior gray horns (cervical spinal cord only)	Brain stem (mesencephalon)	Subconscious regulation of eye, head, neck, and upper limb position in response to visual and auditory stimuli
Reticulospinal tracts	Reticular formation (network of nuclei in brain stem)	Lower motor neurons of anterior gray horns of spinal cord	None (uncrossed)	Subconscious regulation of reflex activity
LATERAL PATHWAY				
Rubrospinal tracts	Red nuclei of mesencephalon	As above	Brain stem (mesencephalon)	Subconscious regulation of upper limb muscle tone and movement

Two distinct populations of neurons exist: one that stimulates neurons by releasing acetylcholine (ACh), and another that inhibits neurons through the release of gamma aminobutyric acid (GABA). Under normal conditions, the excitatory interneurons are kept inactive, and the tracts leaving the basal nuclei have an inhibitory effect on upper motor neurons. In *Parkinson's disease,* the excitatory neurons become more active, leading to problems with the voluntary control of movement.

If the primary motor cortex is damaged, the individual loses the ability to exert fine control over skeletal muscles. However, some voluntary movements can still be controlled by the basal nuclei. In effect, the medial and lateral pathways function as they usually do, but the corticospinal pathway cannot fine-tune the movements. For example, after damage to the primary motor cortex, the basal nuclei can still receive information about planned movements from the prefrontal cortex and can perform preparatory movements of the trunk and limbs. But because the corticospinal pathway is inoperative, precise movements of the forearms, wrists, and hands cannot occur. An individual in this condition can stand, maintain balance, and even walk, but all movements are hesitant, awkward, and poorly controlled.

The Cerebellum

The cerebellum monitors proprioceptive (position) sensations, visual information from the eyes, and vestibular (balance) sensations from the inner ear as movements are underway. Axons within the spinocerebellar tracts deliver proprioceptive information to the cerebellar cortex. Visual information is relayed from the superior colliculi, and balance information is relayed from the vestibular nuclei. The output of the cerebellum affects upper motor neuron activity in the corticospinal, medial, and lateral pathways.

All motor pathways send information to the cerebellum when motor commands are issued. As the movement proceeds, the cerebellum monitors proprioceptive and vestibular information and compares the arriving sensations with those experienced during previous movements. It then adjusts the activities of the upper motor neurons involved. In general, any voluntary movement begins with the activation of far more motor units than are required—or even desirable. The cerebellum acts like a brake, providing the inhibition needed to minimize the number of motor commands used to perform the movement. The pattern and degree of inhibition changes from moment to moment, and this makes the movement efficient, smooth, and precisely controlled.

The patterns of cerebellar activity are learned by trial and error, over many repetitions. Many of the basic patterns are established early in life; examples include the fine balancing adjustments you make while standing and walking. The ability to fine-tune a complex pattern of movement improves with practice, until the movements become fluid and automatic. Consider the relaxed, smooth movements of acrobats, golfers, and sushi chefs. These people move without thinking about the details of their movements. This ability is important, because when you concentrate on voluntary control, the rhythm and pattern of the movement usually fall apart as your primary motor cortex starts overriding the commands of the basal nuclei and cerebellum.

Levels of Processing and Motor Control

All sensory and motor pathways involve a series of synapses, one after the other. Along the way, the information is distributed to processing centers operating at the subconscious level. Consider what happens when you stumble—you often recover your balance even as you become aware that a problem exists. Long before your cerebral cortex could assess the situation, evaluate possible responses (shift weight *here,* move leg *there,* and so on), and issue appropriate motor commands,

Clinical Note

Amyotrophic lateral sclerosis (ALS), commonly known as *Lou Gehrig's disease,* is a progressive, degenerative disorder that affects motor neurons in the spinal cord, brain stem, and cerebral hemispheres. The degeneration affects both upper and lower motor neurons. Because a motor neuron and its dependent muscle fibers are so intimately related, the destruction of CNS neurons causes atrophy of the associated skeletal muscles. Noted physicist Stephen Hawking has this condition.

monosynaptic and polysynaptic reflexes, perhaps adjusted by the brain stem and cerebellum, successfully prevented a fall. This is a general pattern; spinal and cranial reflexes provide rapid, involuntary, preprogrammed responses that preserve homeostasis over the short term. Voluntary responses are more complex and require more time to prepare and execute.

Cranial and spinal reflexes control the most basic motor activities. Integrative centers in the brain perform more elaborate processing, and as we move from the medulla oblongata to the cerebral cortex, the motor patterns become increasingly complex and variable. The most complex and variable motor activities are directed by the primary motor cortex of the cerebral hemispheres.

During development, the spinal and cranial reflexes are the first to appear. More complex reflexes and motor patterns develop as CNS neurons multiply, enlarge, and interconnect. The process proceeds relatively slowly, as billions of neurons establish trillions of synaptic connections. At birth, neither the cerebral nor the cerebellar cortex is fully functional. The behavior of newborn infants is directed primarily by centers in the diencephalon and brain stem.

100 Keys | Neurons of the primary motor cortex innervate motor neurons in the brain and spinal cord responsible for stimulating skeletal muscles. Higher centers in the brain can suppress or facilitate reflex responses; reflexes can complement or increase the complexity of voluntary movements.

Clinical Note

Although it may seem strange, physicians generally take newborn infants into a dark room and shine a light against the skull. They are checking for *anencephaly* (an-en-SEF-uh-lē), a rare condition in which the brain fails to develop at levels above the mesencephalon or lower diencephalon.

In most such cases, the cranium also fails to develop, and diagnosis is easy, but in some cases, a normal skull forms. In such instances, the cranium is empty and translucent enough to transmit light. Unless the condition is discovered right away, the parents may take the infant home, unaware of the problem. All the normal behavior patterns expected of a newborn are present, including suckling, stretching, yawning, crying, kicking, sticking fingers in the mouth, and tracking movements with the eyes. However, death will occur naturally within days or months.

This tragic condition provides a striking demonstration of the role of the brain stem in controlling complex motor patterns. During normal development, these patterns become incorporated into variable and versatile behaviors as control centers and analytical centers appear in the cerebral cortex.

Peripheral Nervous System

The **peripheral nervous system (PNS)** consists of nerves and scattered groups of neuronal cell bodies (ganglia) found outside the CNS. One type of ganglion has already been considered—the dorsal root ganglion of the spinal cord. Others will be covered in the discussion of the autonomic nervous system. Here, we will concern ourselves only with nerves.

Structure of a Nerve

A **nerve** is a bundle of neuron fibers found outside the CNS. Within a nerve, neuron fibers, or processes, are wrapped in protective connective tissue coverings. Each fiber is surrounded by a delicate connective tissue sheath, an **endoneurium** (en"do-nu're-um). Groups of fibers are bound by a coarser connective tissue wrapping, the **perineurium** (per"ĭ-nu're-um), to form fiber bundles, or **fascicles.** Finally, all the fascicles are bound together by a tough fibrous sheath, the **epineurium,** to form the cordlike nerve (Figure 7.37).

Like neurons, nerves are classified according to the direction in which they transmit impulses. Nerves carrying both sensory and motor fibers are called **mixed nerves;** all spinal nerves are mixed nerves. Nerves that carry impulses toward the CNS only are called **sensory,** or **afferent, nerves,** whereas those that carry only motor fibers are **motor,** or **efferent, nerves.**

Cranial Nerves

The 12 pairs of **cranial nerves** primarily serve the head and neck. Only one pair (the vagus nerves) extends to the thoracic and abdominal cavities.

The cranial nerves are numbered in order, and in most cases, their names reveal the most important structures they control. The cranial nerves are described by name, number, course, and major function in Table 7.7. The last column of the table describes how cranial nerves are tested, which is an important part of any neurologic examination. You do not need to memorize these tests, but this information may help you understand cranial nerve function. As you read through the table, also look at Figure 7.38, which shows

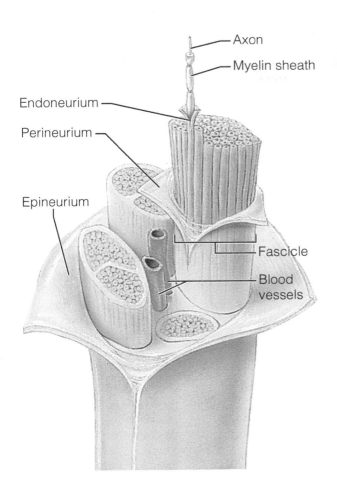

FIGURE 7.37 Structure of a nerve. Three-dimensional view of a portion of a nerve, showing its connective tissue wrappings.

Labels: Axon, Myelin sheath, Endoneurium, Perineurium, Epineurium, Fascicle, Blood vessels

the location of the cranial nerves on the brain's anterior surface.

Most cranial nerves are mixed nerves; however, three pairs, the optic, olfactory, and vestibulocochlear (ves-tib″u-lo-kok′le-ar) nerves, are purely sensory in function. (The older name for the vestibulocochlear nerve is *acoustic nerve,* a name that reveals its role in hearing but not in equilibrium.) I give my students the following little saying as a memory jog to help them remember the cranial nerves in order; perhaps it will help you, too. The first letter of each word in the saying (and both letters of "ah") is the first letter of the cranial nerve to be remembered: "**O**h, **o**h, **o**h, **t**o **t**ouch **a**nd **f**eel **v**ery **g**ood **v**elvet, **ah**."

Spinal Nerves and Nerve Plexuses

The 31 pairs of human **spinal nerves** are formed by the combination of the ventral and dorsal roots of the spinal cord. Although each of the cranial nerves issuing from the brain is named specifically, the spinal nerves are named for the region of the cord from which they arise. Figure 7.39 shows how the nerves are named in this scheme.

Almost immediately after being formed, each spinal nerve divides into **dorsal** and **ventral rami** (ra′mi), making each spinal nerve only about one-half inch long. The rami, like the spinal nerves, contain both motor and sensory fibers. Thus, damage to a spinal nerve or either of its rami results both in loss of sensation and flaccid paralysis of the area of the body served. The smaller dorsal rami serve the skin and muscles of the posterior body trunk. The ventral rami of spinal nerves T_1 through T_{12} form the *intercostal nerves,* which supply the muscles between the ribs and the skin and muscles of the anterior and lateral trunk. The ventral rami of all other spinal nerves form complex networks of nerves called **plexuses,** which serve the motor and sensory needs of the limbs. The four nerve plexuses are described in Table 7.8; three of the four plexuses are shown in Figure 7.40.

Autonomic Nervous System

The **autonomic nervous system (ANS)** is the motor subdivision of the PNS that controls body activities automatically. It is composed of a special group of neurons (or **autonomic plexus**) that regulate cardiac muscle (the heart), smooth muscles (found in the walls of the visceral organs and blood vessels), and glands. Although all body systems contribute to homeostasis, the relative stability of our internal environment depends largely on the workings of the ANS. At every moment, signals flood from the visceral organs into the CNS, and the autonomic nerves make adjustments as necessary to best support body activities. For example, blood flow may be shunted to more "needy" areas, heart and breathing rate may be speeded up or slowed down, blood pressure may be adjusted, and stomach secretions may be increased or decreased. Most of this fine-tuning occurs without our awareness or attention—few of us realize when our pupils dilate

TABLE 7.7	The Cranial Nerves		
Name/Number	**Origin/Course**	**Function**	**Test**
I. Olfactory	Fibers arise from olfactory receptors in the nasal mucosa and synapse with the olfactory bulbs (which, in turn, send fibers to the olfactory cortex)	Purely sensory; carries impulses for the sense of smell	Subject is asked to sniff and identify aromatic substances, such as oil of cloves or vanilla
II. Optic	Fibers arise from the retina of the eye and form the optic nerve. The two optic nerves form the optic chiasma by partial crossover of fibers; the fibers continue to the optic cortex as the optic tracts	Purely sensory; carries impulses for vision	Vision and visual field are tested with an eye chart and by testing the point at which the subject first sees an object (finger) moving into the visual field; eye interior is viewed with an ophthalmoscope
III. Oculomotor	Fibers run from the midbrain to the eye	Supplies motor fibers to four of the six muscles (superior, inferior, and medial rectus, and inferior oblique) that direct the eyeball; to the eyelid; and to the internal eye muscles controlling lens shape and pupil size	Pupils are examined for size, shape, and size equality; pupillary reflex is tested with a penlight (pupils should constrict when illuminated); eye convergence is tested, as is the ability to follow moving objects
IV. Trochlear	Fibers run from the midbrain to the eye	Supplies motor fibers for one external eye muscle (superior oblique)	Tested in common with cranial nerve III for the ability to follow moving objects
V. Trigeminal	Fibers emerge from the pons and form three divisions that run to the face	Conducts sensory impulses from the skin of the face and mucosa of the nose and mouth; also contains motor fibers that activate the chewing muscles	Sensations of pain, touch, and temperature are tested with a safety pin and hot and cold objects; corneal reflex tested with a wisp of cotton; motor branch tested by asking the subject to open mouth against resistance and move jaw from side to side
VI. Abducens	Fibers leave the pons and run to the eye	Supplies motor fibers to the lateral rectus muscle, which rolls the eye laterally	Tested in common with cranial nerve III for the ability to move each eye laterally

(continued)

Name/Number	Origin/Course	Function	Test
TABLE 7.7	*(continued)*		
VII. Facial	Fibers leave the pons and run to the face	Activates the muscles of facial expression and the lacrimal and salivary glands; carries sensory impulses from the taste buds of anterior tongue	Anterior two-thirds of tongue is tested for ability to taste sweet, salty, sour, and bitter substances; subject is asked to close eyes, smile, whistle, etc.; tearing is tested with ammonia fumes
VIII. Vestibulocochlear	Fibers run from the equilibrium and hearing receptors of the inner ear to the brain stem	Purely sensory; vestibular branch transmits impulses for the sense of balance, and cochlear branch transmits impulses for the sense of hearing	Hearing is checked by air and bone conduction, using a tuning fork
IX. Glossopharyngeal	Fibers emerge from the medulla and run to the throat	Supplies motor fibers to the pharynx (throat) that promote swallowing and saliva production; carries sensory impulses from taste buds of the posterior tongue and from pressure receptors of the carotid artery	Gag and swallowing reflexes are checked; subject is asked to speak and cough; posterior tongue may be tested for taste
X. Vagus	Fibers emerge from the medulla and descend into the thorax and abdominal cavity	Fibers carry sensory impulses from and motor impulses to the pharynx, larynx, and the abdominal and thoracic viscera; most motor fibers are parasympathetic fibers that promote digestive activity and help regulate heart activity	Tested in common with cranial nerve IX, since they both serve muscles of the throat
XI. Accessory	Fibers arise from the medulla and superior spinal cord and travel to muscles of the neck and back	Mostly motor fibers that activate the sternocleidomastoid and trapezius muscles	Sternocleidomastoid and trapezius muscles are checked for strength by asking the subject to rotate head and shrug shoulders against resistance
XII. Hypoglossal	Fibers run from the medulla to the tongue	Motor fibers control tongue movements; sensory fibers carry impulses from the tongue	Subject is asked to stick out tongue, and any position abnormalities are noted

Q *If you can't shrug your right shoulder, what cranial nerve is involved?*

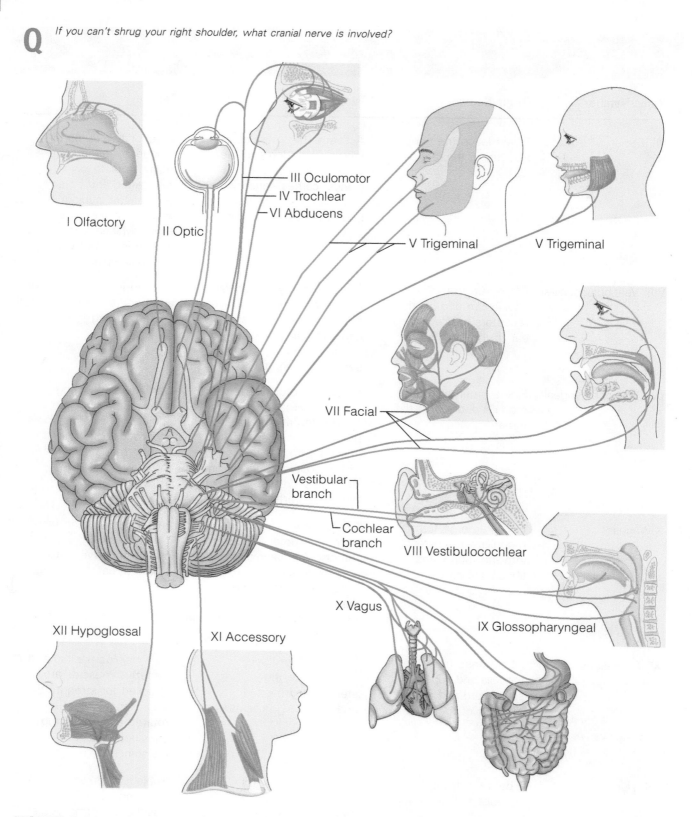

I Olfactory

II Optic

III Oculomotor
IV Trochlear
VI Abducens

V Trigeminal

V Trigeminal

VII Facial

Vestibular branch
Cochlear branch

VIII Vestibulocochlear

XII Hypoglossal

XI Accessory

X Vagus

IX Glossopharyngeal

FIGURE 7.38 Distribution of cranial nerves. Sensory nerves are shown in blue, motor nerves in red. Although cranial nerves III, IV, and VI have sensory fibers, these are not shown because the sensory fibers account for only minor parts of these nerves.

A

Left member of cranial nerve XI.

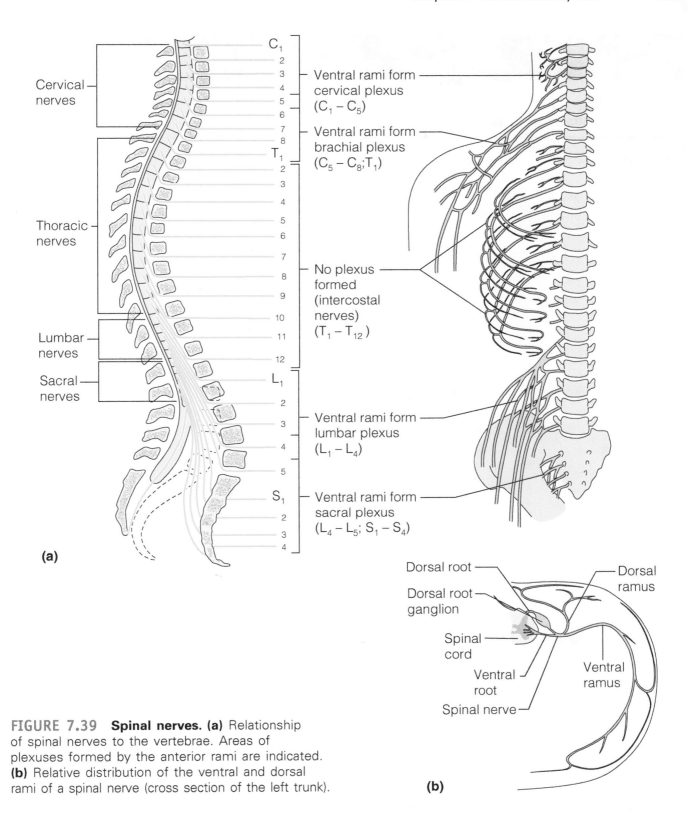

(a)

Cervical nerves

Thoracic nerves

Lumbar nerves

Sacral nerves

C₁ 2 3 4 5 6 7 8
T₁ 2 3 4 5 6 7 8 9 10 11 12
L₁ 2 3 4 5
S₁ 2 3 4

Ventral rami form cervical plexus (C₁ – C₅)

Ventral rami form brachial plexus (C₅ – C₈;T₁)

No plexus formed (intercostal nerves) (T₁ – T₁₂)

Ventral rami form lumbar plexus (L₁ – L₄)

Ventral rami form sacral plexus (L₄ – L₅; S₁ – S₄)

Dorsal root
Dorsal root ganglion
Spinal cord
Ventral root
Spinal nerve
Dorsal ramus
Ventral ramus

(b)

FIGURE 7.39 Spinal nerves. (a) Relationship of spinal nerves to the vertebrae. Areas of plexuses formed by the anterior rami are indicated. **(b)** Relative distribution of the ventral and dorsal rami of a spinal nerve (cross section of the left trunk).

TABLE 7.8   Spinal Nerve Plexuses

Plexus	Origin (from ventral rami)	Important nerves	Body areas served	Result of damage to plexus or its nerves
Cervical	C_1–C_5	Phrenic	Diaphragm and muscles of shoulder and neck	Respiratory paralysis (and death if not treated promptly)
Brachial	C_5–C_8 and T_1	Axillary	Deltoid muscle of shoulder	Paralysis and atrophy of deltoid muscle
		Radial	Triceps and extensor muscles of the forearm	Wristdrop—inability to extend hand at wrist
		Median	Flexor muscles of forearm and some muscles of hand	Decreased ability to flex and abduct hand and flex and abduct thumb and index finger—therefore, inability to pick up small objects
		Musculocutaneous	Flexor muscles of arm	Decreased ability to flex forearm on arm
		Ulnar	Wrist and many hand muscles	Clawhand—inability to spread fingers apart
Lumbar	L_1–L_4	Femoral (including lateral and anterior cutaneous branches)	Lower abdomen, buttocks, anterior thighs, and skin of anteromedial leg and thigh	Inability to extend leg and flex hip; loss of cutaneous sensation
		Obturator	Adductor muscles of medial thigh and small hip muscles; skin of medial thigh and hip joint	Inability to adduct thigh
Sacral	L_4–L_5 and S_1–S_4	Sciatic (largest nerve in body; splits to common fibular and tibial nerves)	Lower trunk and posterior surface of thigh (and leg)	Inability to extend hip and flex knee; sciatica
		• Common fibular (superficial and deep branches)	Lateral aspect of leg and foot	Footdrop—inability to dorsiflex foot
		• Tibial (including sural and plantar branches)	Posterior aspect of leg and foot	Inability to plantar flex and invert foot; shuffling gait
		Superior and inferior gluteal	Gluteus muscles of hip	Inability to extend hip (maximus) or abduct and medially rotate thigh (medius)

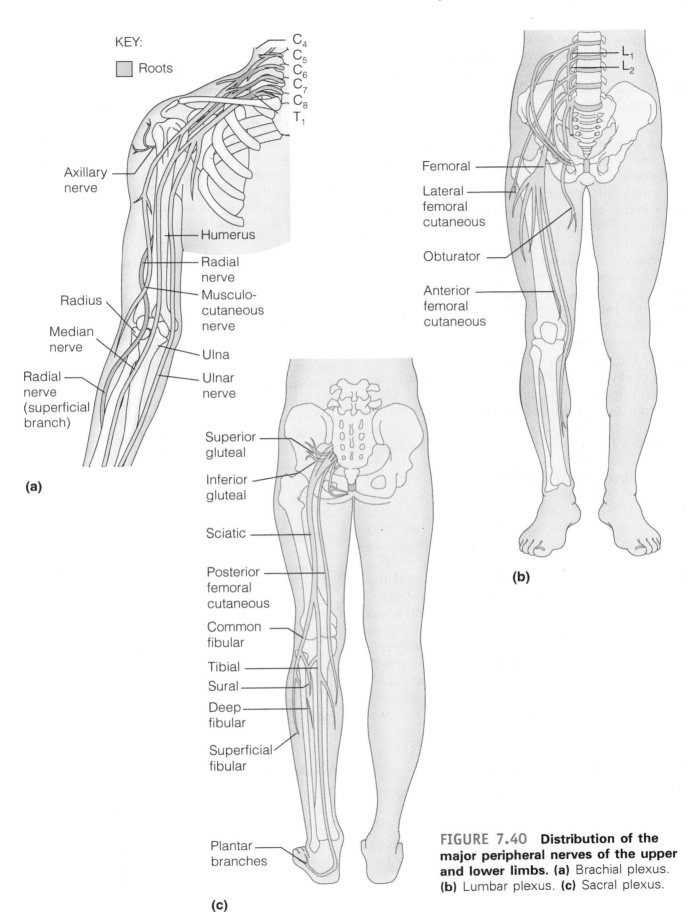

KEY:

Roots

C₄
C₅
C₆
C₇
C₈
T₁

Axillary nerve

Humerus

Radial nerve

Musculo-cutaneous nerve

Radius

Median nerve

Ulna

Ulnar nerve

Radial nerve (superficial branch)

(a)

Femoral

Lateral femoral cutaneous

Obturator

Anterior femoral cutaneous

L₁
L₂

(b)

Superior gluteal

Inferior gluteal

Sciatic

Posterior femoral cutaneous

Common fibular

Tibial

Sural

Deep fibular

Superficial fibular

Plantar branches

(c)

FIGURE 7.40 **Distribution of the major peripheral nerves of the upper and lower limbs. (a)** Brachial plexus. **(b)** Lumbar plexus. **(c)** Sacral plexus.

or our arteries constrict—hence the ANS is also called the **involuntary nervous system.**

Somatic and Autonomic Nervous Systems Compared

Our previous discussions of motor nerves have focused on the activity of the somatic nervous system, the motor subdivision that controls our skeletal muscles. So, before plunging into a description of autonomic nervous system anatomy, we will take the time to point out some important differences between the somatic and autonomic divisions.

Besides differences in their effector organs and in the neurotransmitters released, the patterns of their motor pathways differ. In the somatic division, the cell bodies of the motor neurons are inside the CNS, and their axons (in spinal nerves) extend all the way to the skeletal muscles they serve. The autonomic nervous system, however, has a chain of *two* motor neurons. The first motor neuron of each pair is in the brain or spinal cord. Its axon, the **preganglionic axon** (literally, the "axon before the ganglion"), leaves the CNS to synapse with the second motor neuron in a ganglion outside the CNS. The axon of this neuron, the **postganglionic axon,** then extends to the organ it serves. These differences are summarized in Figure 7.41.

The autonomic nervous system has two arms, the sympathetic and the parasympathetic (Figure 7.42). Both serve the same organs but cause essentially opposite effects, counterbalancing each other's activities to keep body systems running smoothly. The **sympathetic division** mobilizes the body during extreme situations (such as fear, exercise, or rage), whereas the **parasympathetic division** allows us to "unwind" and conserve energy. These differences are examined in more detail shortly, but first we will consider the structural characteristics of the two arms of the ANS.

Anatomy of the Parasympathetic Division

The first neurons of the parasympathetic division are located in brain nuclei of several cranial nerves—III, VII, IX, and X (the vagus being the most important of these) and in the S_2 through S_4 levels of the spinal cord (see Figure 7.42). The neu-

rons of the cranial region send their axons out in cranial nerves to serve the head and neck organs. There they synapse with the second motor neuron in a **terminal ganglion.** From the terminal ganglion, the postganglionic axon extends a short distance to the organ it serves. In the sacral region, the preganglionic axons leave the spinal cord and form the *pelvic splanchnic* (splank'nik) *nerves,* also called the *pelvic nerves,* which travel to the pelvic cavity. In the pelvic cavity, the preganglionic axons synapse with the second motor neurons in terminal ganglia on, or close to, the organs they serve.

Anatomy of the Sympathetic Division

The sympathetic division is also called the *thoracolumbar* (tho"rah-ko-lum'bar) *division* because its first neurons are in the gray matter of the spinal cord from T_1 through L_2 (see Figure 7.42). The preganglionic axons leave the cord in the ventral root, enter the spinal nerve, and then pass through a **ramus communicans,** or small communicating branch, to enter a **sympathetic chain ganglion** (Figure 7.43). The **sympathetic chain,** or **trunk,** lies alongside the vertebral column on each side. After it reaches the ganglion, the axon may synapse with the second neuron in the sympathetic chain at the same or a different level (the postganglionic axon then reenters the spinal nerve to travel to the skin), or the axon may pass through the ganglion without synapsing and form part of the **splanchnic nerves.** The splanchnic nerves travel to the viscera to synapse with the second neuron, found in a **collateral ganglion** anterior to the vertebral column. The major collateral ganglia—the celiac and the superior and inferior mesenteric ganglia—supply the abdominal and pelvic organs. The postganglionic axon then leaves the collateral ganglion and travels to serve a nearby visceral organ.

Now that the anatomical details have been described, we are ready to examine ANS functions in a little more detail.

Autonomic Functioning

Body organs served by the autonomic nervous system receive fibers from both divisions. Exceptions are most blood vessels and most structures of the skin, some glands, and the adrenal medulla, all of which receive only sympathetic

Q *Transmission of nerve impulses along ANS pathways is generally much slower than along somatic fibers. Why?*

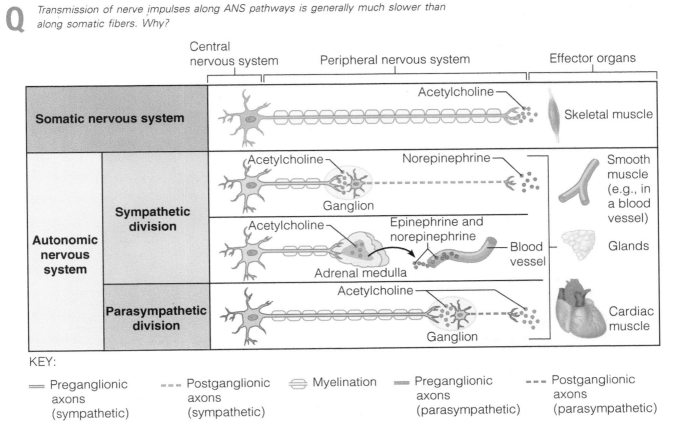

FIGURE 7.41 **Comparison of the somatic and autonomic nervous systems.**

fibers (Table 7.9). When both divisions serve the same organ they cause antagonistic effects, mainly because their postganglionic axons release different neurotransmitters (see Figure 7.41). The parasympathetic fibers, called ***cholinergic*** (ko"lin-er'jik) ***fibers,*** release acetylcholine. The sympathetic postganglionic **fibers,** called **adrenergic** (ad"ren-er'jik) ***fibers,*** release norepinephrine (nor"ep-ĭ-nef'rin). The preganglionic axons of *both* divisions release acetylcholine. To emphasize the *relative* roles of the two arms of the ANS, we will focus briefly on situations in which each division is "in control."

Sympathetic Division The **sympathetic division** is often referred to as the "fight-or-flight" system. Its activity is evident when we are excited or find

ourselves in emergency or threatening situations, such as being frightened by street toughs late at night. A pounding heart; rapid, deep breathing; cold, sweaty skin; a prickly scalp; and dilated eye pupils are sure signs of sympathetic nervous system activity. Under such conditions, the sympathetic nervous system increases heart rate, blood pressure, and blood glucose levels; dilates the bronchioles of the lungs; and brings about many other effects that help the individual cope with the stressor. Dilation of blood vessels in skeletal muscles (so that one can run faster or fight better) and withdrawal of blood from the digestive organs (so that the bulk of the blood can be used to serve the heart, brain, and skeletal muscles) are other examples.

The sympathetic nervous system is working at full speed not only when you are emotionally upset, but also when you are physically stressed. For example, if you have just had surgery or run a marathon, your adrenal glands (activated by the sympathetic nervous system) would be pumping out

A *Postganglionic fibers of the ANS are unmyelinated fibers which conduct much more slowly than the myelinated fibers that are typical of somatic nerve fibers.*

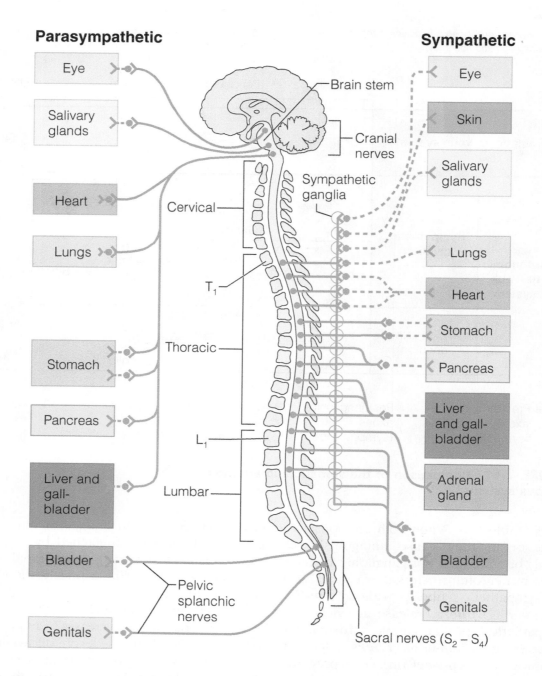

FIGURE 7.42   Anatomy of the autonomic nervous system.
Parasympathetic fibers are shown in purple, sympathetic fibers in green.
Solid lines represent preganglionic fibers; dashed lines indicate
postganglionic fibers.

epinephrine and norepinephrine (see Figure 7.41).
The effects of sympathetic nervous system activation
continue for several minutes until its hormones are
destroyed by the liver. Thus, although sympathetic
nerve impulses themselves may act only briefly, the
hormonal effects they provoke linger. The

widespread and prolonged effects of sympathetic
activation help explain why we need time to "come
down" after an extremely stressful situation.

The sympathetic division generates a head of
steam that enables the body to cope rapidly and
vigorously with situations that threaten homeostasis.

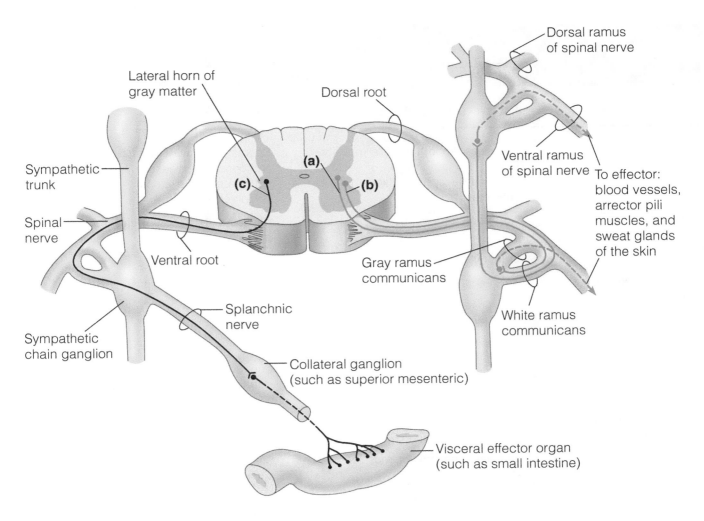

FIGURE 7.43 **Sympathetic pathways. (a)** Synapse in a sympathetic chain ganglion at the same level. **(b)** Synapse in a sympathetic chain ganglion at a different level. **(c)** Synapse in a collateral ganglion anterior to the vertebral column.

Its function is to provide the best conditions for responding to some threat, whether the best response is to run, to see better, or to think more clearly.

Homeostatic Imbalance

Some illnesses or diseases are at least aggravated, if not caused, by excessive sympathetic nervous system stimulation. Certain individuals, called Type A people, always work at breakneck speed and push themselves continually. These are people who are likely to have heart disease, high blood pressure, and ulcers, all of which may result from prolonged sympathetic nervous system activity or the rebound from it. ▲

Parasympathetic Division The **parasympathetic division** is most active when the body is at rest and not threatened in any way. This division, sometimes called the "resting-and-digesting" system, is chiefly concerned with promoting normal digestion and elimination of feces and urine and with conserving body energy, particularly by decreasing demands on the cardiovascular system. (This explains why it is a good idea to relax after a heavy meal so that digestion is not inhibited or disturbed by sympathetic activity.) Its activity is best illustrated by a person who relaxes after a meal and reads the newspaper. Blood pressure and heart and respiratory rates are being regulated at low normal levels, the digestive tract is actively digesting food,

TABLE 7.9   Effects of the Sympathetic and Parasympathetic Divisions of the Autonomic Nervous System

Target organ/system	Parasympathetic effects	Sympathetic effects
Digestive system	Increases smooth muscle mobility (peristalsis) and amount of secretion by digestive system glands; relaxes sphincters	Decreases activity of digestive system and constricts digestive system sphincters (for example, anal sphincter)
Liver	No effect	Causes glucose to be released to blood
Lungs	Constricts bronchioles	Dilates bronchioles
Urinary bladder/urethra	Relaxes sphincters (allows voiding)	Constricts sphincters (prevents voiding)
Kidneys	No effect	Decreases urine output
Heart	Decreases rate; slows and steadies	Increases rate and force of heartbeat
Blood vessels	No effect on most blood vessels	Constricts blood vessels in viscera and skin (dilates those in skeletal muscle and heart); increases blood pressure
Glands—salivary, lacrimal	Stimulates; increases production of saliva and tears	Inhibits; result is dry mouth and dry eyes
Eye (iris)	Stimulates constrictor muscles; constricts pupils	Stimulates dilator muscles; dilates pupils
Eye (ciliary muscle)	Stimulates to increase bulging of lens for close vision	Inhibits; decreases bulging of lens; prepares for distant vision
Adrenal medulla	No effect	Stimulates medulla cells to secrete epinephrine and norepinephrine
Sweat glands of skin	No effect	Stimulates to produce perspiration
Arrector pili muscles attached to hair follicles	No effect	Stimulates; produces "goose bumps"
Penis	Causes erection due to vasodilation	Causes ejaculation (emission of semen)
Cellular metabolism	No effect	Increases metabolic rate; increases blood sugar levels; stimulates fat breakdown

and the skin is warm (indicating that there is no need to divert blood to skeletal muscles or vital organs). The eye pupils are constricted to protect the retinas from excessive damaging light, and the lenses of the eyes are "set" for close vision. We might also consider the parasympathetic division as the "housekeeping" system of the body.

An easy way to remember the most important roles of the two ANS divisions is to think of the parasympathetic division as the **D** (digestion, defecation, and diuresis [urination]) division and the sympathetic division as the **E** (exercise, excitement, emergency, and embarrassment) division. Remember, however, while it is easiest to think of

A Closer Look

Tracking Down CNS Problems

ANYONE who has had a routine physical examination is familiar with the reflex tests done to assess neural function. The doctor taps your patellar (Achilles) tendon with a reflex hammer and your leg muscles contract, resulting in the knee- or ankle-jerk response. These responses show that the spinal cord and brain centers are functioning normally. When reflex tests are abnormal or when brain cancer, intracranial hemorrhage, multiple sclerosis, or hydrocephalus are suspected, more sophisticated neurological tests may be ordered to try to localize and identify the problem.

An "oldie-but-goodie" procedure used to diagnose and localize many different types of brain lesions (such as epileptic lesions, tumors, and abscesses) is *electroencephalography* (e-lek"tro-en-sef-ah-lah'grah-fe). Normal brain function involves the continuous transmission of electrical impulses by neurons. A recording of their activity, called an **electroencephalogram, or EEG,** can be made by placing electrodes at various points on the scalp and connecting these to a recording device (see the figure). The patterns of electrical activity of the neurons are called *brain waves*. Because people differ genetically,

and because everything we have ever experienced has left its imprint in our brain, each of us has a brain wave pattern that is as unique as our fingerprints. The four most commonly seen brain waves are illustrated and described in Figure (b).

As might be expected, brain-wave patterns typical of the alert wide-awake state differ from those that occur during relaxation or deep sleep. Interference with the function of the cerebral cortex is suggested by brain waves that are too fast or too slow, and unconsciousness occurs at both extremes. Sleep and coma result in brain-wave patterns that are slower than normal, whereas fright, epileptic seizures, and some kinds of drug overdose cause abnormally fast brain waves. Since brain waves are seen even during coma, absence of brain waves (a flat EEG) is taken as evidence of clinical death.

Pneumoencephalography (nu"mo-en-sef"ah-lah'grah-fe) provides a fairly clear X-ray picture of the brain ventricles and has long been the procedure of choice for diagnosing hydrocephalus. A small amount of cerebrospinal fluid is withdrawn by lumbar puncture, and air injected into the subarachnoid space floats upward and into the ventricles, allowing them to be

visualized. Although the procedure is remarkably simple, it can cause a blinding headache.

A **cerebral angiogram** (an'je-o-gram) is used to assess the condition of the cerebral arteries serving the brain (or the carotid arteries of the neck, which feed most of those vessels). A dye is injected into an artery, and time is allowed for the dye to become dispersed to the brain. Then, an X-ray is taken of the arteries of interest. The dye allows arteries narrowed by arteriosclerosis to be localized. This procedure is commonly ordered for individuals who have suffered a stroke or who have a history of transient ischemic attacks.

The new imaging techniques described in Chapter 1 have revolutionized the diagnosis of brain lesions. **CT** and **MRI scans** allow most tumors, intracranial lesions, multiple sclerosis plaques, and areas of dead brain tissue *(infarcts)* to be identified quickly. The CT scanner is also becoming an important tool to enhance the precision and safety of brain surgery. **PET scans,** which use high-energy gamma rays to monitor the brain's biochemical activity, can localize lesions that generate epileptic seizures. PET scans are also being used to diagnose Alzheimer's disease. ➤

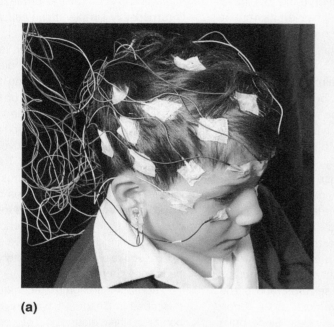

(a)

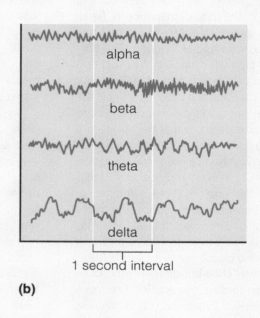

(b)

Electroencephalography and brain waves. (a) To obtain a recording of brain-wave activity (an EEG), electrodes are positioned on the patient's scalp and attached to a recording device called an electroencephalograph. **(b)** Typical EEGs. Alpha waves are typical of the awake, relaxed state; beta waves occur in the awake, alert state; theta waves are common in children but not in normal adults; and delta waves occur during deep sleep.

the sympathetic and parasympathetic divisions as working in an all-or-none fashion, this is rarely the case. A dynamic balance exists between the two divisions, and fine adjustments are continuously made by both. Also, although we have described the parasympathetic division as the "at-rest" system, most blood vessels are controlled only by the sympathetic fibers regardless of whether the body is "on alert" or relaxing. A summary of the major effects of each division appears in Table 7.3.

Developmental Aspects of the Nervous System

Because the nervous system is formed during the first month of embryonic development, any maternal infection early in pregnancy can have extremely harmful effects on the fetal nervous system. For example, maternal measles *(rubella)* often causes deafness and other types of CNS damage. Also, since nervous tissue has the highest metabolic rate in the body, lack of oxygen for even a few minutes leads to death of neurons. (Because smoking decreases the amount of oxygen that can be carried in the blood, a smoking mother may be sentencing her infant to possible brain damage.) Radiation and various drugs (alcohol, opiates, cocaine, and others) can also be very damaging if administered during early fetal development.

Homeostatic Imbalance

In difficult deliveries, a temporary lack of oxygen may lead to *cerebral palsy* (pawl′ze), but this is only one of the suspected causes. Cerebral palsy is a neuromuscular disability in which the voluntary muscles are poorly controlled and spastic due to brain damage. About half of its victims have seizures, are mentally retarded, and/or have impaired hearing or vision. Cerebral palsy is the largest single cause of physical disabilities in children. A number of other congenital malformations, triggered by genetic or environmental factors, also plague the CNS. Most serious are hydrocephalus, *anencephaly*—a failure of the cerebrum to develop, resulting in a child who cannot hear, see, or process sensory inputs—and spina bifida. *Spina bifida* (spi′nah bi′fĭ-dah) results when the vertebrae form incompletely (typically in the lumbosacral region). There are several varieties. In the least serious, a dimple, and perhaps a tuft of hair, appears over the site of

malformation, but no neurological problems occur. In the most serious, meninges, nerve roots, and even parts of the spinal cord protrude from the spine, rendering the lower part of the spinal cord functionless. The child is unable to control the bowels or bladder, and the lower limbs are paralyzed. ▲

One of the last areas of the CNS to mature is the hypothalamus, which contains centers for regulating body temperature. For this reason, premature babies usually have problems in controlling their loss of body heat and must be carefully monitored. Few neurons are formed after birth (because neurons are amitotic), but growth and

Prove It Yourself

Improve Your Memory

Can you improve your ability to learn and remember new information? Yes! The following techniques take advantage of the brain's storage and retrieval mechanisms:

- **Concentrate.** This may seem obvious, but paying attention increases brain activity and epinephrine levels, thereby promoting consolidation of information into long-term memory.
- **Minimize interference.** Go where it is quiet. A noisy environment will impair your ability to concentrate.
- **Break down large amounts of information into smaller topics.** Give yourself time to review each topic, and take a break in between.
- **Rephrase material in your own words.** Restate the information in a way that makes sense to you personally.
- **Test yourself.** Create outlines or diagrams. Try to define key terms before looking up their definitions. Use practice and review questions when they are available.

Short-term memory involves quick bursts of action potentials. Every time you read, think about, or test yourself on a concept, more neurons fire. By studying new material actively and repeatedly, you trigger additional action potentials and improve long-term retention because the neural synapses are reinforced by use.

Systems in Sync

Homeostatic Relationships between the Nervous System and Other Body Systems

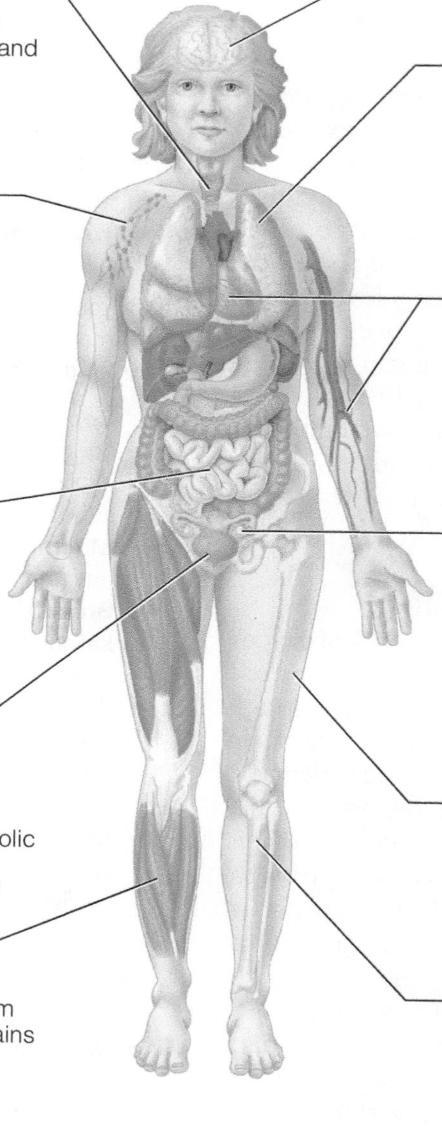

Endocrine System
- Sympathetic division of the ANS activates the adrenal medulla; hypothalamus helps regulate the activity of the anterior pituitary gland and produces two hormones
- Hormones influence metabolism of neurons

Lymphatic System/Immunity
- Nerves innervate lymphoid organs; the brain plays a role in regulating immune function
- Lymphatic vessels carry away leaked tissue fluids from tissues surrounding nervous system structures; immune elements protect all body organs from pathogens (CNS has additional mechanisms)

Digestive System
- ANS (particularly the parasympathetic division) regulates digestive system activity
- Digestive system provides nutrients needed for health of neurons

Urinary System
- ANS regulates bladder emptying and renal blood pressure
- Kidneys help to dispose of metabolic wastes and maintain proper electrolyte composition and pH of blood for neural functioning

Muscular System
- Somatic division of nervous system activates skeletal muscles; maintains muscle health
- Skeletal muscles are the effectors of the somatic division

Nervous System

Respiratory System
- Nervous system regulates respiratory rhythm and depth
- Respiratory system provides life-sustaining oxygen; disposes of carbon dioxide

Cardiovascular System
- ANS helps regulate heart rate and blood pressure
- Cardiovascular system provides blood containing oxygen and nutrients to the nervous system; carries away wastes

Reproductive System
- ANS regulates sexual erection and ejaculation in males; erection of the clitoris in females
- Testosterone masculinizes the brain and underlies sex drive and aggressive behavior

Integumentary System
- Sympathetic division of the ANS regulates sweat glands and blood vessels of skin (therefore heat loss/retention)
- Skin serves as heat/loss surface

Skeletal System
- Nerves innervate bones
- Bones serve as depot for calcium needed for neural function; protect CNS structures

278

maturation of the nervous system continues all through childhood, largely as a result of myelination that goes on during this period. A good indication of the degree of myelination of particular neural pathways is the level of neuromuscular control in that body area. Neuromuscular coordination progresses in a superior to inferior (craniocaudal) direction and in a proximal to distal direction, and we know that myelination occurs in the same sequence.

The brain reaches its maximum weight in the young adult. Over the next 60 years or so, neurons are damaged and die; and our store of neurons continually decreases. However, an unlimited number of neural pathways are always available and ready to be developed. We never run out of "recording tape" and can continue to learn throughout life.

As we grow older, the sympathetic nervous system gradually becomes less and less efficient, particularly in its ability to constrict blood vessels. When elderly people stand up quickly after sitting or lying down, they often become lightheaded or faint. This is because the sympathetic nervous system is not able to react quickly enough to counteract the pull of gravity by activating the vasoconstrictor fibers, and blood pools in the feet. This condition, *orthostatic hypotension,* is a type of low blood pressure resulting from changes in body position as described. Orthostatic hypotension can be prevented to some degree if changes in position are made slowly. This gives the sympathetic nervous system a little more time to adjust and react.

The usual cause of nervous system deterioration is circulatory system problems. For example, *arteriosclerosis* (ar-ter″e-o-skle-ro′sis) and high blood pressure result in a decreasing supply of oxygen to the brain neurons. A gradual lack of oxygen due to the aging process finally leads to *senility,* characterized by forgetfulness, irritability, difficulty in concentrating and thinking clearly, and confusion. A sudden loss of blood and oxygen delivery to the brain results in a CVA, as described earlier. However, many people continue to enjoy intellectual lives and to work at mentally demanding tasks through their entire lives. In fact, fewer than 5 percent of people over the age of 65 demonstrate true senility.

Sadly, many cases of "reversible senility," caused by certain drugs, low blood pressure, constipation, poor nutrition, depression, dehydration, and hormone imbalances, go undiagnosed. The best way to maintain one's mental abilities in old age may be to seek regular medical checkups throughout life.

Although eventual shrinking of the brain is normal, it seems that some individuals (professional boxers and chronic alcoholics, for example) accelerate the process long before aging plays its part. Whether a boxer wins the match or not, the likelihood of brain damage and atrophy increases with each fight as the brain bounces and rebounds within the skull with every blow. The expression "punch drunk" reflects the symptoms of slurred speech, tremors, abnormal gait, and dementia (mental illness) seen in many retired boxers.

Everyone recognizes that alcohol has a profound effect on the mind as well as the body. However, these effects may not be temporary. CT scans of chronic alcoholics reveal reduced brain size at a fairly early age. Like boxers, chronic alcoholics tend to exhibit signs of *senile* (age-related) *dementia* unrelated to the aging process.

The human cerebral hemispheres—our "thinking caps"—are awesome in their complexity. No less amazing are the brain regions that oversee all our subconscious, autonomic body functions—the diencephalon and brain stem—particularly when you consider their relatively insignificant size. The spinal cord, which acts as a reflex center, and the peripheral nerves, which provide communication links between the CNS and body periphery, are equally important to body homeostasis.

A good deal of new terminology has been introduced in this chapter and, as you will see, much of it will come up again in later chapters as we study the other organ systems of the body and examine how the nervous system helps to regulate their activity. The terms *are* essential, so try to learn them as you go along. Use the Glossary at the back of the book as often as you find it helpful.

8

Special Senses

KEY TERMS

People are responsive creatures. Hold freshly baked bread before us, and our mouths water. A sudden clap of thunder makes us jump. These "irritants" (the bread and the thunderclap) and many others are the stimuli that continually greet us and are interpreted by our nervous system.

We are usually told that we have five senses that keep us in touch with what is going on in the external world: touch, taste, smell, sight, and hearing. Actually touch is a mixture of the general senses that the temperature, pressure, and pain receptors of the skin and the proprioceptors of muscles and joints.

Sensory Receptors and Their Classification

Sensory receptors are specialized cells or cell processes that provide your central nervous system with information about conditions inside or outside the body. The term **general senses** is used to describe our sensitivity to temperature, pain, touch, pressure, vibration, and proprioception. General sensory receptors are distributed throughout the body, and they are relatively simple in structure. Some of the information they send to the CNS reaches the primary sensory cortex and our awareness. Sensory information is interpreted on the basis of the frequency of arriving action potentials. For example, when pressure sensations are arriving, the harder the pressure, the higher the frequency of action potentials. The arriving information is called a **sensation.** The conscious awareness of a sensation is called a **perception.**

The **special senses** are **olfaction** (smell), **vision** (sight), **gustation** (taste), **equilibrium** (balance), and **hearing.** These sensations are provided by receptors that are structurally more complex than those of the general senses. Special sensory receptors are located in **sense organs,** such as the eye or ear, where the receptors are protected by surrounding tissues. The information these receptors provide is distributed to specific areas of the cerebral cortex (the auditory cortex, the visual cortex, and so forth) and to centers throughout the brain stem.

Sensory Receptors

Sensory receptors represent the interface between the nervous system and the internal and external environments. A sensory receptor detects an arriving stimulus and translates it into an action potential that can be conducted to the CNS. This translation process is called *transduction.* If transduction does not occur, as far as you are concerned, the stimulus doesn't exist. For example, bees can see ultraviolet light you can't see, and dogs can respond to sounds you can't hear. In each case the stimuli are there—but your receptors cannot detect them.

The Detection of Stimuli

Each receptor has a characteristic sensitivity. For example, a touch receptor is very sensitive to pressure but relatively insensitive to chemical stimuli, whereas a taste receptor is sensitive to dissolved chemicals but insensitive to pressure. This feature is called **receptor specificity.**

Specificity may result from the structure of the receptor cell, or from the presence of accessory cells or structures that shield the receptor cell from other stimuli. The simplest receptors are the dendrites of sensory neurons. The branching tips of these dendrites, called **free nerve endings,** are not protected by accessory structures. Free nerve endings extend through a tissue the way grass roots extend into the soil. They can be stimulated by many different stimuli and therefore exhibit little receptor specificity. For example, free nerve endings that respond to tissue damage by providing pain sensations may be stimulated by chemical stimulation, pressure, temperature changes, or trauma. Complex receptors, such as the eye's visual receptors, are protected by accessory cells and connective tissue layers. These cells are seldom exposed to any stimulus other than light and so provide very specific information.

The area monitored by a single receptor cell is its *receptive field* (Figure 8.1). Whenever a sufficiently strong stimulus arrives in the receptive field, the CNS receives the information "stimulus arriving at receptor X." The larger the receptive field, the poorer your ability to localize a stimulus. A touch receptor on the general body surface, for example, may have a receptive field 7 cm (2.5 in.) in diameter. As a result, you can describe a light touch there as affecting only a general area, not an exact spot. On the tongue or fingertips, where the receptive fields are less than a millimeter in diameter, you can be very precise about the location of a stimulus.

An arriving stimulus can take many forms. It may be a physical force (such as pressure),

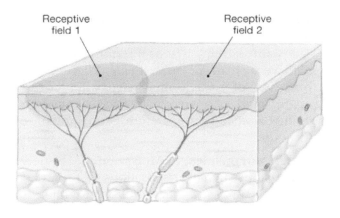

FIGURE 8.1 **Receptors and receptive fields.**
Each receptor cell monitors a specific area known
as the receptive field.

a dissolved chemical, a sound, or light. Regardless of the nature of the stimulus, however, sensory information must be sent to the CNS in the form of action potentials, which are electrical events.

The General Senses

Receptors for the general senses are scattered throughout the body and are relatively simple in structure. Receptors can be classified simply into three categories: exteroceptors, proprioceptors, and interoceptors. **Exteroceptors** provide information about the external environment; **proprioceptors** report the positions of skeletal muscles and joints; **interoceptors** monitor visceral organs and functions.

A more detailed classification system divides the general sensory receptors into four types by the nature of the stimulus that excites them: *nociceptors* (pain), *thermoreceptors* (temperature), *mechanoreceptors* (physical distortion), and *chemoreceptors* (chemical concentration). Each class of receptors has distinct structural and functional characteristics. *The difference between a somatic receptor and a visceral receptor is its location, not its structure.* A pain receptor in the gut looks and acts like a pain receptor in the skin, but the two sensations are delivered to separate locations in the CNS. However, proprioception is a purely somatic sensation—there are no proprioceptors in the visceral organs of the thoracic and abdominopelvic cavities. Your mental map of your body doesn't include these organs; you cannot tell, for example, where your spleen, appendix, or pancreas is at the moment. The visceral organs also have fewer pain, temperature, and touch receptors than one finds elsewhere in the body, and the sensory information

you receive is poorly localized because the receptive fields are very large and may be widely separated.

Although general sensations are widely distributed in the CNS, most of the processing occurs in centers along the sensory pathways in the spinal cord or brain stem. Only about 1 percent of the information provided by afferent fibers reaches the cerebral cortex and our awareness. For example, we usually do not feel the clothes we wear or hear the hum of the engine when riding in a car.

Thermoreceptors

Temperature receptors, or **thermoreceptors,** are free nerve endings located in the dermis, in skeletal muscles, in the liver, and in the hypothalamus. Cold receptors are three or four times more numerous than warm receptors. No structural differences between warm and cold thermoreceptors have been identified.

Temperature sensations are conducted along the same pathways that carry pain sensations. They are sent to the reticular formation, the thalamus, and (to a lesser extent) the primary sensory cortex. Thermoreceptors are phasic receptors: They are very active when the temperature is changing, but they quickly adapt to a stable temperature. When you enter an air-conditioned classroom on a hot summer day or a warm lecture hall on a brisk fall evening, the temperature change seems extreme at first, but you quickly become comfortable as adaptation occurs.

Mechanoreceptors

Mechanoreceptors are sensitive to stimuli that distort their cell membranes. These membranes contain *mechanically regulated ion channels* whose gates open or close in response to stretching, compression, twisting, or other distortions of the membrane. There are three classes of mechanoreceptors:

1. **Tactile receptors** provide the closely related sensations of touch, pressure, and vibration. Touch sensations provide information about shape or texture, whereas pressure sensations indicate the degree of mechanical distortion. Vibration sensations indicate a pulsing or oscillating pressure. The receptors involved may be specialized in some way. For example, rapidly adapting tactile receptors are best suited for detecting vibration. But your interpretation of a sensation as touch rather than pressure is typically a matter of the degree of stimulation, and

not of differences in the type of receptor stimulated.

2. **Baroreceptors** (bar-ō-rē-SEP-torz; *baro-*, pressure) detect pressure changes in the walls of blood vessels and in portions of the digestive, reproductive, and urinary tracts.

3. **Proprioceptors** monitor the positions of joints and muscles. They are the most structurally and functionally complex of the general sensory receptors.

Tactile Receptors **Fine touch and pressure receptors** provide detailed information about a source of stimulation, including its exact location, shape, size, texture, and movement. These receptors are extremely sensitive and have relatively narrow receptive fields. **Crude touch and pressure receptors** provide poor localization and, because they have relatively large receptive fields, give little additional information about the stimulus.

Tactile receptors range in complexity from free nerve endings to specialized sensory complexes with accessory cells and supporting structures. Figure 8.2 shows six types of tactile receptors in the skin:

1. Free nerve endings sensitive to touch and pressure are situated between epidermal cells (Figure 8.2a). There appear to be no structural differences between these receptors and the free nerve endings that provide temperature (such as the Krause nerve endings sensitive to cold mainly found in parts of the eye) or pain sensations. These are the only sensory receptors on the corneal surface of the eye, but in other portions of the body surface, more specialized tactile receptors are probably more important. Free nerve endings that provide touch sensations are tonic receptors with small receptive fields.

2. Wherever hairs are located, the nerve endings of the **root hair plexus** monitor distortions and movements across the body surface (Figure 8.2b). When a hair is displaced, the movement of the follicle distorts the sensory dendrites and produces action potentials. These receptors adapt rapidly, so they are best at detecting initial contact and subsequent movements. Thus, you generally feel your clothing only when you move or when you consciously focus on tactile sensations from the skin.

3. **Tactile discs,** or *Merkel's* (MER-kelz) *discs,* are fine touch and pressure receptors (Figure 8.2c). They are extremely sensitive tonic receptors, with very small receptive fields. The dendritic processes of a single myelinated afferent fiber make close contact with unusually large epithelial cells in the stratum germinativum of the skin.

4. **Tactile corpuscles,** or **Meissner's** (MĪS-nerz) **corpuscles,** perceive sensations of fine touch and pressure and low-frequency vibration. They adapt to stimulation within a second after contact. Tactile corpuscles are fairly large structures, measuring roughly 100 μm in length and 50 μm in width. These receptors are most abundant in the eyelids, lips, fingertips, nipples, and external genitalia. The dendrites are highly coiled and interwoven, and they are surrounded by modified Schwann cells. A fibrous capsule surrounds the entire complex and anchors it within the dermis (Figure 8.2d).

5. **Lamellated** (LAM-e-lāt-ed; *lamella,* a little thin plate) **corpuscles,** or **pacinian** (pa-SIN-ē-an) **corpuscles,** are sensitive to deep pressure. Because they are fast-adapting receptors, they are most sensitive to pulsing or high-frequency vibrating stimuli. A single dendrite lies within a series of concentric layers of collagen fibers and supporting cells (specialized fibroblasts) (Figure 8.2e). The entire corpuscle may reach 4 mm in length and 1 mm in diameter. The concentric layers, separated by interstitial fluid, shield the dendrite from virtually every source of stimulation other than direct pressure. Lamellated corpuscles adapt quickly because distortion of the capsule soon relieves pressure on the sensory process. Somatic sensory information is provided by lamellated corpuscles located throughout the dermis, notably in the fingers, mammary glands, and external genitalia; in the superficial and deep fasciae; and in joint capsules. Visceral sensory information is provided by lamellated corpuscles in mesenteries, in the pancreas, and in the walls of the urethra and urinary bladder.

6. **Ruffini** (roo-FĒ-nē) **corpuscles** are also sensitive to pressure and distortion of the skin, but they are located in the reticular (deep) dermis. These receptors are tonic and show little if any adaptation. The capsule surrounds a core of

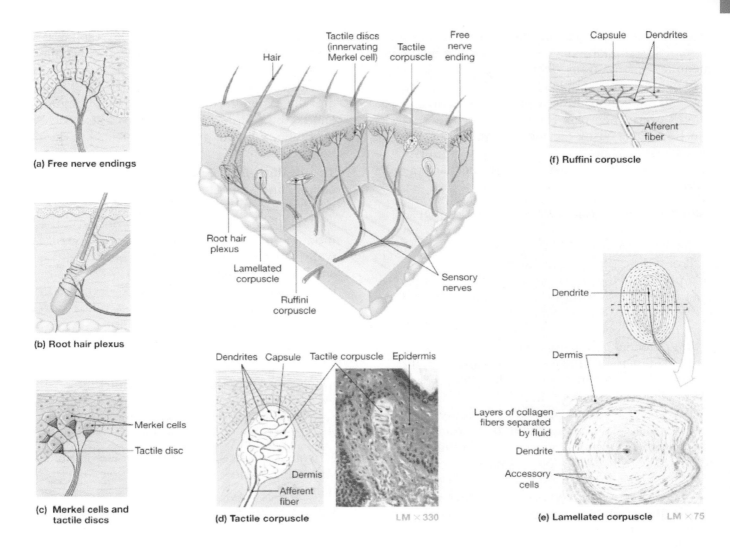

FIGURE 8.2 **Tactile receptors in the skin.**

collagen fibers that are continuous with those of the surrounding dermis (Figure 8.2f). In the capsule, a network of dendrites is intertwined with the collagen fibers. Any tension or distortion of the dermis tugs or twists the capsular fibers, stretching or compressing the attached dendrites and altering the activity in the myelinated afferent fiber.

Our sensitivity to tactile sensations may be altered by infection, disease, or damage to sensory neurons or pathways. As a result, mapping tactile responses can sometimes aid clinical assessment. Sensory losses with clear regional boundaries indicate trauma to spinal nerves. For example, sensory loss within the boundaries of a dermatome can help identify the affected spinal nerve or nerves.

Regional sensitivity to light touch can be checked by gentle contact with a fingertip or a slender wisp of cotton. Vibration receptors are tested by applying the base of a vibrating tuning fork to the skin.

Tickle and itch sensations are closely related to the sensations of touch and pain. The receptors involved are free nerve endings, and the information is carried by unmyelinated Type C fibers. Tickle sensations, which are usually (but not always) described as pleasurable, are produced by a light touch that moves across the skin. Psychological factors are involved in the interpretation of tickle sensations, and tickle sensitivity differs greatly among individuals. Itching is probably produced by the stimulation of the same receptors. Specific "itch spots" can be mapped in the skin, the inner surfaces of the eyelids, and the mucous membrane of the nose. Itch sensations are absent from other mucous membranes and from deep tissues and viscera. Itching is extremely unpleasant, even more unpleasant than pain. Individuals with extreme itching will scratch even when pain is the result. Itch receptors can be stimulated by the injection of histamine or proteolytic enzymes into the epidermis and superficial dermis. The precise receptor mechanism is unknown.

Baroreceptors   Baroreceptors monitor changes in pressure. A baroreceptor consists of free nerve endings that branch within the elastic tissues in the wall of a distensible organ, such as a blood vessel or a portion of the respiratory, digestive, or urinary tract. When the pressure changes, the elastic walls of the tract recoil or expand. This movement distorts the dendritic branches and alters the rate of action potential generation. Baroreceptors respond immediately to a change in pressure, but they adapt rapidly, and the output along the afferent fibers gradually returns to normal.

Baroreceptors monitor blood pressure in the walls of major vessels, including the carotid artery (at the **carotid sinus**) and the aorta (at the **aortic sinus**). The information plays a major role in regulating cardiac function and adjusting blood flow to vital tissues. Baroreceptors in the lungs monitor the degree of lung expansion. This information is relayed to the respiratory rhythmicity centers, which set the pace of respiration. Comparable stretch receptors at various sites in the digestive and urinary tracts trigger a variety of visceral reflexes, including those of urination and defecation.

The Hering–Breuer Reflexes

The **Hering–Breuer reflexes** are named after the physiologists who described them in 1865. The sensory information from these reflexes is distributed to the apneustic centers and the ventral respiratory group. The Hering–Breuer reflexes are not involved in normal quiet breathing (eupnea) or in tidal volumes under 1000 ml. There are two such reflexes:

1. The **inflation reflex** prevents overexpansion of the lungs during forced breathing. Stretch receptors located in the smooth muscle tissue around bronchioles are stimulated by lung expansion. Sensory fibers leaving the stretch receptors of each lung reach the respiratory rhythmicity center on the same side via the vagus nerve. As lung volume increases, the dorsal respiratory group is gradually inhibited, and the expiratory center of the VRG is stimulated. Inhalation stops as the lungs near maximum volume, and active exhalation then begins.

2. The **deflation reflex** inhibits the expiratory centers and stimulates the inspiratory centers when the lungs are deflating. These receptors, which are distinct from those of the inflation reflex, are located in the alveolar wall near the alveolar capillary network. The smaller the volume of the lungs, the greater the degree of inhibition, until exhalation stops and inhalation begins. This reflex normally functions only during forced exhalation, when both the inspiratory and expiratory centers are active.

Proprioceptors   Proprioceptors monitor the position of joints, the tension in tendons and ligaments, and the state of muscular contraction. There are three major groups of proprioceptors:

1. **Muscle spindles.** Muscle spindles monitor skeletal muscle length and trigger stretch reflexes.

2. **Golgi tendon organs. Golgi tendon organs** are similar in function to Ruffini corpuscles but are located at the junction between a skeletal muscle and its tendon. In a Golgi tendon organ, dendrites branch repeatedly and wind around the densely packed collagen fibers of the tendon. These receptors are stimulated by tension in the tendon; they thus monitor the external tension developed during muscle contraction.

3. **Receptors in joint capsules.** Joint capsules are richly innervated by free nerve endings that detect pressure, tension, and movement at the joint. Your sense of body position results from the integration of information from these receptors with information provided by muscle spindles, Golgi tendon organs, and the receptors of the inner ear.

Proprioceptors do not adapt to constant stimulation, and each receptor continuously sends information to the CNS. A relatively small proportion of the arriving proprioceptive information reaches your awareness; most proprioceptive information is processed at subconscious levels.

Chemoreceptors

Specialized chemoreceptive neurons can detect small changes in the concentration of specific chemicals or compounds. In general, **chemoreceptors** respond only to water-soluble and lipid-soluble substances that are dissolved in the surrounding fluid. These receptors exhibit peripheral adaptation over a period of seconds, and central adaptation may also occur.

The chemoreceptors included in the general senses do not send information to the primary sensory cortex, so we are not consciously aware of the sensations they provide. The arriving sensory information is routed to brain stem centers that deal with the autonomic control of respiratory and cardiovascular functions. Neurons in the respiratory centers of the brain respond to the concentration of hydrogen ions (pH) and levels of carbon dioxide molecules in the cerebrospinal fluid. Chemoreceptive neurons are also located in the **carotid bodies,** near the origin of the internal carotid arteries on each side of the neck, and in the **aortic bodies,** between the major branches of the aortic arch. These receptors monitor the pH and the carbon dioxide and oxygen levels in arterial blood. The afferent fibers leaving the carotid or aortic bodies reach the respiratory centers by traveling within cranial nerves IX (glossopharyngeal) and X (vagus).

The Special Senses

Touch is a mixture of the general senses we just discussed. The other four "traditional" senses— *smell, taste, sight,* and *hearing*—are called **special senses.** Receptors for a fifth special sense, *equilibrium,* are housed in the ear, along with the organ of hearing. In contrast to the small and widely distributed general receptors, the **special sense receptors** are either large, complex sensory organs (eyes and ears) or localized clusters of receptors (taste buds and olfactory epithelium).

This chapter focuses on the functional anatomy of each of the special sense organs individually, but keep in mind that sensory inputs are overlapping. What we finally experience—our "feel" of the world—is a blending of stimulus effects.

The Eye and Vision

How we see has captured the curiosity of many researchers. Vision is the sense that has been studied most. Of all the sensory receptors in the body, 70 percent are in the eyes. The optic tracts that carry information from the eyes to the brain are massive bundles, containing over a million nerve fibers. Vision is the sense that requires the most "learning," and the eye appears to delight in being fooled. The old expression "You see what you expect to see" is often very true.

Anatomy of the Eye
External and Accessory Structures

The adult eye is a sphere that measures about 1 inch (2.5 cm) in diameter. Only the anterior one-sixth of the eye's surface can normally be seen. The rest of it is enclosed and protected by a cushion of fat and the walls of the bony orbit. The accessory structures of the eye include the extrinsic eye muscles, eyelids, conjunctiva, and lacrimal apparatus.

Anteriorly the eyes are protected by the **eyelids,** which meet at the medial and lateral corners of the eye, the **medial** and **lateral canthus** respectively (see Figure 8.3b). Projecting from the border of each eyelid are the **eyelashes.** Modified sebaceous glands associated with the eyelid edges are the **tarsal glands.** These glands produce an oily secretion that lubricates the eye (Figure 8.3a). *Ciliary glands,* modified sweat glands, lie between the eyelashes (*cilium* = eyelash).

A delicate membrane, the **conjunctiva** (kon-junk″ti′vah), lines the eyelids and covers part of the outer surface of the eyeball (Figures 8.3a and 8.4). It ends at the edge of the cornea by fusing with the corneal epithelium. The conjunctiva secretes mucus, which helps to lubricate the eyeball and keep it moist.

▲ Homeostatic Imbalance
Inflammation of the conjunctiva, called *conjunctivitis,* results in reddened, irritated eyes. *Pinkeye,* its infectious form caused by bacteria or viruses, is highly contagious. ▲

The **lacrimal apparatus** consists of the lacrimal gland and a number of ducts that drain the lacrimal secretions into the nasal cavity. The

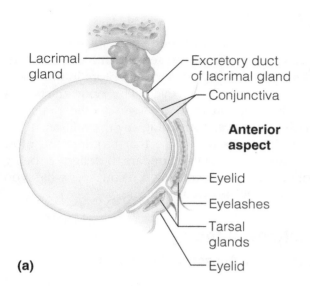

(a)

FIGURE 8.3 **External anatomy of the eye and accessory structures. (a)** Sagittal section of the accessory structures associated with the anterior part of the eye. **(b)** Anterior view of the lacrimal apparatus. The lacrimal gland is shown pulled superiorly by a retractor to expose its ducts.

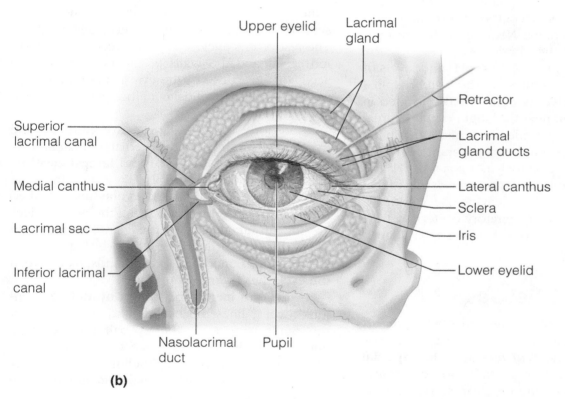

(b)

lacrimal glands are located above the lateral end of each eye. They continually release a dilute salt solution *(tears)* onto the anterior surface of the eyeball through several small ducts (see Figure 8.3). The tears flush across the eyeball into the **lacrimal canals** medially, then into the **lacrimal sac,** and finally into the **nasolacrimal duct,** which empties into the nasal cavity (see Figure 8.3b). Lacrimal secretion also contains anti-

bodies and **lysozyme** (li′so-zīm), an enzyme that destroys bacteria. Thus, it cleanses and protects the eye surface as it moistens and lubricates it. When lacrimal secretion increases substantially, tears spill over the eyelids and fill the nasal cavities, causing congestion and the "sniffles." This happens when the eyes are irritated by foreign objects or chemicals and when we are emotionally upset. In the case of irritation, the enhanced tearing acts to wash away or dilute the irritating substance. The importance of "emotional tears" is poorly understood, but some suspect that crying is important in reducing stress. Anyone who has had a good cry would probably agree, but this has been difficult to prove scientifically.

Homeostatic Imbalance

Because the nasal cavity mucosa is continuous with that of the lacrimal duct system, a cold or nasal inflammation often causes the lacrimal mucosa to become inflamed and swell. This impairs the drainage of tears from the eye surface, causing "watery" eyes. ▲

Six **extrinsic,** or **external, eye muscles** are attached to the outer surface of each eye. These muscles produce gross eye movements and make it possible for the eyes to follow a moving object. The names, locations, actions, and cranial nerve serving each of the extrinsic muscles are given in Figure 8.4.

Internal Structures: The Eyeball

The eye itself, commonly called the **eyeball,** is a hollow sphere (Figure 8.5). Its wall is composed of three *tunics,* or coats, and its interior is filled with

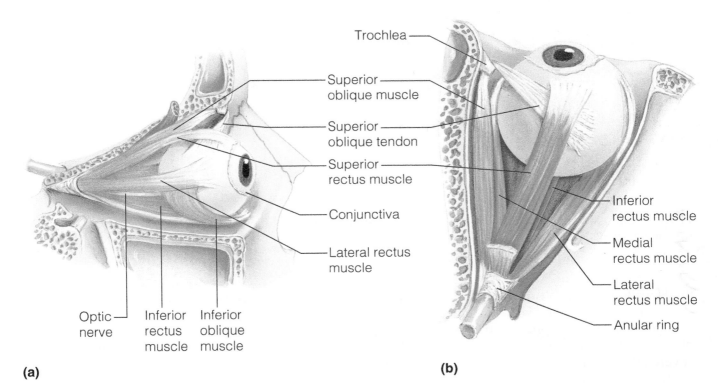

(a)

(b)

Name	Action	Controlling cranial nerve
Lateral rectus	Moves eye laterally	VI (abducens)
Medial rectus	Moves eye medially	III (oculomotor)
Superior rectus	Elevates eye	III (oculomotor)
Inferior rectus	Depresses eye	III (oculomotor)
Inferior oblique	Elevates eye and turns it laterally	III (oculomotor)
Superior oblique	Depresses eye and turns it laterally	IV (trochlear)

(c)

FIGURE 8.4 Extrinsic muscles of the eye.
(a) Lateral view of the right eye. **(b)** Superior view of the right eye. The four rectus muscles originate from the anular ring, a ringlike tendon at the back of the eye socket. **(c)** Summary of cranial nerve supply and actions of the extrinsic eye muscles.

Q   *Which layer of the eye would be the first to be affected by deficient tear production?*

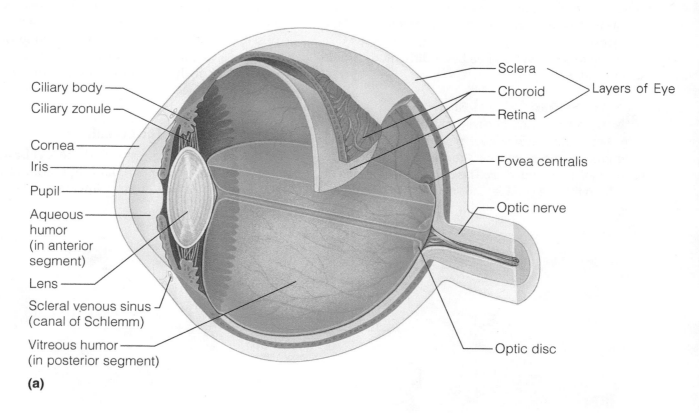

Ciliary body
Ciliary zonule
Cornea
Iris
Pupil
Aqueous humor (in anterior segment)
Lens
Scleral venous sinus (canal of Schlemm)
Vitreous humor (in posterior segment)

Sclera
Choroid — Layers of Eye
Retina
Fovea centralis
Optic nerve
Optic disc

(a)

FIGURE 8.5   Internal anatomy of the eye (sagittal section).
(a) Diagrammatic view.

fluids called *humors* that help to maintain its shape. The lens, the main focusing apparatus of the eye, is supported upright within the eye cavity, dividing it into two chambers. Now that we have covered the general anatomy of the eyeball, we are ready to get specific.

Tunics of the Eyeball   The outermost tunic, the protective **sclera** (skle′rah), is thick, white connective tissue. Also called the *fibrous tunic,* the sclera is seen anteriorly as the "white of the eye." Its central anterior portion is modified so that it is crystal clear. This transparent "window" is the **cornea** (kor′ne-ah) through which light enters the eye. The cornea is well supplied with nerve endings. Most are pain fibers, and when the cornea is touched, blinking and increased tearing occur.

Even so, the cornea is the most exposed part of the eye, and it is very vulnerable to damage. Luckily, its ability to repair itself is extraordinary. Furthermore, the cornea is the only tissue in the body that can be transplanted from one person to another without the worry of rejection. Since it has no blood vessels, it is beyond the reach of the immune system.

The middle coat of the eyeball is the *vascular tunic* which has three distinguishable regions. Most posteriorly is the **choroid** (ko′roid), a blood-rich nutritive tunic that contains a dark pigment. The pigment prevents light from scattering inside the eye. Moving anteriorly, the choroid is modified to form two smooth muscle structures, the **ciliary** (sil′e-er-e) **body,** to which the **lens** is attached by a suspensory ligament called the **ciliary zonule,** and then the **iris.** The pigmented iris has a rounded opening, the **pupil,** through which light passes. Circularly and radially arranged smooth

A   *The outermost sclera (mostly its cornea), which is normally continuously washed by tears.*

FIGURE 8.5 (*continued*)
Internal anatomy of the eye (sagittal section). (b) Photograph.

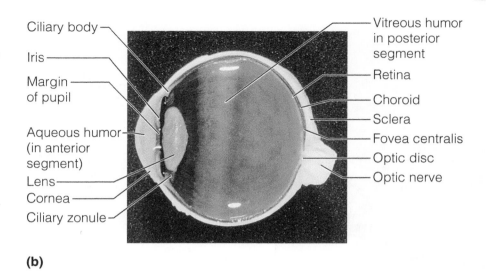

(b)

muscle fibers form the iris, which acts like the diaphragm of a camera. That is, it regulates the amount of light entering the eye so that one can see as clearly as possible in the available light. In close vision and bright light, the circular muscles contract, and the pupil constricts. In distant vision and dim light, the radial fibers contract to enlarge (dilate) the pupil, which allows more light to enter the eye.

The innermost *sensory tunic* of the eye is the delicate white **retina** (ret′ĭ-nah), which extends anteriorly only to the ciliary body. The retina contains millions of receptor cells, the **rods** and **cones.** Rods and cones are called **photoreceptors** because they respond to light. Electrical signals pass from the photoreceptors via a two-neuron chain—**bipolar cells** and then **ganglion cells**—before leaving the retina via the **optic nerve** as nerve impulses that are transmitted to the optic cortex. The result is vision.

The photoreceptor cells are distributed over the entire retina, except where the **optic nerve** (composed of ganglion cell axons) leaves the eyeball; this site is called the **optic disc,** or **blind spot.** When light from an object is focused on the optic disc, it disappears from our view and we cannot see it. To illustrate this, perform the blind spot demonstration by holding Figure 8.7 about 18 inches (45 cm) from your eyes. Close your left eye and stare at the X with your right eye. Move the figure slowly toward your face, keeping your right eye focused on the X. When the dot focuses on your blind spot, which lacks photoreceptors, the dot will disappear. Repeat the test for your left

eye. This time close your right eye and stare at the dot with your left eye. Move the page as before until the X disappears.

The rods and cones are not evenly distributed in the retina. The rods are most dense at the periphery, or edge, of the retina and decrease in number as the center of the retina is approached. The rods allow us to see in gray tones in dim light, and they provide for our peripheral vision.

Homeostatic Imbalance

Anything that interferes with rod function hinders our ability to see at night, a condition called *night blindness*. Night blindness dangerously impairs the ability to drive safely at night. Its most common cause is prolonged vitamin A deficiency, which eventually results in deterioration of much of the neural retina. As described in the "A Closer Look" box on Visual Pigment, vitamin A is one of the building blocks of the pigments the photoreceptor cells need to respond to light. Vitamin A supplements will restore function if taken before degenerative changes occur. ▲

Cones are discriminatory receptors that allow us to see the details of our world in color under bright light conditions. They are densest in the center of the retina and decrease in number toward the retinal edge. Lateral to each blind spot is the **fovea centralis** (fo′ve-ah sen-tra′lis), a tiny pit that contains only cones (see Figure 8.5). Consequently, this is the area of greatest **visual acuity,** or point of sharpest vision, and anything we wish to view critically is focused on the fovea centralis.

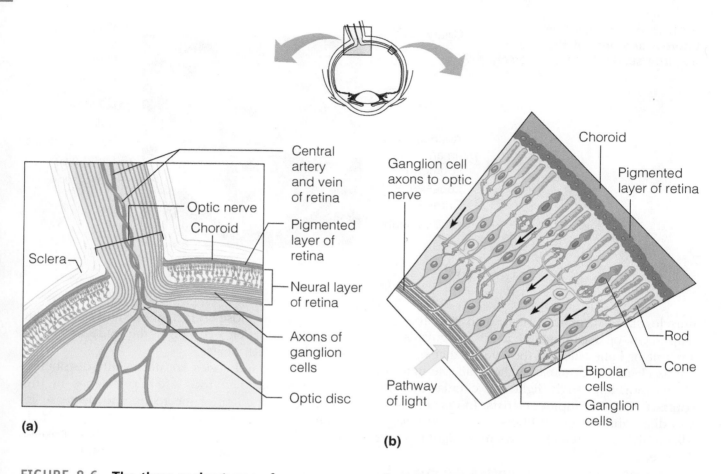

FIGURE 8.6 **The three major types of neurons composing the retina.**
(a) Schematic view of the posterior part of the eyeball illustrating how the axons of the ganglion cells form the optic nerve, which leaves the back of the eyeball at the optic disc. **(b)** Notice in this schematic view of the neural layer of the retina that light passes through the thickness of the retina to excite the rods and cones. The flow of electrical signals (black arrows) occurs in the opposite direction: from the rods and cones to the bipolar cells and finally to the ganglion cells. The ganglion cells generate the nerve impulses that leave the eye via the optic nerve.

There are three varieties of cones. Each type is most sensitive to particular wavelengths of visible light (Figure 8.8). One type responds most vigorously to blue light, another to green light. The third cone variety responds to a range including both green and red wavelengths of light. However, this is the only cone population to respond to red light at all, so these are called the "red cones." Impulses received at the same time from more than one type of cone by the visual cortex are interpreted as *intermediate* colors. For example, simultaneous impulses from blue and red color receptors are seen as purple or violet tones. When all three cone types are being stimulated, we see white. If someone shines red light into one of your eyes and

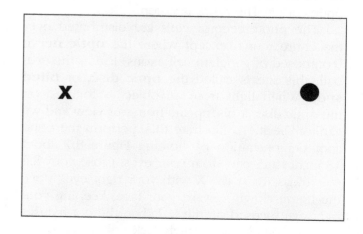

FIGURE 8.7 **Figure for blind spot test.**

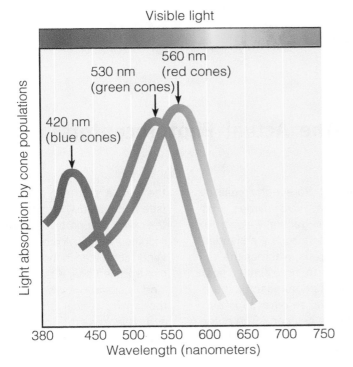

FIGURE 8.8   Sensitivities of the three cone types to the different wavelengths of visible light.

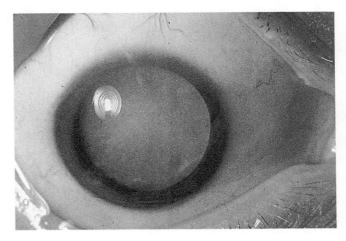

FIGURE 8.9   Photograph of a cataract. The cataract appears as a milky structure that seems to fill the pupil.

green into the other, you will see yellow, indicating that the "mixing" and interpretation of colors occurs in the brain, not in the retina.

Homeostatic Imbalance

Lack of all three cone types results in total *color blindness,* whereas lack of one cone type leads to partial color blindness. Most common is the lack of red or green receptors, which leads to two varieties of red-green color blindness. Red and green are seen as the same color—either red or green, depending on the cone type *present.* Many color-blind people are unaware of their condition because they have learned to rely on other cues—such as differences in intensities of the same color—to distinguish something green from something red, for example on traffic signals. Since the genes regulating color vision are on the X (female) sex chromosome, color blindness is a sex-linked condition. It occurs almost exclusively in males. ▲

Lens   Light entering the eye is focused on the retina by the lens, a flexible biconvex crystal-like structure. The **lens** is held upright in the eye by a suspensory ligament, the ciliary zonule, attached to the ciliary body (see Figure 8.5).

Homeostatic Imbalance

In youth, the lens is perfectly transparent and has the consistency of hardened jelly, but as we age it becomes increasingly hard and opaque. **Cataracts,** which result from this process, cause vision to become hazy and eventually cause blindness in the affected eye (Figure 8.9). Current treatment of cataracts is either surgical removal of the lens and replacement with a lens implant or special cataract glasses. ▲

The lens divides the eye into two segments or chambers. The *anterior (aqueous) segment,* anterior to the lens, contains a clear watery fluid called **aqueous humor.** The *posterior (vitreous) segment,* posterior to the lens, is filled with a gel-like substance called **vitreous** (vit′re-us) **humor,** or the **vitreous body** (see Figure 8.5). Vitreous humor helps prevent the eyeball from collapsing inward by reinforcing it internally. Aqueous humor is similar to blood plasma and is continually secreted by a special area of the choroid. Like the vitreous humor, it helps maintain *intraocular* (in″trah-ok′u-lar) *pressure,* or the pressure inside the eye. It also provides nutrients for the lens and cornea, which lack a blood supply. Aqueous humor is reabsorbed into the venous blood through the **scleral venous sinus (canal of Schlemm** [shlĕm]**),** which is located at the junction of the sclera and cornea.

A Closer Look

Visual Pigments—The Actual Photoreceptors

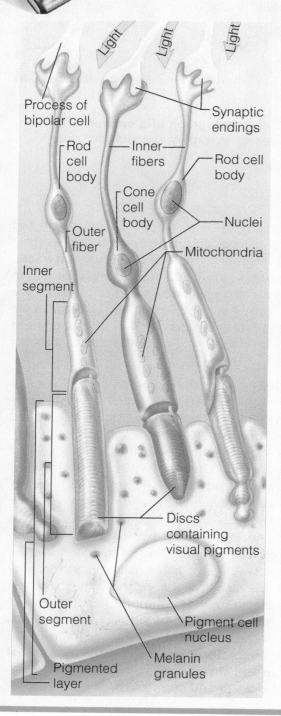

Process of bipolar cell
Synaptic endings
Rod cell body
Inner fibers
Rod cell body
Cone cell body
Nuclei
Outer fiber
Mitochondria
Inner segment
Discs containing visual pigments
Outer segment
Pigment cell nucleus
Melanin granules
Pigmented layer

THE tiny photoreceptor cells of the retina have names that reflect their general shapes. As shown to the left, rods are slender, elongated neurons, whereas the fatter cones taper to more pointed tips. In each type of photoreceptor, there is a region called an *outer segment,* attached to the cell body. The outer segment corresponds to a light-trapping dendrite, in which the discs containing the visual pigments are stacked like a row of pennies.

The behavior of the visual pigments is dramatic. When light strikes them, they lose their color, or are "bleached"; shortly afterward, they regenerate their pigment. Absorption of light and pigment bleaching cause electrical changes in the photoreceptor cells that ultimately cause nerve impulses to be transmitted to the brain for visual interpretation. Pigment regeneration ensures that one is not blinded and unable to see in bright sunlight.

A good deal is known about the structure and function of **rhodopsin,** the purple pigment found in rods (see figure below). It is formed from the union of a protein **(opsin)** and a modified vitamin A product **(retinal)**. When combined in rhodopsin, retinal has a kinked shape that allows it to bind to opsin. But when light strikes rhodopsin, retinal straightens out and releases the protein. Once straightened out, the retinal continues its conversion until it is once again vitamin A. As these changes occur, the purple color of rhodopsin changes to the yellow of retinal and finally becomes colorless as the change to vitamin A occurs. Thus the term "bleaching of the pigment" accurately describes the color changes that occur when light hits the pigment. Regeneration of rhodopsin occurs as vitamin A is again converted to the kinked form of retinal and recombined with opsin in an ATP-requiring process. The cone pigments, while similar to rhodopsin, differ in the specific kinds of proteins they contain.

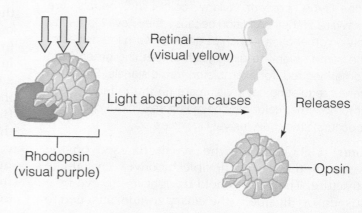

Rhodopsin (visual purple)
Light absorption causes
Retinal (visual yellow)
Releases
Opsin

Homeostatic Imbalance

If drainage of aqueous humor is blocked, pressure within the eye increases dramatically and begins to compress the delicate retina and optic nerve. The resulting condition, **glaucoma** (glaw-ko'mah), eventually causes pain and possibly blindness. Glaucoma is a common cause of blindness in elderly persons. Since it progresses slowly and has almost no symptoms at first, it tends to occur without obvious signs. Later signs include seeing halos around lights, headaches, and blurred vision. A simple instrument called a *tonometer* (to-nom'e-ter) is used to measure the intraocular pressure. This examination should be performed yearly in people over 40. Glaucoma is treated with eyedrops (miotics), which increase the rate of aqueous humor drainage, or with surgical enlargement of the drainage channel. ▲

The *ophthalmoscope* (of-thal'mo-skōp) is an instrument that illuminates the interior of the eyeball, allowing the retina, optic disc, and internal blood vessels to be viewed and examined. Certain pathological conditions such as diabetes, arteriosclerosis, and degeneration of the optic nerve and retina can be detected by such an examination. When the ophthalmoscope is correctly set, the **fundus,** or posterior wall, of the healthy eye should appear as shown in Figure 8.10.

Pathway of Light through the Eye and Light Refraction

When light passes from one substance to another substance that has a different density, its speed changes and its rays are bent, or **refracted.** Light rays are bent in the eye as they encounter the cornea, aqueous humor, lens, and vitreous humor.

The refractive, or bending, power of the cornea and humors is constant. However, that of the lens can be changed by changing its shape—that is, by making it more or less convex, so that light can be properly focused on the retina. The greater the lens convexity, or bulge, the more it bends the light. On the other hand, the flatter the lens, the less it bends the light.

The resting eye is "set" for distant vision. In general, light from a distant source (over 20 feet away) approaches the eye as parallel rays (Figure 8.11a), and no change in lens shape is necessary for it to be focused properly on the retina. However, light from a close object tends to scatter and to *diverge,* or

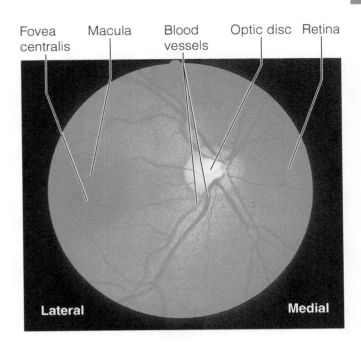

FIGURE 8.10   The posterior wall (fundus) of the retina as seen with an ophthalmoscope. Notice the optic disc, from which the blood vessels radiate.

spread out, and the lens must bulge more to make close vision possible (Figure 8.11b). To achieve this, the ciliary body contracts, allowing the lens to become more convex. This ability of the eye to focus specifically for close objects (those less than 20 feet away) is called **accommodation.** The image formed on the retina as a result of the light-bending activity of the lens is a *real image*—that is, it is reversed from left to right, upside down (inverted), and smaller than the object (Figure 8.12). The normal eye is able to accommodate properly. However, vision problems occur when a lens is too strong or too weak (overconverging and underconverging, respectively) or from structural problems of the eyeball (as described in the "A Closer Look" box on near- and farsightedness).

Visual Fields and Visual Pathways to the Brain

Axons carrying impulses from the retina are bundled together at the posterior aspect of the eyeball and issue from the back of the eye as the optic nerve. At the **optic chiasma** (ki-as'mah; *chiasm* = cross) the fibers from the medial side of each eye cross over to the opposite side. The fiber tracts that

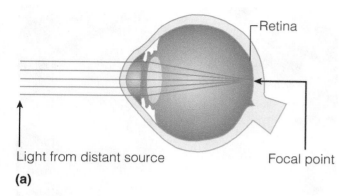

Light from distant source   Focal point

(a)

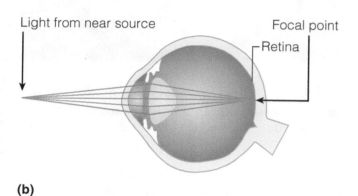

Light from near source   Focal point

(b)

FIGURE 8.11   Relative convexity of the lens during focusing for distant and close vision. **(a)** Light rays from a distant object are nearly parallel as they reach the eye and can be focused without requiring changes in lens convexity. **(b)** Diverging light rays from close objects require that the lens bulge more to focus the image sharply on the retina.

result are the **optic tracts.** Each optic tract contains fibers from the lateral side of the eye on the same side and the medial side of the opposite eye. The optic tract fibers synapse with neurons in the thalamus, whose axons form the **optic radiation,** which runs to the occipital lobe of the brain. There they synapse with the cortical cells, and visual interpretation, or seeing, occurs. The visual pathway from the eye to the brain is shown in Figure 8.13. As you can see, each side of the brain receives

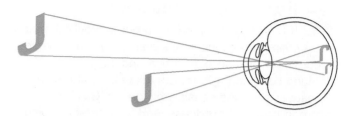

FIGURE 8.12   Real image (reversed left to right, and upside down) formed on the retina. Notice that the farther away the object, the smaller its image on the retina.

visual input from both eyes—from the lateral field of vision of the eye on its own side and the medial field of the other eye. Also notice that each eye "sees" a slightly different view, but their *visual fields* overlap quite a bit. As a result of these two facts, humans have *binocular vision.* Binocular vision, literally "two-eyed vision," provides for depth perception, also called "three-dimensional" vision, as our visual cortex fuses the two slightly different images delivered by the two eyes.

Homeostatic Imbalance

Hemianopia (hem″e-ah-no′pe-ah) is the loss of the same side of the visual field of both eyes, which results from damage to the visual cortex on one side only (as occurs in some CVAs). Thus, the person would not be able to see things past the middle of his or her visual field on either the right or left side, depending on the site of the CVA. Such individuals should be carefully attended and warned of objects in the nonfunctional (nonseeing) side of the visual field. Their food and personal objects should always be placed on their functional side, or they might miss them. ▲

Eye Reflexes

Both the internal and the external eye muscles are necessary for proper eye function. The internal muscles are controlled by the autonomic nervous system. These muscles include those of the ciliary body, which alters lens curvature, and the radial and circular muscles of the iris, which control pupil size. The external muscles are the rectus and oblique muscles attached to the eyeball exterior. The external (extrinsic) muscles control eyemovements and make it possible to follow moving objects. They are also responsible for **convergence,** which is the reflexive movement of the eyes medially when we view close objects. When convergence occurs, both eyes are aimed toward the near object being viewed. The extrinsic muscles are controlled by somatic fibers of cranial nerves III, IV, and VI, as shown in Figure 8.4.

When the eyes are suddenly exposed to bright light, the pupils immediately constrict; this is the **photopupillary reflex.** This protective reflex prevents excessively bright light from damaging the delicate photoreceptors. The pupils also constrict reflexively when we view close objects; this **accommodation pupillary reflex** provides for more acute vision.

Reading requires almost continuous work by both sets of muscles. The muscles of the ciliary body bring about the lens bulge, and the circular (or *constrictor*) muscles of the iris produce the accommodation pupillary reflex. In addition, the extrinsic muscles must converge the eyes as well as move them to follow the printed lines. This is why long periods of reading tire the eyes and often result in what is commonly called *eyestrain.* When you read for an extended time, it is helpful to look up from time to time and stare into the distance. This temporarily relaxes all the eye muscles.

The Ear: Hearing and Balance

At first glance, the machinery for hearing and balance appears very crude. Fluids must be stirred to stimulate the receptors of the ear: sound vibrations move fluid to stimulate hearing receptors, whereas gross movements of the head disturb fluids surrounding the balance organs. Receptors that respond to such physical forces are called **mechanoreceptors** (mek″ah-no-re-sep′terz). Our hearing apparatus allows us to hear an extraordinary range of sound, and our highly sensitive equilibrium receptors keep our nervous system continually up to date on the position and movements of the head. Without this information, it would be difficult, if not impossible, to maintain our balance. Although these two sense organs are housed together in the ear, their receptors respond to different stimuli and are activated independently of one another.

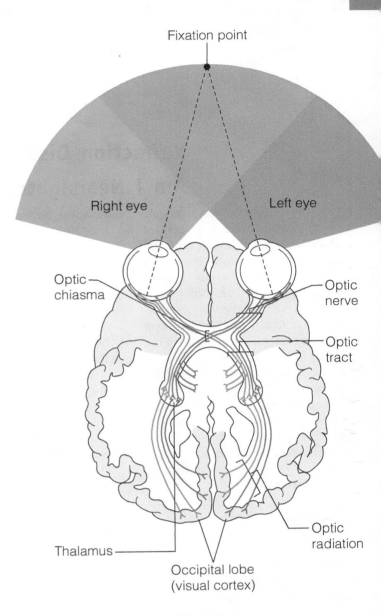

FIGURE 8.13 Visual fields of the eyes and visual pathway to the brain. Notice that the visual fields overlap considerably (area of binocular vision). Notice also the retinal sites at which a real image would be focused when both eyes are fixed on a close, pointlike object.

Anatomy of the Ear

Anatomically, the ear is divided into three major areas: the outer, or external, ear; the middle ear; and the inner, or internal, ear (Figure 8.14). The outer and middle ear structures are involved with hearing *only*. The inner ear functions in both equilibrium and hearing.

A Closer Look

Refraction Disorders = Errors in Refraction: Am I Nearsighted or Farsighted?

IT seems that whenever people who wear glasses or contact lenses get together and discuss their vision, one of them says something like, "Nearby objects appear blurry to me, but I can't remember if that means I'm nearsighted or farsighted." Or, someone else may say, "My glasses allow me to see faraway objects more clearly, so does that mean I am farsighted?" Here we will explain the meaning of nearsightedness and farsightedness as we explore the basis of eye-focusing disorders.

The eye that focuses images correctly on the retina is said to have **emmetropia** (em″ ē-tro′pe-ah), literally, "harmonious vision." Such an eye is shown in part (a) of the figure.

Nearsightedness is formally called **myopia** (mi″o′pe-ah; "short vision"). It occurs when the parallel light rays from distant objects fail to reach the retina and instead are focused in front of it; see part (b) in the figure. Therefore, *distant* objects appear blurry to myopic people. Nearby objects are in focus,

however, because the lens "accommodates" (bulges) to focus the image properly on the retina. Myopia results from an eyeball that is too long, a lens that is too strong, or a cornea that is too curved. Correction requires *concave* corrective lenses that diverge the light rays before they enter the eye, so that they converge farther back. To answer the first question posed above, *near*sighted people see *near* objects clearly and need corrective lenses to focus distant objects.

Farsightedness is formally called **hyperopia** (hi″per-o′pe-ah; "far vision"). It occurs when the parallel light rays from distant objects are focused *behind* the retina—at least in the resting eye in which the lens is flat and the ciliary muscle is relaxed; see part (c) in the figure. Hyperopia usually results from an eyeball that is too short or a "lazy" lens. People with hyperopia can see distant objects clearly because their ciliary muscles contract continuously to increase the light-bending power of the lens, which moves the focal point forward onto the retina. However, the

diverging rays from *nearby* objects are focused so far behind the retina that even at full "bulge," the lens cannot focus the image on the retina. Therefore, nearby objects appear blurry. Furthermore, hyperopic individuals are subject to eyestrain as their endlessly contracting ciliary muscles tire from overwork. Correction of hyperopia requires *convex* corrective lenses that converge the light rays before they enter the eye. To answer the second question posed at the beginning of this essay, *far*sighted people can see *far*away objects clearly and require corrective lenses to focus on nearby objects. Unequal curvatures in different parts of the cornea or lens cause **astigmatism** (ah-stig′mah-tizm). In this condition, blurry images occur because points of light are focused not as points on the retina but as lines (*astigma* = not a point). Special cylindrically ground lenses or contacts are used to correct this problem. Eyes that are myopic or hyperopic *and* astigmatic require a more complex correction.

Refraction Disorders = Errors in Refraction: Am I Nearsighted or Farsighted? *(continued)*

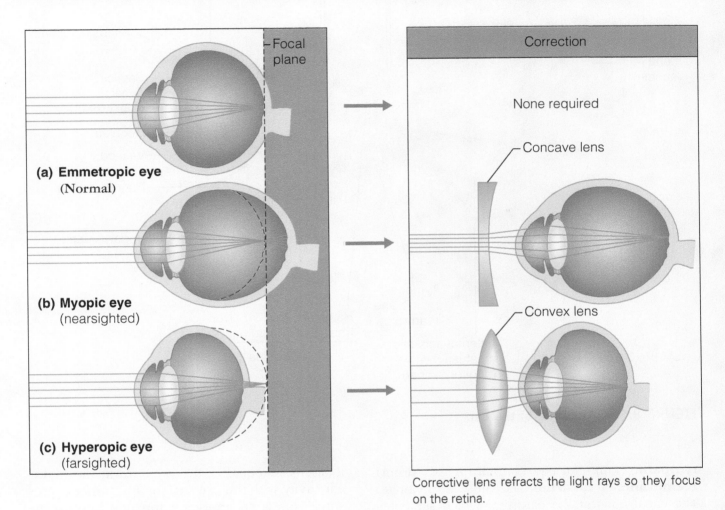

Corrective lens refracts the light rays so they focus on the retina.

Outer (External) Ear

The **outer ear** is composed of the pinna and the external acoustic meatus. The **pinna** (pin′nah), or **auricle** (aw′ri-kul), is what most people call the "ear"—the shell-shaped structure surrounding the auditory canal opening. In many animals, it collects and directs sound waves into the auditory canal, but in humans this function is largely lost.

The **external acoustic meatus** (or **external auditory canal**) is a short, narrow chamber (about 1 inch long by one-quarter inch wide) carved into the temporal bone of the skull. In its skin-lined walls are the **ceruminous** (sĕ-roo′mĭ-nus) **glands,** which secrete a waxy yellow substance called **earwax,** or **cerumen.** Sound waves entering the external auditory canal eventually hit the

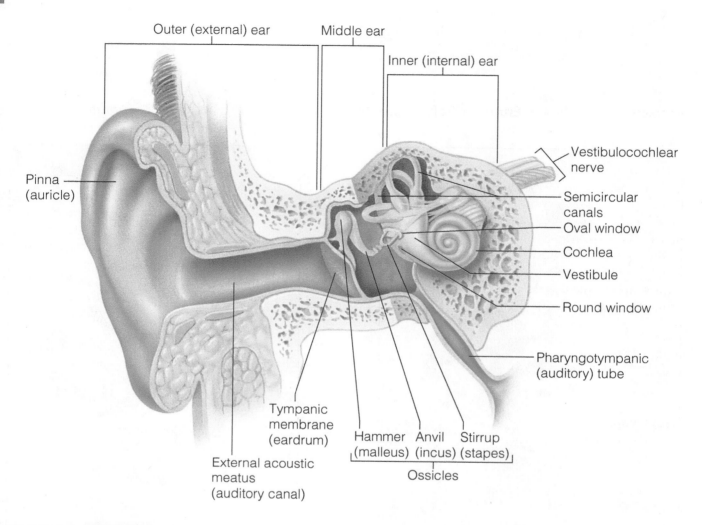

Outer (external) ear   Middle ear

Inner (internal) ear

Pinna
(auricle)

Vestibulocochlear
nerve

Semicircular
canals

Oval window

Cochlea

Vestibule

Round window

Pharyngotympanic
(auditory) tube

Tympanic
membrane
(eardrum)

Hammer   Anvil   Stirrup
(malleus) (incus) (stapes)

Ossicles

External acoustic
meatus
(auditory canal)

FIGURE 8.14 Anatomy of the ear.

tympanic (tim-pan'ik; *tympanum* = drum) **membrane,** or **eardrum,** and cause it to vibrate. The canal ends at the eardrum, which separates the outer from the middle ear.

Middle Ear

The **middle ear,** or **tympanic cavity,** is a small, air-filled cavity within the temporal bone. It is flanked laterally by the eardrum and medially by a bony wall with two openings, the **oval window** and the inferior, membrane-covered **round window.** The **pharyngotympanic** (or **auditory**) **tube** runs obliquely downward to link the middle ear cavity with the throat, and the mucosae lining the two regions are continuous. Normally, the pharyngotympanic tube is flattened and closed, but swallowing or yawning can open

it briefly to equalize the pressure in the middle ear cavity with the external, or atmospheric, pressure. This is an important function because the eardrum does not vibrate freely unless the pressure on both of its surfaces is the same. When the pressures are unequal, the eardrum bulges inward or outward, causing hearing difficulty (voices may sound far away) and sometimes earaches. The ear-popping sensation of the pressures equalizing is familiar to anyone who has flown in an airplane.

▲ Homeostatic Imbalance

Inflammation of the middle ear, *otitis media* (o-ti'tis me'de-ah), is a fairly common result of a sore throat, especially in children, whose pharyngotympanic tubes run more horizontally. In otitis media, the eardrum bulges and often becomes inflamed. When large amounts of fluid or pus accumulate in the cavity, an emergency *myringotomy* (lancing of the eardrum) may be required to relieve the pressure. During myringotomy, a tiny tube is implanted in the eardrum that allows pus formed in the middle ear to continue to drain into the external ear canal. The tube usually falls out by itself within the year. ▲

The more horizontal course of the pharyngo-tympanic tube in infants also explains why it is never a good idea to "prop" a bottle or feed them when they are lying flat (a condition that favors the entry of the food into that tube).

The tympanic cavity is spanned by the three smallest bones in the body, the **ossicles** (os'sĭ-kulz), which transmit the vibratory motion of the eardrum to the fluids of the inner ear (see Figure 8.12). These bones, named for their shape, are the **hammer,** or **malleus** (mă'le-us), the **anvil,** or **incus** (in'kus), and the **stirrup,** or **stapes** (sta'pēz). When the eardrum moves, the hammer moves with it and transfers the vibration to the anvil. The anvil, in turn, passes it on to the stirrup, which presses on the oval window of the inner ear. The movement at the oval window sets the fluids of the inner ear into motion, eventually exciting the hearing receptors.

Inner (Internal) Ear

The **inner ear** is a maze of bony chambers called the **osseous,** or **bony, labyrinth** (lab'ĭ-rinth), located deep within the temporal bone, and just behind the eye socket. The three subdivisions of the bony labyrinth are the **cochlea** (kok'le-ah), the **vestibule** (ves'ti-būl), and the **semicircular canals.** The vestibule is situated between the semicircular canals and the cochlea. The views of the bony labyrinth typically seen in textbooks, including this one, are somewhat misleading because we are really talking about a cavity. The view seen in Figure 8.14 can be compared to a *cast* of the bony labyrinth; that is, a labyrinth that was filled with plaster of paris and then had the bony walls removed after the plaster hardened. The shape of the plaster then reveals the shape of the *cavity* that worms through the temporal bone.

The bony labyrinth is filled with a plasmalike fluid called **perilymph** (per'ĭ-limf). Suspended in the perilymph is a **membranous labyrinth,** a system of membrane sacs that more or less follows the shape of the bony labyrinth. The membranous labyrinth itself contains a thicker fluid called **endolymph** (en'do-limf).

Mechanisms of Equilibrium

If a cat is released upside down from a certain height, it will land on its feet. If an infant is tilted backward, its eyes will roll downward so that its gaze remains fixed (the *doll's-eye reflex*). Both of these reactions, and countless others, are compensations for a disturbance in balance, reflexes that depend on the sensory receptors within the vestibule and semicircular canals.

The equilibrium sense is not easy to describe because it does not see, hear, or feel. What it *does* is respond (frequently without our awareness) to the various movements of our head. The equilibrium receptors of the inner ear, sometimes called the **vestibular apparatus,** can be divided into two functional arms—one arm responsible for monitoring *static equilibrium,* and the other involved with *dynamic equilibrium.*

Static Equilibrium

Within the membrane sacs of the vestibule are receptors called **maculae** (mak'u-le; "spots") that are essential to our sense of **static equilibrium** (Figure 8.15). The maculae report on the position of the head with respect to the pull of gravity when the body is not moving (*static* = at rest). Since they provide information on which way is up or down, they help us keep our head erect. They are extremely important to divers swimming in the dark depths (where most other orienting cues are absent), enabling them to tell which way is up (to the surface). Each macula is a patch of receptor cells with their "hairs" embedded in the **otolithic membrane,** a gel or jellylike material containing **otoliths** (o'to-lithz), tiny stones made of calcium salts. As the head moves, the otoliths roll in response to changes in the pull of gravity. This movement creates a pull on the gel, which in turn slides like a greased plate over the hair cells, bending their hairs. This event activates the hair cells, which send impulses along the **vestibular nerve** (a division of cranial nerve VIII) to the cerebellum of the brain, informing it of the position of the head in space.

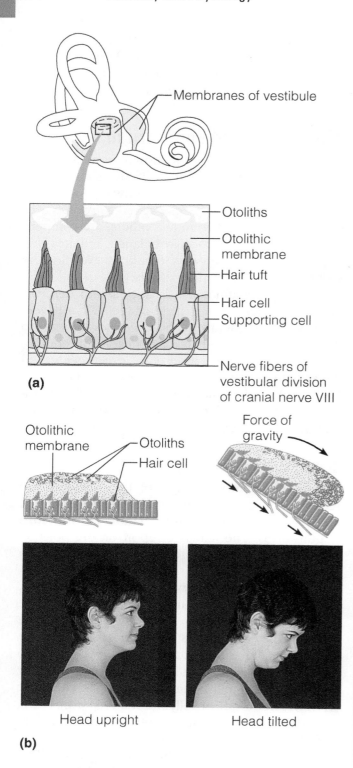

(a)

Membranes of vestibule

Otoliths

Otolithic membrane

Hair tuft

Hair cell

Supporting cell

Nerve fibers of vestibular division of cranial nerve VIII

Otolithic membrane

Otoliths

Hair cell

Force of gravity

Head upright

Head tilted

(b)

FIGURE 8.15   Structure and function of maculae (static equilibrium receptors). (a) Diagrammatic view of part of a macula. **(b)** When the head is tipped, the maculae are stimulated by movement of the otoliths in the gelatinous otolithic membrane in the direction of gravitational pull, which creates a pull on the hair cells.

Dynamic Equilibrium

The **dynamic equilibrium** receptors, found in the semicircular canals, respond to angular or rotatory movements of the head, rather than to straight-line movements. When you twirl on the dance floor or suffer through a rough boat ride, these receptors are working overtime. The semicircular canals (each about one-half inch, or 1.3 cm, around) are oriented in the three planes of space. Thus, regardless of which plane one moves in, there will be receptors to detect the movement.

Within each membranous semicircular canal is a receptor region called a **crista ampullaris** (kris′tah am″pu-lar′is), which consists of a tuft of hair cells covered with a gelatinous cap called the **cupula** (ku′pu-lah) (Figure 8.16). When your head moves in an arclike or angular direction, the endolymph in the canal lags behind. Then, as the cupula drags against the stationary endolymph, the cupula bends—like a swinging door—with the body's motion. This stimulates the hair cells, and impulses are transmitted up the **vestibular nerve** to the cerebellum. When you are moving at a constant rate, the receptors gradually stop sending impulses, and you no longer have the sensation of motion until your speed or direction of movement changes.

Prove It Yourself

Fluids Move in the Semicircular Canals in Response to Head Movement

You can easily demonstrate that fluids move in the semicircular canals as you move your head. First, fill a glass half-full with water and place a few objects in it, such as peppercorns or peas. Now twist the glass a half-turn or so. Notice that the objects (and the water) move more slowly than the glass, especially if the movement of the glass is rapid. The water and the objects appear to be flowing in the opposite direction from the glass, but in fact they are just slow to get started.

When you stop rotating the glass, the opposite happens. The water and the objects continue to spin for a short time.

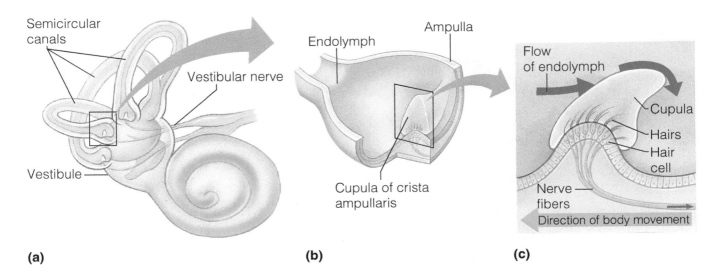

Semicircular canals

Vestibular nerve

Vestibule

Endolymph

Ampulla

Cupula of crista ampullaris

Flow of endolymph

Cupula

Hairs

Hair cell

Nerve fibers

Direction of body movement

(a) **(b)** **(c)**

FIGURE 8.16 **Structure and function of the crista ampullaris** (dynamic equilibrium receptor region). **(a)** Arranged in the three spatial planes, the semicircular ducts in the semicircular canals each have a swelling called an ampulla at their base. **(b)** Each ampulla contains a crista ampullaris, a receptor that is essentially a cluster of hair cells with hairs projecting into a gelatinous cap called the cupula. **(c)** When head position changes in an angular direction, inertia causes the endolymph in the semicircular ducts to lag behind, and as the cupula moves it drags across the endolymph bending the hair cells in the opposite direction. The bending results in increased impulse transmission in the sensory neurons. This mechanism adjusts quickly if the angular motion (or rotation) continues at a constant speed.

Although the receptors of the semicircular canals and vestibule are responsible for dynamic and static equilibrium, respectively, they usually act together. Besides these equilibrium senses, sight and the proprioceptors of the muscles and tendons are also important in providing information used to control balance to the cerebellum.

Mechanism of Hearing

Within the **cochlear duct,** the endolymph-containing membranous labyrinth of the snail-like cochlea is the **organ of Corti** (kor'te), which contains the hearing receptors, or **hair cells** (Figure 8.17a). The chambers (scalae) above and below the cochlear duct contain perilymph. Sound waves that reach the cochlea through vibrations of the eardrum, ossicles, and oval window set the cochlear fluids into motion (Figure 8.18). As the sound waves are transmitted by the ossicles from the eardrum to the oval window, their force

(amplitude) is increased by the lever activity of the ossicles. In this way, nearly the total force exerted on the much larger eardrum reaches the tiny oval window, which in turn sets the fluids of the inner ear into motion, and these pressure waves set up vibrations in the **basilar membrane.** The receptor cells, positioned on the basilar membrane in the organ of Corti, are stimulated when their "hairs" are bent or tweaked by the movement of the gel-like **tectorial** (tek-to're-al) **membrane** that lies over them (Figure 8.17b). The length of the fibers spanning the basilar membrane "tunes" specific regions to vibrate at specific frequencies. In general, high-pitch sounds disturb the shorter fibers of the basilar membrane and stimulate receptor cells close to the oval window, whereas low-pitch sounds affect longer fibers and activate specific hair cells further along the cochlea. Once stimulated, the hair cells transmit impulses along the **cochlear nerve** (a division of cranial nerve VIII— the vestibulocochlear nerve) to the auditory cortex

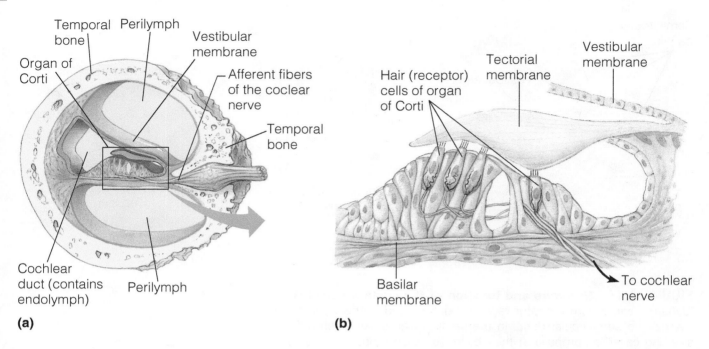

FIGURE 8.17 Anatomy of the cochlea. (a) A cross-sectional view of one turn of the cochlea, showing the position of the organ of Corti in the cochlear duct. The cavities of the bony labyrinth contain perilymph. The cochlear duct contains endolymph. **(b)** Detailed structure of the organ of Corti. The receptor cells (hair cells) rest on the basilar membrane.

in the temporal lobe, where interpretation of the sound, or hearing, occurs. Since sound usually reaches the two ears at different times, we could say that we hear "in stereo." Functionally, this helps us to determine where sounds are coming from in our environment.

When the same sounds, or tones, keep reaching the ears, the auditory receptors tend to *adapt* or stop responding to those sounds, and we are no longer aware of them. This is why the drone of a continually running motor does not demand our attention after the first few seconds. However, hearing is the last sense to leave our awareness when we fall asleep or receive anesthesia (or die) and is the first to return as we awaken.

Hearing and Equilibrium Deficits

Homeostatic Imbalance

Children with ear problems or hearing deficits often pull on their ears or fail to respond when spoken to. Under such conditions, tuning fork or audiometry testing is done to try to diagnose the problem.

Deafness is defined as *hearing loss of any degree*— from a slight loss to a total inability to hear sound. Generally speaking, there are two kinds of deafness: conduction and sensorineural. Temporary or permanent *conduction deafness* results when something interferes with the conduction of sound vibrations to the fluids of the inner ear. Something as simple as a buildup of earwax may be the cause. Other causes of conduction deafness include fusion of the ossicles (a problem called *otosclerosis* [o"to-sklě-ro'sis]), a ruptured eardrum, and *otitis media.*

Sensorineural deafness occurs when there is degeneration or damage to the receptor cells in the organ of Corti, to the cochlear nerve, or to neurons of the auditory cortex. This often results from extended listening to excessively loud sounds. Thus, whereas conduction deafness results from mechanical factors, sensorineural deafness is a problem of nervous system structures.

A person who has a hearing loss due to conduction deafness will still be able to hear by bone conduction, even though his or her ability to hear air-conducted sounds (the normal conduction route) is decreased or lost. On the other hand, individuals with

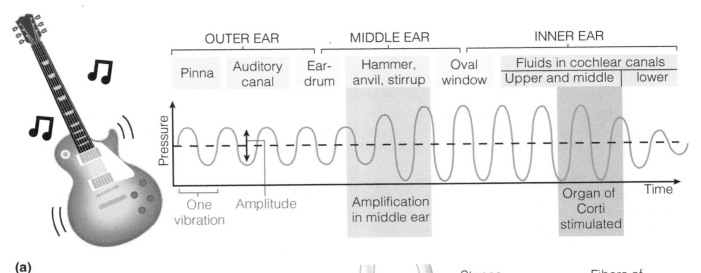

(a)

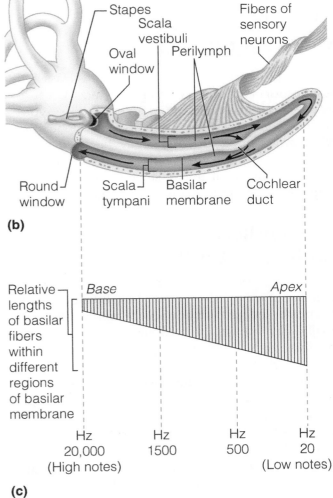

(b)

FIGURE 8.18 Route of sound waves through the ear and activation of the cochlear hair cells.
(a) To excite the hair cells in the organ of Corti in the inner ear, sound wave vibrations must pass through air, membranes, bone, and fluid. **(b)** The cochlea is drawn as if it is uncoiled to make the events of sound transmission occurring there easier to follow. Sound waves of low frequency that are below the level of hearing travel entirely around the cochlear duct without exciting hair cells. But sounds of higher frequency result in pressure waves that penetrate through the cochlear duct and basilar membrane to reach the scala tympani. This causes the basilar membrane to vibrate maximally in certain areas in response to certain frequencies of sound, stimulating particular hair cells and sensory neurons. The differential stimulation of hair cells is perceived in the brain as sound of a certain pitch. **(c)** The length of the fibers spanning the basilar membrane tune specific regions to vibrate at specific frequencies. The higher notes—20,000 Hertz (Hz)—are detected by shorter hair cells along the base of the basilar membrane.

(c)

sensorineural deafness cannot hear better by *either* conduction route. Hearing aids, which use skull bones to conduct sound vibrations to the inner ear, are generally very successful in helping those with conduction deafness to hear. They are less helpful for sensorineural deafness.

Equilibrium problems are usually obvious. Nausea, dizziness, and problems in maintaining balance are common symptoms, particularly when impulses from the vestibular apparatus "disagree" with what we see (visual input). There also may be strange (jerky or rolling) eye movements.

A serious pathology of the inner ear is *Ménière's* (mān"e-airz') *disease*. The exact cause of this condition is not fully known, but suspected causes are arteriosclerosis, degeneration of cranial nerve VIII, and increased pressure of the inner ear fluids. In Ménière's disease, progressive deafness occurs. Affected individuals become nauseated and often have *vertigo* (a sensation of spinning) that is so severe that they cannot stand up without extreme discomfort. Anti-motion sickness drugs are often prescribed to decrease the discomfort. ▲

Chemical Senses: Taste and Smell

The receptors for taste and olfaction are classified as **chemoreceptors** (ke"mo-re-sep'terz) because they respond to chemicals in solution. Five types of taste receptors have been identified, but the olfactory receptors (for smell) are believed to be sensitive to a much wider range of chemicals. The receptors for smell and taste complement each other and respond to many of the same stimuli.

Olfactory Receptors and the Sense of Smell

Even though our sense of smell is far less acute than that of many other animals, the human nose is still much keener than any machine in picking up small differences in odors. Some people capitalize on this ability by becoming tea and coffee blenders, perfumers, or wine tasters.

The thousands of **olfactory receptors,** receptors for the sense of smell, occupy a postage stamp–sized area in the roof of each nasal cavity (Figure 8.19). Air entering the nasal cavities must make a hairpin turn to enter the respiratory passageway below, so sniffing, which causes more air to flow superiorly across the olfactory receptors, intensifies the sense of smell.

The **olfactory receptor cells** are neurons equipped with **olfactory hairs,** long cilia that protrude from the nasal epithelium (called the olfactory membrane) and are continually bathed by a layer of mucus secreted by underlying glands.

When the receptors are stimulated by chemicals dissolved in the mucus, they transmit impulses along the **olfactory filaments,** which collectively make up the **olfactory nerve** (cranial nerve I), to the olfactory cortex of the brain. There interpretation of the odor occurs, and an "odor snapshot" is made. The olfactory pathways are closely tied into the limbic system (emotional-visceral part of the brain). Thus, olfactory impressions are long-lasting and very much a part of our memories and emotions. For example, the smell of chocolate chip cookies may remind you of your grandmother, and the smell of a special pipe tobacco may make you think of your father. There are hospital smells, school smells, baby smells, travel smells. The list can be continued almost without end. Our reactions to odors are rarely neutral. We tend to either like or dislike certain odors, and we change, avoid, or add odors according to our preferences.

The olfactory receptors are exquisitely sensitive—just a few molecules can activate them. Like the auditory receptors, the olfactory neurons tend to adapt rather quickly when they are exposed to an unchanging stimulus, in this case, an odor. This is why a woman stops smelling her own perfume after a while but will quickly pick up the scent of another perfume on someone else.

▲ Homeostatic Imbalance

While it is possible to have either taste or smell deficits, most people seeking medical help for loss of chemical senses have olfactory disorders, or *anosmias* (ah-noz'me-uz). Most anosmias result from head injuries, the aftereffects of nasal cavity inflammation (due to a cold, an allergy, or smoking), or aging. Some brain disorders can destroy the sense of smell or mimic it. For example, *olfactory auras* (olfactory hallucinations) are experienced by some epileptics just before they go into seizures. ▲

Taste Buds and the Sense of Taste

The word *taste* comes from the Latin word *taxare,* which means "to touch, estimate, or judge." When we taste things, we are, in fact, testing or judging our environment in an intimate way, and the sense of taste is considered by many to be the most pleasurable of our special senses. There is no question that what does not taste good to us will usually not be allowed to enter the body.

Q   *How does sniffing help to identify scents?*

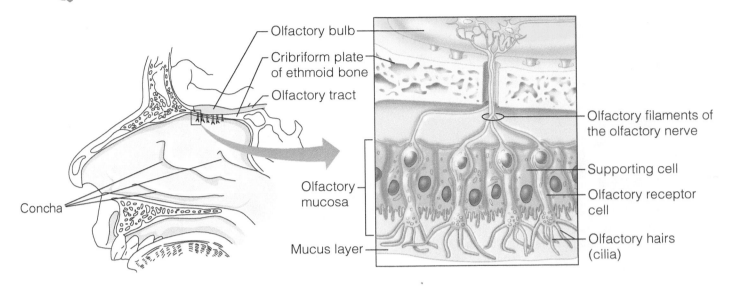

FIGURE 8.19   **Location and cellular makeup of the olfactory epithelium.**

The **taste buds,** or specific receptors for the sense of taste, are widely scattered in the oral cavity. Of the 10,000 or so taste buds that we have, most are located on the tongue. A few are found on the soft palate and inner surface of the cheeks.

The dorsal tongue surface is covered with small peglike projections, or **papillae** (pah-pil′e), of three types: sharp *filiform* (fil′ĭ-form) papillae and the rounded *fungiform* (fun′jĭ-form) and *circumvallate* (ser″kum-val′at) papillae. The taste buds are found on the sides of the circumvallate papillae and on the more numerous fungiform papillae (Figure 8.20). The specific cells that respond to chemicals dissolved in the saliva are epithelial cells called **gustatory cells,** which are surrounded by supporting cells in the taste bud. Their long microvilli—the **gustatory hairs**—protrude through the **taste pore,** and when they are stimulated, they depolarize and impulses are transmitted to the brain. Three cranial nerves—VII, IX, and X—carry taste impulses from the various taste buds to the gustatory cortex. The **facial nerve** (VII) serves the anterior part of the tongue. The other two cranial nerves—the **glossopharyngeal**

and **vagus,** respectively—serve the other taste bud–containing areas.

There are five basic taste sensations, each corresponding to stimulation of one of the five major types of taste buds. The *sweet receptors* respond to substances such as sugars, saccharine, and some amino acids. Some believe that the common factor is the hydroxyl (OH⁻) group. *Sour receptors* respond to hydrogen ions (H⁺), or the acidity of the solution; *bitter receptors* to alkaloids; and *salty receptors* to metal ions in solution. *Umami* (u-mah′me; "delicious"), a taste discovered by the Japanese, is elicited by the amino acid glutamate which appears to be responsible for the "beef taste" of steak and the flavor of monosodium glutamate, a food additive. Historically, the tip of the tongue was believed to be most sensitive to sweet and salty substances, its sides to sour, the back of the tongue to bitter, and the pharynx to umami. Actually there are only slight differences in the locations of the taste receptors in different regions of the tongue, and most taste buds respond to two, three, four, or even all five taste modalities.

Taste likes and dislikes have homeostatic value. A liking for sugar and salt will satisfy the body's need for carbohydrates and minerals (as well as some amino acids). Many sour, naturally acidic foods (such as oranges, lemons, and

A   *It brings more odor-containing air into contact with the olfactory receptors in the superior part of the nasal cavity.*

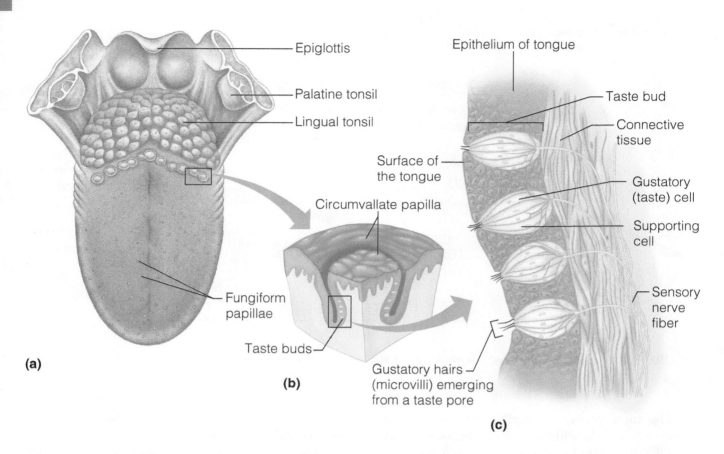

FIGURE 8.20   Location and structure of taste buds. (a) Taste buds on the tongue are associated with papillae, projections of the tongue mucosa. **(b)** A sectioned circumvallate papilla shows the position of the taste buds in its lateral walls. **(c)** An enlarged view of four taste buds.

tomatoes) are rich sources of vitamin C, an essential vitamin. Umami guides the intake of proteins; and, since many natural poisons and spoiled foods are bitter, our dislike for bitterness is protective. (The position of large numbers of bitter receptors on the most posterior part of the tongue seems strange, however, because usually by the time we actually taste a bitter substance, we have swallowed some of it.)

Taste is affected by many factors, and what is commonly referred to as our sense of taste depends heavily on stimulation of our olfactory receptors by aromas. Think of how bland food is when your nasal passages are congested by a cold. Without the sense of smell, our morning coffee would simply taste bitter. In addition, the temperature and texture of food can enhance or spoil its taste for us. For example, some people will not eat foods that have a pasty texture (avocados) or that are gritty (pears), and almost everyone considers a

cold greasy hamburger unfit to eat. "Hot" foods like chili peppers actually excite pain receptors in the mouth.

Developmental Aspects of the Special Senses

The special sense organs, essentially part of the nervous system, are formed very early in embryonic development. For example, the eyes, which are literally outgrowths of the brain, are developing by the fourth week. All of the special senses are functional, to a greater or lesser degree, at birth.

Homeostatic Imbalance

Congenital eye problems are relatively uncommon, but some examples can be given. *Strabismus* (strah-biz'mus), commonly called "crossed eyes," results from unequal pulls by the external eye muscles that prevent the baby from coordinating movement of the two eyes. First, exercises are used to strengthen the weaker eye muscles and/or the stronger eye may be covered with an eye patch to force the weaker muscles to become stronger. If these measures are not successful, surgery is always used to correct the condition because, if it is allowed to persist, the brain may stop recognizing signals from the deviating eye, causing that eye to become functionally blind.

Maternal infections, particularly *rubella* (measles), that occur during early pregnancy may lead to congenital blindness or cataracts. If the mother has a type of sexually transmitted disease called *gonorrhea* (gon"o-re'ah), the baby's eyes will be infected by the bacteria during delivery. In the resulting *conjunctivitis*, specifically called *ophthalmia neonatorum* (of-thal'me-ah ne"o-na-to'rum), the baby's eyelids become red and swollen, and pus is produced. All states legally require that all newborn babies' eyes be routinely treated with silver nitrate or antibiotics shortly after birth. ▲

Generally speaking, vision is the only special sense that is not fully functional when the baby is born, and many years of "learning" are needed before the eyes are fully mature. The eyeballs continue to enlarge until the age of 8 or 9, but the lens grows throughout life. At birth, the eyeballs are foreshortened, and all babies are hyperopic (farsighted). As the eyes grow, this condition usually corrects itself. The newborn infant sees only in gray tones, eye movements are uncoordinated, and often only one eye at a time is used. Because the lacrimal glands are not fully developed until about two weeks after birth, the baby is tearless for this period, even though he or she may cry lustily.

By 5 months, the infant is able to focus on articles within easy reach and to follow moving objects, but visual acuity is still poor (the infant sees an object that is 20 feet away clearly that someone with mature vision would see clearly when it is 200 feet away—such vision is said to be 20/200). By the time the child is 5 years old, color vision is well developed, visual acuity has improved to about 20/30, and depth perception is present, providing a readiness to begin reading. By school age, the earlier hyperopia has usually been replaced by emmetropia. This condition continues until about age 40, when **presbyopia** (pres"be-o'pe-ah) begins to set in. Presbyopia (literally, "old vision") results from decreasing lens

elasticity that accompanies aging. This condition makes it difficult to focus for close vision; it is basically farsightedness. The person who holds the newspaper at arm's length to read it provides the most familiar example of this developmental change in vision.

As aging occurs, the lacrimal glands become less active and the eyes tend to become dry and more vulnerable to bacterial infection and irritation. The lens loses its crystal clarity and becomes discolored. The dilator muscles of the iris become less efficient; thus, the pupils are always somewhat constricted. These last two conditions work together to decrease by half the amount of light reaching the retina, so that visual acuity is dramatically lower by one's 70s. In addition to these changes, elderly people are susceptible to certain conditions that may result in blindness, such as glaucoma and cataracts. Other common aging-related problems, such as arteriosclerosis and diabetes, may lead to the death of the delicate photoreceptors because of an increasing lack of oxygen and nutrients.

▲ Homeostatic Imbalance

Congenital abnormalities of the ears are fairly common. Examples include partly or completely missing pinnas and closed or absent external acoustic meatuses. Maternal infections can have a devastating effect on ear development, and maternal rubella during the early weeks of pregnancy results in sensorineural deafness. ▲

A newborn infant can hear after his or her first cry, but early responses to sound are mostly reflexive—for example, crying and clenching the eyelids in response to a loud noise. By the age of 3 or 4 months, the infant is able to localize sounds and will turn to the voices of family members. Critical listening occurs in the toddler as he or she begins to imitate sounds, and good language skills are very closely tied to an ability to hear well.

Except for ear inflammations *(otitis)* resulting from bacterial infections or allergies, few problems affect the ears during childhood and adult life. By the 60s, however, a gradual deterioration and atrophy of the organ of Corti begins and leads to a loss in the ability to hear high tones and speech sounds. This condition, **presbycusis** (pres"bĭ-ku'sis), is a type of sensorineural deafness. In some cases, the ear ossicles fuse *(otosclerosis)*, which compounds the hearing problem by interfering with sound conduction to the inner ear. Because many elderly people refuse to accept their hearing loss and resist using hearing aids, they begin to rely more and more on their vision for clues as to what is going on around them and may be accused of ignoring people. Although presbycusis was once considered a disability of old age, it is becoming much more common in younger people as our world grows noisier day by day. Noise pollution has become a major health problem, and the damage caused by excessively loud sounds is progressive and cumulative. Each insult causes a bit more damage. Music played and heard at deafening levels is definitely a contributing factor to the deterioration of the hearing receptors.

The chemical senses, taste and smell, are sharp at birth, and infants relish some food that adults consider bland or tasteless. Some researchers claim the sense of smell is just as important as the sense of touch in guiding a newborn baby to its mother's breast. However, very young children seem indifferent to odors and can play happily with their own feces. As they get older, their emotional responses to specific odors increase.

There appear to be few problems with the chemical senses throughout childhood and young adulthood. Beginning in the mid-40s, our ability to taste and smell diminishes, which reflects the gradual decrease in the number of these receptor cells. Almost half of people over the age of 80 cannot smell at all, and their sense of taste is poor. This may explain their inattention to formerly disagreeable odors, and why older adults often prefer highly seasoned (although not necessarily spicy) foods or lose their appetite entirely.

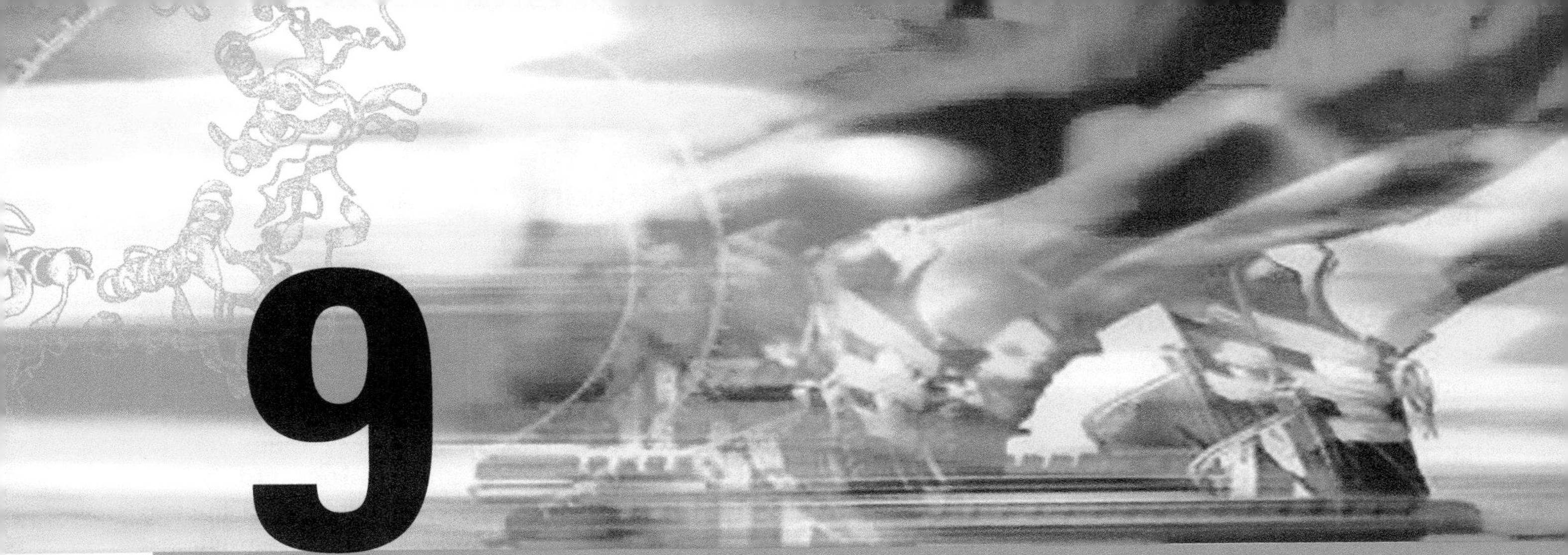

9

The Endocrine System

KEY TERMS

- hormone, p. 312
- target cells, p. 314
- negative feedback, p. 322
- exocrine gland, p. 323

When insulin molecules, carried passively along in the blood, leave the blood and bind tightly to protein receptors of nearby cells, the response is dramatic: bloodborne glucose molecules begin to disappear into the cells, and cellular activity accelerates. Such is the power of the second great controlling system of the body, the **endocrine system.** Along with the nervous system, it coordinates and directs the activity of the body's cells. However, the speed of control in these two great regulating systems is very different. The nervous system is "built for speed." It uses nerve impulses to prod the muscles and glands into immediate action so that rapid adjustments can be made in response to changes occurring both inside and outside the body. On the other hand, the more slowly acting endocrine system uses chemical messengers called **hormones,** which are released into the blood to be transported leisurely throughout the body.

Although hormones have widespread and varied effects, the major processes controlled by hormones are reproduction; growth and development; mobilizing body defenses against stressors; maintaining electrolyte, water, and nutrient balance of the blood; and regulating cellular metabolism and energy balance. As you can see, the endocrine system regulates processes that go on for relatively long periods and, in some cases, continuously.

The Endocrine System and Hormone Function— An Overview

Compared to other organs of the body, the organs of the endocrine system are small and unimpressive. Indeed, to collect 1 kg (about 2.2 pounds) of hormone-producing tissue, you would need to collect *all* the endocrine tissue from eight or nine adults! The endocrine organs also lack the structural or anatomical continuity typical of most organ systems. Instead, bits and pieces of endocrine tissue are tucked away in widely separated regions of the body (see Figure 9.6). However, functionally, the endocrine organs are very impressive, and when their role in maintaining body homeostasis is considered, they are true giants.

The Chemistry of Hormones

The key to the incredible power of the endocrine glands is the hormones they produce and secrete. *Hormones* may be defined as chemical substances that are secreted by cells into the extracellular fluids and regulate the metabolic activity of other cells in the body. Although many different hormones are produced, nearly all of them can be classified chemically as either **amino acid–based molecules** (including proteins, peptides, and amines) or **steroids.** Steroid hormones (made from cholesterol) include the sex hormones made by the gonads (ovaries and testes) and the hormones produced by the adrenal cortex. All others are nonsteroidal amino acid derivatives. If we also consider the local hormones called **prostaglandins** (pros"tah-glan'dinz), described later in the chapter (see Table 9.3), we must add a third chemical class, because the prostaglandins are made from highly active lipids found in the cells' plasma membranes.

Mechanisms of Hormone Action

Although the bloodborne hormones circulate to all the organs of the body, a given hormone affects only certain tissue cells or organs, referred to as its **target cells** or **target organs.** In order for a target cell to respond to a hormone, specific protein receptors must be present on its plasma membrane or in its interior to which *that* hormone can attach. Only when this binding occurs can the hormone influence the workings of a cell.

The term *hormone* comes from a Greek word meaning "to arouse." In fact, the body's hormones do just that. They "arouse" or bring about their effects on the body's cells primarily by *altering* cellular activity—that is, by increasing or decreasing the rate of a normal, or usual, metabolic process rather than by stimulating a new one. The precise changes that follow hormone binding depend on the specific hormone and the target cell type, but typically one or more of the following occurs:

1. Changes in plasma membrane permeability or electrical state.

2. Synthesis of proteins or certain regulatory molecules (such as enzymes) in the cell.

3. Activation or inactivation of enzymes.

4. Stimulation of mitosis.

Q *What determines if a hormone will influence a given body cell?*

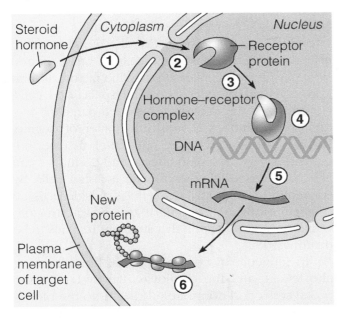

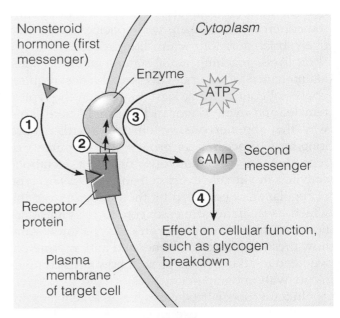

(a) Steroid hormone action

(b) Nonsteroid hormone action

FIGURE 9.1 Mechanisms of hormone action. (a) Direct gene activation: the steroid hormone mechanism. **(b)** A second messenger system: the nonsteroid (amino acid–based) hormone mechanism.

Despite the huge variety of hormones, there are really only two mechanisms by which hormones trigger changes in cells. Steroidal hormones (and, strangely, thyroid hormone) use the mechanism shown in Figure 9.1a. Being lipid-soluble molecules, the steroid hormones can (1) diffuse through the plasma membranes of their target cells. Once inside, the steroid hormone (2) enters the nucleus, and (3) binds to a specific receptor protein there. The hormone-receptor complex then (4) binds to specific sites on the cell's DNA, (5) activating certain genes to transcribe messenger RNA (mRNA). The mRNA then (6) is translated in the cytoplasm, resulting in the synthesis of new proteins.

Nonsteroidal hormones—protein and peptide hormones—are unable to enter the target cells. Instead they bind to receptors situated on the target cell's plasma membrane and utilize a **second-messenger system.** In these cases

(Figure 9.1b), (1) the hormone binds to the membrane receptor, (2) setting off a series of reactions that activates an enzyme. The enzyme, in turn, (3) catalyzes a reaction that produces a second messenger molecule (in this case, *cyclic AMP*, also known as *cAMP* or cyclic adenine monophosphate) that (4) oversees additional intracellular changes that promote the typical response of the target cell to the hormone. As you might guess, there are a variety of possible second messengers (including *G proteins* and *calcium ions*) and many possible target cell responses to the same hormone, depending on the tissue type stimulated.

Let's look a little closer at how the body uses intercellular communication to preserve homeostasis.

Intercellular Communication

To preserve homeostasis, cellular activities must be coordinated throughout the body. Neurons monitor

A *A hormone can only influence a body cell if that cell has receptors for that hormone on its plasma membrane or internally.*

or control specific cells or groups of cells. However, the number of cells innervated is only a small fraction of the total number of cells in the body, and the commands issued are very specific and of relatively brief duration. Many life processes are not short-lived; reaching adult stature takes decades. Maintenance of reproductive capabilities requires continual control for at least 30 years in the typical female, and even longer in the male. There is no way that the nervous system can regulate such long-term processes as growth, development, or reproduction, which involve or affect metabolic activities in virtually every cell and tissue. This type of regulation is provided by the endocrine system, which uses chemical messengers to relay information and instructions between cells. To understand how these messages are generated and interpreted, we need to take a closer look at how cells communicate with one another.

In a few specialized cases, cellular activities are coordinated by the exchange of ions and molecules between adjacent cells across gap junctions. This **direct communication** occurs between two cells of the same type, and the cells must be in extensive physical contact. The two cells communicate so closely that they function as a single entity. Gap junctions (1) coordinate ciliary movement among epithelial cells, (2) coordinate the contractions of cardiac muscle cells, and (3) facilitate the propagation of action potentials from one neuron to the next at electrical synapses.

Direct communication is highly specialized and relatively rare. Most of the communication between cells involves the release and receipt of chemical messages. Each cell continuously "talks" to its neighbors by releasing chemicals into the extracellular fluid. These chemicals tell cells what their neighbors are doing at any moment. The result is the coordination of tissue function at the local level. The use of chemical messengers to transfer information from cell to cell within a single tissue is called **paracrine communication.** The chemicals involved are called paracrine factors, also known as *local hormones*. Examples of paracrine factors include the prostaglandins and the various growth factors.

Paracrine factors enter the bloodstream, but their concentrations are usually so low that distant cells and tissues are not affected. However, some paracrine factors, including several of the prostaglandins and related chemicals, have primary effects in their tissues of origin and secondary effects in other tissues and organs. When secondary effects occur, the paracrine factors are also acting as **hormones**—chemical messengers that are released in one tissue and transported in the bloodstream to alter the activities of specific cells in other tissues. Whereas most cells release paracrine factors, typical hormones are produced only by specialized cells. Nevertheless, the difference between paracrine factors and hormones is mostly a matter of degree. Paracrine factors can diffuse out of their tissue of origin and have widespread effects, and hormones can affect their tissues of origin as well as distant cells. By convention, a substance with effects outside its tissue of origin is called a *hormone* if its chemical structure is known, and a *factor* if that structure remains to be determined.

In intercellular communication, hormones are like letters, and the cardiovascular system is the postal service. A hormone released into the bloodstream is distributed throughout the body. Each hormone has **target cells,** specific cells that possess the receptors needed to bind and "read" the hormonal message when it arrives. But hormones are really like bulk mail advertisements—cells throughout the body are exposed to them whether or not they have the necessary receptors. At any moment, each individual cell can respond to only a few of the hormones present. The other hormones are ignored, because the cell lacks the receptors to read the messages they contain. The activity of hormones in coordinating cellular activities in tissues in distant portions of the body is called **endocrine communication.**

Hormones alter the operations of target cells by changing the types, quantities, or activities of important enzymes and structural proteins. In other words, a hormone may:

- stimulate the synthesis of an enzyme or a structural protein not already present in the cytoplasm by activating appropriate genes in the cell nucleus;

- increase or decrease the rate of synthesis of a particular enzyme or other protein by changing the rate of transcription or translation; or

- turn an existing enzyme or membrane channel "on" or "off" by changing its shape or structure.

Through one or more of these mechanisms, a hormone can modify the physical structure or biochemical properties of its target cells. Because the target cells can be anywhere in the body, a single hormone can alter the metabolic activities of multiple tissues and organs simultaneously. These effects may be slow to appear, but they typically persist for days. Consequently, hormones are effective in coordinating cell, tissue, and organ activities on a sustained, long-term basis. For example, circulating hormones keep body water content and levels of electrolytes and organic nutrients within normal limits 24 hours a day throughout our entire lives.

Cells can respond to several different hormones simultaneously. Gradual changes in the quantities and identities of circulating hormones can therefore produce complex changes in the body's physical structure and physiological capabilities. Examples include the processes of embryological and fetal development, growth, and puberty. Hormonal regulation is thus quite suitable for directing gradual, coordinated processes, but it is totally unable to handle situations requiring split-second responses. That kind of crisis management is the job of the nervous system.

Although the nervous system also relies primarily on chemical communication, it does not send messages through the bloodstream. Instead, neurons release a neurotransmitter at a synapse very close to target cells that bear the appropriate receptors. The command to release the neurotransmitter rapidly travels from one location to another in the form of action potentials propagated along axons. The nervous system thus acts like a telephone company, with a cable network carrying high-speed "messages" to specific destinations throughout the body. The effects of neural stimulation are generally short-lived, and they tend to be restricted to specific target cells—primarily because the neurotransmitter is rapidly broken down or recycled. This form of **synaptic communication** is ideal for crisis management: If you are in danger of being hit by a speeding bus, the nervous system can coordinate and direct your leap to safety. Once the crisis is over and the neural circuits quiet down, things soon return to normal.

Table 9.1 summarizes the ways cells and tissues communicate with one another. Viewed from a general perspective, the differences between the nervous and endocrine systems seem relatively clear. In fact, these broad organizational and functional distinctions are the basis for treating them as two separate systems. Yet when we consider them in detail, we see that the two systems are similarly organized:

- Both systems rely on the release of chemicals that bind to specific receptors on their target cells.

- The two systems share many chemical messengers; for example, norepinephrine and epinephrine are called *hormones* when released into the bloodstream, but *neurotransmitters* when released across synapses.

- Both systems are regulated primarily by negative feedback control mechanisms.

- The two systems share a common goal: to preserve homeostasis by coordinating and regulating the activities of other cells, tissues, organs, and systems.

Next we introduce the components and functions of the endocrine system and explore the interactions between the nervous and endocrine systems.

An Overview of the Endocrine System

The **endocrine system** includes all the endocrine cells and tissues of the body that produce hormones or paracrine factors with effects beyond their tissues of origin. *Endocrine cells* are glandular secretory cells that release their secretions into the extracellular fluid. This characteristic distinguishes them from *exocrine cells,* which secrete their products onto epithelial surfaces, generally by way of ducts. The chemicals released by endocrine cells may affect only adjacent cells, as in the case of most paracrine factors, or they may affect cells throughout the body.

The tissues, organs, and hormones of the endocrine system are introduced in Figure 9.2. Some of these organs, such as the pituitary gland, have endocrine secretion as a primary function. Others, such as the pancreas, have many other functions in addition to endocrine secretion.

Classes of Hormones

Hormones can be divided into three groups on the basis of their chemical structure: (1) *amino acid derivatives,* (2) *peptide hormones,* and (3) *lipid derivatives.*

TABLE 9.1   Mechanisms of Intercellular Communication

Mechanism	Transmission	Chemical Mediators	Distribution of Effects
Direct communication	Through gap junctions	Ions, small solutes, lipid-soluble materials	Usually limited to adjacent cells of the same type that are interconnected by connexons
Paracrine communication	Through extracellular fluid	Paracrine factors	Primarily limited to local area, where concentrations are relatively high. Target cells must have appropriate receptors
Endocrine communication	Through the circulatory system	Hormones	Target cells are primarily in other tissues and organs and must have appropriate receptors
Synaptic communication	Across synaptic clefts	Neurotransmitters	Limited to very specific area. Target cells must have appropriate receptors

Amino Acid Derivatives

Amino acid derivatives are relatively small molecules that are structurally related to amino acids, the building blocks of proteins. This group of hormones, sometimes known as the *biogenic amines,* are synthesized from the amino acids *tyrosine* (TĪ-rō-sēn) and *tryptophan* (TRIP-tō-fan). Tyrosine derivatives include (1) thyroid hormones, produced by the thyroid gland, and (2) the compounds epinephrine (E), norepinephrine (NE), and dopamine, which are sometimes called *catecholamines* (kat-e-KŌ-la-mēnz). The primary hormone derivative of tryptophan is melatonin (mel-a-TŌ-nin), produced by the pineal gland.

Peptide Hormones

Peptide hormones are chains of amino acids. In general, peptide hormones are synthesized as prohormones—inactive molecules that are converted to active hormones either before or after they are secreted.

Peptide hormones can be divided into two groups. One group consists of glycoproteins. These proteins are more than 200 amino acids long and have carbohydrate side chains. The glycoproteins include *thyroid-stimulating hormone (TSH), luteinizing hormone (LH),* and *follicle-stimulating hormone (FSH)* from the anterior lobe of the pituitary gland, as well as several hormones produced in other organs.

The second group of peptide hormones is large and diverse; it includes hormones that range from short polypeptide chains, such as *antidiuretic hormone (ADH)* and *oxytocin* (9 amino acids apiece), to small proteins, such as *growth hormone* (GH; 191 amino acids) and *prolactin* (PRL; 198 amino acids). This group includes all the hormones secreted by the hypothalamus, heart, thymus, digestive tract, pancreas, and posterior lobe of the pituitary gland, as well as

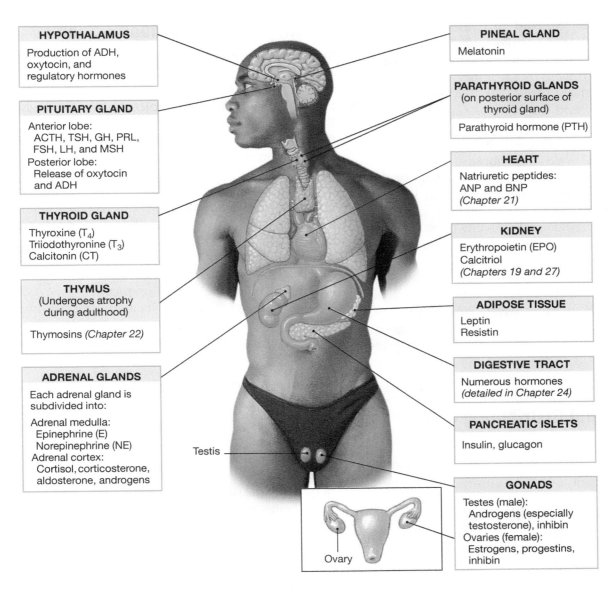

HYPOTHALAMUS

Production of ADH, oxytocin, and regulatory hormones

PITUITARY GLAND

Anterior lobe:
  ACTH, TSH, GH, PRL, FSH, LH, and MSH
Posterior lobe:
  Release of oxytocin and ADH

THYROID GLAND

Thyroxine (T$_4$)
Triiodothyronine (T$_3$)
Calcitonin (CT)

THYMUS
(Undergoes atrophy during adulthood)

Thymosins *(Chapter 22)*

ADRENAL GLANDS

Each adrenal gland is subdivided into:

Adrenal medulla:
  Epinephrine (E)
  Norepinephrine (NE)
Adrenal cortex:
  Cortisol, corticosterone, aldosterone, androgens

Testis

PINEAL GLAND

Melatonin

PARATHYROID GLANDS
(on posterior surface of thyroid gland)

Parathyroid hormone (PTH)

HEART

Natriuretic peptides: ANP and BNP
(Chapter 21)

KIDNEY

Erythropoietin (EPO)
Calcitriol
(Chapters 19 and 27)

ADIPOSE TISSUE

Leptin
Resistin

DIGESTIVE TRACT

Numerous hormones
(detailed in Chapter 24)

PANCREATIC ISLETS

Insulin, glucagon

GONADS

Testes (male):
  Androgens (especially testosterone), inhibin
Ovaries (female):
  Estrogens, progestins, inhibin

Ovary

FIGURE 9.2   Organs and tissues of the endocrine system.

most of the hormones secreted by the anterior lobe of the pituitary gland.

Lipid Derivatives

There are two classes of *lipid derivatives:* (1) *eicosanoids,* derived from *arachidonic* (a-rak-i-DON-ik) *acid,* a 20-carbon fatty acid, and (2) *steroid hormones,* derived from cholesterol.

Eicosanoids Eicosanoids (ī-KŌ-sa-noydz) are small molecules with a five-carbon ring at one end. These compounds are important paracrine factors that coordinate cellular activities and affect enzymatic processes (such as blood clotting) in extracellular fluids. Some of the eicosanoids also have secondary roles as hormones.

Leukotrienes (loo-kō-TRĪ-ēns) are eicosanoids released by activated white blood cells, or *leukocytes.* Leukotrienes are important in coordinating tissue responses to injury or disease. **Prostaglandins,** a second group of eicosanoids, are produced in most tissues of the body. Within each tissue, the prostaglandins released are involved primarily in coordinating local cellular activities. In some tissues, prostaglandins are converted to **thromboxanes** (throm-BOX-ānz) and **prostacyclins** (pros-ta-SĪ-klinz), which also have strong paracrine effects.

Steroid Hormones   **Steroid hormones** are lipids structurally similar to cholesterol. Steroid hormones are released by male and female reproductive organs (*androgens* by the testes, *estrogens* and *progestins* by the ovaries), the adrenal glands (*corticosteroids*), and the kidneys (*calcitriol*). The individual hormones differ in the side chains attached to the basic ring structure.

In the blood, steroid hormones are bound to specific transport proteins in the plasma. For this reason, they remain in circulation longer than do secreted peptide hormones. The liver gradually absorbs these steroids and converts them to a soluble form that can be excreted in the bile or urine.

Our focus in this chapter is on circulating hormones whose primary functions are the coordination of activities in many tissues and organs. We will consider eicosanoids in chapters that discuss individual tissues and organs, including Chapters 10 (the blood), 12 (the lymphatic system), and 16 (the reproductive system).

Secretion and Distribution of Hormones

Hormone release typically occurs where capillaries are abundant, and the hormones quickly enter the bloodstream for distribution throughout the body. Within the blood, hormones may circulate freely or bound to special carrier proteins. A freely circulating hormone remains functional for less than one hour, and sometimes for as little as two minutes. It is inactivated when (1) it diffuses out of the bloodstream and binds to receptors on target cells, (2) it is absorbed and broken down by cells of the liver or kidneys, or (3) it is broken down by enzymes in the plasma or interstitial fluids.

Thyroid hormones and steroid hormones remain in circulation much longer, because when these hormones enter the bloodstream, more than 99 percent of them become attached to special transport proteins. For each hormone an equilibrium state exists between the free and bound forms: As the free hormones are removed and inactivated, they are replaced by the release of bound hormones. At any given time, the bloodstream contains a substantial reserve (several weeks' supply) of bound hormones.

Mechanisms of Hormone Action

To affect a target cell, a hormone must first interact with an appropriate receptor. A hormone receptor, like a neurotransmitter receptor, is a protein molecule to which a particular molecule binds strongly. Each cell has receptors for responding to several different hormones, but cells in different tissues have different combinations of receptors. This arrangement is one reason hormones have differential effects on specific tissues. For every cell, the presence or absence of a specific receptor determines the cell's hormonal sensitivities. If a cell has a receptor that can bind a particular hormone, that cell will respond to the hormone's presence. If a cell lacks the proper receptor for that hormone, the hormone will have no effect on that cell.

Hormone receptors are located either on the cell membrane or inside the cell. Using a few specific examples, we will now introduce the basic mechanisms involved.

Hormones and Cell Membrane Receptors

The receptors for catecholamines (E, NE, and dopamine), peptide hormones, and eicosanoids are in the cell membranes of their respective target cells. Because catecholamines and peptide hormones are not lipid soluble, they are unable to penetrate a cell membrane. Instead, these hormones bind to receptor proteins at the *outer* surface of the cell membrane (extracellular receptors). Eicosanoids, which *are* lipid soluble, diffuse across the membrane to reach receptor proteins on the *inner* surface of the membrane (intracellular receptors).

First and Second Messengers   A hormone that binds to receptors in the cell membrane cannot have a direct effect on the activities under way inside the target cell. Such a hormone cannot, for example, begin building a protein or catalyzing a specific reaction. Instead, the hormone uses an intracellular intermediary to exert its effects. The hormone, or **first messenger**, does something that leads to the appearance of a **second messenger** in the cytoplasm. The second messenger may act as an enzyme activator, inhibitor, or cofactor, but the net result is a change in the rates of various metabolic reactions. The most important second messengers are (1) *cyclic-AMP (cAMP),* a derivative of ATP; (2) *cyclic-GMP (cGMP),* a derivative of GTP, another high-energy compound; and (3) calcium ions.

The binding of a small number of hormone molecules to membrane receptors may lead to the appearance of thousands of second messengers in a cell. This process, which magnifies the effect of a hormone on the target cell, is called *amplification*. Moreover, the arrival of a single hormone may promote the release of more than one type of second messenger, or the production of a linked sequence of enzymatic reactions known as a *receptor cascade*. Through such mechanisms, the hormone can alter many aspects of cell function simultaneously.

The presence or absence of a hormone can also affect the nature and number of hormone receptor proteins in the cell membrane. **Down-regulation** is a process in which the presence of a hormone triggers a decrease in the number of hormone receptors. In down-regulation, when levels of a particular hormone are high, cells become less sensitive to it. Conversely, **up-regulation** is a process in which the absence of a hormone triggers an increase in the number of hormone receptors. In up-regulation, when levels of a particular hormone are low, cells become *more* sensitive to it.

The link between the first messenger and the second messenger generally involves a **G protein**, an enzyme complex coupled to a membrane receptor. The name *G protein* refers to the fact that these proteins bind GTP. A G protein is activated when a hormone binds to its receptor at the membrane surface. What happens next depends on the nature of the G protein and its effects on second messengers in the cytoplasm; Figure 9.3 diagrams the major patterns of response to G protein activation.

G Proteins and cAMP   Many G proteins, once activated, exert their effects by changing the concentration of the second messenger *cyclic-AMP* (cAMP) within the cell. In most cases, the result is an increase in cAMP levels, and this accelerates metabolic activity within the cell.

The steps involved in increasing cAMP levels are diagrammed in Figure 9.3 (left):

- The activated G protein activates the enzyme adenylate cyclase, also called *adenylyl cyclase.*

- Adenylate cyclase converts ATP to the ring-shaped molecule *cyclic-AMP.*

- Cyclic-AMP then functions as a second messenger, typically by activating a *kinase.* A kinase is

an enzyme that performs *phosphorylation,* the attachment of a high-energy phosphate group ($\sim PO_4^{3-}$) to another molecule.

- Generally, the kinases activated by cyclic-AMP phosphorylate proteins. The effect on the target cell depends on the nature of the proteins affected. The phosphorylation of membrane proteins, for example, can open ion channels. In the cytoplasm, many important enzymes can be activated only by phosphorylation; one important example is the enzyme that releases glucose from glycogen reserves in skeletal muscles and the liver.

The hormones calcitonin, parathyroid hormone, ADH, ACTH, epinephrine, FSH, LH, TSH, and glucagon all produce their effects by this mechanism. The increase is usually short-lived, because the cytoplasm contains another enzyme, **phosphodiesterase (PDE)**, which inactivates cyclic-AMP by converting it to AMP (adenosine monophosphate).

Figure 9.3 (center) depicts one way the activation of a G protein can *lower* the concentration of cAMP within the cell. In this case, the activated G protein stimulates PDE activity and inhibits adenylate cyclase activity. Levels of cAMP then decline, because cAMP breakdown accelerates while cAMP synthesis is prevented. The decline has an inhibitory effect on the cell, because without phosphorylation, key enzymes remain inactive. This is the mechanism respon-sible for the inhibitory effects that follow the stimulation of α_2 adrenergic receptors by catecholamines.

G Proteins and Calcium Ions   An activated G protein can trigger either the opening of calcium ion channels in the membrane or the release of calcium ions from intracellular stores. The steps involved are diagrammed in Figure 9.3 (right panel). The G protein first activates the enzyme *phospholipase C (PLC)*. This enzyme triggers a receptor cascade that begins with the production of **diacylglycerol (DAG)** and **inositol triphosphate (IP$_3$)** from membrane phospholipids. The cascade then proceeds as follows:

- IP$_3$ diffuses into the cytoplasm and triggers the release of Ca^{2+} from intracellular reserves, such as those in the smooth endoplasmic reticulum of many cells.

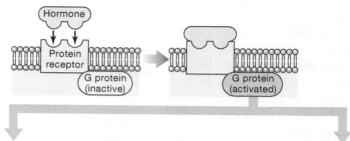

EFFECTS ON cAMP LEVELS

ACTIVATION OF ADENYLATE CYCLASE

INHIBITION OF ADENYLATE CYCLASE; ACTIVATION OF PDE

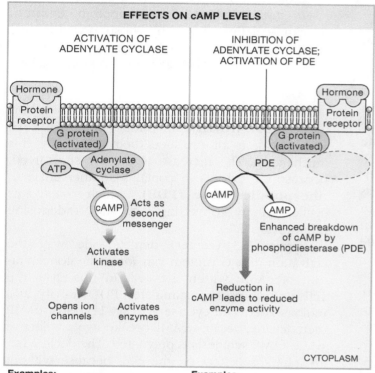

Examples:
- Epinephrine and norepinephrine (β receptors)
- Calcitonin
- Parathyroid hormone
- ADH, ACTH, FSH, LH, TSH
- Glucagon

Examples:
- Epinephrine and norepinephrine (α_2 receptors)

EFFECTS ON Ca²⁺ LEVELS

ACTIVATION OF PHOSPHOLIPASE C

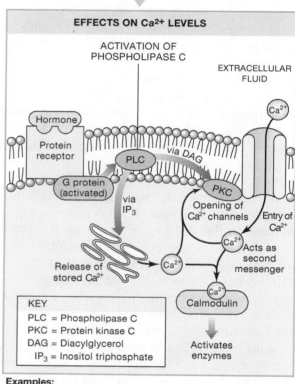

KEY
PLC = Phospholipase C
PKC = Protein kinase C
DAG = Diacylglycerol
IP_3 = Inositol triphosphate

Examples:
- Epinephrine and norepinephrine (α_1 receptors)
- Oxytocin
- Regulatory hormones of hypothalamus
- Several eicosanoids

FIGURE 9.3 **G proteins and hormone activity.** Peptide hormones, catecholamines, and eicosanoids bind to membrane receptors and activate G proteins. G protein activation may involve effects on cAMP levels (at left), or effects on Ca²⁺ levels (at right).

- The combination of DAG and intracellular calcium ions activates another membrane protein: protein kinase C (PKC). The activation of PKC leads to the phosphorylation of calcium channel proteins, a process that opens the channels and permits the entry of extracellular Ca²⁺ This sets up a positive feedback loop that rapidly elevates intracellular calcium ion concentrations.

- The calcium ions themselves serve as messengers, generally in combination with an intracellular protein called calmodulin. Once it has bound calcium ions, calmodulin can activate specific cytoplasmic enzymes. This chain of events is responsible for the stimulatory effects that follow the activation of α_1 receptors by epinephrine or norepinephrine. Calmodulin activation is also involved in the responses to oxytocin and to several regulatory hormones secreted by the hypothalamus.

Hormones and Intracellular Receptors

Steroid hormones diffuse across the lipid part of the cell membrane and bind to receptors in the cytoplasm or nucleus. The hormone–receptor complexes then activate or deactivate specific genes (Figure 9.4a). By this mechanism, steroid hormones can alter the rate of DNA transcription in the nucleus, and thus change the pattern of protein synthesis. Alterations in the synthesis of enzymes or structural proteins will directly affect both the metabolic activity and the structure of the target cell. For example, the sex hormone *testosterone* stimulates the production of enzymes and structural proteins in skeletal muscle fibers, causing an increase in muscle size and strength.

Thyroid hormones cross the cell membrane primarily by a transport mechanism. Once in the cytosol, these hormones bind to receptors within the nucleus and on mitochondria (Figure 9.4b). The hormone–receptor complexes in the nucleus activate specific genes or change the rate of transcription. The change in rate affects the metabolic

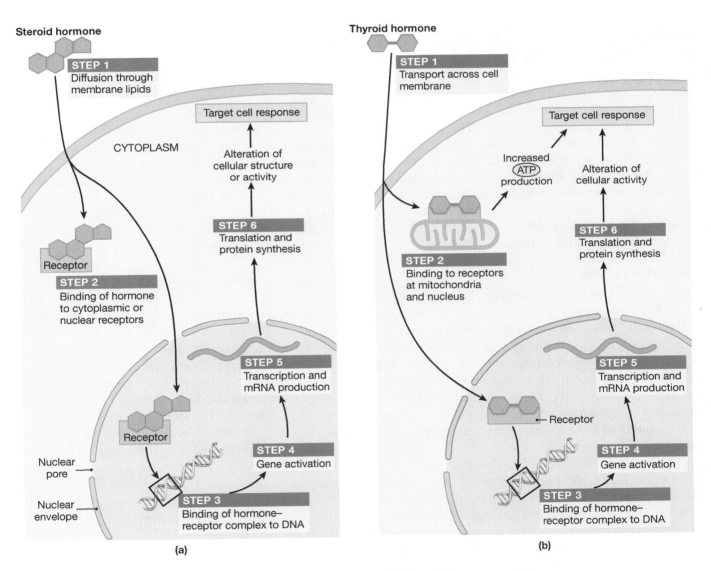

(a)

(b)

FIGURE 9.4   Effects of intracellular hormone binding. (a) Steroid hormones diffuse through the membrane lipids and bind to receptors in the cytoplasm or nucleus. The complex then binds to DNA in the nucleus, activating specific genes. **(b)** Thyroid hormones enter the cytoplasm and bind to receptors in the nucleus to activate specific genes. They also bind to receptors on mitochondria and accelerate ATP production.

activities of the cell by increasing or decreasing the concentration of specific enzymes. Thyroid hormones bound to mitochondria increase the mitochondrial rates of ATP production.

100 Keys | Hormones coordinate cell, tissue, and organ activities on a sustained basis. They circulate in the extracellular fluid and bind to specific receptors on or in target cells. They then modify cellular activities by altering membrane permeability, activating or inacti-vating key enzymes, or changing genetic activity.

Control of Endocrine Activity

The functional organization of the nervous system parallels that of the endocrine system in many ways. In Chapter 7, we considered the basic operation of neural reflex arcs, the simplest organizational units in the nervous system. The most direct arrangement was a monosynaptic reflex, such as the stretch reflex. Polysynaptic reflexes provide more complex and variable responses to stimuli, and higher centers, which integrate multiple inputs, can facilitate or inhibit these reflexes as needed. **Endocrine reflexes** are the functional counterparts of neural reflexes.

Endocrine Reflexes

Endocrine reflexes can be triggered by (1) *humoral stimuli* (changes in the composition of the extracellular fluid), (2) *hormonal stimuli* (the arrival or removal of a specific hormone), or (3) *neural stimuli* (the arrival of neurotransmitters at neuroglandular junctions). In most cases, endocrine reflexes are controlled by negative feedback mechanisms: A stimulus triggers the production of a hormone whose direct or indirect effects reduce the intensity of the stimulus.

A simple endocrine reflex involves only one hormone. The endocrine cells involved respond directly to changes in the composition of the extracellular fluid. The secreted hormone adjusts the activities of target cells and restores homeostasis. Simple endocrine reflexes control hormone secretion by the heart, pancreas, parathyroid gland, and digestive tract.

More complex endocrine reflexes involve one or more intermediary steps and two or more hormones.

Control of Hormone Release

Now that we've discussed *how* hormones work, the next question is, "What prompts the endocrine glands to release or not release their hormones?" Let's take a look.

Negative feedback mechanisms are the chief means of regulating blood levels of nearly all hormones. In such systems, hormone secretion is triggered by some internal or external stimulus; then rising hormone levels inhibit further hormone release (even while promoting responses in their target organs). As a result, blood levels of many hormones vary only within a very narrow range.

The stimuli that activate the endocrine organs fall into three major categories—hormonal, humoral, and neural (Figure 9.5). The most common stimulus is a *hormonal stimulus,* in which endocrine organs are prodded into action by other hormones. For example, hypothalamic hormones stimulate the anterior pituitary gland to secrete its hormones, and many anterior pituitary hormones stimulate other endocrine organs to release their hormones into the blood (Figure 9.5a). As the hormones produced by the final target glands increase in the blood, they "feed back" to inhibit the release of anterior pituitary hormones and thus their own release. Hormone release promoted by this mechanism tends to be rhythmic, with hormone blood levels rising and falling again and again.

Changing blood levels of certain ions and nutrients may also stimulate hormone release. Such stimuli are referred to as *humoral* (hyoo-mor'al) *stimuli* to distinguish them from hormonal stimuli, which are also bloodborne chemicals. The term *humoral* refers to the ancient use of the word *humor* to indicate the various body fluids (blood, bile, and others). For example, the release of parathyroid hormone (PTH) by cells of the parathyroid glands is prompted by decreasing blood calcium levels. Because PTH acts by several routes to reverse that decline, blood Ca^{2+} levels soon rise, ending the stimulus for PTH release (Figure 9.5b). Other hormones released in response to humoral stimuli include calcitonin, released by the thyroid gland, and insulin, produced by the pancreas.

In isolated cases, nerve fibers stimulate hormone release and the target cells are said to respond to *neural stimuli*. The classic example is sympathetic nervous system stimulation of the

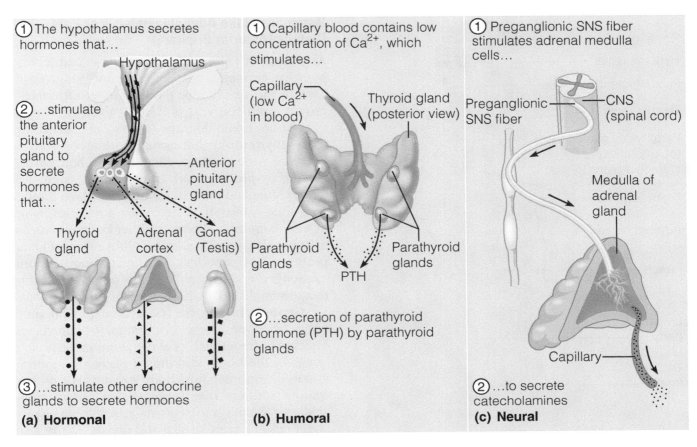

① The hypothalamus secretes hormones that...

Hypothalamus

② ...stimulate the anterior pituitary gland to secrete hormones that...

Anterior pituitary gland

Thyroid gland

Adrenal cortex

Gonad (Testis)

③ ...stimulate other endocrine glands to secrete hormones

(a) Hormonal

① Capillary blood contains low concentration of Ca^{2+}, which stimulates...

Capillary (low Ca^{2+} in blood)

Thyroid gland (posterior view)

Parathyroid glands

Parathyroid glands

PTH

② ...secretion of parathyroid hormone (PTH) by parathyroid glands

(b) Humoral

① Preganglionic SNS fiber stimulates adrenal medulla cells...

Preganglionic SNS fiber

CNS (spinal cord)

Medulla of adrenal gland

Capillary

② ...to secrete catecholamines

(c) Neural

FIGURE 9.5 **Endocrine gland stimuli. (a)** Hormonal stimulus. In this example, hormones released by the hypothalamus stimulate the anterior pituitary to release hormones that stimulate other endocrine organs to secrete hormones. **(b)** Humoral stimulus. Low blood calcium levels trigger parathyroid hormone (PTH) release from the parathyroid glands. PTH causes blood calcium levels to rise by stimulating release of Ca^{2+} from bone. Consequently, the stimulus for PTH secretion ends. **(c)** Neural stimulus. The stimulation of adrenal medullary cells by sympathetic nervous system (SNS) fibers triggers the release of catecholamines (epinephrine and norepinephrine) to the blood.

adrenal medulla to release norepinephrine and epinephrine during periods of stress (Figure 9.5c). Although these three mechanisms typify most systems that control hormone release, they by no means explain all of them, and some endocrine organs respond to many different stimuli.

The Major Endocrine Organs

The major endocrine organs of the body include the **pituitary, thyroid, parathyroid, adrenal, pineal,** and **thymus glands,** the **pancreas,** and the gonads (**ovaries** and **testes**) (Figure 9.6). The **hypothalamus,** which is part of the nervous system, is also recognized as a major endocrine organ because it produces several hormones. Although the function of some hormone-producing glands (the anterior pituitary, thyroid, adrenals, and parathyroids) is purely endocrine, the function of others (pancreas and gonads) is mixed—both endocrine and exocrine. Both types of glands are formed from epithelial tissue, but the endocrine glands are **ductless glands** that produce hormones that they release into the blood or lymph. (As you might expect, the endocrine glands have a very rich blood supply.) Conversely, the exocrine glands

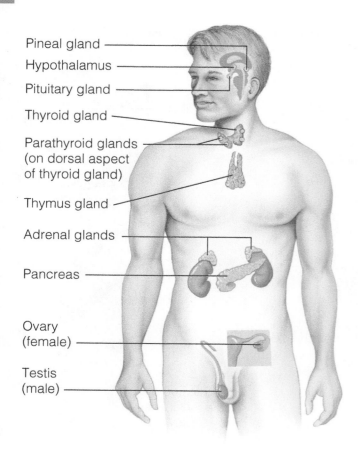

Pineal gland

Hypothalamus

Pituitary gland

Thyroid gland

Parathyroid glands
(on dorsal aspect
of thyroid gland)

Thymus gland

Adrenal glands

Pancreas

Ovary
(female)

Testis
(male)

FIGURE 9.6   Location of the major endocrine organs of the body. (The parathyroid glands, which appear to be on the anterior surface of the thyroid gland in this illustration, are actually located on its posterior aspect in most cases.)

release their products at the body's surface or into body cavities through ducts. Here we direct our attention to the endocrine glands only.

Besides the more detailed descriptions of the endocrine organs provided next, a summary of their hormones' main actions and regulatory factors appears in Table 9.2.

Pituitary Gland (Also Called Hypophysis Cerebri)

The **pituitary** (pǐ-tu'ǐ-tār"e) **gland** is approximately the size of a grape. It hangs by a stalk from the inferior surface of the hypothalamus of the brain, where it is snugly surrounded by the "Turk's saddle" of the sphenoid bone. It has two functional lobes—the anterior pituitary (glandular tissue) and the posterior pituitary (nervous tissue).

Hormones of the Adenohypophysis or Pars Distalis (Anterior Pituitary)

As shown in Figure 9.7, there are several anterior pituitary hormones that affect many body organs. Two of the six anterior pituitary lobe hormones— growth hormone and prolactin—exert their major effects on nonendocrine targets. The remaining four—thyrotropic hormone, adrenocorticotropic hormone, and the two gonadotropic hormones— are all **tropic** (tro'pik) **hormones.** Tropic hormones stimulate their target organs, which are also endocrine glands, to secrete their hormones, which in turn exert their effects on other body organs and tissues. All anterior pituitary hormones (1) are proteins (or peptides), (2) act through second-messenger systems, and (3) are regulated by hormonal stimuli and, in most cases, negative feedback.

Growth hormone (GH) is a general metabolic hormone. However, its major effects are directed to the growth of skeletal muscles and long bones of the body, and thus it plays an important role in determining final body size. GH is a protein-sparing and anabolic hormone that causes amino acids to be built into proteins and stimulates most target cells to grow in size and divide. At the same time, it causes fats to be broken down and used for energy while it spares glucose, helping to maintain blood sugar homeostasis.

Homeostatic Imbalance

If untreated, both deficits and excesses of GH may result in structural abnormalities. Hyposecretion, or lack of GH during childhood, leads to *pituitary dwarfism*. Body proportions are fairly normal, but the person as a whole is a living miniature (with a maximum adult height of 4 feet). Hypersecretion (oversecretion) during childhood results in *gigantism*. The individual becomes extremely tall; 8 to 9 feet is common. Again, body proportions are fairly normal. If hypersecretion occurs after long-bone growth has ended, **acromegaly** (ak"ro-meg'ah-le) results. The facial bones, particularly the lower jaw and the bony ridges underlying the eyebrows, enlarge tremendously, as do the feet and hands. Thickening of soft tissues leads to coarse or malformed facial features. Most cases of hypersecretion by endocrine organs (the pituitary and the other endocrine organs) result from tumors of the affected gland. The tumor cells act in much the same way as the normal glandular cells do; that is, they produce the hormones normally made by that gland. The use of pharmacological doses of GH to reverse some of the effects of aging is

Q What effect would elevated levels of thyroid hormone in the blood have on TSH secretion?

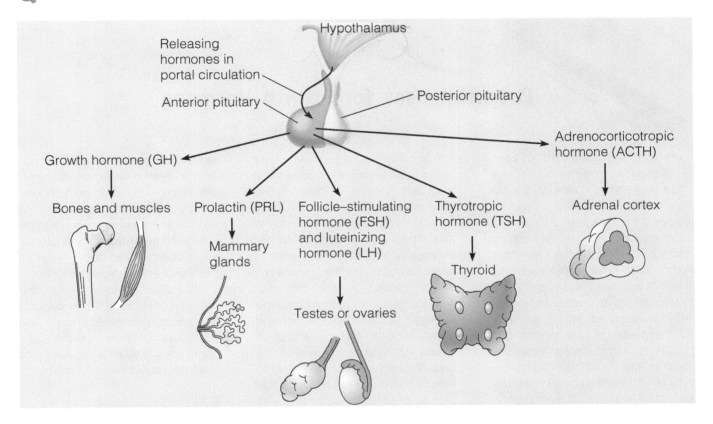

FIGURE 9.7 **Hormones of the anterior pituitary and their major target organs.** Secretion of anterior pituitary hormones is stimulated by releasing hormones secreted by hypothalamic neurons. The releasing hormones are secreted into a capillary network that connects via portal veins to a second capillary bed in the anterior lobe of the pituitary gland.

highlighted in the "A Closer Look" box on potential uses for the growth hormone. ▲

Prolactin (PRL) is a protein hormone structurally similar to growth hormone. Its only known target in humans is the breast (*pro* = for; *lact* = milk). After childbirth, it stimulates and maintains milk production by the mother's breasts. Its function in males is not known.

Adrenocorticotropic (ad-re″no-kor″tĭ-ko-tro′pik) **hormone (ACTH)** affects glucose metabolism as it regulates the endocrine activity of the cortex portion of the adrenal gland. **Thyroid-stimulating hormone (TSH)**, also called **thyrotropic hormone (TH)**, influences the growth and activity of the thyroid gland.

The **gonadotropic** (gon″ă-do-trop′ik) **hormones** regulate the hormonal activity of the **gonads** (ovaries and testes). In females, **follicle-stimulating hormone (FSH)** stimulates follicle development in the ovaries. As the follicles mature, they produce estrogen, and eggs are readied for ovulation. In males, FSH stimulates sperm development by the testes. **Luteinizing** (lu′te-in-īz″ing) **hormone (LH)** triggers ovulation of an egg from the female ovary and causes the ruptured follicle to produce progesterone and some estrogen. In men, LH is also referred to as **interstitial cell–stimulating hormone (ICSH)** because it stimulates testosterone production by the interstitial cells of the testes.

A   *It would inhibit TSH secretion by the anterior pituitary.*

A Closer Look

Potential Uses for Growth Hormone

GROWTH hormone (GH) has been used for pharmaceutical purposes (that is, as a drug) since its discovery in the 1950s. Originally obtained from the pituitary glands of cadavers, it is now biosynthesized and administered by injection. Although GH is widely used in clinical trials, its use as a prescription drug is restricted until its helpful and harmful effects—many of which are very intriguing—can be fully documented.

GH is administered legally to children who do not produce it naturally or who have chronic kidney failure, to allow these children to grow to near-normal heights. Unfortunately, some physicians succumb to parental pressures to prescribe GH to children who *do* produce it but are extremely short.

When GH is administered to *adults* with a growth-hormone deficiency, body fat decreases and lean body mass, bone density, and muscle mass increase. It also appears to increase the performance and muscle mass of the heart, and it decreases blood cholesterol, boosts the immune system, and perhaps improves one's psychological outlook. Such effects (particularly those involving increased muscle mass and decreased body fat) have led to abuse of GH by bodybuilders and athletes, which is one reason why this substance remains restricted.

Because GH may also reverse some effects of aging, anti-aging clinics using GH injections to delay aging are springing up. Many people naturally stop producing GH after age 60, and this may explain why their ratio of lean-to-fat mass declines and their skin thins. GH already is the drug treatment of choice for many aging Hollywood stars who dread the loss of their youth and vitality. Administration of GH to elderly patients reverses these declines. However, clinical studies reveal that the administered GH does not increase strength or exercise tolerance in elderly patients, and a careful study of very sick patients in intensive care units (where GH is routinely given to restore nitrogen balance) found that high doses of GH are associated with increased mortality. For these reasons, earlier media claims that GH is a "youth potion" have proven to be dangerously misleading, and GH should not be administered to the very old or the critically ill.

GH may help AIDS patients. Because of improved antibiotics, fewer AIDS patients are dying from opportunistic infections. The other side of this picture is that more die from the weight loss called "wasting." It has been shown that injections of GH can actually reverse wasting during AIDS, leading to weight gain—a gain of lean muscle. In 1996, the U.S. Food and Drug Administration approved the use of GH to treat such wasting.

GH is not a wonder drug, even in cases where it is clearly beneficial. GH treatment is expensive and has undesirable side effects. It can lead to fluid retention and edema, joint and muscle pain, high blood sugar, glucose intolerance, and gynecomastia (breast enlargement in males). Hypertension, heart enlargement, diabetes, and cancer of the colon are other possible results of high doses of GH, and edema and headaches accompany even the lowest doses. Carefully tailored dosages can avoid most of these side effects, however.

Intensive research into the potential benefits of GH is ongoing and should keep this hormone in the public eye for years to come. Let's hope its unbridled use does not become a public health problem.

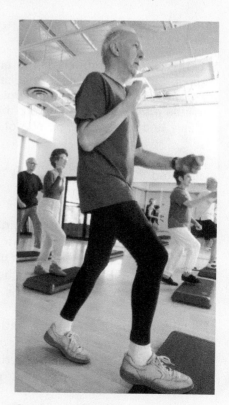

Can growth hormone help elderly patients?

Homeostatic Imbalance

Hyposecretion of FSH or LH leads to sterility in both males and females. In general, hypersecretion does not appear to cause any problems. However, some drugs used to promote fertility stimulate the release of the gonadotropic hormones, and multiple births (indicating multiple ovulations at the same time rather than the usual single ovulation each month) are fairly common after their use. ▲

Pituitary-Hypothalamus Relationship

Despite its insignificant size, the anterior pituitary gland controls the activity of so many other endocrine glands that it has often been called the **"master endocrine gland."** Its removal or destruction has a dramatic effect on the body. The adrenal and thyroid glands and gonads atrophy, and results of hyposecretion by those glands quickly become obvious. However, the anterior pituitary is not as all-powerful in its control as it might appear because the release of each of its hormones is controlled by **releasing** and **inhibiting hormones** produced by the hypothalamus. The hypothalamus liberates these regulatory hormones into the blood of the portal circulation, which connects the blood supply of the hypothalamus with that of the anterior pituitary. [In a *portal circulation*, two capillary beds are connected by vein(s); in this case, the capillaries of the hypothalamus are drained by veins which empty into the capillaries of the anterior pituitary, giving direct, one-way communication between the two glands.]

The hypothalamus also makes two additional hormones, oxytocin and antidiuretic hormone, which are transported along the axons of the hypothalamic **neurosecretory cells** to the posterior pituitary for storage (Figure 9.8). They are later released into the blood in response to nerve impulses from the hypothalamus. Figure 9.9 shows how the hypothalamus provides feedback control of endocrine secretion.

Hormones of the Neurohypophysis or Pars Nervosa (Posterior Pituitary Lobe)

The posterior pituitary is not an endocrine gland in the strict sense because it *does not make* the peptide hormones it releases. Instead, as mentioned above, it simply acts as a storage area for hormones made by hypothalamic neurons.

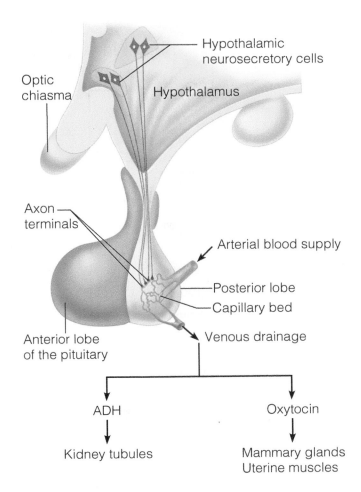

FIGURE 9.8 Hormones released by the posterior lobe of the pituitary and the target organs of such hormones. Neurosecretory cells in the hypothalamus synthesize oxytocin and antidiuretic hormone (ADH) and transport them down their axons to the posterior pituitary. There, the hormones are stored until their release is triggered by nerve impulses from the hypothalamus.

Oxytocin (ok″se-to′sin) is released in significant amounts only during childbirth and in nursing women. It stimulates powerful contractions of the uterine muscle during labor, during sexual relations, and when a woman breast-feeds her baby. It also causes milk ejection (the *let-down reflex*) in a nursing woman. Both natural and synthetic oxytocic drugs (Pitocin and others) are used to induce labor or to hasten labor that is progressing normally but at a slow pace. Less frequently, oxytocics are used to stop postpartum bleeding (by causing constriction of the ruptured blood vessels at the placental site) and to stimulate the milk ejection reflex.

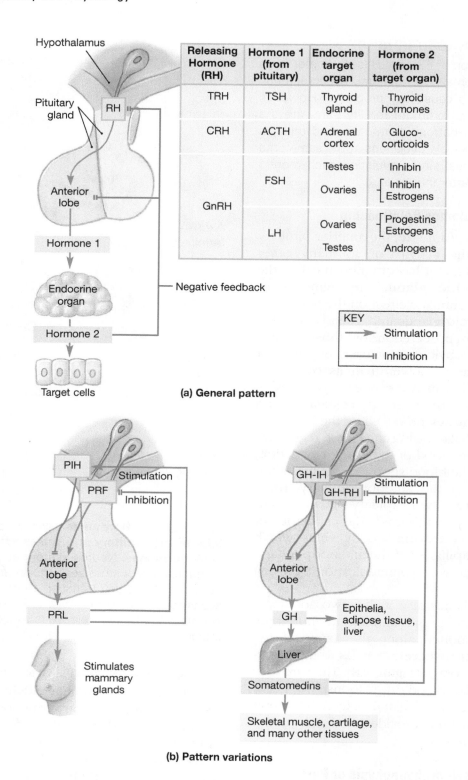

Releasing Hormone (RH)	Hormone 1 (from pituitary)	Endocrine target organ	Hormone 2 (from target organ)
TRH	TSH	Thyroid gland	Thyroid hormones
CRH	ACTH	Adrenal cortex	Gluco-corticoids
GnRH	FSH	Testes	Inhibin
		Ovaries	Inhibin Estrogens
	LH	Ovaries	Progestins Estrogens
		Testes	Androgens

(a) General pattern

KEY
→ Stimulation
⊣ Inhibition

(b) Pattern variations

FIGURE 9.9   Feedback control of endocrine secretion. (a) A typical pattern of regulation when multiple endocrine organs are involved. The hypothalamus produces a releasing hormone (RH) to stimulate hormone production by other glands; control occurs via negative feedback. **(b)** Variations on the theme outlined in part (a). Left: The regulation of prolactin (PRL) production by the anterior lobe. In this case, the hypothalamus produces both a releasing factor (PRF) and an inhibiting hormone (PIH); when one is stimulated, the other is inhibited. Right: The regulation of growth hormone (GH) production by the anterior lobe; when GH–RH release is inhibited, GH–IH release is stimulated.

The second hormone released by the posterior pituitary is **antidiuretic** (an"ti-di"u-ret'ik) **hormone (ADH).** *Diuresis* is urine production. Thus, an antidiuretic is a chemical that inhibits or prevents urine production. ADH causes the kidneys to reabsorb more water from the forming urine; as a result, urine volume decreases and blood volume increases. In larger amounts, ADH also increases blood pressure by causing constriction of the arterioles (small arteries). For this reason, it is sometimes referred to as **vasopressin** (vas"o-pres'in).

Drinking alcoholic beverages inhibits ADH secretion and results in output of large amounts of urine. The dry mouth and intense thirst experienced "the morning after" reflect this dehydrating effect of alcohol. Certain drugs, classed together as *diuretics,* antagonize the effects of ADH, causing water to be flushed from the body. These drugs are used to manage the edema (water retention in tissues) typical of congestive heart failure.

100 Keys | The hypothalamus produces regulatory factors that adjust the activities of the anterior lobe of the pituitary gland, which produces seven hormones. Most of these hormones control other endocrine organs, including the thyroid gland, adrenal gland, and gonads. The anterior lobe also produces growth hormone, which stimulates cell growth and protein synthesis. The posterior lobe of the pituitary gland releases two hormones produced in the hypothalamus; ADH restricts water loss and promotes thirst, and oxytocin stimulates smooth muscle contractions in the mammary glands and uterus (in females) and the prostate gland (in males).

Thyroid Gland

The **thyroid gland** is a hormone-producing gland that is familiar to most people primarily because many obese individuals blame their overweight condition on their "glands" (meaning the thyroid). Actually, the effect of thyroid hormones on body weight is not as great as many believe it to be.

The thyroid gland is located at the base of the throat, just inferior to the Adam's apple, where it is easily palpated during a physical examination. It is a fairly large gland consisting of two lobes joined by a central mass, or *isthmus* (Figure 9.10). The thyroid gland makes two hormones, one called *thyroid hormone,* the other called *calcitonin.*

Internally, the thyroid gland is composed of hollow structures called **follicles,** which store a sticky colloidal material (Figure 9.10b). Thyroid hormone is derived from this colloid.

Thyroid hormone, often referred to as the body's major metabolic hormone, is actually two active iodine-containing hormones, **thyroxine** (thi-rok'sin), or **T₄,** and **triiodothyronine** (tri"i'o-do-thi'ro-nēn), or **T₃.** Thyroxine is the major hormone secreted by the thyroid follicles. Most triiodothyronine is formed at the target tissues by conversion of thyroxine to triiodothyronine. These two hormones are very much alike. Each is constructed from two tyrosine amino acids linked together, but thyroxine has four bound iodine atoms, whereas triiodothyronine has three (thus, T_4 and T_3, respectively).

Thyroid hormone controls the rate at which glucose is "burned," or oxidized, and converted to body heat and chemical energy. Since all body cells depend on a continuous supply of chemical energy to power their activities, every cell in the body is a target. Thyroid hormone is also important for normal tissue growth and development, especially in the reproductive and nervous systems.

Homeostatic Imbalance

Without iodine, functional hormones cannot be made. The source of iodine is our diet, and the foods richest in iodine are seafoods. Years ago, many people who lived in the Midwest, in areas with iodine-deficient soil that were far from the seashore (and a supply of fresh seafood), developed **goiters** (goy'terz). That region of the country came to be known as the "goiter belt." A goiter is an enlargement of the thyroid gland (Figure 9.11) that results when the diet is deficient in iodine. TSH keeps "calling" for thyroxine, and the thyroid gland continues to enlarge so that it can put out more thyroxine. Without iodine, however, the thyroid makes only the peptide part of the molecule, which is nonfunctional and thus fails to provide negative feedback to inhibit TSH release. Simple goiter is uncommon in the United States today because most of our salt is iodized, but it is still a problem in some other areas of the world.

Hyposecretion of thyroxine may indicate problems other than iodine deficiency, such as lack of stimulation by TSH. If it occurs in early childhood, the result is *cretinism* (kre'tin-izm). Cretinism results in dwarfism in which adult body proportions remain childlike. Together the head and trunk are about 1½ times the length of the legs rather than approximately the same length, as in normal adults. Untreated cretins are

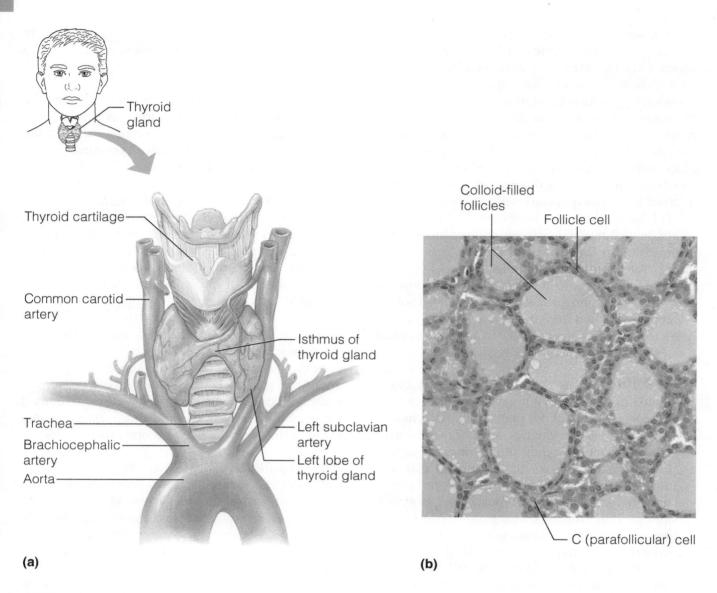

(a)

(b)

FIGURE 9.10   Anatomy of the thyroid gland. (a) Location of the thyroid gland, anterior view. **(b)** Photomicrograph of the thyroid gland (250×).

mentally retarded. Their hair is scanty, and their skin is dry. If the hyposecretion problem is discovered early, hormone replacement will prevent mental retardation and other signs and symptoms of the deficiency. Hypothyroidism occurring in adults results in *myxedema* (mik"se-de'mah), in which there is both physical and mental sluggishness (however, mental retardation does not occur). Other signs are a puffiness of the face, fatigue, poor muscle tone, low body temperature (the person is always cold), obesity, and dry skin. Oral thyroxine is prescribed to treat this condition.

Hyperthyroidism generally results from a tumor of the thyroid gland. Extreme overproduction of

thyroxine results in a high basal metabolic rate, intolerance of heat, rapid heartbeat, weight loss, nervous and agitated behavior, and a general inability to relax. *Graves' disease* is one form of hyperthyroidism. In addition to the symptoms of hyperthyroidism given earlier, the thyroid gland enlarges and the eyes may bulge, or protrude anteriorly (a condition called *exophthalmos* (ek"sof-thal'mos) (Figure 9.12). Hyperthyroidism may be treated surgically by removal of part of the thyroid (and/or a tumor if present) or chemically by administering thyroid-blocking drugs or radioactive iodine, which destroy some of the thyroid cells. ▲

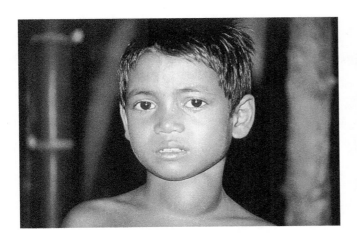

FIGURE 9.11   Goiter. An enlarged thyroid (goiter) of a boy from Bangladesh.

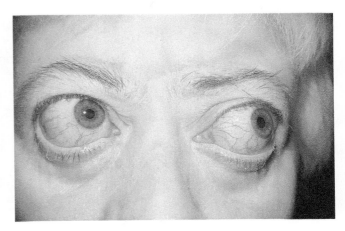

FIGURE 9.12   The exophthalmos of Graves' disease.

The second important hormone product of the thyroid gland, **calcitonin**, or **thyrocalcitonin**, decreases blood calcium levels by causing calcium to be deposited in the bones. It acts antagonistically to parathyroid hormone, the hormone produced by the parathyroid glands. Whereas thyroxine is made and stored in follicles before it is released to the blood, calcitonin is made by the so-called **C (parafollicular) cells** found in the connective tissue *between* the follicles (Figure 9.10b). It is released directly to the blood in response to increasing levels of blood calcium. Few effects of hypo- or hypersecretion of calcitonin are known, but it is believed that calcitonin production is meager or ceases in elderly adults. This may help to explain (at least in part) the progressive decalcification of bones that accompanies aging.

Parathyroid Glands

The **parathyroid glands** are tiny masses of glandular tissue most often found on the posterior surface of the thyroid gland (see Figure 9.6). Typically, there are two glands on each thyroid lobe; that is, a total of four, but as many as eight have been reported, and some may be in other regions of the neck. The parathyroids secrete **parathyroid hormone (PTH),** or **parathormone** (par″ah-thor′mōn), which is the most important regulator of calcium ion (Ca^{2+}) homeostasis of the blood. When blood calcium levels drop below a certain level, the parathyroids release PTH, which stimulates bone destruction cells (osteoclasts) to break down bone matrix and release calcium into the blood. Thus, PTH is a *hypercalcemic*

hormone (that is, it acts to increase blood levels of calcium), whereas calcitonin is a *hypocalcemic* hormone. The negative feedback interaction between these two hormones as they control blood calcium level is illustrated in Figure 9.13. Although the skeleton is the major PTH target, PTH also stimulates the kidneys and intestine to absorb more calcium (from urinary filtrate and foodstuffs, respectively).

Homeostatic Imbalance

If blood calcium levels fall too low, neurons become extremely irritable and overactive. They deliver impulses to the muscles at such a rapid rate that the muscles go into uncontrollable spasms *(tetany),* which may be fatal. Before surgeons knew the importance of these tiny glands on the backside of the thyroid, they would remove a hyperthyroid patient's gland entirely. Many times this resulted in death. Once it was revealed that the parathyroids are functionally very different from the thyroid gland, surgeons began to leave at least some parathyroid-containing tissue (if at all possible) to take care of blood calcium homeostasis.

Severe hyperparathyroidism causes massive bone destruction—an X-ray examination of the bones shows large punched-out holes in the bony matrix. The bones become very fragile, and spontaneous fractures begin to occur. ▲

Adrenal Glands (Suprarenal)

As illustrated in Figure 9.6, the two bean-shaped **adrenal glands** curve over the top of the kidneys.

Q *What effect would removal of the parathyroid glands have on blood calcium levels?*

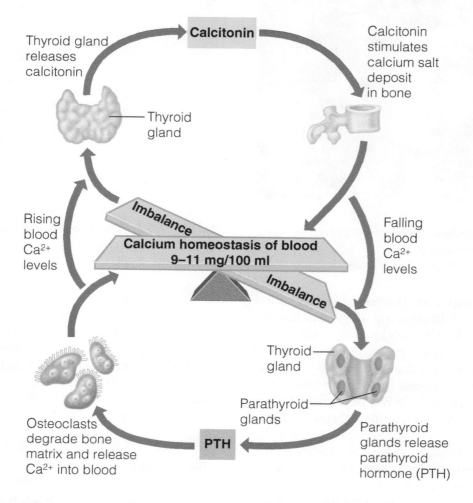

FIGURE 9.13 **Hormonal controls of ionic calcium levels in the blood.** PTH and calcitonin operate in negative feedback control systems that influence each other.

Although the adrenal gland looks like a single organ, it is structurally and functionally two endocrine organs in one. Much like the pituitary gland, it has glandular (cortex) and neural tissue (medulla) parts. The central medulla region is enclosed by the adrenal cortex, which contains three separate layers of cells.

Hormones of the Adrenal Cortex

The **adrenal cortex** produces three major groups of steroid hormones collectively called **cortico-** **steroids** (kor″ti-ko-ster′oidz)—mineralocorticoids, glucocorticoids, and sex hormones.

The **mineralocorticoids**, mainly **aldosterone** (al″dos-ter′ōn), are produced by the outermost adrenal cortex cell layer. As their name suggests, the mineralocorticoids are important in regulating the mineral (or salt) content of the blood, particularly the concentrations of sodium and potassium ions. Their target is the kidney tubules that selectively reabsorb the minerals or allow them to be flushed out of the body in urine. When blood levels of aldosterone rise, the kidney tubule cells reclaim increasing amounts of sodium ions and secrete more potassium ions into the urine. When sodium is reabsorbed, water follows. Thus, the mineralocorticoids help regulate both water and

A *Blood calcium levels would drop because the bones would no longer be exposed to the bone-digesting stimulus of PTH.*

electrolyte balance in body fluids. As shown in Figure 9.14, the release of aldosterone is stimulated by humoral factors such as fewer sodium ions or more potassium ions in the blood (and by ACTH to a lesser degree). **Renin,** an enzyme produced by the kidneys when blood pressure drops, also causes the release of aldosterone by triggering a series of reactions that form **angiostensin II,** a potent stimulator of aldosterone release. A hormone released by the heart, **atrial natriuretic (na″tre-u-ret′ik) peptide (ANP),** prevents aldosterone release, its goal being to *reduce* blood volume and blood pressure.

The middle cortical layer produces **glucocorticoids,** which include **cortisone** and **cortisol.** Glucocorticoids promote normal cell metabolism and help the body to resist *long-term stressors,*

primarily by increasing blood glucose levels. When blood levels of glucocorticoids are high, fats and even proteins are broken down by body cells and converted to glucose, which is released to the blood. For this reason, glucocorticoids are said to be *hyperglycemic hormones.* Glucocorticoids also seem to control the more unpleasant effects of inflammation by decreasing edema, and they reduce pain by inhibiting some pain-causing molecules called *prostaglandins* (see Table 9.3). Because of their anti-inflammatory properties, glucocorticoids are often prescribed as drugs to suppress inflammation for patients with rheumatoid arthritis and poison ivy. Glucocorticoids are released from the adrenal cortex in response to rising blood levels of ACTH.

Regardless of one's gender, both male and female **sex hormones** are produced by the adrenal

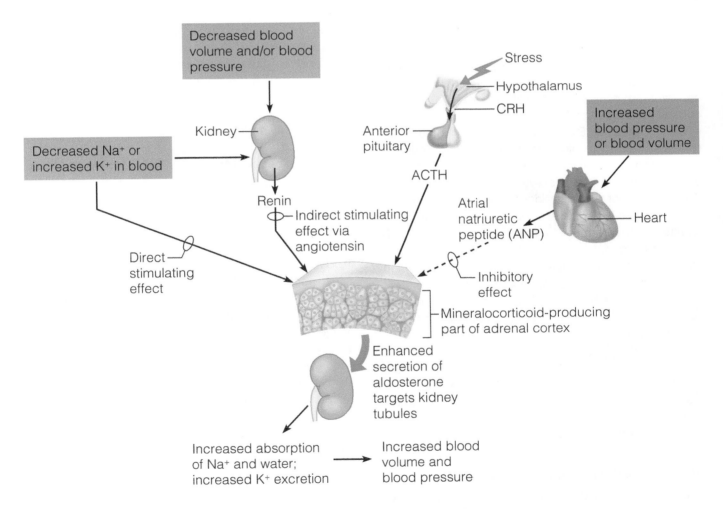

FIGURE 9.14 Major mechanisms controlling aldosterone release from the adrenal cortex. Solid arrows indicate factors that stimulate aldosterone release; dashed arrow indicates an inhibitory factor.

cortex throughout life in relatively small amounts. Although the bulk of the sex hormones produced by the innermost cortex layer are **androgens** (male sex hormones), some **estrogens** (female sex hormones) are also formed.

Homeostatic Imbalance

A generalized hyposecretion of all the adrenal cortex hormones leads to *Addison's disease*. A major sign of Addison's disease is a peculiar bronze tone of the skin. Because aldosterone levels are low, sodium and water are lost from the body, which leads to problems with electrolyte and water balance. This, in turn, causes the muscles to become weak, and shock is a possibility. Other signs and symptoms of Addison's disease include those resulting from deficient levels of glucocorticoids, such as hypoglycemia, a lessened ability to cope with stress (burnout), and suppression of the immune system (and thereby increased susceptibility to infection). A complete lack of glucocorticoids is incompatible with life.

Hypersecretion problems are generally the result of tumors, and the resulting condition depends on the cortical area involved. Hyperactivity of the outermost cortical area results in *hyperaldosteronism* (hi"per-al"dos-ter'on-izm). Excessive water and sodium are retained, leading to high blood pressure and edema, and potassium is lost to such an extent that the activity of the heart and nervous system may be disrupted. When the tumor is in the middle cortical area, *Cushing's syndrome* occurs. Excessive output of glucocorticoids results in a "moon face" and the appearance of a "buffalo hump" of fat on the upper back (Figure 9.15). Other common and undesirable effects include high blood pressure, hyperglycemia and possible diabetes, weakening of the bones (as protein is withdrawn to be converted to glucose), and severe depression of the immune system.

Hypersecretion of the sex hormones leads to *masculinization*, regardless of sex. In adult males, these effects may be masked, but in females, the results are often dramatic. A beard develops, and a masculine pattern of body hair distribution occurs, among other things. ▲

Hormones of the Adrenal Medulla

The **adrenal medulla,** like the posterior pituitary, develops from a knot of nervous tissue. When the medulla is stimulated by sympathetic nervous system neurons, its cells release two similar hormones, **epinephrine** (ep"ĭ-nef'rin), also called **adrenaline,** and **norepinephrine (noradrenaline),** into the bloodstream. Collectively, these hormones are referred to as **catecholamines** (kat"ĕ-kol-ah'menz). Since some sympathetic neurons also release norepinephrine as a neurotransmitter, the adrenal medulla is often thought of as a "misplaced sympathetic nervous system ganglion."

When you are (or feel) threatened physically or emotionally, your sympathetic nervous system brings about the "fight-or-flight" response to help you cope with the stressful situation. One of the organs it stimulates is the adrenal medulla, which literally pumps its hormones into the bloodstream to enhance and prolong the effects of the neurotransmitters of the sympathetic nervous system. Basically, the catecholamines increase heart rate, blood pressure, and blood glucose levels and dilate the small passageways of the lungs. These events result in more oxygen and glucose in the blood and a faster circulation of blood to the body organs (most importantly, to the brain, muscles, and heart). Thus, the body is better able to deal with a short-term stressor, whether the job at hand is to fight, begin the inflammatory process, or make you more alert so you think more clearly.

The catecholamines of the adrenal medulla prepare the body to cope with a brief or short-term stressful situation and cause the so-called *alarm stage* of the stress response. Glucocorticoids, by contrast, are produced by the adrenal cortex and are more important in helping the body to cope with prolonged or continuing stressors, such as dealing with the death of a family member or having a major operation. Glucocorticoids operate primarily during the *resistance stage* of the stress response. If they are successful in protecting the body, the problem will eventually be resolved without lasting damage to the body. When the stress continues on and on, the adrenal cortex may simply "burn out," which is usually fatal. The relationship of catecholamines and glucocorticoids in the stress response is shown in Figure 9.16.

Homeostatic Imbalance

Damage or destruction of the adrenal medulla has no major effects as long as the sympathetic nervous system neurons continue to function normally. However, hypersecretion of catecholamines leads to

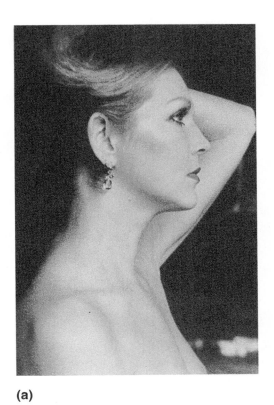

(a)

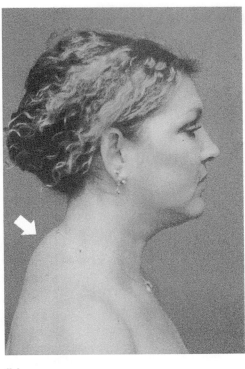

(b)

FIGURE 9.15 **Appearance of a woman (a) before and (b) during Cushing's disease.** The characteristic "buffalo hump" of fat on the woman's upper back is indicated by a white arrow.

symptoms typical of excessive sympathetic nervous system activity—a rapidly beating heart, high blood pressure, and a tendency to perspire and be very irritable. Surgical removal of the catecholamine-secreting cells corrects this condition. ▲

Pancreatic Islets

The **pancreas,** located close to the stomach in the abdominal cavity (see Figure 9.6), is a mixed gland. Probably the best-hidden endocrine glands in the body are the **pancreatic islets,** formerly called the *islets of Langerhans* (lahng'er-hanz). These little masses of hormone-producing tissue are scattered among the enzyme-producing acinar tissue of the pancreas. The **exocrine** (enzyme-producing) part of the pancreas, which acts as part of the digestive system, will be discussed later; only the pancreatic islets will be considered here.

Although there are more than a million islets, separated by exocrine cells, each of these tiny clumps of cells busily manufactures its hormones and works like an organ within an organ. Two important hormones produced by the islet cells are **insulin** and **glucagon** (gloo'kah-gon). The islets also produce small amounts of other hormones, but those will not be discussed here.

High levels of glucose in the blood stimulate the release of insulin from the **beta** (ba'tah) **cells** (Figure 9.17) of the islets. Insulin acts on just about all body cells and increases their ability to transport glucose across their plasma membranes. Once inside the cells, glucose is oxidized for energy or converted to glycogen for energy or fat for storage. These activities are also speeded up by insulin. Since insulin sweeps the glucose out of the blood, its effect is said to be *hypoglycemic.* As blood glucose levels fall, the stimulus for insulin release ends—another classic case of negative feedback control. Many hormones have hyperglycemic effects (glucagon, glucocorticoids, and epinephrine, to name a few), but insulin is the only hormone that decreases blood glucose levels. Insulin is absolutely necessary for the use of glucose by the body cells. Without it, essentially no glucose can get into the cells to be used.

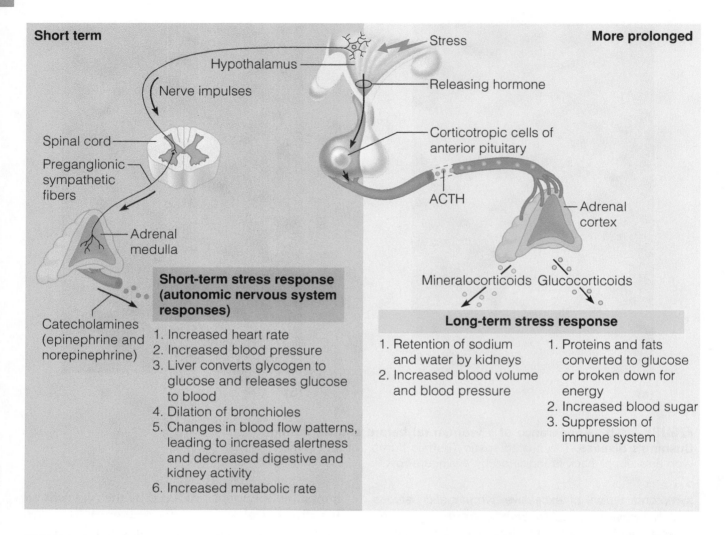

Short term

Stress

Hypothalamus

Nerve impulses

Releasing hormone

Spinal cord

Corticotropic cells of anterior pituitary

Preganglionic sympathetic fibers

ACTH

More prolonged

Adrenal medulla

Adrenal cortex

Catecholamines (epinephrine and norepinephrine)

Mineralocorticoids   Glucocorticoids

Short-term stress response (autonomic nervous system responses)

1. Increased heart rate
2. Increased blood pressure
3. Liver converts glycogen to glucose and releases glucose to blood
4. Dilation of bronchioles
5. Changes in blood flow patterns, leading to increased alertness and decreased digestive and kidney activity
6. Increased metabolic rate

Long-term stress response

1. Retention of sodium and water by kidneys
2. Increased blood volume and blood pressure

1. Proteins and fats converted to glucose or broken down for energy
2. Increased blood sugar
3. Suppression of immune system

FIGURE 9.16 Roles of the hypothalamus, adrenal medulla, and adrenal cortex in the stress response. (Note that ACTH is only a weak stimulator of mineralocorticoid release under normal conditions.)

Homeostatic Imbalance

Without insulin, blood levels of glucose (which normally range from 80 to 120 mg/100 ml of blood) rise to dramatically high levels (for example, 600 mg/100 ml of blood). In such instances, glucose begins to spill into the urine because the kidney tubule cells cannot reabsorb it fast enough. As glucose flushes from the body, water follows, leading to dehydration. The clinical name for this condition is **diabetes mellitus** (me-li′tus), which literally means that something sweet (*mel* = honey) is passing through or siphoning (*diabetes* = Greek "siphon") from the body. Because cells cannot use glucose, fats and even proteins are broken down and used to meet the energy requirements of the body. As a result, body weight begins to decline. Loss of body proteins leads to a decreased ability to fight infections,

so diabetics must be careful with their hygiene and in caring for even small cuts and bruises. When large amounts of fats (instead of sugars) are used for energy, the blood becomes very acidic (**acidosis** [as″ĭ-do′sis]) as ketones (intermediate products of fat breakdown) appear in the blood. On the basis of cause, this condition of acidosis (as″i-do′sis) is referred to as **ketosis.** Unless corrected, coma and death result. The three cardinal signs of diabetes mellitus are (1) *polyuria* (pol″e-u′re-ah)—excessive urination to flush out the glucose and ketones; (2) *polydipsia* (pol″e-dip′se-ah)—excessive thirst resulting from water loss; and (3) *polyphagia* (pol″e-fa′je-ah)—hunger due to inability to use sugars and the loss of fat and proteins from the body.

Those with mild cases of diabetes mellitus (most cases of type II, or adult-onset, diabetes) produce

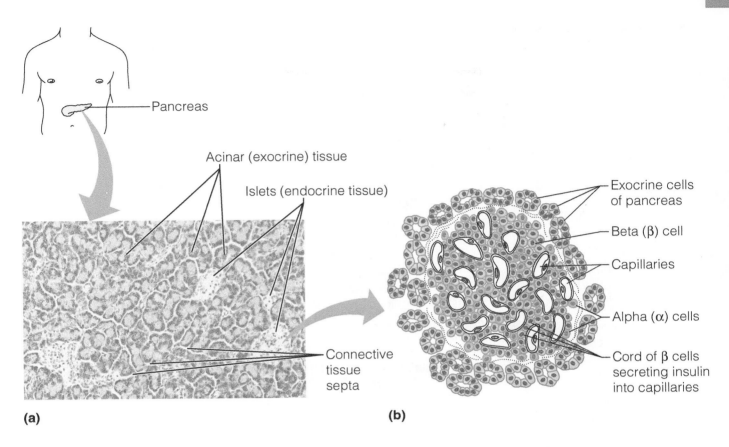

(a)

(b)

FIGURE 9.17 **Pancreatic tissue. (a)** Photomicrograph of pancreas with exocrine and endocrine (islets) areas clearly visible (110×). **(b)** Diagrammatic view of a pancreatic islet. Beta cells produce insulin, which aids cells in taking up glucose from the blood. Alpha cells produce glucagon, which stimulates liver cells to release glucose to the blood.

insulin, but for some reason, their insulin receptors are unable to respond to it, a situation called **insulin resistance.** Type II diabetics are treated with special diets or oral hypoglycemic medications that prod the sluggish islets into action and increase the sensitivity of the target tissues to insulin and of beta cells to the stimulating effects of glucose. To regulate blood glucose levels in the more severe type I (juvenile, or brittle) diabetic, insulin is infused continuously by an insulin pump worn externally, or a regimen of carefully planned insulin injections is administered throughout the day. ▲

Glucagon acts as an antagonist of insulin; that is, it helps to regulate blood glucose levels but in a way opposite to that of insulin (Figure 9.18). Its release by the **alpha** (al′fah) **cells** (see Figure 9.17b) of the islets is stimulated by low blood levels of glucose. Its action is basically hyperglycemic. Its

primary target organ is the liver, which it stimulates to break down stored glycogen to glucose and to release the glucose into the blood. No important disorders resulting from hypo- or hypersecretion of glucagon are known.

Pineal Gland

The **pineal** (pin′e-al) **body,** also called the **pineal gland,** is a small, cone-shaped gland found in the roof of the third ventricle of the brain (see Figure 9.6). The endocrine function of this tiny gland is still somewhat of a mystery. Although many chemical substances have been identified in the pineal gland, only the hormone **melatonin** (mel″ah-to′nin) appears to be secreted in substantial amounts. The levels of melatonin rise and fall during the course of the day and night. Peak levels

Q *What happens to the liver's ability to synthesize and store glycogen when glucagon blood levels rise?*

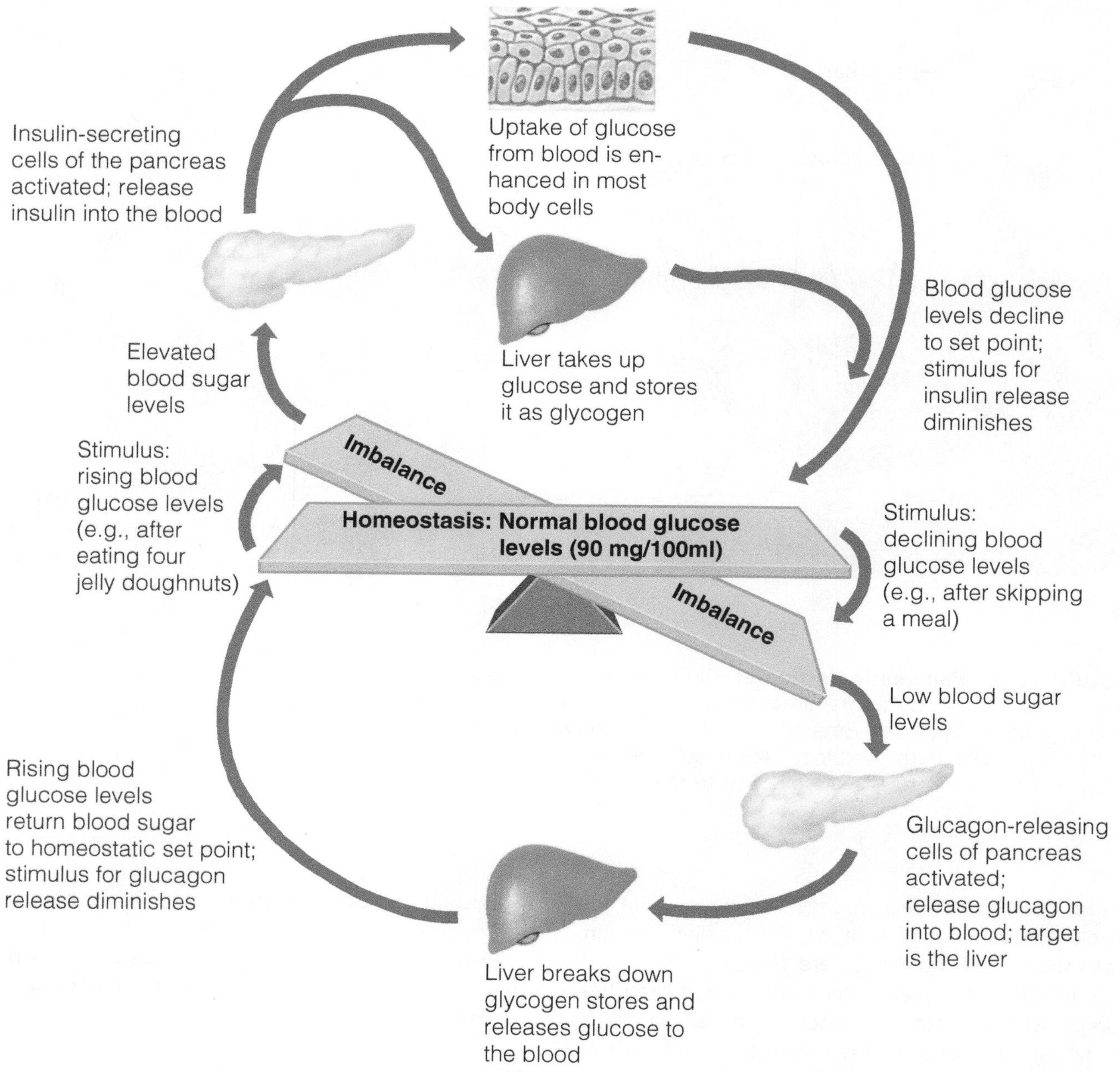

Insulin-secreting cells of the pancreas activated; release insulin into the blood

Uptake of glucose from blood is enhanced in most body cells

Elevated blood sugar levels

Liver takes up glucose and stores it as glycogen

Blood glucose levels decline to set point; stimulus for insulin release diminishes

Stimulus: rising blood glucose levels (e.g., after eating four jelly doughnuts)

Imbalance

Homeostasis: Normal blood glucose levels (90 mg/100ml)

Imbalance

Stimulus: declining blood glucose levels (e.g., after skipping a meal)

Low blood sugar levels

Rising blood glucose levels return blood sugar to homeostatic set point; stimulus for glucagon release diminishes

Glucagon-releasing cells of pancreas activated; release glucagon into blood; target is the liver

Liver breaks down glycogen stores and releases glucose to the blood

FIGURE 9.18 Regulation of blood glucose levels by a negative feedback mechanism involving pancreatic hormones.

occur at night and make us drowsy; the lowest levels occur during daylight around noon. Melatonin is believed to be a "sleep trigger" that plays an important role in establishing the body's day-night cycle. In some animals, melatonin also helps regulate mating behavior and rhythms. In humans, it is believed to coordinate the hormones of fertility and to inhibit the reproductive system (especially the ovaries of females) so that sexual maturation is prevented from occurring before adult body size has been reached.

A *Glucagon inhibits those activities in the liver, so the liver's ability to perform them would decrease as glucagon levels rise.*

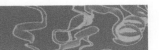

TABLE 9.2	Major Endocrine Glands and Some of Their Hormones

Gland		Hormone	Chemical class	Representative actions	Regulated by
Pineal body		Melatonin	Amine	Involved in biological rhythms (daily and seasonal)	Light/dark cycles
Hypothalamus		Hormones released by the posterior pituitary; releasing and inhibiting hormones that regulate the anterior pituitary (see below)			
Pituitary gland					
• Posterior lobe (releases hormones made by the hypothalamus)		Oxytocin	Peptide	Stimulates contraction of uterus and the milk "let-down" reflex	Nervous system (hypothalamus) in response to uterine stretching and/or suckling of a baby
		Antidiuretic hormone (ADH)	Peptide	Promotes retention of water by kidneys	Hypothalamus in response to water/salt imbalance
• Anterior lobe		Growth hormone (GH)	Protein	Stimulates growth (especially of bones and muscles) and metabolism	Hypothalamic releasing and inhibiting hormones
		Prolactin (PRL)	Protein	Stimulates milk production	Hypothalamic hormones
		Follicle-stimulating hormone (FSH)	Protein	Stimulates production of ova and sperm	Hypothalamic hormones
		Luteinizing hormone (LH), also called interstitial cell stimulating hormone (ICSH)	Protein	Stimulates ovaries and testes	Hypothalamic hormones
		Thyroid-stimulating hormone (TSH)	Protein	Stimulates thyroid gland	Thyroxine in blood; hypothalamic hormones
		Adrenocorticotropic hormone (ACTH)	Protein	Stimulates adrenal cortex to secrete glucocorticoids	Glucocorticoids; hypothalamic hormones
Thyroid gland		Thyroxine (T_4) and triiodothyronine (T_3)	Amine	Stimulates metabolism	TSH

(continued)

TABLE 9.2   *(continued)*

Gland	Hormone	Chemical class	Representative actions	Regulated by
Thyroid gland	Calcitonin	Peptide	Reduces blood calcium level	Calcium level in blood
Parathyroid glands	Parathyroid hormone (PTH)	Peptide	Raises blood calcium level	Calcium level in blood
Thymus gland	Thymosin	Peptide	"Programs" T lymphocytes	Not known
Adrenal glands				
• Adrenal medulla	Epinephrine and norepinephrine	Amines	Raise blood glucose level; increase rate of metabolism; constrict certain blood vessels	Nervous system (sympathetic division)
• Adrenal cortex	Glucocorticoids	Steroids	Increase blood glucose	ACTH
	Mineralocorticoids	Steroids	Promote reabsorption of Na^+ and excretion of K^+ in kidneys	Changes in blood volume or blood pressure; K^+ (potassium) or Na^+ levels in blood
Pancreas	Insulin	Protein	Reduces blood glucose	Glucose level in blood
	Glucagon	Protein	Raises blood glucose	Glucose level in blood
Gonads				
• Testes	Androgens	Steroids	Support sperm formation; development and maintenance of male secondary sex characteristics	FSH and LH
• Ovaries	Estrogens	Steroids	Stimulate uterine lining growth; development and maintenance of female secondary sex characteristics	FSH and LH
	Progesterone	Steroids	Promotes growth of uterine lining	FSH and LH

Thymus Gland

The **thymus gland** is located in the upper thorax, posterior to the sternum. Large in infants and children, it decreases in size throughout adulthood. By old age, it is composed mostly of fibrous connective tissue and fat. The thymus produces a hormone called **thymosin** (thi′mo-sin), and during childhood the thymus acts as an incubator for the maturation of a special group of white blood cells (*T lymphocytes,* or *T cells*) that are important in the immune response. The role of the thymus (and its hormones) in immunity is described along with the lymphatic system in Chapter 12.

Gonads

The female and male gonads (see Figure 9.6) produce sex hormones that are identical to those produced by adrenal cortex cells. The major differences are the source and relative amounts produced.

Hormones of the Ovaries

The female *gonads* (go′nadz), or **ovaries,** are paired, almond-sized organs located in the pelvic cavity. Besides producing female sex cells (ova, or eggs), ovaries produce two groups of steroid hormones, *estrogens* and *progesterone*. The ovaries do not really begin to function until puberty, when the anterior pituitary gonadotropic hormones stimulate them into activity. This results in the rhythmic ovarian cycles in which ova develop and blood levels of ovarian hormones rise and fall.

Estrogens, primarily **estrone** (es′trōn) and **estradiol** (es″trah-di′ol), produced by the **Graafian follicles** of the ovaries, stimulate the development of the secondary sex characteristics in females (primarily growth and maturation of the reproductive organs and the appearance of hair in the pubic and axillary regions). In addition, the estrogens work with progesterone to prepare the uterus to receive a fertilized egg. This results in cyclic changes in the uterine lining, which is called the **menstrual cycle.** Estrogens also help maintain pregnancy and prepare the breasts to produce milk (lactation). However, the placenta and not the ovaries is the source of the estrogens at this time.

Progesterone (pro-jes′tĕ-rōn), as already noted, acts with estrogen to bring about the menstrual cycle. During pregnancy, it quiets the muscles of the uterus so that an implanted embryo will not be aborted and helps prepare breast tissue for lactation. Progesterone is produced by another glandular structure of the ovaries, the **corpus luteum** (lu′te-um). The corpus luteum produces both estrogen and progesterone, but progesterone is secreted in larger amounts.

Ovaries are stimulated to release their estrogens and progesterone in a cyclic way by the anterior pituitary gonadotropic hormones. More detail on this feedback cycle and on the structure and function of the ovaries is given in Chapter 16 on reproduction but it should be obvious that hyposecretion of the ovarian hormones severely hampers the ability of a woman to conceive and bear children.

Hormones of the Testes

The paired oval **testes** of the male are suspended in a sac, the *scrotum,* outside the pelvic cavity. In addition to male sex cells, or *sperm,* the testes also produce male sex hormones, or **androgens,** of which **testosterone** (tes-tos′tĕ-rōn) is the most important. Testosterone, made by the **interstitial cells** of the testes, causes development of the adult male sex characteristics. It promotes the growth and maturation of the reproductive system organs to prepare the young man for reproduction. It also causes the male's secondary sex characteristics (growth of facial hair, development of heavy bones and muscles, and lowering of the voice) to appear and stimulates the male sex drive.

In adults, testosterone is necessary for continuous production of sperm. In cases of hyposecretion, the man becomes sterile; such cases are usually treated by testosterone injections. Both the endocrine and exocrine functions of the testes begin at puberty under the influence of the anterior pituitary gonadotropic hormones. Testosterone production is specifically stimulated by LH. Chapter 16, which deals with the reproductive system, contains more information on the structure and exocrine function of the testes.

Other Hormone-Producing Tissues and Organs

Besides the major endocrine organs, pockets of hormone-producing cells are found in fatty tissue and in the walls of the small intestine, stomach, kidneys, and heart—organs whose chief functions have little to do with hormone production. The placenta, a temporary organ formed during pregnancy, produces hormones generally thought of as ovarian hormones (estrogen and progesterone). Additionally, certain tumor cells, such as those of some lung and pancreatic cancers, make hormones identical to those made in normal endocrine glands but in an excessive and uncontrolled fashion.

Because most of these hormones are described in later chapters, their chief characteristics are only summarized in Table 9.3. Only the placenta is considered further here.

Placenta

The **placenta** (plah-sen'tah) is a remarkable organ formed temporarily in the uterus of pregnant women. In addition to its roles as the respiratory, excretory, and nutrition-delivery systems for the fetus, it also produces hormones that help to maintain the pregnancy and pave the way for delivery of the baby.

During very early pregnancy, a hormone called **human chorionic** (ko"re-on'ik) **gonadotropin (hCG)** is produced by the developing embryo and then by the fetal part of the placenta. Similar to LH (luteinizing hormone), hCG stimulates the corpus luteum of the ovary to *continue* producing estrogen and progesterone so that the lining of the uterus is not sloughed off in menses. (The home pregnancy tests sold over the counter test for the presence of hCG in the woman's urine.) In the third month, the placenta assumes the job of producing *estrogen* and *progesterone*, and the ovaries become inactive for the rest of the pregnancy. The high estrogen and progesterone blood levels maintain the lining of the uterus (thus, the pregnancy) and prepare the breasts for producing milk. *Human placental lactogen (hPL)* works cooperatively with estrogen and progesterone in preparing the breasts for lactation, and *relaxin,* another placental hormone, causes the mother's pelvic ligaments and the pubic symphysis to relax and become more flexible, which eases birth passage.

TABLE 9.3	Hormones Produced by Organs Other Than the Major Endocrine Organs			
Hormone	**Chemical composition**	**Source**	**Stimulus for secretion**	**Target organ/Effects**
Prostaglandins (PGs); several groups indicated by letters A–I (PGA–PGI)	Derived from fatty acid molecules	Plasma membranes of virtually all body cells	Various (local irritation, hormones, etc.)	Have many targets, but act locally at site of release. Examples of effects include: increase blood pressure by acting as vasoconstrictors; cause constriction of respiratory passageways; stimulate muscle of the uterus promoting labor; enhance blood clotting; promote inflammation and pain; increase output of digestive secretions by stomach; cause fever
Gastrin	Peptide	Stomach	Food	*Stomach:* stimulates glands to release hydrochloric acid (HCl)
Intestinal gastrin	Peptide	Duodenum of small intestine (enteroendocrine glands)	Food, especially fats	*Stomach:* inhibits HCl secretion and gastrointestinal tract mobility

(continued)

TABLE 9.3 *(continued)*

Hormone	Chemical composition	Source	Stimulus for secretion	Target organ/Effects
Secretin	Peptide	Duodenum (enteroendocrine glands in walls of duodenum)	Food	*Pancreas:* stimulates release of bicarbonate-rich juice *Liver:* increases release of bile *Stomach:* inhibits secretory activity
Cholecystokinin (CCK)	Peptide	Duodenum (enteroendocrine glands)	Food	*Pancreas:* stimulates release of enzyme-rich juice *Gallbladder:* stimulates expulsion of stored bile *Duodenal papilla:* causes sphincter to relax, allowing bile and pancreatic juice to enter duodenum
Erythropoietin	Glycoprotein	Kidney	Hypoxia	*Bone marrow:* stimulates production of red blood cells
Renin		Kidney		Increase blood flow and pressure
Active vitamin D_3	Steroid	Kidney (activates vitamin D made by epidermal cells of skin)	PTH	*Intestine:* stimulates active transport of dietary calcium across intestinal cell membranes
Atrial natriuretic peptide (ANP)	Peptide	Heart	Stretching of heart	*Kidney:* inhibits sodium ion reabsorption and renin release *Adrenal cortex:* inhibits secretion of aldosterone
Leptin	Peptide	Adipose tissue	Fatty foods	*Brain:* suppresses appetite and increases energy expenditure

Systems in Sync

Homeostatic Relationships between the Endocrine System and Other Body Systems

Endocrine System

Nervous System
- Many hormones (growth hormone, thyroxine, sex hormones) influence normal maturation and function of the nervous system
- Hypothalamus controls anterior pituitary function

Respiratory System
- Epinephrine influences ventilation (dilates bronchioles)
- Respiratory system provides oxygen; disposes of carbon dioxide; converting enzyme in lungs converts angiotensin I to angiotensin II

Lymphatic System/Immunity
- Lymphocytes "programmed" by thymic hormones seed the lymph nodes; glucocorticoids depress the immune response and inflammation
- Lymph provides a route for transport of hormones

Cardiovascular System
- Several hormones influence blood volume, blood pressure, and heart contractility; erythropoietin stimulates red blood cell production
- Blood is the main transport medium of hormones; heart produces atrial natriuretic peptide

Digestive System
- Local gastro-intestinal (GI) hormones influence GI function; activated vitamin D necessary to absorb calcium from diet; catecholamines influence digestive system activity
- Digestive system provides nutrients to endocrine organs

Reproductive System
- Hypothalamic, anterior pituitary, and gonadal hormones direct reproductive system development and function; oxytocin and prolactin involved in birth and breastfeeding
- Gonadal hormones feed back to influence endocrine system function

Urinary System
- Aldosterone and ADH influence renal function; erythropoietin released by kidneys promotes red blood cell formation
- Kidneys activate vitamin D (considered a hormone)

Integumentary System
- Androgens activate sebaceous glands; estrogen increases skin hydration
- Skin produces a precursor of vitamin D (cholecalciferol or provitamin D)

Muscular System
- Growth hormone is essential for normal muscular development; other hormones (thyroxine and catecholamines) influence muscle metabolism
- Muscular system mechanically protects some endocrine glands; muscular activity promotes catecholamine release

Skeletal System
- PTH and calcitonin regulate calcium blood levels; growth hormone, T_3, T_4, and sex hormones are necessary for normal skeletal development
- The skeleton protects some endocrine organs, especially those in brain, chest, and pelvis

Unit 5

Maintenance of the Human Body

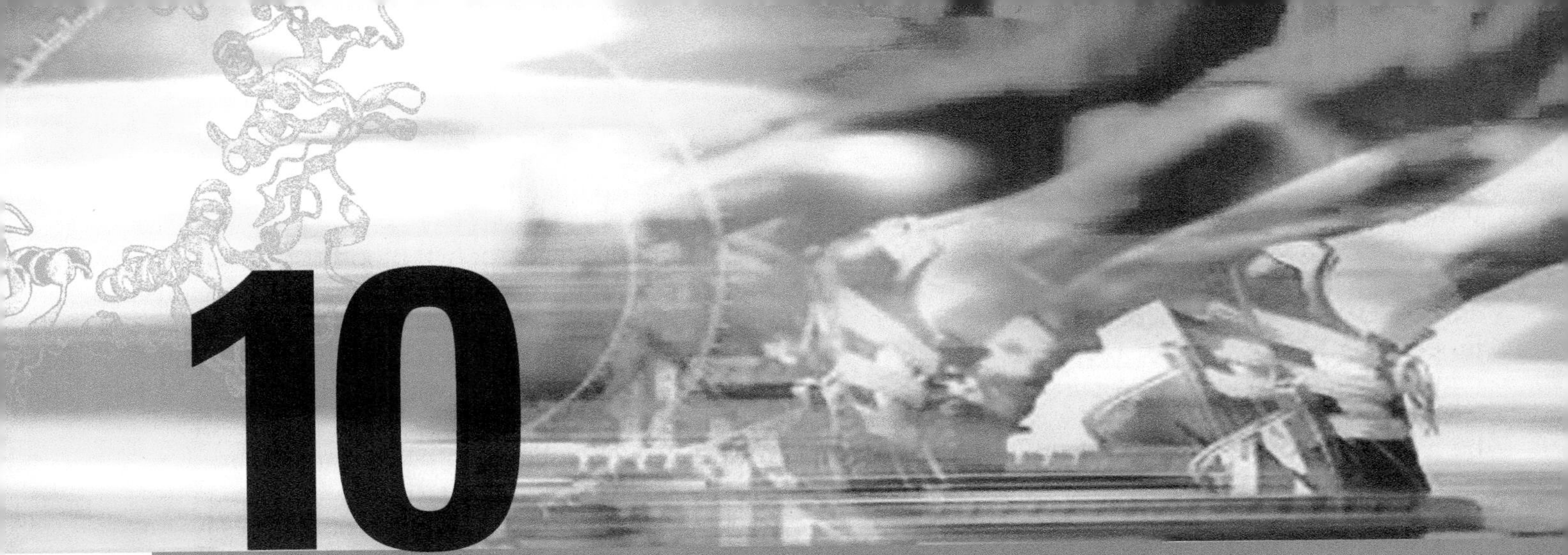

10

The Cardiovascular System: The Blood

KEY TERMS

- plasma, p. 346
- coagulation, p. 353
- serum, p. 354

Blood is the "river of life" that surges within us. It transports everything that must be carried from one place to another within the body—nutrients, wastes (headed for elimination from the body), and body heat—through blood vessels. For centuries, long before modern medicine, people recognized that blood was vital (some believed "magical"), and its loss was always considered to be a possible cause of death. In this chapter, we consider the composition and function of this life-sustaining fluid.

Composition and Functions of Blood

Components

Among all of the body's tissues, blood is unique: It is the only *fluid* tissue. Although blood appears to be a thick, homogeneous liquid, the microscope reveals it has both solid and liquid components. Essentially, blood is a complex connective tissue in which living blood cells, the **formed elements,** are suspended in a nonliving fluid of the blood called **plasma** (plaz'muh).

If a sample of blood is spun in a centrifuge, the heavier formed elements are packed down by centrifugal force and the plasma rises to the top (Figure 10.1). Most of the reddish mass at the bottom of the tube consists of *erythrocytes* (eh-rith'ro-sīts), the red blood cells that function in oxygen transport. Although it is barely visible in Figure 10.1, there is a thin, whitish layer called the **buffy coat** at the junction between the formed elements and the plasma. This layer contains *leukocytes* (lu'ko-sīts; *leuko* = white), the white blood cells that act in various ways to protect the body, and *platelets,* cell fragments that function in the blood-clotting process. Erythrocytes normally account for about 45 percent of the total volume of a blood sample, a percentage known as the **hematocrit.** White blood cells and platelets contribute less than 1 percent, and plasma makes up most of the remaining 55 percent of whole blood.

Physical Characteristics and Volume

Blood is a sticky opaque fluid with a characteristic metallic taste. As children, we discover its saltiness the first time we stick a cut finger into our mouth.

Depending on the amount of oxygen it is carrying, the color of blood varies from scarlet (oxygen-rich) to a dull red (oxygen-poor). Blood is heavier than water and about five times thicker, or more viscous, largely because of its formed elements, with a specific gravity of 1.057 for adults and 1.066 for infants. Blood is slightly alkaline, with a pH between 7.35 and 7.45. Its temperature (38°C, or 100.4°F) is always slightly higher than body temperature.

Blood accounts for approximately 8 percent of body weight, and its volume in healthy males is 5 to 6 liters, or approximately 6 quarts.

Plasma

Plasma, which is approximately 90 percent water, is the liquid part of the blood. Over 100 different substances are dissolved in this straw-colored fluid. Examples of dissolved substances include nutrients, salts (electrolytes), respiratory gases, hormones, plasma proteins, and various wastes and products of cell metabolism.

Plasma proteins are the most abundant solutes in plasma. Except for antibodies and protein-based hormones, most plasma proteins are made by the liver. The plasma proteins serve a variety of functions. For instance, **albumin** (al-bu'min) contributes to the osmotic pressure of blood, which acts to keep water in the bloodstream; clotting proteins help stem blood loss when a blood vessel is injured; and antibodies help protect the body from pathogens. Plasma proteins are *not* taken up by cells to be used as food fuels or metabolic nutrients, as are other solutes such as glucose, fatty acids, and oxygen.

The composition of plasma varies continuously as cells remove or add substances to the blood. Assuming a healthy diet, however, the composition of plasma is kept relatively constant by various homeostatic mechanisms of the body. For example, when blood proteins drop to undesirable levels, the liver is stimulated to make more proteins; when the blood starts to become too acid **(acidosis)** or too basic **(alkalosis),** both the respiratory system and the kidneys are called into action to restore it to its normal, slightly alkaline pH range of 7.35 to 7.45. Various body organs make literally dozens of adjustments day in and day out to maintain the many plasma solutes at life-sustaining levels. Besides transporting various substances around the body, plasma helps to distribute body heat evenly throughout the body.

Q *How would a decrease in the amount of plasma proteins affect plasma volume?*

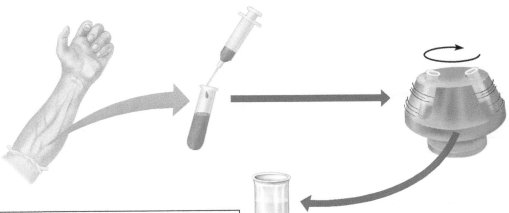

Plasma 55%	
Constituent	**Major Functions**
Water	Solvent for carrying other substances; absorbs heat
Salts (electrolytes) Sodium Potassium Calcium Magnesium Chloride Bicarbonate	Osmotic balance, pH buffering, regulation of membrane permeability
Plasma proteins Albumin—10%	Osmotic balance, pH buffering
Fibrinogen—4% Globulins—35%	Clotting of blood Defense (antibodies), hormones and lipid transport
Substances transported by blood Nutrients (glucose, fatty acids, amino acids, vitamins)	
Waste products of metabolism (urea, uric acid)	
Respiratory gases (O_2 and CO_2) Hormones	

Formed elements (cells) 45%		
Cell Type	**Number (per mm³ of blood)**	**Functions**
Erythrocytes (red blood cells)	4 – 6 million	Transport oxygen and help transport carbon dioxide
Leukocytes (white blood cells)	4000 – 11,000	Defense and immunity
Basophil		Lymphocyte
	Eosinophil	
Neutrophil		Monocyte
Platelets	250,000 – 500,000	Blood clotting

FIGURE 10.1 **The composition of blood.**

Formed Elements

If you observe a stained smear of human blood under a light microscope, you will see smooth, disc-shaped red blood cells, a variety of gaudily stained white blood cells, and, most likely, some scattered platelets that look like debris (Figure 10.2). However, erythrocytes vastly outnumber the other types of formed elements. Table 10.2 provides a summary of the important characteristics of the various formed elements that make up about 45 percent of whole blood.

Erythrocytes

Erythrocytes, or **red blood cells (RBCs),** function primarily to ferry oxygen in blood to all cells of the body. They are superb examples of the "fit" between cell structure and function. RBCs differ from other blood cells because they are *anucleate* (a-nu′kle-at); that is, they lack a nucleus. They also contain very few organelles. In fact, mature RBCs circulating in the blood are literally sacs of hemoglobin molecules.

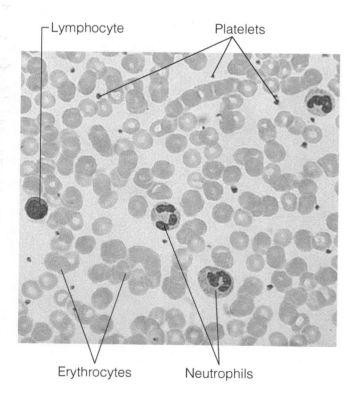

Lymphocyte   Platelets

Erythrocytes   Neutrophils

FIGURE 10.2 Photomicrograph of a blood smear. Most of the cells in this view are erythrocytes (red blood cells). Two kinds of leukocytes (white blood cells) are also present: lymphocytes and neutrophils. Also note the platelets.

Hemoglobin (he″mo-glo′bin) **(Hb),** an iron-bearing protein, transports the bulk of the oxygen that is carried in the blood. (It also binds with a small amount of carbon dioxide.) Moreover, because erythrocytes lack mitochondria and make ATP by anaerobic mechanisms, they do not use up any of the oxygen they are transporting, making them very efficient oxygen transporters indeed.

Erythrocytes are small cells shaped like biconcave discs—flattened discs with depressed centers on both sides (see Figures 10.2 and 10.3a). Because of their thinner centers, they look like miniature doughnuts when viewed with a microscope. Their small size and peculiar shape provide a large surface area relative to their volume, making them ideally suited for gas exchange.

RBCs outnumber white blood cells by about 1000 to 1 and are the major factor contributing to blood viscosity. Although the numbers of RBCs in the circulation do vary, there are normally about 5 million cells per cubic millimeter of blood. (A cubic millimeter [mm^3] is a very tiny drop of blood, almost not enough to be seen.) When the number of RBC/mm^3 increases, blood viscosity increases. Similarly, as the number of RBCs decreases, blood thins and flows more rapidly. However, let's not get carried away talking about RBC *numbers*. Although their numbers are important, it is the amount of hemoglobin in the bloodstream at any time that really determines how well the erythrocytes are performing their role of oxygen transport.

The more hemoglobin molecules the RBCs contain, the more oxygen they will be able to carry. Perhaps the most accurate way of measuring the oxygen-carrying capacity of the blood is to determine how much hemoglobin it contains. Since a single red blood cell contains about 250 million hemoglobin molecules, each capable of binding 4 molecules of oxygen, each of these tiny cells can carry about 1 billion molecules of oxygen! This information is astounding but not very practical. Much more important clinically is the fact that normal blood contains 12–18 grams (g) hemoglobin per 100 milliliters (ml) blood. The hemoglobin content is slightly higher in men (13–18 g) than in women (12–16 g).

Homeostatic Imbalance

A decrease in the oxygen-carrying ability of the blood, whatever the reason, is **anemia** (ah-ne′me-ah).

Anemia may be the result of (1) a lower-than-normal *number* of RBCs, or (2) abnormal or deficient *hemoglobin content* in the RBCs. Several types of anemia are classified and described briefly in Table 10.1, but one of these, *sickle cell anemia*, deserves a little more attention because people with this genetic disorder are frequently seen in hospital emergency rooms.

In sickle cell anemia (SCA), the abnormal hemoglobin formed becomes spiky and sharp (Figure 10.3b) when the RBCs unload oxygen molecules or when the oxygen content of the blood is lower than normal, as during vigorous exercise, anxiety, or other stressful situations. The deformed (crescent-shaped) erythrocytes rupture easily and dam up in small blood vessels. These events interfere with oxygen delivery and cause extreme pain. It is amazing that this havoc results from a change in just *one* of the amino acids in each of the beta chains of the globin molecule!

Sickle cell anemia occurs chiefly in black people who live in the malaria belt of Africa and among their descendants. Apparently, the same gene that causes sickling makes red blood cells infected by the malaria-causing parasite stick to the capillary walls and then lose potassium, an essential nutrient for survival of the parasite. Hence, the malaria-causing parasite is prevented from multiplying within the red blood cells, and individuals with the sickle cell gene have a better chance of surviving where malaria is prevalent. Only those carrying two copies of the defective gene have sickle cell anemia. Those carrying just one sickling gene have *sickle cell trait (SCT)*; they generally do not display the symptoms but can pass on the sickling gene to their offspring.

An excessive or abnormal increase in the number of erythrocytes is **polycythemia** (pol"e-si-the'me-ah). Polycythemia may result from bone marrow cancer *(polycythemia vera)*. It may also be a normal physiologic (homeostatic) response to living at high altitudes where the air is thinner and less oxygen is available *(secondary polycythemia)*. The major problem that results from excessive numbers of RBCs is increased blood viscosity, which causes it to flow sluggishly in the body and impairs circulation. ▲

Leukocytes

Although **leukocytes,** or **white blood cells (WBCs),** are far less numerous than red blood cells, they are crucial to body defense against disease. On average, there are 4000 to 11,000 WBCs/mm³, and they account for less than 1 percent of total blood volume. White blood cells are the only

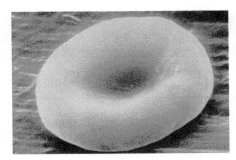

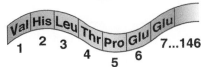

(a) Normal hemoglobin

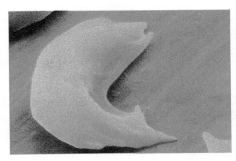

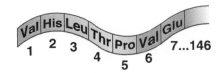

(b) Sickle cell hemoglobin

FIGURE 10.3 Comparison of (a) normal erythrocyte to a (b) sickled erythrocyte (31,500×).

complete cells in blood; that is, they contain nuclei and the usual organelles.

Leukocytes form a protective, movable army that helps defend the body against damage by bacteria, viruses, parasites, and tumor cells. As such, they have some very special characteristics. Red blood cells are confined to the bloodstream and carry out their functions in the blood. White blood cells, by contrast, are able to slip into and out of the blood vessels—a process called *diapedesis* (di"ah-peh-de'sis; "leaping across"). The circulatory system is simply their means of transportation to areas of the body where their services are needed for inflammatory or immune responses.

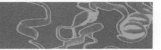

TABLE 10.1 Types of Anemia		
Direct cause	**Resulting from**	**Leading to**
Decrease in RBC number	Sudden hemorrhage	Hemorrhagic anemia
	Lysis of RBCs as a result of bacterial infections	Hemolytic (he"mo-lit'ik) anemia
	Lack of vitamin B_{12} (usually due to lack of intrinsic factor required for absorption of the vitamin; intrinsic factor is formed by stomach mucosa cells)	Pernicious (per-nish'us) anemia
	Depression/destruction of bone marrow by cancer, radiation, or certain medications	Aplastic anemia
Inadequate hemoglobin content in RBCs	Lack of iron in diet or slow/prolonged bleeding (such as heavy menstrual flow or bleeding ulcer), which depletes iron reserves needed to make hemoglobin; RBCs are small and pale because they lack hemoglobin	Iron deficiency anemia
Abnormal hemoglobin in RBCs	Genetic defect leads to abnormal hemoglobin, which becomes sharp and sickle-shaped under conditions of increased oxygen use by body; occurs mainly in people of African descent	Sickle cell anemia

In addition, WBCs can locate areas of tissue damage and infection in the body by responding to certain chemicals that diffuse from the damaged cells. This capability is called *positive chemotaxis* (ke"mo-tax'is). Once they have "caught the scent," the WBCs move through the tissue spaces by *ameboid* (ah-me'boid) *motion* (they form flowing cytoplasmic extensions that help move them along). By following the diffusion gradient, they pinpoint areas of tissue damage and rally round in large numbers to destroy microorganisms or dead cells.

Whenever WBCs mobilize for action, the body speeds up their production, and as many as twice the normal number of WBCs may appear in the blood within a few hours. A total WBC count above 11,000 cells/mm^3 is referred to as **leukocytosis** (lu"ko-si-to'sis). Leukocytosis generally indicates that a bacterial or viral infection is stewing in the body. The opposite condition, **leukopenia** (lu"ko-pe'ne-ah), is an abnormally low WBC count. It is commonly caused by certain drugs, such as corticosteroids and anticancer agents.

Homeostatic Imbalance

Leukocytosis is a normal and desirable response to infectious threats to the body. By contrast, the excessive production of abnormal WBCs that occurs in infectious mononucleosis and leukemia is distinctly pathological. In **leukemia** (lu-ke'me-ah), literally "white blood," the bone marrow becomes cancerous, and huge numbers of WBCs are turned out rapidly. Although this might not appear to present a problem, the "newborn" WBCs are immature and incapable of carrying out their normal protective functions. Consequently, the body becomes the easy prey of disease-causing bacteria and viruses. ▲

WBCs are classified into two major groups, depending on whether or not they contain visible granules in their cytoplasm. Specific characteristics of the leukocytes are listed in Table 10.2. Microscopic views can be seen in Figure 10.1.

Granulocytes (gran'u-lo-sītz") are granule-containing WBCs. They have lobed nuclei, which typically consist of several rounded nuclear areas

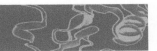

TABLE 10.2   Characteristics of Formed Elements of the Blood

Cell type	Occurrence in blood (per mm³)	Cell anatomy*	Function
Erythrocytes (red blood cells, or RBCs)	4–6 million	Salmon-colored biconcave disks; anucleate; literally, sacs of hemoglobin; most organelles have been ejected	Transport oxygen bound to hemoglobin molecules; also transport small amount of carbon dioxide
Leukocytes (white blood cells, or WBCs)	4000–11,000		
Granulocytes			
• Neutrophils	3000–7000 (40–70% of WBCs)	Cytoplasm stains pale pink and contains fine granules, which are difficult to see; deep purple nucleus consists of three to seven lobes connected by thin strands of nucleoplasm	Active phagocytes; number increases rapidly during short-term or acute infections
• Eosinophils	100–400 (1–4% of WBCs)	Red coarse cytoplasmic granules; figure-8 or bilobed nucleus stains blue-red	Kill parasitic worms; increase during allergy attacks; might phagocytize antigen-antibody complexes and inactivate some inflammatory chemicals
• Basophils	20–50 (0–1% of WBCs)	Cytoplasm has a few large blue-purple granules; U- or S-shaped nucleus with constrictions, stains dark blue	Granules contain histamine (vasodilator chemical), which is discharged at sites of inflammation
Agranulocytes			
• Lymphocytes	1500–3000 (20–45% of WBCs)	Cytoplasm pale blue and appears as thin rim around nucleus; spherical (or slightly indented) dark purple-blue nucleus	Part of immune system; one group (B lymphocytes) produces antibodies; other group (T lymphocytes) involved in graft rejection, fighting tumors and viruses, and activating B lymphocytes
• Monocytes	100–700 (4–8% of WBCs)	Abundant gray-blue cytoplasm; dark blue-purple nucleus often kidney-shaped	Active phagocytes that become macrophages in the tissues; long-term "clean-up team"; increase in number during chronic infections such as tuberculosis
Platelets	250,000–500,000	Essentially irregularly shaped cell fragments; stain deep purple	Needed for normal blood clotting; initiate clotting cascade by clinging to broken area; help to control blood loss from broken blood vessels

*Appearance when stained with Wright's stain.

connected by thin strands of nuclear material. The granules in their cytoplasm stain specifically with Wright's stain. The granulocytes include the neutrophils (nu'tro-filz), eosinophils (e"o-sin'o-filz), and basophils (ba'so-filz).

1. **Neutrophils** have a multilobed nucleus and very fine granules that respond to both acid and basic stains. Consequently, the cytoplasm as a whole stains pink. Neutrophils are avid phagocytes at sites of acute infection.

2. **Eosinophils** have a blue-red nucleus that resembles an old-fashioned telephone receiver and sport large brick-red cytoplasmic granules. Their number increases rapidly during allergies and infections by parasitic worms (flatworms, tapeworms, etc.).

3. **Basophils,** the rarest of the WBCs, contain large histamine-containing granules that stain dark blue. **Histamine** is an inflammatory chemical that makes blood vessels leaky and attracts other WBCs to the inflammatory site.

The second group, **agranulocytes,** lack visible cytoplasmic granules. Their nuclei are closer to the norm—that is, they are spherical, oval, or kidney-shaped. The agranulocytes include lymphocytes (lim'fo-sīts) and monocytes (mon'o-sīts).

1. **Lymphocytes** have a large dark purple nucleus that occupies most of the cell volume. Only slightly larger than RBCs, lymphocytes tend to take up residence in lymphatic tissues, where they play an important role in the immune response.

2. **Monocytes** are the largest of the WBCs. Except for their more abundant cytoplasm and indented nucleus, they resemble large lymphocytes. When they migrate into the tissues, they change into macrophages with huge appetites. Macrophages are very important in fighting chronic infections, such as tuberculosis.

Platelets (Thrombocytes)

Platelets are not cells in the strict sense. They are fragments of bizarre multinucleate cells called **megakaryocytes** (meg"ah-kar'e-o-sīts), which pinch off thousands of anucleate platelet "pieces" that quickly seal themselves off from the surrounding fluids. The platelets appear as darkly staining, irregularly shaped bodies scattered among the other blood cells. The normal platelet count in blood is about 300,000/mm^3. As indicated in Table 10.2, platelets are needed for the clotting process that occurs in plasma when blood vessels are ruptured or broken. (This process is explained in the section on hemostasis later in this chapter.)

Hematopoiesis (Blood Cell Formation)

Blood cell formation, or **hematopoiesis** (hem"ah-to-poi-e'sis), occurs in red bone marrow, or *myeloid* tissue. In adults, this tissue is found chiefly in the flat bones of the skull and pelvis, the ribs, sternum, and proximal epiphyses of the humerus and femur. Each type of blood cell is produced in different numbers in response to changing body needs and different stimuli. After they mature, they are discharged into the blood vessels surrounding the area.

All the formed elements arise from a common type of *stem cell,* the **hemocytoblast** (he"mo-si'to-blast), which resides in the red bone marrow. Their development differs, however, and once a cell is committed to a specific blood pathway, it cannot change. As indicated in the flowchart in Figure 10.4, the hemocytoblast forms two types of descendants— the *lymphoid stem cell,* which produces lymphocytes, and the *myeloid stem cell,* which can produce all other classes of formed elements.

Because they are anucleate, RBCs are unable to synthesize proteins, grow, or divide. As they age, RBCs become more rigid and begin to fragment, or fall apart, in 100 to 120 days. Their remains are eliminated by phagocytes in the spleen, liver, and other body tissues. Lost cells are replaced more or less continuously by the division of hemocytoblasts in the red bone marrow. The developing RBCs divide many times and then begin synthesizing huge amounts of hemoglobin. Suddenly, when enough hemoglobin has been accumulated, the nucleus and most organelles are ejected and the cell collapses inward. The result is the young RBC, called a *reticulocyte* (rĕ-tik'u-lo-sīt) because it still contains some rough endoplasmic reticulum (ER). The reticulocytes enter the bloodstream to begin their task of transporting oxygen. Within 2 days of release, they have ejected the remaining ER and have become fully functioning erythrocytes. The entire developmental process from hemocytoblast to mature RBC takes 3 to 5 days.

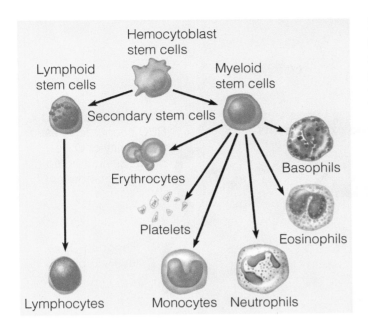

FIGURE 10.4   The development of blood cells.
All blood cells differentiate from a common source, hemocytoblast stem cells in red bone marrow. The population of stem cells renews itself by mitosis. Some of these cells become lymphoid stem cells, which then develop into two classes of lymphocytes that function in the immune response. All other blood cells differentiate from myeloid stem cells, which are also derived from the stem cells.

The rate of erythrocyte production is controlled by a hormone called **erythropoietin** (ĕ-rith″ro-poi-e′tin). Normally a small amount of erythropoietin circulates in the blood at all times, and red blood cells are formed at a fairly constant rate. Although the liver produces some, the kidneys play the major role in producing this hormone. When blood levels of oxygen begin to decline for any reason, the kidneys step up their release of erythropoietin (Figure 10.5). Erythropoietin targets the bone marrow, prodding it into "high gear" to turn out more RBCs. As you might expect, an overabundance of erythrocytes, or an excessive amount of oxygen in the bloodstream, depresses erythropoietin release and red blood cell production. An important point to remember is that it is *not* the relative number of RBCs in the blood that controls RBC production. Control is based on their ability to transport enough oxygen to meet the body's demands.

Like erythrocyte production, the formation of leukocytes and platelets is stimulated by hormones. These *colony stimulating factors (CSFs)* and *interleukins* not only prompt red bone marrow to turn out leukocytes, but also marshal up an army of WBCs to ward off attacks by enhancing the ability of mature leukocytes to protect the body. Apparently, they are released in response to specific chemical signals in the environment such as inflammatory chemicals and certain bacteria or their toxins. The hormone *thrombopoietin* accelerates the production of platelets, but little is known about how that process is regulated.

When bone marrow problems or disease conditions such as aplastic anemia or leukemia are suspected, a special needle is used to withdraw a small sample of red marrow from one of the flat bones (ilium or sternum) close to the body surface. This procedure provides cells for a microscopic examination called a *bone marrow biopsy.*

Hemostasis

Normally, blood flows smoothly past the intact lining (endothelium) of blood vessel walls. But if a blood vessel wall breaks, a series of reactions is set in motion to accomplish **hemostasis** (*hem* = blood; *stasis* = standing still), or stoppage of blood flow. This response, which is fast and localized, involves many substances normally present in plasma, as well as some that are released by platelets and injured tissue cells.

Hemostasis involves three major phases, which occur in rapid sequence: **platelet plug formation, vascular spasms,** and **coagulation,** or **blood clotting.** Blood loss at the site is permanently prevented when fibrous tissue grows into the clot and seals the hole in the blood vessel.

Basically, hemostasis occurs as follows (Figure 10.6):

1. **Platelet plug forms.** Platelets are repelled by an intact endothelium, but when it is broken so that the underlying collagen fibers are exposed, the platelets become "sticky" and cling to the damaged site. Anchored platelets release chemicals that attract more platelets to the site, and as more and more platelets pile up, a small mass called a *platelet plug,* or *white thrombus,* is formed.

2. **Vascular spasms occur.** The anchored platelets also release **serotonin** (ser″o-to′nin), which causes that blood vessel to go into spasms. The spasms narrow the blood vessel at that point,

Q *Why do many people with advanced kidney disease become anemic?*

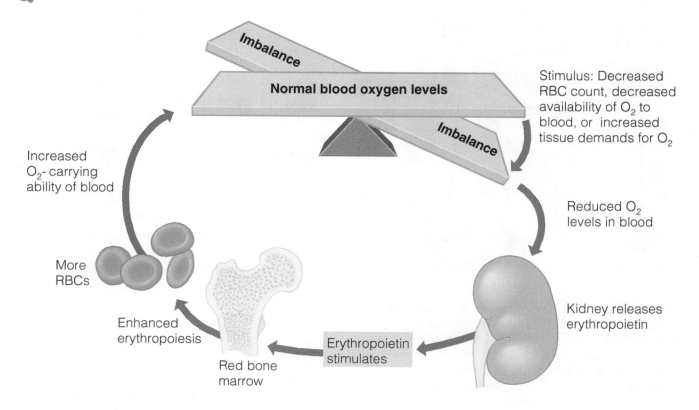

FIGURE 10.5   Mechanism for regulating the rate of RBC production.
Increased erythropoietin release, which stimulates RBC production in bone marrow, occurs when oxygen levels in the blood become inadequate to support normal cellular activity, whatever the cause.

decreasing blood loss until clotting can occur. (Other factors causing vessel spasms include direct injury to the smooth muscle cells and stimulation of local pain receptors.)

3. Coagulation events occur.

a. At the same time, the injured tissues are quickly releasing **tissue factor (TF),** a substance that plays an important role in clotting following the extrinsic pathway.

b. **PF₃,** a phospholipid that coats the surfaces of the platelets, interacts with TF, vitamin K and other blood protein clotting factors, and calcium ions (Ca²⁺) to form over time an activator that triggers the *clotting cascade* following the intrinsic pathway.

c. This **prothrombin activator** converts **prothrombin** (pro-throm'bin), present in the plasma, to **thrombin,** an enzyme.

d. Thrombin then joins soluble **fibrinogen** (fi-brin'o-jen) proteins into long hairlike molecules of insoluble **fibrin,** which forms a meshwork that traps the RBCs and forms the basis of the clot (Figure 10.7). Within the hour, the clot begins to retract, squeezing **serum** (plasma minus the clotting proteins) from the mass and pulling the ruptured edges of the blood vessel closer together.

Normally, blood clots within 3 to 6 minutes. As a rule, once the clotting cascade has started, the triggering factors are rapidly inactivated to prevent widespread clotting ("solid blood"). Eventually, the endothelium regenerates, and the clot is broken down. Once these events of the clotting cascade were understood, it became clear that placing a

A   *The kidneys produce most of the erythropoietin that stimulates red blood cell production by the bone marrow.*

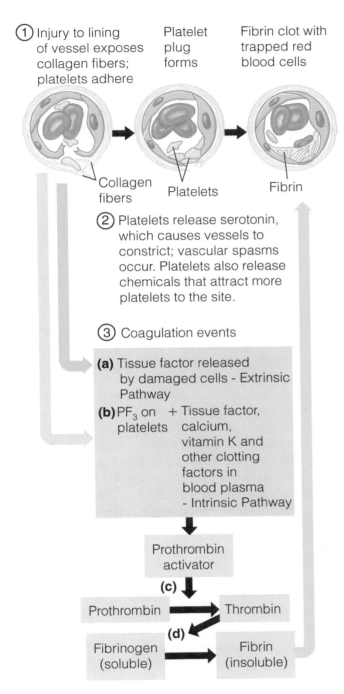

① Injury to lining of vessel exposes collagen fibers; platelets adhere

Platelet plug forms

Fibrin clot with trapped red blood cells

Collagen fibers   Platelets   Fibrin

② Platelets release serotonin, which causes vessels to constrict; vascular spasms occur. Platelets also release chemicals that attract more platelets to the site.

③ Coagulation events

(a) Tissue factor released by damaged cells - Extrinsic Pathway

(b) PF₃ on platelets + Tissue factor, calcium, vitamin K and other clotting factors in blood plasma - Intrinsic Pathway

Prothrombin activator

(c)

Prothrombin ➡ Thrombin

(d)

Fibrinogen (soluble) ➡ Fibrin (insoluble)

FIGURE 10.6   Hemostasis. The multistep process, detailed in the text, begins when a blood vessel is damaged and connective tissue in the vessel wall is exposed to blood.

sterile gauze over a cut or applying pressure to a wound would speed up the clotting process. The gauze provides a rough surface to which the platelets can adhere, and the pressure fractures cells, increasing the release of tissue factor locally.

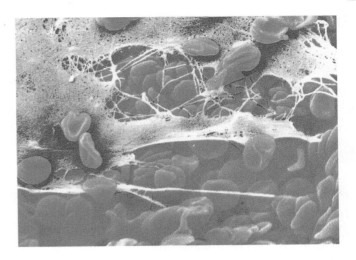

FIGURE 10.7   Fibrin clot. Scanning electron micrograph (artificially colored) of red blood cells trapped in a mesh of fibrin threads.

Disorders of Hemostasis

Homeostatic Imbalance

The two major disorders of hemostasis—undesirable clot formation and bleeding disorders—are at opposite poles.

Undesirable Clotting

Despite the body's safeguards against abnormal clotting, undesirable clots sometimes form in intact blood vessels, particularly in the legs. A clot that develops and persists in an unbroken blood vessel is called a **thrombus** (throm′bus). If large enough, it may prevent blood flow to the cells beyond the blockage. For example, if a thrombus forms in the blood vessels serving the heart *(coronary thrombosis)*, the consequences may be death of heart muscle and a fatal heart attack. If a thrombus breaks away from the vessel wall and floats freely in the bloodstream, it becomes an **embolus** (em′bo-lus; plural, *emboli*). An embolus is usually no problem unless or until it lodges in a blood vessel too narrow for it to pass through. For example, a *cerebral embolus* may cause a stroke.

Undesirable clotting may be caused by anything that roughens the endothelium of a blood vessel and encourages clinging of platelets, such as severe burns, physical blows, or an accumulation of fatty material. Slowly flowing blood, or blood pooling, is another risk factor, especially in immobilized patients. In this case, clotting factors are not washed away as usual and accumulate so that clot formation becomes possible. A number of anticoagulants, most importantly aspirin, heparin, and dicumarol, are used clinically for thrombus-prone patients.

Bleeding Disorders

The most common causes of abnormal bleeding are platelet deficiency (thrombocytopenia) and deficits of some of the clotting factors, such as might result from impaired liver function or certain genetic conditions.

Thrombocytopenia results from an insufficient number of circulating platelets. Even normal movements cause spontaneous bleeding from small blood vessels. This is evidenced by many small purplish blotches, called *petechiae* (pe-te'ke-e), on the skin. It can arise from any condition that suppresses myeloid tissue, such as bone marrow cancer, radiation, or certain drugs.

When the liver is unable to synthesize its usual supply of clotting factors, abnormal and often severe bleeding episodes occur. If vitamin K (needed by the liver cells to produce the clotting factors) is deficient, the problem is easily corrected with vitamin K supplements. However, when liver function is severely impaired (as in hepatitis and cirrhosis), only whole blood transfusions are helpful.

The term **hemophilia** (he"mo-fil'e-ah) applies to several different hereditary bleeding disorders that result from a lack of any of the factors needed for clotting. Commonly called "bleeder's disease," the hemophilias have similar signs and symptoms that begin early in life. Even minor tissue trauma results in prolonged bleeding and can be life-threatening. Repeated bleeding into joints causes them to become disabled and painful. When a bleeding episode occurs, hemophiliacs are given a transfusion of fresh plasma or injections of the purified clotting factor they lack. Because hemophiliacs are absolutely dependent on one or the other of these therapies, some have become the victims of blood-transmitted viral diseases such as hepatitis and AIDS. These problems have been largely resolved because of the availability of genetically engineered clotting factors. ▲

Blood Groups and Transfusions

As we have seen, blood is vital for transporting substances through the body. When blood loss occurs, the blood vessels constrict and the bone marrow steps up blood cell formation in an attempt to keep the circulation going. However, the body can compensate for a loss of blood volume only up to a certain limit. Losses of 15 to 30 percent lead to

pallor and weakness. Losses of over 30 percent cause severe shock, which can be fatal. Whole blood transfusions are routinely given to replace substantial blood loss and to treat severe anemia or thrombocytopenia. The usual blood bank procedure involves collecting blood from a donor and mixing it with an anticoagulant to prevent clotting. The treated blood can be stored (refrigerated at 4°C, or 39.2°F) for about 35 days until needed.

Human Blood Groups

Although whole blood transfusion can save lives, people have different blood groups, and transfusing incompatible or mismatched blood can be fatal. How so? The plasma membranes of RBCs, like those of all body cells, bear genetically determined proteins (antigens), called **agglutinogens,** which identify each person as unique. An **antigen** (an'tĭ-jen) is a substance that the body recognizes as foreign; it stimulates the immune system to release antibodies or use other means to mount a defense against it. Most antigens are foreign proteins, such as those that are part of viruses or bacteria that have managed to invade the body. Although each of us tolerates our own cellular (self) antigens, one person's RBC proteins will be recognized as foreign if transfused into another person with different RBC antigens. The "recognizers" are **antibodies,** called **agglutinins,** present in the plasma that attach to RBCs bearing surface antigens different from those on the patient's (blood recipient's) RBCs. Binding of the antibodies causes the RBCs to clump, a phenomenon called **agglutination*** (ah-gloo"tĭ-na'shun), which leads to the clogging of small blood vessels throughout the body. During the next few hours, the foreign RBCs are lysed (ruptured) and their hemoglobin is released into the bloodstream. Although the transfused blood is unable to deliver the increased oxygen-carrying capacity hoped for and some tissue areas may be deprived of blood, the most devastating consequence of severe transfusion reactions is that the freed hemoglobin molecules may block the kidney tubules and cause kidney failure. Transfusion reactions can also cause fever, chills, nausea, and vomiting, but in the absence of

---

*The RBC antigens that promote this clumping are sometimes called **agglutinogens** (ag"loo-tin'o-jenz), and the antibodies that bind them together are called **agglutinins** (ag"loo'tĭ-ninz).

kidney shutdown these reactions are rarely fatal. Treatment is aimed at preventing kidney damage by infusing alkaline fluids to dilute and dissolve the hemoglobin and diuretics to flush it out of the body in urine.

There are over 30 common RBC antigens in humans, allowing each person's blood cells to be classified into different blood groups. However, it is the antigens of the ABO and Rh blood groups that cause the most vigorous transfusion reactions. These two blood groups are described here.

As shown in Table 10.3, the **ABO blood groups** are based on which of two antigens, type A or type B, a person inherits. Absence of both antigens results in type O blood, presence of both antigens leads to type AB, and the possession of either A or B antigen yields type A or B blood, respectively. In the ABO blood group, antibodies are formed during infancy against the ABO antigens *not* present on your own RBCs. As shown in the table, a baby with neither the A nor the B antigen (group O) forms both anti-A and anti-B antibodies, while those with type A antigens (group A) form anti-B antibodies, and so on.

The **Rh blood groups** are so named because one of the eight Rh antigens (agglutinogen D) was originally identified in **Rh**esus monkeys. Later the same antigen was discovered in human beings. Most Americans are Rh$^+$ (Rh positive), meaning that their RBCs carry the Rh antigen. Unlike the antibodies of the ABO system, anti-Rh antibodies are *not* automatically formed and present in the blood of Rh$^-$ (Rh negative) individuals. However, if an Rh$^-$ person receives mismatched blood (that is, Rh$^+$), shortly after the transfusion, his or her immune system becomes sensitized and begins producing antibodies (anti-Rh$^+$ antibodies) against the foreign blood type. **Hemolysis** (rupture of RBCs) does not occur with the first transfusion because it takes time for the body to react and start making antibodies. However, the second time and every time thereafter, a typical transfusion reaction occurs in which the patient's antibodies attack and rupture the donor's Rh$^+$ RBCs.

An important Rh-related problem occurs in pregnant Rh$^-$ women who are carrying Rh$^+$ babies. The *first* such pregnancy usually results in the delivery of a healthy baby. But because the

TABLE 10.3 ABO Blood Groups

Blood group	Frequency (% U.S. population) White	Black	Asian	RBC antigens Present (agglutinogens)	Illustration	Plasma antibodies (agglutinins)	Blood that can be received without reaction
AB	4	4	5	A B		None	A, B, AB, O Universal recipient
B	11	20	27	B		Anti-A	B, O
A	40	27	28	A		Anti-B	A, O
O	45	49	40	None		Anti-A Anti-B	O Universal donor

mother is sensitized by Rh⁺ antigens that have passed through the placenta into her bloodstream, she will form anti-Rh⁺ antibodies unless treated with RhoGAM shortly after giving birth. RhoGAM is an immune serum that prevents this sensitization and her subsequent immune response. If she is not treated and becomes pregnant again with an Rh⁺ baby, her antibodies will cross through the placenta and destroy the baby's RBCs, producing a condition known as *hemolytic disease of the newborn*. The baby is anemic and becomes hypoxic and cyanotic (the skin takes on a blue cast). Brain damage and even death may result unless fetal transfusions are done before birth to provide more RBCs for oxygen transport.

Blood Typing

The importance of determining the blood group of both the donor and the recipient *before* blood is transfused is glaringly obvious. The general procedure for determining ABO blood type is briefly outlined in Figure 10.8. Essentially, it involves testing the blood by mixing it with two different types of immune serum—anti-A and anti-B. Agglutination occurs when RBCs of a group A person are mixed with the anti-A serum but not when they are mixed with the anti-B serum. Likewise, RBCs of type B blood are clumped by anti-B serum but not by anti-A serum. Because it is critical that blood groups be compatible, cross matching is also done. *Cross matching* involves testing for agglutination of donor RBCs by the recipient's serum and of the recipient's RBCs by the donor serum. Typing for the Rh factors is done in the same manner as ABO blood typing.

Developmental Aspects of Blood

In the young embryo, development of the entire circulatory system occurs early. Before birth, there are many sites of blood cell formation—the fetal liver and spleen, among others—but by the seventh month of development, the red marrow has become the chief site of hematopoiesis, and it remains so throughout life. Generally, embryonic blood cells are circulating in the newly formed blood vessels by day 28 of development. Fetal hemoglobin (HbF) differs from the hemoglobin formed after birth. It has a greater ability to pick up

Q *Which blood types can be transfused into a person with type B blood?*

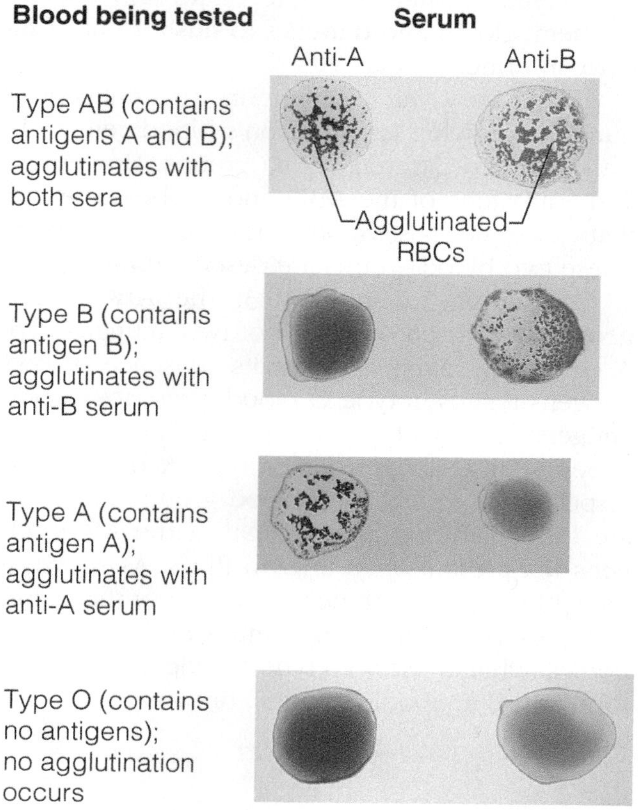

FIGURE 10.8 Blood typing of ABO blood groups. When serum containing anti-A or anti-B antibodies is added to a blood sample diluted with saline, agglutination will occur between the antibody and the corresponding antigen (if present).

oxygen, a characteristic that is highly desirable since fetal blood is less oxygen rich than that of the mother. After birth, fetal blood cells are gradually replaced by RBCs that contain the more typical hemoglobin A (HbA). In situations in which the fetal RBCs are destroyed at such a rapid rate that the immature infant liver cannot rid the body of hemoglobin breakdown products in the bile fast enough, the infant becomes *jaundiced* (jawn'dist). This type of jaundice generally causes no major problems and is referred to as *physiologic jaundice*, to distinguish it from more serious disease conditions that result in jaundiced, or yellowed, tissues.

A   *Types B and O.*

Homeostatic Imbalance

Various congenital diseases result from genetic factors (such as hemophilia and sickle cell anemia) and from interactions with maternal blood factors (such as hemolytic disease of the newborn). Dietary factors can lead to abnormalities in blood cell formation as well as hemoglobin production. Iron deficiency anemia is especially common in women because of their monthly blood loss during menses.

The young and the old are particularly at risk for leukemia. With increasing age, chronic types of leukemias, anemias, and diseases involving undesirable clot formation are more prevalent. However, these are usually secondary to disorders of the heart, blood vessels, or immune system. The elderly are particularly at risk for pernicious anemia because the stomach mucosa (which produces intrinsic factor) atrophies with age. ▲

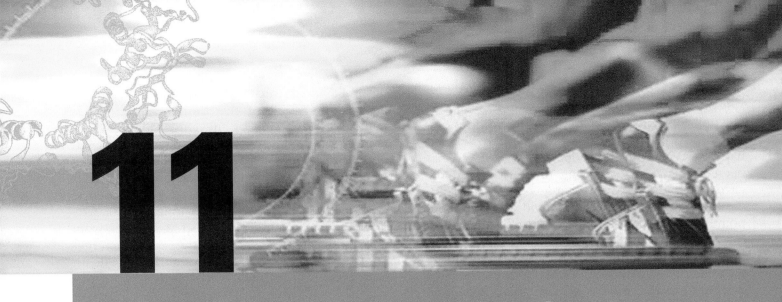

11

The Cardiovascular System: The Heart and Blood Vessels

KEY TERM

When most people hear the term *cardiovascular system,* they immediately think of the heart. We have all felt our own heart "pound" from time to time, and we tend to get a bit nervous when this happens. The crucial importance of the heart has been recognized for a long time. However, the **cardiovascular system** is much more than just the heart, and from a scientific and medical standpoint, it is important to understand *why* this system is so vital to life.

The almost continuous traffic into and out of a busy factory at rush hour occurs at a snail's pace compared to the endless activity going on within our bodies. Night and day, minute after minute, our trillions of cells take up nutrients and excrete wastes. Although the pace of these exchanges slows during sleep, they must go on continuously, because when they stop, we die. Cells can make such exchanges only with the tissue fluid in their immediate vicinity. Thus, some means of changing and "refreshing" these fluids is necessary to renew the nutrients and prevent pollution caused by the buildup of wastes. Like the bustling factory, the body must have a transportation system to carry its various "cargos" back and forth. Instead of roads, railway tracks, and airways, the body's delivery routes are its hollow blood vessels.

Most simply stated, the major function of the cardiovascular system is transportation. Using blood as the transport vehicle, the system carries oxygen, nutrients, cell wastes, hormones, and many other substances vital for body homeostasis to and from the cells. The force to move the blood around the body is provided by the beating heart.

The cardiovascular system can be compared to a muscular pump equipped with one-way valves and a system of large and small plumbing tubes within which the blood travels. Blood (the substance transported) was discussed in Chapter 10. Here we will consider the heart (the pump) and the blood vessels (the network of tubes).

The Heart

Anatomy of the Heart

Location and Size

The relative size and weight of the heart give few hints of its incredible strength. Approximately the size of a person's fist, the hollow, cone-shaped heart weighs less than a pound. Snugly enclosed within the inferior **mediastinum** (me″de-ah-sti′num), the middle cavity of the thorax, the heart is flanked on each side by the lungs (Figure 11.1). Its more pointed **apex** is directed toward the left hip and rests on the diaphragm, approximately at the level of the fifth intercostal space. (This is exactly where one would place a stethoscope to count the heart rate for an apical pulse.) Its broader posterosuperior aspect, or **base,** from which the great vessels of the body emerge, points toward the right shoulder and lies beneath the second rib.

Coverings and Wall

The heart is enclosed by a double sac of serous membrane, the **pericardium** (per″i-kar′de-um). The thin **epicardium,** or **visceral pericardium,** tightly hugs the external surface of the heart and is actually part of the heart wall (Figure 11.2b). It is continuous at the heart base with the loosely applied **parietal pericardium,** which is reinforced on its superficial face by dense connective tissue, referred to as the **fibrous pericardium.** This fibrous layer helps protect the heart and anchors it to surrounding structures, such as the diaphragm and sternum. A slippery lubricating fluid (serous fluid) is produced by the serous pericardial membranes. This fluid allows the heart to beat easily in a relatively frictionless environment as the pericardial layers slide smoothly across each other.

Homeostatic Imbalance

Inflammation of the pericardium, *pericarditis* (per″ĭ-kar-di′tis), often results in a decrease in the amount of serous fluid. This causes the pericardial layers to bind and stick to each other, forming painful *adhesions* that interfere with heart movements. ▲

The heart walls are composed of three layers: the outer *epicardium* (the visceral pericardium described above), the *myocardium,* and the innermost *endocardium* (Figure 11.2b). The **myocardium** (mi″o-kar′de-um) consists of thick bundles of cardiac muscle twisted and whorled into ringlike arrangements (see Figure 11.3). It is the layer that actually contracts. The myocardium is reinforced internally by a dense, fibrous connective tissue network called the "skeleton of the heart." The **endocardium** (en″do-kar′de-um) is a thin, glistening sheet of endothelium that lines the heart chambers. It is continuous with the linings

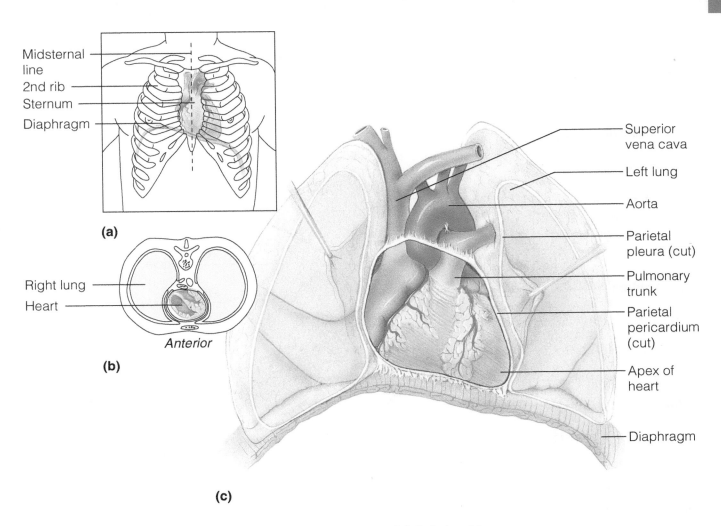

Midsternal line
2nd rib
Sternum
Diaphragm

(a)

Right lung
Heart

Anterior

(b)

Superior vena cava
Left lung
Aorta
Parietal pleura (cut)
Pulmonary trunk
Parietal pericardium (cut)
Apex of heart
Diaphragm

(c)

FIGURE 11.1   Location of the heart within the thorax. (a) Relationship of the heart to the sternum and ribs. **(b)** Cross-sectional view showing relative position of the heart in the thorax. **(c)** Relationship of the heart and great vessels to the lungs.

of the blood vessels leaving and entering the heart. Figure 11.2 shows two views of the heart—an external anterior view and a frontal section. As the anatomical areas of the heart are described in the next section, keep referring to Figure 11.2 to locate each of the heart structures or regions. Figure 11.3 shows a closer view of the layers of the heart wall: the epicardium, myocardium, and endocardium.

Chambers and Associated Great Vessels

The heart has four hollow chambers or cavities—two **atria** (a′tre-ah, singular *atrium*) and two **ventricles** (ven′trĭ-kulz). Each of these chambers is lined with endocardium, which helps blood flow smoothly through the heart. *The superior atria are primarily receiving chambers.* As a rule, they are not important in the pumping activity of the heart. Blood flows into the atria under low pressure from the veins of the body and then continues on to fill the ventricles. *The inferior, thick-walled ventricles are the discharging chambers,* or actual pumps of the heart. When they contract, blood is propelled out of the heart and into the circulation. As illustrated in Figure 11.2a, the right ventricle forms most of the heart's anterior surface; the left ventricle forms its apex. The septum that divides the heart longitudinally is referred to as the **interventricular** or **interatrial septum,** depending on which chamber it divides and separates.

Q *Which heart chamber has the thickest walls? What is the functional significance of this structural difference?*

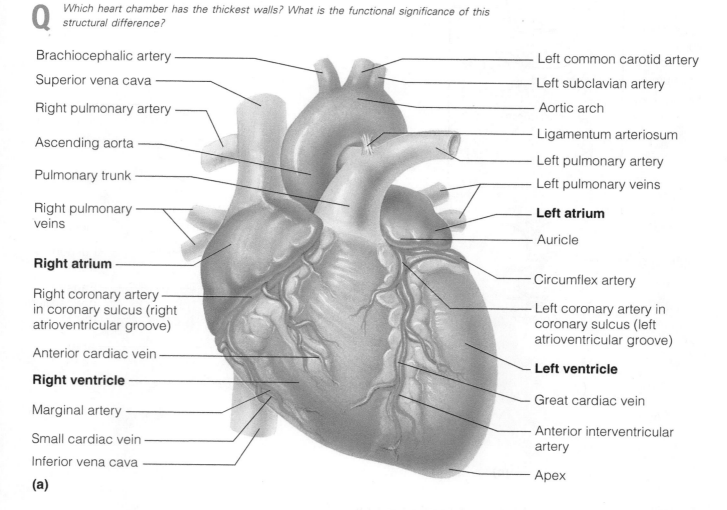

Brachiocephalic artery

Superior vena cava

Right pulmonary artery

Ascending aorta

Pulmonary trunk

Right pulmonary veins

Right atrium

Right coronary artery in coronary sulcus (right atrioventricular groove)

Anterior cardiac vein

Right ventricle

Marginal artery

Small cardiac vein

Inferior vena cava

(a)

Left common carotid artery

Left subclavian artery

Aortic arch

Ligamentum arteriosum

Left pulmonary artery

Left pulmonary veins

Left atrium

Auricle

Circumflex artery

Left coronary artery in coronary sulcus (left atrioventricular groove)

Left ventricle

Great cardiac vein

Anterior interventricular artery

Apex

FIGURE 11.2 Gross anatomy of the heart. (a) Anterior surface view.

Although it is a single organ, the heart functions as a double pump. The right side works as the pulmonary circuit pump. It receives relatively oxygen-poor blood from the veins of the body through the large **superior** and **inferior venae cavae** (ka′ve) and pumps it out through the **pulmonary trunk.** The pulmonary trunk splits into the right and left **pulmonary arteries,** which carry blood to the lungs, where oxygen is picked up and carbon dioxide is unloaded. Oxygen-rich blood drains from the lungs and is returned to the left side of the heart through the four **pulmonary veins.** The circulation just described, from the right side of

the heart to the lungs and back to the left side of the heart, is called the **pulmonary circulation** (Figure 11.4). Its only function is to carry blood to the lungs for gas exchange and then return it to the heart.

Blood returned to the left side of the heart is pumped out of the heart into the **aorta** (a-or′tah), from which the systemic arteries branch to supply essentially all body tissues. Oxygen-poor blood circulates from the tissues back to the right atrium via the systemic veins, which finally empty their cargo into either the superior or inferior vena cava. This second circuit, from the left side of the heart through the body tissues and back to the right side of the heart, is called the **systemic circulation** (see Figure 11.4). It supplies oxygen- and nutrient-rich blood to all body organs. Because the left ventricle is the systemic pump that pumps blood over a much longer pathway through the body, its walls are

A *The left ventricle's walls are the thickest; that chamber pumps blood throughout the entire body and back to the heart; the right ventricle serves a short circuit through the lungs and back to the heart, so does not require as much muscle tissue.*

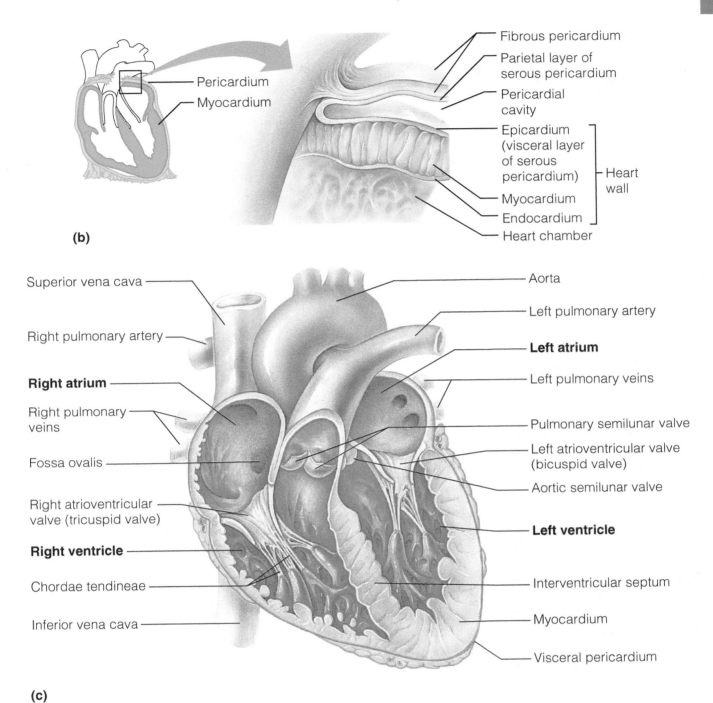

(b)

(c)

FIGURE 11.2 (*Continued*) **(b)** Heart wall and coverings layers.
(c) Frontal section showing interior chambers and valves.

substantially thicker than those of the right ventricle, and it is a much more powerful pump.

Valves

The heart is equipped with four valves, which allow blood to flow in only one direction through the heart chambers—from the atria through the ventricles and out the great arteries leaving the heart (see Figure 11.2a). The **atrioventricular** (a″tre-o-ven-trik′u-lar), or **AV, valves** are located between the atrial and ventricular chambers on each side. The AV valves prevent backflow into

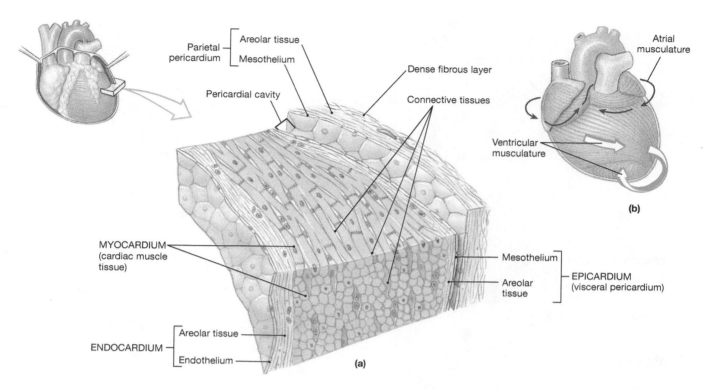

FIGURE 11.3   The heart wall. (a) A diagrammatic section through the heart wall, showing the relative positions of the epicardium, myocardium, and endocardium. The proportions are not to scale; the relative thickness of the myocardial wall has been greatly reduced. **(b)** Cardiac muscle tissue forms concentric layers that wrap around the atria or spiral within the walls of the ventricles.

the atria when the ventricles contract. The left AV valve—the **bicuspid,** or **mitral** (mi′tral), **valve**—consists of two flaps, or cusps, of endocardium. The right AV valve, the **tricuspid valve,** has three flaps. Tiny white cords, the **chordae tendineae** (kor′de ten-din′e)—literally, "tendinous cords" (but I like to think of them as the "heart strings" of song)—anchor the flaps to the walls of the ventricles. When the heart is relaxed and blood is passively filling its chambers, the AV-valve flaps hang limply into the ventricles (Figure 11.5a). As the ventricles contract, they press on the blood in their chambers, and the intraventricular pressure (pressure inside the ventricles) begins to rise. This causes the AV-valve flaps to be forced upward, closing the valves. At this point, the chordae tendineae are working to anchor the flaps in a closed position. If the flaps were unanchored, they would blow upward into the atria like an umbrella being turned inside out by a gusty wind. In this manner, the AV valves prevent backflow into the atria when the ventricles are contracting.

The second set of valves, the **semilunar** (sem″e-lu′nar) **valves,** guards the bases of the two large arteries leaving the ventricular chambers. Thus, they are known as the **pulmonary** and **aortic semilunar valves** (see Figure 11.2b). Each semilunar valve has three leaflets that fit tightly together when the valves are closed. When the ventricles are contracting and forcing blood out of the heart, the leaflets are forced open and flattened against the walls of the arteries by the tremendous force of rushing blood (Figure 11.5b). Then, when the ventricles relax, the blood begins to flow backward toward the heart, and the leaflets fill with blood, closing the valves. This prevents arterial blood from reentering the heart.

Each set of valves operates at a different time. The AV valves are open during heart relaxation and closed when the ventricles are contracting. The semilunar valves are closed during heart relaxation and are forced open when the ventricles contract. As they open and close in response to pressure changes in the heart, the valves force blood to continually move forward in its journey through the heart.

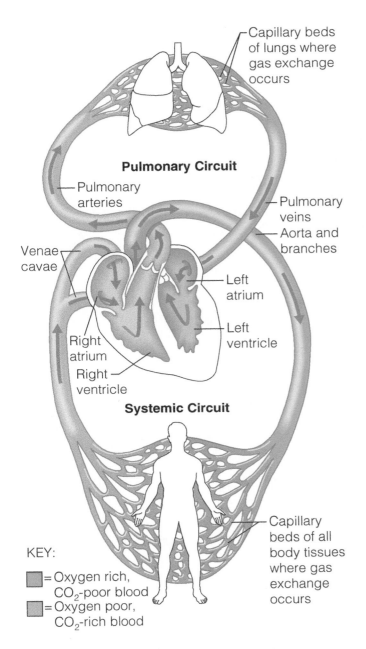

Pulmonary Circuit

Capillary beds of lungs where gas exchange occurs

Pulmonary arteries

Pulmonary veins

Aorta and branches

Venae cavae

Left atrium

Left ventricle

Right atrium

Right ventricle

Systemic Circuit

Capillary beds of all body tissues where gas exchange occurs

KEY:

☐ = Oxygen rich, CO_2-poor blood
☐ = Oxygen poor, CO_2-rich blood

FIGURE 11.4 The systemic and pulmonary circulations. The left side of the heart is the systemic pump; the right side is the pulmonary circuit pump. (Although there are two pulmonary arteries, one each to the right and left lung, for simplicity only one is shown.)

▲ Homeostatic Imbalance

Heart valves are basically simple devices, and the heart—like any mechanical pump—can function with "leaky" valves as long as the damage is not too great. However, severely deformed valves can seriously hamper cardiac function. For example, an *incompetent valve* forces the heart to pump and repump the same blood because the valve does not close properly and blood backflows. In *valvular stenosis,* the valve flaps become stiff, often because of repeated bacterial infection of the endocardium **(endocarditis).** This forces the heart to contract more vigorously than normal. In each case, the heart's workload increases, and ultimately, the heart weakens and may fail. Under such conditions, the faulty valve is replaced with a synthetic valve or a valve taken from a pig heart. ▲

Cardiac Muscle Tissue

Cardiac muscle cells are interconnected by **intercalated discs** (Figure 11.6a, b). At an intercalated disc, the interlocking membranes of adjacent cells are held together by desmosomes and linked by gap junctions (Figure 11. 6c). The tiny connections between cells allow communication to flow between cells, giving the signal for all to contract at once. Intercalated discs convey the force of contraction from cell to cell and propagate action potentials. Table 11.1 provides a quick review of the structural and functional differences between cardiac muscle cells and skeletal muscle fibers. Among the histological characteristics of cardiac muscle cells that differ from those of skeletal muscle fibers are (1) small size; (2) a single, centrally located nucleus; (3) branching interconnections between cells; and (4) the presence of intercalated discs.

Internal Anatomy and Organization

In this section, we examine the major landmarks and structures visible on the interior surface of the heart. We've briefly discussed the atria and ventricles already, but now let's take a closer look. In a sectional view, you can see that the right atrium communicates with the right ventricle, and the left atrium with the left ventricle. The atria are separated by the **interatrial septum** (*septum,* wall); the ventricles are separated by the much thicker **interventricular septum.** Each septum is a muscular partition. **Atrioventricular (AV) valves,** folds of fibrous tissue, extend into the openings between the atria and ventricles. These valves permit blood flow in one direction only: from the atria to the ventricles.

The Right Atrium

The right atrium receives blood from the systemic circuit through the two great veins: the **superior**

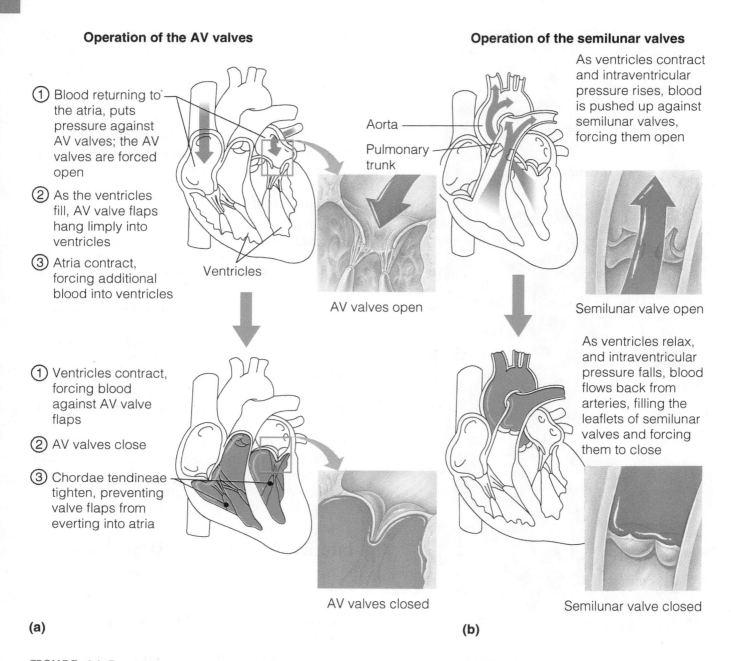

Operation of the AV valves

① Blood returning to the atria, puts pressure against AV valves; the AV valves are forced open

② As the ventricles fill, AV valve flaps hang limply into ventricles

③ Atria contract, forcing additional blood into ventricles

Ventricles

AV valves open

① Ventricles contract, forcing blood against AV valve flaps

② AV valves close

③ Chordae tendineae tighten, preventing valve flaps from everting into atria

AV valves closed

(a)

Operation of the semilunar valves

As ventricles contract and intraventricular pressure rises, blood is pushed up against semilunar valves, forcing them open

Aorta

Pulmonary trunk

Semilunar valve open

As ventricles relax, and intraventricular pressure falls, blood flows back from arteries, filling the leaflets of semilunar valves and forcing them to close

Semilunar valve closed

(b)

FIGURE 11.5 Operation of the heart valves. (a) Atrioventricular (AV) valves. **(b)** Semilunar valves.

vena cava (VĒ-na KĀ-vuh; plural, *venae cavae*) and the **inferior vena cava.** The superior vena cava, which opens into the posterior and superior portion of the right atrium, delivers blood to the right atrium from the head, neck, upper limbs, and chest. The inferior vena cava, which opens into the posterior and inferior portion of the right atrium, carries blood to the right atrium from the rest of the trunk, the viscera, and the lower limbs. The

cardiac veins of the heart return blood to the **coronary sinus,** a large, thin-walled vein that opens into the right atrium inferior to the connection with the superior vena cava.

The opening of the coronary sinus lies near the posterior edge of the interatrial septum. From the fifth week of embryonic development until birth, the **foramen ovale,** an oval opening, penetrates the interatrial septum and connects

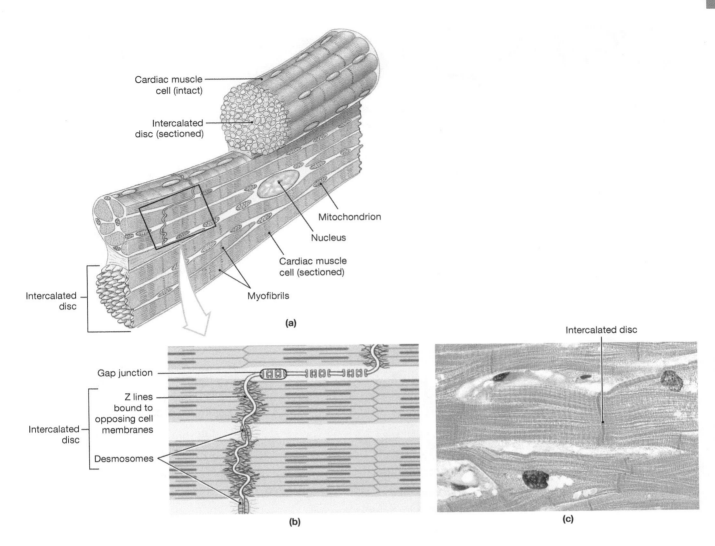

FIGURE 11.6   Cardiac muscle cells. (a) A diagrammatic view of cardiac muscle tissue. **(b)** The structure of an intercalated disc. **(c)** A sectional view of cardiac muscle tissue.

the two atria of the fetal heart. Before birth, the foramen ovale permits blood flow from the right atrium to the left atrium while the lungs are developing. At birth, the foramen ovale closes, and the opening is permanently sealed off within three months of delivery. (If the foramen ovale does not close, serious cardiovascular problems result. The **fossa ovalis,** a small, shallow depression, persists at this site in the adult heart.)

The posterior wall of the right atrium and the interatrial septum have smooth surfaces. In contrast, the anterior atrial wall and the inner surface of the auricle contain prominent muscular ridges called the **pectinate muscles** (*pectin,* comb), or *musculi pectinati.*

Structural Differences between the Left and Right Ventricles

The function of an atrium is to collect blood that is returning to the heart and convey it to the attached ventricle. The functional demands on the right and left atria are similar, and the two chambers look almost identical. The demands on the right and left ventricles, however, are very different, and the two have significant structural differences.

Anatomical differences between the left and right ventricles are best seen in a three-dimensional view (Figure 11.7a). The lungs are close to the heart, and the pulmonary blood vessels are relatively short and wide. Thus, the right ventricle normally does not need to work very hard to push blood through the pulmonary circuit. Accordingly,

| TABLE 11.1 | Structural and Functional Differences between Cardiac Muscle Cells and Skeletal Muscle Fibers | |

Feature	Cardiac Muscle Cells	Skeletal Muscle Fibers
Size	$10 - 20 \mu m \times 50 - 100 \mu m$	$100 \mu m \times$ up to 40 cm
Nuclei	Typically 1 (rarely 2–5)	Multiple (hundreds)
Contractile proteins	Sarcomeres along myofibrils	Sarcomeres along myofibrils
Internal membranes	Short T tubules; no triads formed with sarcoplasmic reticulum	Long T tubules form triads with cisternae of the sarcoplasmic reticulum
Mitochondria	Abundant (25% of cell volume)	Much less abundant
Inclusions	Myoglobin, lipids, glycogen	Little myoglobin, few lipids, but extensive glycogen reserves
Blood supply	Very extensive	More extensive than in most connective tissues, but sparse compared with supply to cardiac muscle cells
Metabolism (resting)	Not applicable	Aerobic, primarily lipid-based
Metabolism (active)	Aerobic, primarily using lipids and carbohydrates	Anaerobic, through breakdown of glycogen reserves
Contractions	Twitches with brief relaxation periods; long refractory period prevents tetanic contractions	Usually sustained contractions
Stimulus for contraction	Autorhythmicity of pacemaker cells generates action potentials	Activity of somatic motor neuron generates action potentials in sarcolemma
Trigger for contraction	Calcium entry from the ECF and calcium release from the sarcoplasmic reticulum	Calcium release from the sarcoplasmic reticulum
Intercellular connections	Branching network with cell membranes locked together at intercalated discs; connective tissue fibers tie adjacent layers together	Adjacent fibers tied together by connective tissue fibers

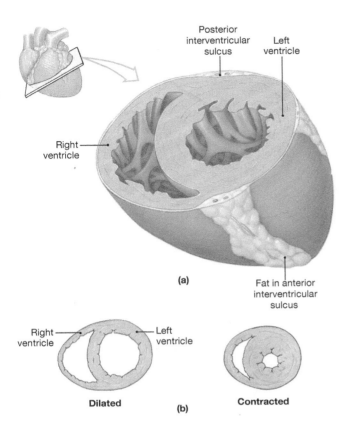

(a)

Posterior interventricular sulcus

Left ventricle

Right ventricle

Fat in anterior interventricular sulcus

Right ventricle — Left ventricle

Dilated   **(b)**   Contracted

FIGURE 11.7 Structural differences between the left and right ventricles. (a) A diagrammatic sectional view through the heart, showing the relative thicknesses of the two ventricles. Notice the pouchlike shape of the right ventricle and the thickness of the left ventricle. **(b)** Diagrammatic views of the ventricles just before a contraction (dilated) and just after a contraction (contracted). ATLAS: Plate 45d.

the wall of the right ventricle is relatively thin. In sectional view, it resembles a pouch attached to the massive wall of the left ventricle. When it contracts, the right ventricle acts like a bellows, squeezing the blood against the thick wall of the left ventricle. This mechanism moves blood very efficiently with minimal effort, but it develops relatively low pressures.

A comparable pumping arrangement would not be suitable for the left ventricle, because four to six times as much pressure must be exerted to push blood around the systemic circuit as around the pulmonary circuit. The left ventricle has an extremely thick muscular wall and is round in cross section (Figure 11.7a). When this ventricle contracts, (1) the distance between the base and apex

decreases, and (2) the diameter of the ventricular chamber decreases. The effect is similar to simultaneously squeezing and rolling up the end of a toothpaste tube. The pressure generated is more than enough to open the aortic valve and eject blood into the ascending aorta.

As the powerful left ventricle contracts, it also bulges into the right ventricular cavity (Figure 11.7b). This action improves the efficiency of the right ventricle's efforts. Individuals whose right ventricular musculature has been severely damaged may survive, because the contraction of the left ventricle helps push blood into the pulmonary circuit.

The Heart Valves

The heart has a series of one-way valves that prevent the backflow of blood as the chambers contract. We will now consider the structure and function of these heart valves.

The Atrioventricular Valves   The atrioventricular (AV) valves prevent the backflow of blood from the ventricles to the atria when the ventricles are contracting. The chordae tendineae and papillary muscles play important roles in the normal function of the AV valves. When the ventricles are relaxed, the chordae tendineae are loose, and the AV valves offer no resistance to the flow of blood from the atria into the ventricles (Figure 11.8a). When the ventricles contract, blood moving back toward the atria swings the cusps together, closing the valves (Figure 11.8b). At the same time, the contraction of the papillary muscles tenses the chordae tendineae, stopping the cusps before they swing into the atria. If the chordae tendineae are cut or the papillary muscles are damaged, backflow **(regurgitation)** of blood into the atria occurs each time the ventricles contract.

The Semilunar Valves   The pulmonary and aortic valves prevent the backflow of blood from the pulmonary trunk and aorta into the right and left ventricles, respectively. Unlike the AV valves, the semilunar valves do not require muscular braces, because the arterial walls do not contract and the relative positions of the cusps are stable. When the semilunar valves close, the three symmetrical cusps support one another like the legs of a tripod (Figure 11.8a,c).

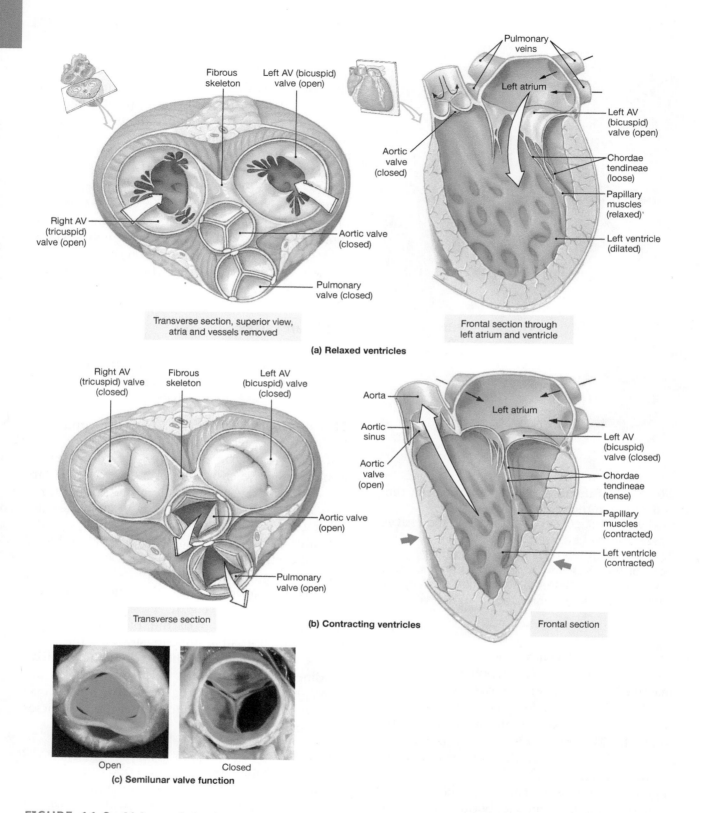

(a) Relaxed ventricles

Fibrous skeleton

Left AV (bicuspid) valve (open)

Right AV (tricuspid) valve (open)

Aortic valve (closed)

Pulmonary valve (closed)

Transverse section, superior view, atria and vessels removed

Pulmonary veins

Left atrium

Left AV (bicuspid) valve (open)

Aortic valve (closed)

Chordae tendineae (loose)

Papillary muscles (relaxed)

Left ventricle (dilated)

Frontal section through left atrium and ventricle

(b) Contracting ventricles

Right AV (tricuspid) valve (closed)

Fibrous skeleton

Left AV (bicuspid) valve (closed)

Aortic valve (open)

Pulmonary valve (open)

Transverse section

Aorta

Aortic sinus

Aortic valve (open)

Left atrium

Left AV (bicuspid) valve (closed)

Chordae tendineae (tense)

Papillary muscles (contracted)

Left ventricle (contracted)

Frontal section

(c) Semilunar valve function

Open

Closed

FIGURE 11.8 Valves of the heart. White arrows indicate blood flow into or out of a ventricle; black arrows, blood flow into an atrium; and green arrows, ventricular contraction. **(a)** When the ventricles are relaxed, the AV valves are open and the semilunar valves are closed. The chordae tendineae are loose, and the papillary muscles are relaxed. **(b)** When the ventricles are contracting, the AV valves are closed and the semilunar valves are open. In the frontal section, notice the attachment of the left AV valve to the chordae tendineae and papillary muscles. **(c)** The aortic valve in the open (left) and closed (right) positions. The individual cusps brace one another in the closed position.

Saclike dilations of the base of the ascending aorta are adjacent to each cusp of the aortic valve. These sacs, called **aortic sinuses,** prevent the individual cusps from sticking to the wall of the aorta when the valve opens. The *right* and *left coronary arteries,* which deliver blood to the myocardium, originate at the aortic sinuses.

Serious valve problems can interfere with cardiac function. If valve function deteriorates to the point at which the heart cannot maintain adequate circulatory flow, symptoms of **valvular heart disease (VHD)** appear. Congenital malformations may be responsible, but in many cases, the condition develops after carditis, an inflammation of the heart, occurs. One relatively common cause of carditis is **rheumatic** (roo-MAT-ik) **fever,** an acute childhood reaction to infection by streptococcal bacteria.

100 Keys | The heart has four chambers, two associated with the pulmonary circuit (right atrium and right ventricle) and two with the systemic circuit (left atrium and left ventricle). The left ventricle has a greater workload and is much more massive than the right ventricle, but the two chambers pump equal amounts of blood. AV valves prevent backflow from the ventricles into the atria, and semilunar valves prevent backflow from the aortic and pulmonary trunks into the ventricles.

Connective Tissues and the Fibrous Skeleton

The connective tissues of the heart include large numbers of collagen and elastic fibers. Each cardiac muscle cell is wrapped in a strong, but elastic, sheath, and adjacent cells are tied together by fibrous cross-links, or "struts." These fibers are, in turn, interwoven into sheets that separate the superficial and deep muscle layers. The connective-tissue fibers (1) provide physical support for the cardiac muscle fibers, blood vessels, and nerves of the myocardium; (2) help distribute the forces of contraction; (3) add strength and prevent overexpansion of the heart; and (4) provide elasticity that helps return the heart to its original size and shape after a contraction.

The **fibrous skeleton** of the heart consists of four dense bands of tough elastic tissue that encircle the heart valves and the bases of the pulmonary trunk and aorta (see Figure 11.8). These bands

stabilize the positions of the heart valves and ventricular muscle cells and electrically insulate the ventricular cells from the atrial cells.

The Blood Supply to the Heart

The heart works continuously, so cardiac muscle cells require reliable supplies of oxygen and nutrients. Although a great volume of blood flows through the chambers of the heart, the myocardium needs its own, separate blood supply. The **coronary circulation** supplies blood to the muscle tissue of the heart. During maximum exertion, the demand for oxygen rises considerably. The blood flow to the myocardium may then increase to nine times that of resting levels. The coronary circulation includes an extensive network of coronary blood vessels (Figure 11.9).

The Coronary Arteries

The left and right **coronary arteries** originate at the base of the ascending aorta, at the aortic sinuses (see Figure 11.9a). Blood pressure here is the highest in the systemic circuit. Each time the left ventricle contracts, it forces blood into the aorta. The arrival of additional blood at elevated pressures stretches the elastic walls of the aorta. When the left ventricle relaxes, blood no longer flows into the aorta, pressure declines, and the walls of the aorta recoil. This recoil, called *elastic rebound,* pushes blood both forward, into the systemic circuit, and backward, through the aortic sinus and then into the coronary arteries. Thus, the combination of elevated blood pressure and elastic rebound ensures a continuous flow of blood to meet the demands of active cardiac muscle tissue. However, myocardial blood flow is not steady; it peaks while the heart muscle is relaxed, and almost ceases while it contracts.

The **right coronary artery,** which follows the coronary sulcus around the heart, supplies blood to (1) the right atrium, (2) portions of both ventricles, and (3) portions of the conducting system of the heart, including the *sinoatrial (SA)* and *atrioventricular (AV) nodes.* The cells of these nodes are essential to establishing the normal heart rate. We will focus on their functions and their part in regulating the heart rate in a later section.

Inferior to the right atrium, the right coronary artery generally gives rise to one or more **marginal arteries,** which extend across the

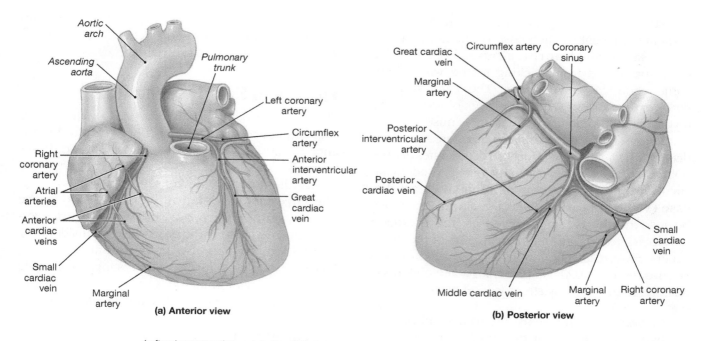

Aortic arch
Ascending aorta
Right coronary artery
Atrial arteries
Anterior cardiac veins
Small cardiac vein
Marginal artery
Pulmonary trunk
Left coronary artery
Circumflex artery
Anterior interventricular artery
Great cardiac vein

(a) Anterior view

Great cardiac vein
Marginal artery
Posterior interventricular artery
Posterior cardiac vein
Circumflex artery
Coronary sinus
Middle cardiac vein
Marginal artery
Right coronary artery
Small cardiac vein

(b) Posterior view

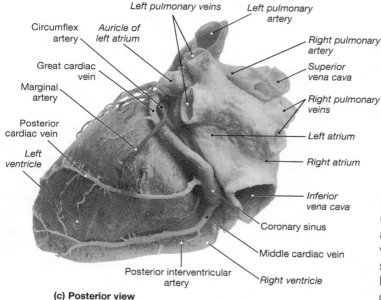

Circumflex artery
Auricle of left atrium
Great cardiac vein
Marginal artery
Posterior cardiac vein
Left ventricle
Left pulmonary veins
Left pulmonary artery
Right pulmonary artery
Superior vena cava
Right pulmonary veins
Left atrium
Right atrium
Inferior vena cava
Coronary sinus
Middle cardiac vein
Right ventricle
Posterior interventricular artery

(c) Posterior view

FIGURE 11.9 Coronary circulation.
(a) Coronary vessels supplying and draining the anterior surface of the heart. **(b)** Coronary vessels supplying and draining the posterior surface of the heart. **(c)** A posterior view of the heart; the vessels have been injected with colored latex (liquid rubber). ATLAS: Plate 45b,c.

surface of the right ventricle (see Figure 11.9a,b). The right coronary artery then continues across the posterior surface of the heart, supplying the **posterior interventricular artery,** or *posterior descending artery,* which runs toward the apex within the posterior interventricular sulcus (see Figure 11.9b,c). The posterior interventricular artery supplies blood to the interventricular septum and adjacent portions of the ventricles.

The **left coronary artery** supplies blood to the left ventricle, left atrium, and interventricular

septum. As it reaches the anterior surface of the heart, it gives rise to a circumflex branch and an anterior interventricular branch. The **circumflex artery** curves to the left around the coronary sulcus, eventually meeting and fusing with small branches of the right coronary artery (see Figure 11.9a–c). The much larger **anterior interventricular artery,** or *left anterior descending artery,* swings around the pulmonary trunk and runs along the surface within the anterior interventricular sulcus (see Figure 11.9a).

The anterior interventricular artery supplies small tributaries continuous with those of the posterior interventricular artery. Such interconnections between arteries are called **arterial anastomoses** (a-nas-tō-MŌ-sēz; *anastomosis,* outlet). Because the arteries are interconnected in this way, the blood supply to the cardiac muscle remains relatively constant despite pressure fluctuations in the left and right coronary arteries as the heart beats.

The Cardiac Veins

The various cardiac veins are shown in Figure 11.9. The **great cardiac vein** begins on the anterior surface of the ventricles, along the interventricular sulcus. This vein drains blood from the region supplied by the anterior interventricular artery, a branch of the left coronary artery. The great cardiac vein reaches the level of the atria and then curves around the left side of the heart within the coronary sulcus. The vein empties into the coronary sinus, which lies in the posterior portion of the coronary sulcus. The coronary sinus opens into the right atrium near the base of the inferior vena cava.

Other cardiac veins that empty into the great cardiac vein or the coronary sinus include (1) the **posterior cardiac vein,** draining the area served by the circumflex artery, (2) the **middle cardiac vein,** draining the area supplied by the posterior interventricular artery, and (3) the **small cardiac vein,** which receives blood from the posterior surfaces of the right atrium and ventricle. The **anterior cardiac veins,** which drain the anterior surface of the right ventricle, empty directly into the right atrium.

Clinical Note

Coronary Artery Disease

The term **coronary artery disease (CAD)** refers to areas of partial or complete blockage of coronary circulation. Cardiac muscle cells need a constant supply of oxygen and nutrients, so any reduction in blood flow to the heart muscle produces a corresponding reduction in cardiac performance. Such reduced circulatory supply, known as **coronary ischemia** (is-KE-me-uh), generally results from partial or complete blockage of the coronary arteries. The usual cause is the formation of a fatty deposit, or *atherosclerotic plaque,* in the wall of a coronary vessel. The plaque, or an associated *thrombus* (clot), then narrows the passageway and reduces blood flow. Spasms in the smooth muscles of the vessel wall can further decrease or even stop blood flow. Plaques may be visible by *angiography* or high-resolution ultrasound, and the metabolic effects can be detected in digital subtraction angiography (DSA) scans of the heart (Figure 11.10a,b).

One of the first symptoms of CAD is commonly **angina pectoris** (an-JT-nuh PEK-tor-is; *angina,* pain spasm + *pectoris,* of the chest). In its most common form, a temporary ischemia develops when the workload of the heart increases. Although the individual may feel comfortable at rest, exertion or emotional stress can produce a sensation of pressure, chest constriction, and pain that may radiate from the sternal area to the arms, back, and neck.

Angina can typically be controlled by a combination of drug treatment and changes in lifestyle, including (1) limiting activities known to trigger angina attacks (such as strenuous exercise) and avoiding stressful situations, (2) stopping smoking, and (3) lowering fat consumption. Among the medications used to control angina are drugs that block sympathetic stimulation (*propranolol* or *metoprolol*), vasodilators such as nitroglycerin (nT-tro-GLIS-er-in), and drugs that block calcium movement into the cardiac and vascular smooth muscle cells (*calcium channel blockers*).

Angina can also be treated surgically. Blockage by a single, soft plaque may be reduced with the aid of a long, slender **catheter** (KATH-e-ter), a small-diameter tube. The catheter is inserted into a large peripheral artery and guided into a coronary artery to the plaque. A variety of surgical tools can be slid into the catheter, and the plaque can then be removed using laser beams or chewed to pieces by a device that resembles a miniature version of a Roto-Rooter drain cleaner. Debris created during the destruction of a plaque could block smaller vessels, so the pieces are sucked up through the catheter (an *atherectomy*).

In **balloon angioplasty** (AN-je-o-plas-te; *angeion,* vessel), the tip of the catheter contains an inflatable balloon. Once in position, the balloon is inflated, pressing the plaque against the vessel walls. This procedure works best for small (under 10 mm), soft plaques. Several factors make angioplasty a highly attractive treatment: (1) The mortality rate during angioplasty is

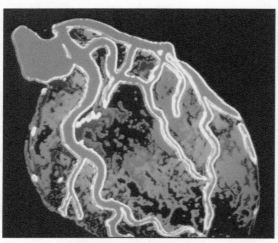

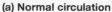

(a) Normal circulation

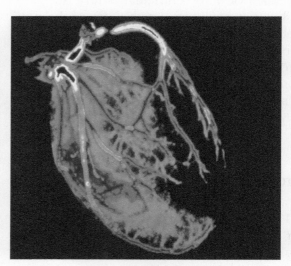

(b) Restricted circulation

FIGURE 11.10   Coronary Circulation and Clinical Testing. (a) A color-enhanced digital subtraction angiography (DSA) image of a healthy heart. The ventricular walls have an extensive circulatory supply. (The atria are not shown.) **(b)** A color-enhanced DSA image of a damaged heart. Most of the ventricular myocardium is deprived of circulation.

only about 1 percent; (2) the success rate is more than 90 percent; and (3) the procedure can be performed on an outpatient basis. Because plaques commonly redevelop after angioplasty, a fine tubular wire mesh called a *stent* may be inserted into the vessel, holding it open. Stents are now part of the standard protocol for many cardiac specialists, as the long-term success rate and incidence of complications are significantly lower than those of balloon angioplasty alone. If the circulatory blockage is too large for a single stent, multiple stents can be inserted along the length of the vessel.

When angioplasty and stents are not advisable, coronary bypass surgery may be done. In a **coronary artery bypass graft (CABG)**, a small section is removed from either a small artery (commonly the *internal thoracic artery*) or a peripheral vein (such as the *great saphenous vein* of the leg) and is used to create a detour around the obstructed portion of a coronary artery. As many as four coronary arteries can be rerouted this way during a single operation. The procedures are named according to the number of vessels repaired, so we speak of single, double, triple, or quadruple coronary bypasses. The mortality rate during surgery for such operations—when they are performed before significant heart damage has occurred—is 1–2 percent. Under these conditions, the procedure eliminates angina symptoms in 70 percent of the cases and provides partial relief in another 20 percent.

Although coronary bypass surgery offers certain advantages, recent studies have shown that for mild angina, it does not yield significantly better results than drug therapy. Current guidelines recommend that coronary bypass surgery be reserved for cases of severe angina that do not respond to other treatment.

Physiology of the Heart

As the heart beats or contracts, the blood makes continuous round trips—into and out of the heart, through the rest of the body, and then back to the heart—only to be sent out again. The amount of work that a heart does is almost too incredible to believe. In one day it pushes the body's supply of 6 quarts or so of blood (6 liters [L]) through the blood vessels over 1000 times, meaning that it actually pumps about 6000 quarts of blood in a single day!

Intrinsic Conduction System of the Heart: Setting the Basic Rhythm

Unlike skeletal muscle cells that must be stimulated by nerve impulses before they will contract, cardiac muscle cells can and do contract spontaneously and independently, even if all nervous connections are severed. Moreover, these spontaneous contractions occur in a regular and continuous way. Although cardiac muscle *can* beat independently, the muscle cells in different areas of the heart have different rhythms. The atrial cells beat about 60 times per minute, but the ventricular cells contract much more slowly (20–40/min). Therefore, without some type of unifying control system, the heart would be an uncoordinated and inefficient pump.

Two systems act to regulate heart activity. One of these involves the nerves of the autonomic nervous system that act like brakes and accelerators to decrease or increase the heart rate depending on which division is activated. This topic is considered later in this chapter. The second system is the **intrinsic conduction system,** or **nodal system,** that is built into the heart tissue (Figure 11.11) and sets its basic rhythm. The intrinsic conduction system is composed of a special tissue found nowhere else in the body; it is much like a cross between muscle and nervous tissue. This system causes heart muscle depolarization in only one direction—from the atria to the ventricles. In addition, it enforces a contraction rate of approximately 75 beats per minute on the heart; thus, the heart beats as a coordinated unit.

One of the most important parts of the intrinsic conduction system is a crescent-shaped node of tissue called the **sinoatrial** (si"no-a'tre-al) **(SA) node,** located in the right atrium. Other components include the **atrioventricular (AV) node** at the junction of the atria and ventricles, the **atrioventricular (AV) bundle (bundle of His)** and the right and left **bundle branches** located in the interventricular septum, and finally the **Purkinje** (pur-kin'je) **fibers,** which spread within the muscle of the ventricle walls.

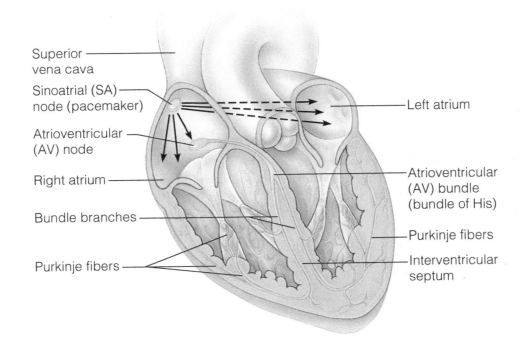

FIGURE 11.11 The intrinsic conduction system of the heart. The depolarization wave is initiated by the sinoatrial (SA) node and then passes successively through the atrial myocardium to the atrioventricular (AV) node, the AV bundle, the right and left bundle branches, and the Purkinje fibers in the ventricular walls.

The SA node is a tiny cell mass with a mammoth job. Because it has the highest rate of depolarization in the whole system, it starts each heartbeat and sets the pace for the whole heart. Consequently, the SA node is often called the **pacemaker.** From the SA node, the impulse spreads through the atria to the AV node, and then the atria contract. At the AV node, the impulse is delayed briefly to give the atria time to finish contracting. It then passes rapidly through the AV bundle, the bundle branches, and the Purkinje fibers, resulting in a "wringing" contraction of the ventricles that begins at the heart apex and moves toward the atria. This contraction effectively ejects blood superiorly into the large arteries leaving the heart. The next "A Closer Look" box and a brief section on electrocardiography that appear shortly in this chapter describe this clinical procedure for mapping the electrical activity of the heart.

Modifying the Basic Rhythm: Extrinsic Innervation of the Heart

Although the basic heart rate is set by the intrinsic conduction system, fibers of the autonomic nervous system modulate the marchlike beat and introduce a subtle variability from one beat to the next. The sympathetic nervous system (the "accelerator") increases both the rate and the force of heartbeat; parasympathetic activation (the "brakes") slows the heart. These neural controls are explained later. Here we discuss the anatomy of the nerve supply to the heart.

The cardiac centers are located in the medulla oblongata. The sympathetic **cardioacceleratory center** projects to motor neurons in the T_1–T_5 level of the spinal cord. These neurons, in turn, synapse with ganglionic neurons in the cervical and upper thoracic sympathetic chain ganglia (Figure 11.12). From there, postganglionic fibers run through the cardiac plexus to the heart where they innervate the SA and AV nodes, heart muscle, and the coronary arteries. The parasympathetic or **cardioinhibitory center** sends impulses to the dorsal vagus nucleus in the medulla, which in turn sends inhibitory impulses to the heart via branches of the **vagus nerves.** Most parasympathetic ganglionic motor neurons lie in ganglia in the heart wall and their fibers project most heavily to the SA and AV nodes.

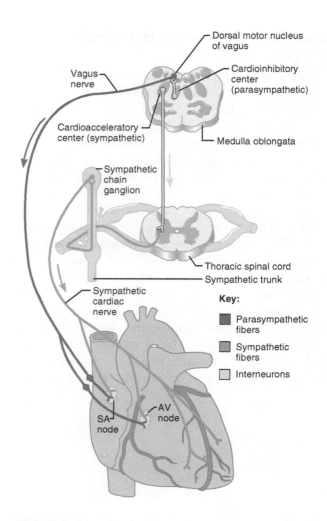

FIGURE 11.12   Autonomic innervation of the heart.

Electrocardiography

The electrical currents generated in and transmitted through the heart spread throughout the body and can be amplified with an **electrocardiograph.** The graphic recording of heart activity obtained is called an **electrocardiogram** (**ECG** or **EKG;** *kardio* is German for "heart"). An ECG is a composite of all of the APs generated by nodal and contractile cells at a given time and *not,* as sometimes assumed, a tracing of a single AP. Recording electrodes (leads) are positioned at various sites on the body surface; typically in a clinical setting, 12 leads are used. Three are bipolar leads that measure the voltage difference either between the arms or between an arm and a leg, and nine are unipolar leads. Together the 12 leads provide a fairly comprehensive picture of the heart's electrical activity.

A Closer Look

Electrocardiography: (Don't) Be Still My Heart

WHEN impulses pass through the heart, electrical currents are generated that spread throughout the body. These impulses can be detected on the body surface and recorded with an *electrocardiograph*. The recording that is made, the **electrocardiogram (ECG)**, traces the flow of current through the heart. The illustration shows a normal ECG tracing.

The typical ECG has three recognizable waves. The first wave, the **P wave**, is small and signals the depolarization of the atria immediately before they contract. The large **QRS complex**, which results from the depolarization of the ventricles, has a complicated shape. It precedes the contraction of the ventricles. The **T wave** results from currents flowing during the repolarization of the ventricles. (Atrial repolarization is generally hidden by the large QRS complex, which is being recorded at the same time.)

Abnormalities in the shape of the waves and changes in their timing send signals that something may be wrong with the intrinsic conduction system or may indicate a *myocardial infarct* (present or past). A myocardial infarct is an area of heart tissue

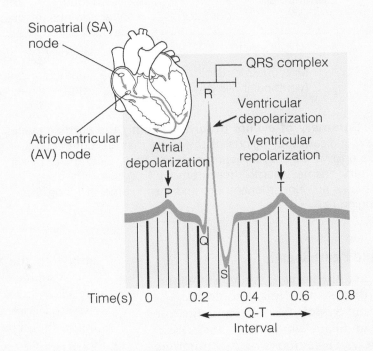

This electrocardiogram tracing shows the three normally recognizable deflection waves—P, QRS, and T.

in which the cardiac cells have died; it is generally a result of *ischemia.* During *fibrillation,* the normal pattern of the ECG is totally lost, and the heart ceases to act as a functioning pump.

Tachycardia (tak"e-kar'de-ah) is a rapid heart rate (over 100 beats per minute). **Bradycardia** (brad" e-kar'de-ah) is a heart rate that is substantially slower than normal (less than 60 beats per minute). Neither condition is pathological, but prolonged tachycardia may progress to fibrillation.

Q *Are the ventricular cardiac cells contracting isometrically or isotonically during the first part of phase 2?*

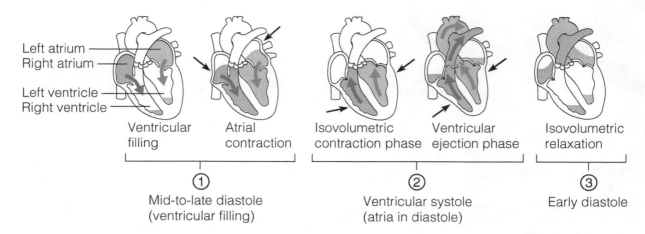

Left atrium
Right atrium
Left ventricle
Right ventricle

Ventricular filling   Atrial contraction   Isovolumetric contraction phase   Ventricular ejection phase   Isovolumetric relaxation

① Mid-to-late diastole (ventricular filling)   ② Ventricular systole (atria in diastole)   ③ Early diastole

FIGURE 11.13   Summary of events occurring during the cardiac cycle.
(Small black arrows indicate the regions of the heart that are contracting; thick red and blue arrows indicate direction of blood flow. During the *isovolumetric* (literally "same volume measurement") phases in periods 2 and 3, the ventricles are closed chambers and the volume of blood they contain is unchanging.)

Cardiac Cycle and Heart Sounds

In a healthy heart, the atria contract simultaneously. Then, as they start to relax, contraction of the ventricles begins. **Systole** (sis′to-le) and **diastole** (di-as′to-le) mean heart *contraction* and *relaxation,* respectively. Since most of the pumping work is done by the ventricles, these terms always refer to the contraction and relaxation of the *ventricles* unless otherwise stated.

The term **cardiac cycle** refers to the events of one complete heartbeat, during which both atria and ventricles contract and then relax. Since the average heart beats approximately 75 times per minute, the length of the cardiac cycle is normally about 0.8 second. We will consider the cardiac cycle in terms of events occurring during three periods—*mid-to-late diastole, ventricular systole,* and *early diastole* (Figure 11.13).

1. **Mid-to-late diastole.** Our discussion begins with the heart in complete relaxation. At this point, the pressure in the heart is low, and blood is flowing passively into and through the atria into the ventricles from the pulmonary and systemic circulations. The semilunar valves are closed, and the AV valves are open. Then the atria contract and force the blood remaining in their chambers into the ventricles.

2. **Ventricular systole.** Shortly after, ventricular contraction (systole) begins and the pressure within the ventricles increases rapidly, closing the AV valves. When the intraventricular pressure (pressure in the ventricles) is higher than the pressure in the large arteries leaving the heart, the semilunar valves are forced open, and blood rushes through them out of the ventricles. During ventricular systole, the atria are relaxed, and their chambers are again filling with blood.

3. **Early diastole.** At the end of systole, the ventricles relax, the semilunar valves snap shut (preventing backflow), and for a moment, the ventricles are completely closed chambers. During early diastole, the intraventricular pressure drops. When it drops below the pressure in the atria (which has been increasing as blood has been filling their chambers), the AV valves are forced open, and the ventricles again begin to refill rapidly with blood, completing the cycle.

A *Isometrically until they have enough force to overcome the back pressure of the blood against the semilunar valves, at which point their contraction becomes isotonic.*

When using a stethoscope, you can hear two distinct sounds during each cardiac cycle. These **heart sounds** are often described by the two syllables "lub" and "dup," and the sequence is lub-dup, pause, lub-dup, pause, and so on. The first heart sound (lub) is caused by the closing of the AV valves. The second heart sound (dup) occurs when the semilunar valves close at the end of systole. The first heart sound is longer and louder than the second heart sound, which tends to be short and sharp.

Homeostatic Imbalance

Abnormal or unusual heart sounds are called *murmurs*. Blood flows silently as long as the flow is smooth and uninterrupted. If it strikes obstructions, its flow becomes turbulent and generates sounds, such as heart murmurs, that can be heard with a stethoscope. Heart murmurs are fairly common in young children (and some elderly people) with perfectly healthy hearts, probably because their heart walls are relatively thin and vibrate with rushing blood. However, most often, murmurs indicate valve problems. For example, if a valve does not close tightly (is *incompetent*), a swishing sound will be heard *after* that valve has (supposedly) closed, as the blood flows back through the partially open valve. Distinct sounds also can be heard when blood flows turbulently through *stenosed* (narrowed) valves.

Cardiac Output of a Dual Pressure Pump

Cardiac output (CO) is the amount of blood pumped out by *each* side of the heart (actually each ventricle) in 1 minute. It is the product of the **heart rate (HR)** and the **stroke volume (SV).** Stroke volume is the volume of blood pumped out by a ventricle with each heartbeat. In general, stroke volume increases as the force of ventricular contraction increases. If we use the normal resting values for heart rate (75 beats per minute) and stroke volume (70 ml per beat), the average adult cardiac output can be easily figured:

CO = HR (75 beats/min) × SV (70 ml/beat)

CO = 5250 ml/min

Since the normal adult blood volume is about 5000 ml, the entire blood supply passes through the body once each minute. Cardiac output varies with the demands of the body. It rises when the stroke volume is increased or the heart beats faster

or both; it drops when either or both of these factors decrease. Since this is so, let's take a look at how stroke volume and heart rate are regulated.

Regulation of Stroke Volume A healthy heart pumps out about 60 percent of the blood present in its ventricles. As noted above, this is approximately 70 ml (about 2 ounces) with each heartbeat. According to *Starling's law of the heart,* the critical factor controlling stroke volume is how much the cardiac muscle cells are stretched just before they contract. The more they are stretched, the stronger the contraction will be. The important factor stretching the heart muscle is *venous return,* the amount of blood entering the heart and distending its ventricles. If one side of the heart suddenly begins to pump more blood than the other, the increased venous return to the opposite ventricle will force it to pump out an equal amount, thus preventing backup of blood in the circulation.

Anything that increases the volume or speed of venous return also increases stroke volume and force of contraction (Figure 11.14). For example, a slow heartbeat allows more time for the ventricles to fill. Exercise speeds venous return because it results in increased heart rate and force. The enhanced squeezing action of active skeletal muscles on the veins returning blood to the heart, the so-called muscular pump, also plays a major role in increasing the venous return. On the other hand, low venous return, such as might result from severe blood loss or an extremely rapid heart rate, decreases stroke volume, causing the heart to beat less forcefully.

Factors Modifying Basic Heart Rate In healthy people, stroke volume tends to be relatively constant. However, when blood volume drops suddenly or when the heart has been seriously weakened, stroke volume declines, and cardiac output is maintained by a faster heartbeat. Although heart contraction does not depend on the nervous system, its rate *can* be changed temporarily by the autonomic nerves. Indeed, the most important external influence on heart rate is the activity of the autonomic nervous system. Heart rate is also modified by various chemicals, hormones, and ions. Some of these factors are summarized in Figure 11.14.

Neural (ANS) Controls During times of physical or emotional stress, the nerves of the *sympathetic division* of the autonomic nervous system more strongly stimulate the SA and AV nodes and the

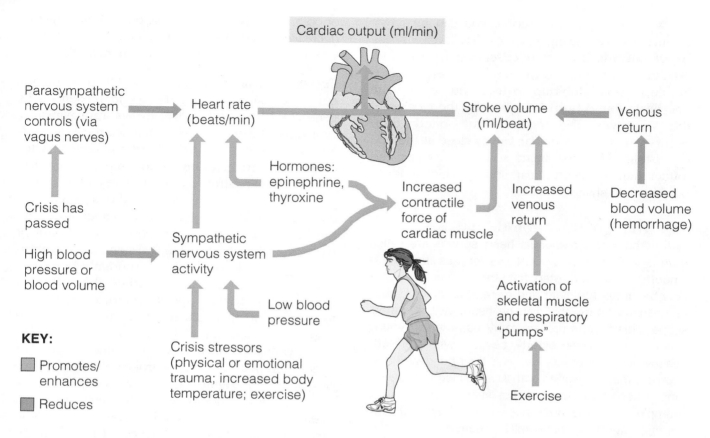

FIGURE 11.14 **Influence of selected factors on cardiac output.** Note that the direction of the flowchart is from the bottom up.

cardiac muscle itself. As a result, the heart beats more rapidly. This is a familiar phenomenon to anyone who has ever been frightened or has had to run to catch a bus. As fast as the heart pumps under ordinary conditions, it really speeds up when special demands are placed on it. Since a faster blood flow increases the rate at which fresh blood reaches body cells, more oxygen and glucose are made available to them during periods of stress. When demand declines, the heart adjusts. *Parasympathetic nerves,* primarily the **vagus nerves,** slow and steady the heart, giving it more time to rest during noncrisis times. In patients with *congestive heart failure,* a condition in which the heart is nearly "worn out" due to age, hypertensive heart disease, or another pathological process, the heart pumps weakly. For those patients, the drug digitalis is routinely prescribed. It enhances contractile force and stroke volume of the heart resulting in greater cardiac output.

Various hormones and ions can have a dramatic effect on heart activity. *Epinephrine,* which

mimics the effect of the sympathetic nerves, and *thyroxine* both increase heart rate. Electrolyte imbalances pose a real threat to the heart. For example, reduced levels of ionic calcium in the blood depress the heart, whereas excessive blood calcium causes such prolonged contractions that the heart may stop entirely. Excesses or a lack of needed ions such as sodium and potassium also modify heart activity. A deficit of potassium ions in the blood, for example, causes the heart to beat feebly, and abnormal heart rhythms appear.

Physical Factors   A number of physical factors, including age, gender, exercise, and body temperature, influence heart rate. Resting heart rate is fastest in the fetus (140–160 beats per minute) and then gradually decreases throughout life. The average heart rate is faster in females (72–80 beats per minute) than in males (64–72 beats per minute). Heat increases heart rate by boosting the metabolic rate of heart cells. This explains the rapid, pounding heartbeat you feel when you have a high fever and accounts in part for the effect of exercise on heart rate (remember, working muscles generate heat). Cold has the opposite effect; it directly decreases heart rate. As noted above, exercise acts through nervous system controls (sympathetic division) to increase heart rate (and also, through the action of the muscular pump, to increase stroke volume).

Overview: The Control of Cardiac Output

Figure 11.15 summarizes the factors involved in the normal regulation of cardiac output. As we've discussed, cardiac output can be adjusted by changes in either heart rate or stroke volume, but now let's look at these processes in more detail. For convenience, we will consider these independently as we discuss the individual factors involved. However, changes in cardiac output generally reflect changes in both heart rate and stroke volume.

The heart rate can be adjusted by the activities of the autonomic nervous system or by circulating hormones. The stroke volume can be adjusted by changing the end-diastolic volume (how full the ventricles are when they start to contract), the end-systolic volume (how much blood remains in the ventricle after it contracts), or both. Stroke volume

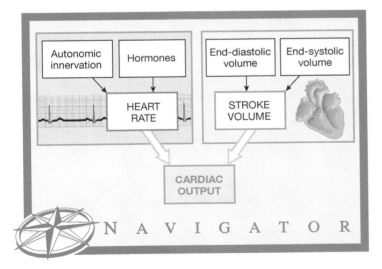

FIGURE 11.15 Factors affecting cardiac output. A simplified version of this figure will appear as a Navigator icon in key figures as we move from one topic to the next.

peaks when EDV is highest and ESV is lowest. A variety of other factors can influence cardiac output under abnormal circumstances; we will consider several examples in a separate section.

Factors Affecting the Heart Rate

Under normal circumstances, autonomic activity and circulating hormones are responsible for making delicate adjustments to the heart rate as circulatory demands change. These factors act by modifying the natural rhythm of the heart. Even a heart removed for a heart transplant will continue to beat unless steps are taken to prevent it from doing so.

Autonomic Innervation

The sympathetic and parasympathetic divisions of the autonomic nervous system innervate the heart by means of the *cardiac plexus* (Figure 11.16). Postganglionic sympathetic neurons are located in the cervical and upper thoracic ganglia. The vagus nerves (X) carry parasympathetic preganglionic fibers to small ganglia in the cardiac plexus. Both ANS divisions innervate the SA and AV nodes and the atrial muscle cells. Although ventricular muscle cells are also innervated by both divisions, sympathetic fibers far outnumber parasympathetic fibers there.

The *cardiac centers* of the medulla oblongata contain the autonomic headquarters for cardiac control. The **cardioacceleratory center** controls sympathetic neurons that increase the heart rate; the adjacent **cardioinhibitory center** controls the parasympathetic neurons that slow the heart rate. The activities of the cardiac centers are regulated by reflex pathways and through input from higher centers, especially from the parasympathetic and sympathetic headquarters in the hypothalamus.

Cardiac Reflexes Information about the status of the cardiovascular system arrives over visceral sensory fibers accompanying the vagus nerve and the sympathetic nerves of the cardiac plexus. The cardiac centers monitor **baroreceptors** and **chemoreceptors** innervated by the glossopharyngeal (IX) and vagus (X) nerves. On the basis of the information received, the centers adjust cardiac performance to maintain adequate circulation to vital organs, such as the brain. The centers respond to changes in blood pressure as reported

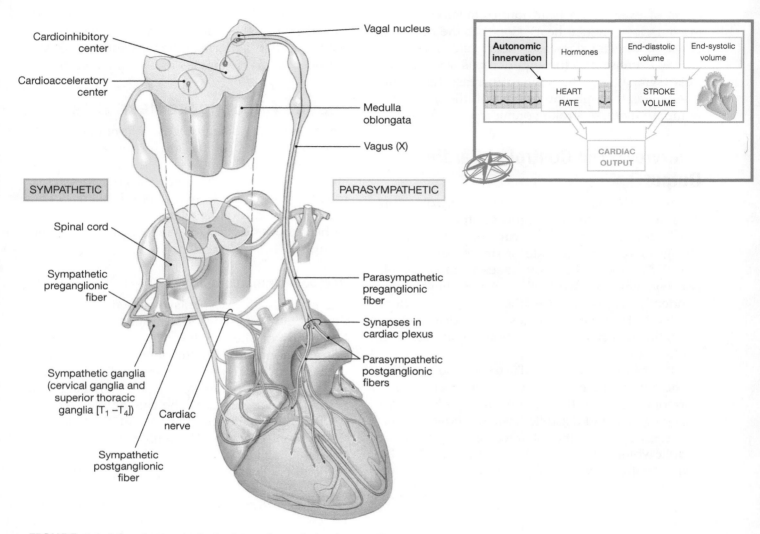

FIGURE 11.16   Autonomic innervation of the heart. The Navigator icon
in the shadow box highlights the topic we will consider in this section.

by baroreceptors and in arterial concentrations of
dissolved oxygen and carbon dioxide as reported
by chemoreceptors. For example, a decline in
blood pressure or oxygen concentrations or an
increase in carbon dioxide levels generally indicates that the heart must work harder to meet the
demands of peripheral tissues. The cardiac centers
then call for an increase in cardiac activity.

Autonomic Tone   As is the case in other organs
with dual innervation, the heart has a resting autonomic tone. Both autonomic divisions are
normally active at a steady background level,
releasing ACh and NE at the nodes and into the
myocardium. Thus, cutting the vagus nerves
increases the heart rate, and sympathetic blocking
agents slow the heart rate.

Effects on the SA Node   The sympathetic and
parasympathetic divisions alter the heart rate by
changing the ionic permeabilities of cells in the
conducting system. The most dramatic effects
are seen at the SA node, where changes in the
rate at which impulses are generated affect the
heart rate.

Consider the SA node of a resting individual
whose heart is beating at 75 bpm. Any factor that
changes the rate of spontaneous depolarization or
the duration of repolarization will alter the heart
rate by changing the time required to reach threshold. Acetylcholine released by parasympathetic
neurons opens chemically regulated K^+ channels
in the cell membrane, thereby dramatically slowing
the rate of spontaneous depolarization and also

slightly extending the duration of repolarization. The result is a decline in heart rate.

NE released by sympathetic neurons binds to beta-1 receptors, leading to the opening of sodium-calcium ion channels. The subsequent influx of positively charged ions increases the rate of depolarization and shortens the period of repolarization. The nodal cells reach threshold more quickly, and the heart rate increases.

The Atrial Reflex The **atrial reflex,** or **Bainbridge reflex,** involves adjustments in heart rate in response to an increase in the venous return. When the walls of the right atrium are stretched, the stimulation of stretch receptors in the atrial walls triggers a reflexive increase in heart rate caused by increased sympathetic activity. Thus, when the rate of venous return to the heart increases, the heart rate, and hence the cardiac output, rises as well.

Hormones

Epinephrine, norepinephrine, and thyroid hormone increase the heart rate by their effect on the SA node. The effects of epinephrine on the SA node are similar to those of norepinephrine. Epinephrine also affects the contractile cells; after massive sympathetic stimulation of the adrenal medullae, the myocardium may become so excitable that abnormal contractions occur.

▲ Homeostatic Imbalance

The pumping action of the healthy heart maintains a balance between cardiac output and venous return. But when the pumping efficiency of the heart is depressed so that circulation is inadequate to meet tissue needs, **congestive heart failure (CHF)** occurs. Congestive heart failure is usually a progressive condition that reflects weakening of the heart by *coronary atherosclerosis* (clogging of the coronary vessels with fatty buildup), persistent high blood pressure, or multiple myocardial infarctions (leading to repair with noncontracting scar tissue).

Because the heart is a double pump, each side can fail independently of the other. If the left heart fails, *pulmonary congestion* occurs. The right side of the heart continues to propel blood to the lungs, but the left side is unable to eject the returning blood into the systemic circulation. As blood vessels within the lungs become swollen with blood, the pressure within them increases, and fluid leaks from the circulation into the lung tissue, causing **pulmonary edema.** If untreated, the person suffocates.

If the right side of the heart fails, *peripheral congestion* occurs as blood backs up in the systemic circulation. Edema is most noticeable in the distal parts of the body: The feet, ankles, and fingers become swollen and puffy. Failure of one side of the heart puts a greater strain on the opposite side, and eventually, the whole heart fails. ▲

Blood Vessels

Blood circulates inside the blood vessels, which form a closed transport system, the so-called **vascular system.** The idea that blood circulates, or "makes rounds," through the body is only about 300 years old. The ancient Greeks believed that blood moved through the body like an ocean tide, first moving out from the heart and then ebbing back to it in the same vessels to get rid of its impurities in the lungs. It was not until the seventeenth century that William Harvey, an English physician, proved that blood did, in fact, move in circles.

Like a system of roads, the vascular system has its freeways, secondary roads, and alleys. As the heart beats, blood is propelled into the large **arteries** leaving the heart. It then moves into successively smaller and smaller arteries and then into the **arterioles** (ar-ter′e-ōlz), which feed the **capillary** (kap′ĭ-lar″e) **beds** in the tissues. Capillary beds are drained by **venules** (ven′ulz), which in turn empty into **veins** that finally empty into the great veins (venae cavae) entering the heart. Thus arteries, which carry blood away from the heart, and veins, which drain the tissues and return the blood to the heart, are simply conducting vessels—the freeways and secondary roads. Only the tiny hairlike capillaries, which extend and branch through the tissues and connect the smallest arteries (arterioles) to the smallest veins (venules), directly serve the needs of the body cells. The capillaries are the side streets or alleys that intimately intertwine among the body cells and provide access to individual "homes." It is only through their walls that exchanges between the tissue cells and the blood can occur.

Notice that this book routinely depicts arteries red and veins blue because, by convention, red indicates oxygen-rich blood and blue indicates relatively oxygen-depleted, carbon dioxide-rich blood, the normal status of blood in most of the body's arteries and veins. However, there are exceptions to this convention which will be pointed out as they are encountered.

Microscopic Anatomy of Blood Vessels

Tunics

Except for the microscopic capillaries, the walls of blood vessels have three coats, or tunics (Figure 11.17). The **tunica intima** (tu'nĭ-kah in-tim'ah), which lines the lumen or interior of the vessels, is a thin layer of **endothelium** (squamous epithelial cells) resting on a basement membrane. Its cells fit closely together and form a slick surface that decreases friction as blood flows through the vessel lumen.

The **tunica media** (me'de-ah) is the bulky middle coat. It is mostly smooth muscle and elastic tissue. Some of the larger arteries have *elastic laminae,* complete sheets of elastic tissue in addition to the scattered elastic fibers. The smooth muscle, which is controlled by the sympathetic nervous system, is active in changing the diameter of the vessels. As the vessels constrict or dilate, blood pressure increases or decreases, respectively.

The **tunica externa** (eks'tern-ah) is the outermost tunic; it is composed largely of fibrous connective tissue. Its function is basically to support and protect the vessels.

Structural Differences between Arteries, Veins, and Capillaries

The walls of arteries are usually much thicker than the walls of veins. Their tunica media, in particular, tends to be much heavier. This structural difference is related to a difference in function of these two types of vessels. Arteries, which are closer to the pumping action of the heart, must be able to expand as blood is forced into them and then recoil passively as the blood flows off into the circulation during diastole. Their walls must be strong and stretchy enough to take these continuous changes in pressure (see Figure 11.17).

On the other hand, veins are far from the heart in the circulatory pathway, and the pressure in them tends to be low all the time. Thus veins have thinner walls. However, since the blood pressure in veins is usually too low to force the blood back to the heart and blood returning to the heart often

flows against gravity, veins are modified to ensure that the amount of blood returning to the heart *(venous return)* equals the amount being pumped out of the heart *(cardiac output)* at any time. The lumens of veins tend to be much larger than those of corresponding arteries, and the larger veins have **valves** that prevent backflow of blood (see Figure 11.17). Skeletal muscle activity also enhances venous return. As the muscles surrounding the veins contract and relax, the blood is forced or squeezed through the veins toward the heart (Figure 11.18). Finally, when we inhale, the drop in pressure that occurs in the thorax causes the large veins near the heart to expand and fill. Thus, the "respiratory pump" also helps return blood to the heart (see Figure 11.14).

The transparent walls of the capillaries are only one cell layer thick—just the tunica intima. Because of this exceptional thinness, exchanges are easily made between the blood and the tissue cells. The tiny capillaries tend to form interweaving networks called **capillary beds.** The flow of blood from an arteriole to a venule—that is, through a capillary bed—is called **microcirculation.** In most body regions, a capillary bed consists of two types of vessels: (1) a **vascular shunt,** a vessel that directly connects the arteriole and venule at opposite ends of the bed, and (2) **true capillaries,** the actual *exchange vessels* (Figure 11.19).

The *true capillaries* number 10 to 100 per capillary bed, depending on the organ or tissues served. They usually branch off the proximal end of the shunt and return to the distal end, but occasionally they spring from the **terminal arteriole** and empty directly into the **postcapillary venule.** A cuff of smooth muscle fibers, called a **precapillary sphincter,** surrounds the root of each true capillary and acts as a valve to regulate the flow of blood into the capillary. Blood flowing through a terminal arteriole may take one of two routes: through the true capillaries or through the shunt. When the precapillary sphincters are relaxed (open), blood flows through the true capillaries and takes part in exchanges with tissue cells. When the sphincters are contracted (closed), blood flows through the shunts and bypasses the tissue cells.

The walls of larger veins and arteries even contain small vessels that supply blood to the smooth muscle cells and fibroblasts of the tunica. These blood vessels are called the vasa vasorum.

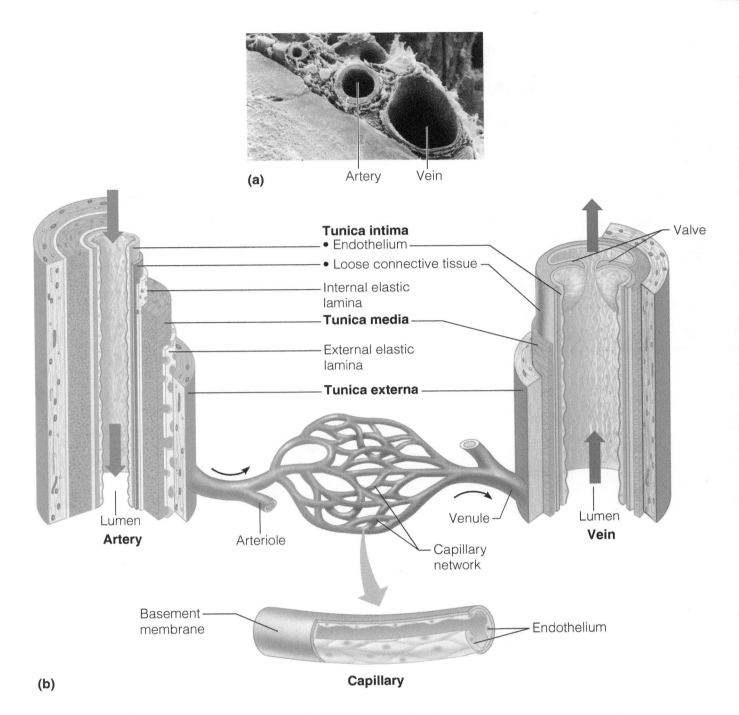

(a) Artery   Vein

Tunica intima
• Endothelium
• Loose connective tissue
Internal elastic lamina
Tunica media
External elastic lamina
Tunica externa

Valve

Lumen
Artery

Arteriole

Capillary network

Venule

Lumen
Vein

Basement membrane

Endothelium

Capillary

(b)

FIGURE 11.17 Structure of blood vessels. (a) Scanning electron micrograph of an artery and vein in cross section (120×). **(b)** The walls of arteries and veins are composed of three tunics: the tunica intima (endothelium underlain by a basement membrane), tunica media (smooth muscle and elastic fibers), and tunica externa (largely collagen fibers). Capillaries—between arteries and veins in the circulatory pathway—are composed only of the tunica intima. Notice that the tunica media is thick in arteries and relatively thin in veins. Part **(a)**: Copyright by R.G. Kessel and R.H. Kardon, *Tissues and Organs: A Text-Atlas of Scanning Electron Microscopy,* W.H. Freeman and Company, 1979, all rights reserved.

Prove It Yourself

Venous Valves Prevent Backflow

To demonstrate the efficiency of the venous valves in preventing backflow of blood, perform the following simple experiment.

Allow one hand to hang by your side for a minute or two, until the blood vessels on its dorsal aspect become distended (swollen) with blood. Place two fingertips side by side against one of the distended veins. Then, pressing firmly, move your proximal finger along the vein toward your heart. Now release that finger. As you can see, the vein remains collapsed in spite of gravity. Now remove your distal finger, and watch the vein fill rapidly with blood.

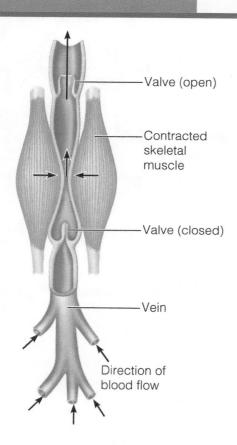

FIGURE 11.18 **Operation of the muscular pump.** When skeletal muscles contract and press against the flexible veins, the valves proximal to the area of contraction are forced open, and blood is squeezed toward the heart. The valves distal to the point of contraction are closed by the backflowing blood.

Q *Assume the capillary bed depicted here is in the biceps brachii muscle of your arm. What condition would the capillary bed be in (a or b) if you were doing push-ups at the gym?*

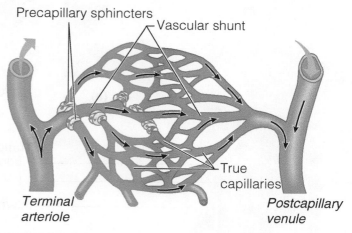

(a) Sphincters open

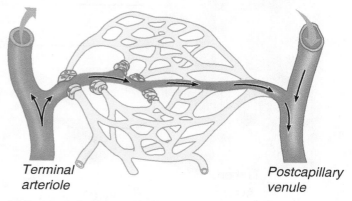

(b) Sphincters closed

FIGURE 11.19 **Anatomy of a capillary bed.** The vascular shunt bypasses the true capillaries when precapillary sphincters controlling blood entry into the true capillaries are constricted.

Gross Anatomy of Blood Vessels

Major Arteries of the Systemic Circulation

The **aorta** is the largest artery of the body, and it is a truly splendid vessel. In adults, the aorta is about the size of a garden hose (with an internal diameter the size of your thumb); it issues from the left ventricle of the heart. It decreases only slightly in

A   *a. The true capillaries would be flushed with blood to serve the working muscle cells.*

size as it runs to its terminus. Different parts of the aorta are named for their location or shape. The aorta springs upward from the left ventricle of the heart as the **ascending aorta,** arches to the left as the **aortic arch,** and then plunges downward through the thorax following the spine **(thoracic aorta)** to finally pass through the diaphragm into the abdominopelvic cavity, where it becomes the **abdominal aorta** (Figure 11.20).

The major branches of the aorta and the organs they serve are listed next in sequence from the heart. Figure 11.20 shows the course of the aorta and its major branches. As you locate the arteries on the figure, be aware of ways to make your learning easier. In many cases, the name of the artery tells you the body region or organs served (renal artery, brachial artery, and coronary artery) or the bone followed (femoral artery and ulnar artery).

Arterial Branches of the Ascending Aorta

- The only branches of the ascending aorta are the **right [R.]** and **left [L.] coronary arteries,** which serve the heart.

Arterial Branches of the Aortic Arch

- The **brachiocephalic** (bra″ke-o-se-fal′ik) **trunk** (the first branch off the aortic arch) splits into the **R. common carotid** (kah-ro′tid) **artery** and **R. subclavian** (sub-kla′ve-an) **artery.** (See same-named vessels on left side of body for organs served.)

- The **L. common carotid artery** is the second branch off the aortic arch. It divides, forming the **L. internal carotid,** which serves the brain, and the **L. external carotid,** which serves the skin and muscles of the head and neck.

- The third branch of the aortic arch, the **L. subclavian artery,** gives off an important branch—the **vertebral artery,** which serves part of the brain. In the axilla, the subclavian artery becomes the **axillary artery** and then continues into the arm as the **brachial artery,** which supplies the arm. At the elbow, the brachial artery splits to form the **radial** and **ulnar arteries,** which serve the forearm.

Arterial Branches of the Thoracic Aorta

- The *intercostal arteries* (ten pairs) supply the muscles of the thorax wall. Other branches of the thoracic aorta supply the lungs *(bronchial*

arteries), the esophagus *(esophageal arteries),* and the diaphragm *(phrenic arteries).* These arteries are not illustrated in Figure 11.20.

Arterial Branches of the Abdominal Aorta

- The **celiac trunk** is the first branch of the abdominal aorta. It is a single vessel that has three branches: (1) the **L. gastric artery** supplies the stomach, (2) the **splenic artery** supplies the spleen, and (3) the **common hepatic artery** supplies the liver.

- The unpaired **superior mesenteric** (mes″en-ter′ik) **artery** supplies most of the small intestine and the first half of the large intestine, or colon.

- The **renal** (R. and L.) **arteries** serve the kidneys.

- The **gonadal** (R. and L.) **arteries** supply the gonads. They are called the *ovarian arteries* in females (serving the ovaries) and the *testicular arteries* in males (serving the testes).

- The *lumbar arteries* (not illustrated in Figure 11.20) are several pairs of arteries serving the heavy muscles of the abdomen and trunk walls.

- The **inferior mesenteric artery** is a small, unpaired artery supplying the second half of the large intestine.

- The **common iliac** (R. and L.) **arteries** are the final branches of the abdominal aorta. Each divides into an **internal iliac artery,** which supplies the pelvic organs (bladder, rectum, and so on), and an **external iliac artery,** which enters the thigh, where it becomes the **femoral artery.** The femoral artery and its branch, the **deep femoral artery,** serve the thigh. At the knee, the femoral artery becomes the **popliteal artery,** which then splits into the **anterior** and **posterior tibial arteries,** which supply the leg and foot. The anterior tibial artery terminates in the **dorsalis pedis artery,** which supplies the dorsum of the foot. (The dorsalis pedis is often palpated in patients with circulatory problems of the legs to determine if the distal part of the leg has adequate circulation.)

Major Veins of the Systemic Circulation

Although arteries are generally located in deep, well-protected body areas, many veins are more superficial and some are easily seen and palpated on the body surface. Most deep veins follow the course

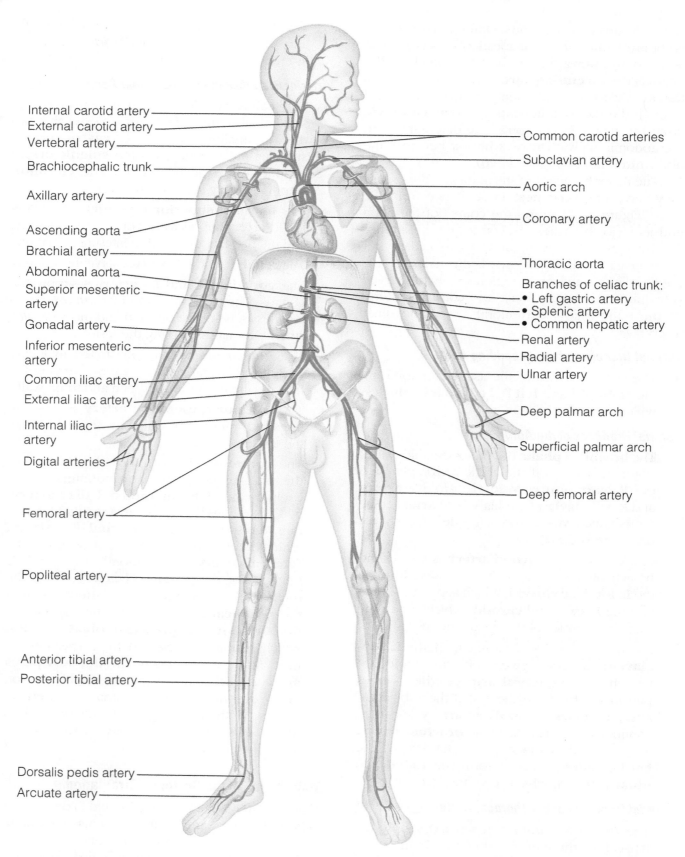

Internal carotid artery

External carotid artery

Vertebral artery

Brachiocephalic trunk

Axillary artery

Ascending aorta

Brachial artery

Abdominal aorta

Superior mesenteric artery

Gonadal artery

Inferior mesenteric artery

Common iliac artery

External iliac artery

Internal iliac artery

Digital arteries

Femoral artery

Popliteal artery

Anterior tibial artery

Posterior tibial artery

Dorsalis pedis artery

Arcuate artery

Common carotid arteries

Subclavian artery

Aortic arch

Coronary artery

Thoracic aorta

Branches of celiac trunk:
• Left gastric artery
• Splenic artery
• Common hepatic artery

Renal artery

Radial artery

Ulnar artery

Deep palmar arch

Superficial palmar arch

Deep femoral artery

FIGURE 11.20 Major arteries of the systemic circulation, anterior view.

of the major arteries; and, with a few exceptions, the naming of these veins is identical to that of their companion arteries. Major systemic arteries branch off the aorta, whereas the veins converge on the venae cavae, which enter the right atrium of the heart. Veins draining the head and arms empty into the **superior vena cava** and those draining the lower body empty into the **inferior vena cava.** These veins are described next and shown in Figure 11.21. As before, locate the veins on the figure as you read their descriptions.

Veins Draining into the Superior Vena Cava

Veins draining into the superior vena cava are named in a distal to proximal direction; that is, in the same direction the blood flows into the superior vena cava.

- The **radial** and **ulnar veins** are deep veins draining the forearm. They unite to form the deep **brachial vein,** which drains the arm and empties into the **axillary vein** in the axillary region.

- The **cephalic** (se-fal′ik) **vein** provides for the superficial drainage of the lateral aspect of the arm and empties into the axillary vein.

- The **basilic** (bah-sil′ik) **vein** is a superficial vein that drains the medial aspect of the arm and empties into the brachial vein proximally. The basilic and cephalic veins are joined at the anterior aspect of the elbow by the **median cubital vein.** (The median cubital vein is often chosen as the site for blood removal for the purpose of blood testing.)

- The **subclavian vein** receives venous blood from the arm through the axillary vein and from the skin and muscles of the head through the **external jugular vein.**

- The **vertebral vein** drains the posterior part of the head.

- The **internal jugular vein** drains the dural sinuses of the brain.

- The **brachiocephalic** (R. and L.) **veins** are large veins that receive venous drainage from the subclavian, vertebral, and internal jugular veins on their respective sides. The brachiocephalic veins join to form the superior vena cava, which enters the heart.

- The *azygos* (az′ĭ-gos) *vein* is a single vein that drains the thorax and enters the superior vena

cava just before it joins the heart. (This vein is not illustrated in Figure 11.21.)

Veins Draining into the Inferior Vena Cava

The inferior vena cava, which is much longer than the superior vena cava, returns blood to the heart from all body regions below the diaphragm. As before, we will trace the venous drainage in a distal to proximal direction.

- The **anterior** and **posterior tibial veins** and the **fibular vein** drain the leg (calf and foot). The posterior tibial vein becomes the **popliteal vein** at the knee and then the **femoral vein** in the thigh. The femoral vein becomes the **external iliac vein** as it enters the pelvis.

- The **great saphenous** (sah-fe′nus) **veins** are the longest veins in the body. They receive the superficial drainage of the leg. They begin at the **dorsal venous arch** in the foot and travel up the medial aspect of the leg to empty into the femoral vein in the thigh.

- Each **common iliac** (R. and L.) **vein** is formed by the union of the **external iliac vein** and the **internal iliac vein** (which drains the pelvis) on its own side. The common iliac veins join to form the inferior vena cava, which then ascends superiorly in the abdominal cavity.

- The *R. gonadal vein* drains the right ovary in females and the right testicle in males. (The *L. gonadal vein* empties into the left renal vein superiorly.) (The gonadal veins are not illustrated in Figure 11.21.)

- The **renal** (R. and L.) **veins** drain the kidneys.

- The **hepatic portal vein** is a single vein that drains the digestive tract organs and carries this blood through the liver before it enters the systemic circulation. (The hepatic portal circulation is discussed in the next section.)

- The **hepatic** (R. and L.) **veins** drain the liver.

Special Circulations

Arterial Supply of the Brain and the Circle of Willis

A continuous blood supply to the brain is crucial, since a lack of blood for even a few minutes causes the delicate brain cells to die. The brain is supplied

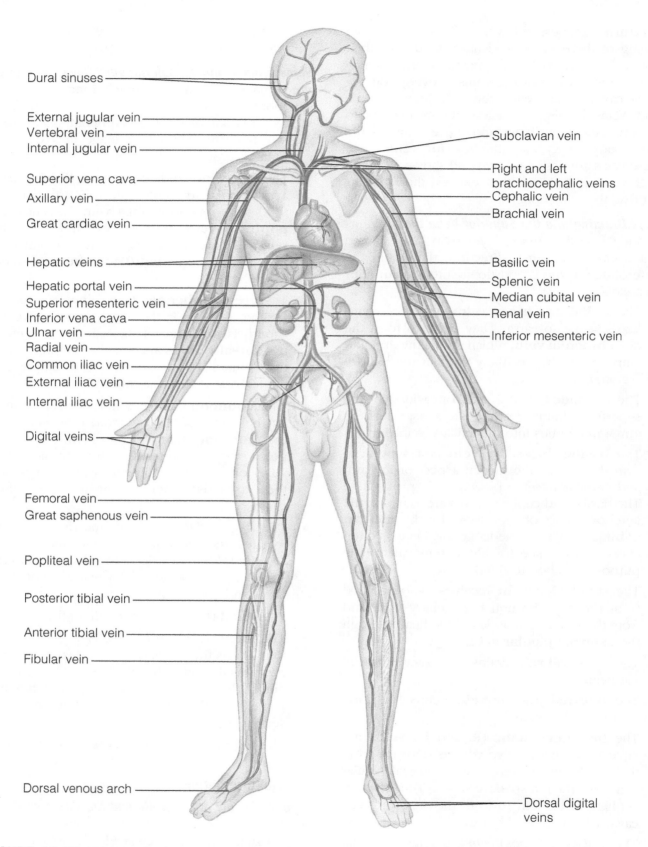

Dural sinuses

External jugular vein
Vertebral vein
Internal jugular vein

Superior vena cava

Axillary vein

Great cardiac vein

Hepatic veins

Hepatic portal vein
Superior mesenteric vein
Inferior vena cava
Ulnar vein
Radial vein
Common iliac vein
External iliac vein
Internal iliac vein

Digital veins

Femoral vein
Great saphenous vein

Popliteal vein

Posterior tibial vein

Anterior tibial vein

Fibular vein

Dorsal venous arch

Subclavian vein

Right and left
brachiocephalic veins
Cephalic vein
Brachial vein

Basilic vein
Splenic vein
Median cubital vein
Renal vein
Inferior mesenteric vein

Dorsal digital
veins

FIGURE 11.21   Major veins of the systemic circulation, anterior view. The vessels of the pulmonary circulation are not illustrated, accounting for the incomplete appearance of the circulation from the heart.

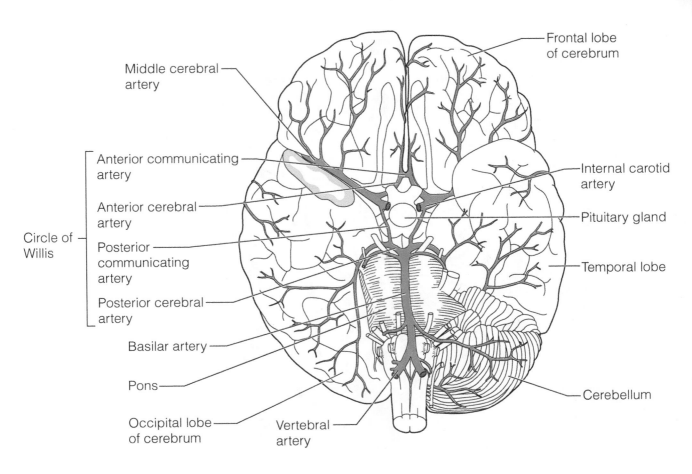

Middle cerebral artery

Anterior communicating artery

Anterior cerebral artery

Circle of Willis

Posterior communicating artery

Posterior cerebral artery

Basilar artery

Pons

Occipital lobe of cerebrum

Vertebral artery

Frontal lobe of cerebrum

Internal carotid artery

Pituitary gland

Temporal lobe

Cerebellum

FIGURE 11.22 Arterial supply of the brain. (Cerebellum is shown only on the left side of the brain.)

by two pairs of arteries, the internal carotid arteries and the vertebral arteries (Figure 11.22).

The **internal carotid arteries,** branches of the common carotid arteries, run through the neck and enter the skull through the temporal bone. Once inside the cranium, each divides into the **anterior** and **middle cerebral arteries,** which supply most of the cerebrum.

The paired **vertebral arteries** pass upward from the subclavian arteries at the base of the neck. Within the skull, the vertebral arteries join to form the single **basilar artery,** which serves the brain stem and cerebellum as it travels upward. At the base of the cerebrum, the basilar artery divides to form the **posterior cerebral arteries,** which supply the posterior part of the cerebrum.

The anterior and posterior blood supplies of the brain are united by small *communicating arterial branches.* The result is a complete circle of connecting blood vessels called the **circle of**

Willis, which surrounds the base of the brain. The circle of Willis protects the brain by providing more than one route for blood to reach brain tissue in case of a clot or impaired blood flow anywhere in the system.

Hepatic Portal Circulation The veins of the **hepatic portal circulation** drain the digestive organs, spleen, and pancreas and deliver this blood to the liver through the **hepatic portal vein** (Figure 11.23). When you have just eaten, the hepatic portal blood contains large amounts of nutrients. Since the liver is a key body organ involved in maintaining the proper glucose, fat, and protein concentrations in the blood, this system "takes a detour" to ensure that the liver processes these substances before they enter the systemic circulation. As blood flows slowly through the liver, some of the nutrients are removed to be stored or processed in various

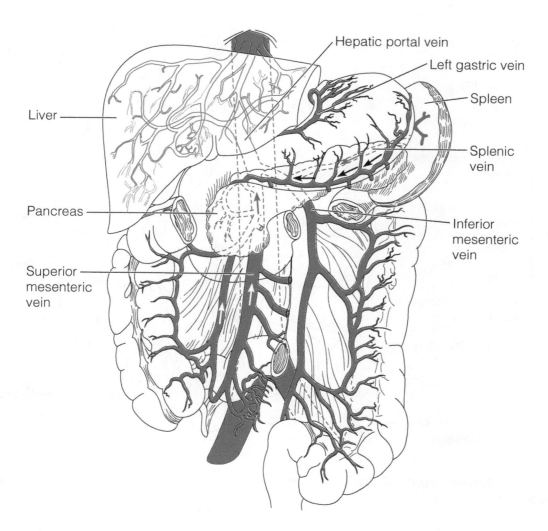

FIGURE 11.23   **The hepatic portal circulation.**

ways for later release to the blood. The liver is drained by the hepatic veins that enter the inferior vena cava. Like the portal circulation that links the hypothalamus of the brain and the anterior pituitary gland, the hepatic portal circulation is a unique and unusual circulation. Normally, arteries feed capillary beds, which in turn drain into veins. Here we see *veins* feeding the liver circulation.

The **inferior mesenteric vein,** draining the terminal part of the large intestine, drains into the **splenic vein,** which itself drains the spleen, pancreas, and the left side of the stomach. The splenic vein and **superior mesenteric vein** (which drains the small intestine and the first part of the colon) join to form the hepatic portal vein.

The **L. gastric vein,** which drains the right side of the stomach, drains directly into the hepatic portal vein.

Circulation to the Heart

The coronary arteries arise at the base of the ascending aorta, where systemic pressures are highest. Each time the heart contracts, it squeezes the coronary vessels, so blood flow is reduced. In the left ventricle, systolic pressures are high enough that blood can flow into the myocardium only during diastole; over this period, elastic rebound helps drive blood along the coronary vessels. Normal cardiac muscle cells can tolerate these brief circulatory interruptions because they have substantial oxygen reserves.

When you are at rest, coronary blood flow is about 250 ml/min. When the workload on your heart increases, local factors, such as reduced O_2 levels and lactic acid production, dilate the coronary vessels and increase blood flow. Epinephrine released during sympathetic stimulation promotes the vasodilation of coronary vessels while increasing heart rate and the strength of cardiac contractions. As a result, coronary blood flow increases while vasoconstriction occurs in other tissues.

For unclear reasons, some individuals experience *coronary spasms,* which can temporarily restrict coronary circulation and produce symptoms of angina. A permanent restriction or blockage of coronary vessels (as in coronary artery disease) and tissue damage (as caused by a myocardial infarction) can limit the heart's ability to increase its output, even under maximal stimulation. Individuals with these conditions experience signs and symptoms of heart failure when the cardiac workload increases much above resting levels.

Circulation to the Lungs

The lungs contain roughly 300 million *alveoli* (al-VĒ-ō-lī; *alveolus,* sac), delicate epithelial pockets where gas exchange occurs. Each alveolus is surrounded by an extensive capillary network. Blood flow through the lungs is regulated primarily by local responses to oxygen levels within individual alveoli. When an alveolus contains oxygen in abundance, the associated vessels dilate, so blood flow increases, promoting the absorption of oxygen from the alveolar air. When the oxygen content of the air is very low, the vessels constrict, so blood is shunted to alveoli that still contain significant levels of oxygen. This mechanism maximizes the efficiency of the respiratory system, because the circulation of blood through the capillaries of an alveolus has no benefit unless that alveolus contains oxygen.

This mechanism is precisely the opposite of that in other tissues, where a decline in oxygen levels causes local vasodilation rather than vasoconstriction. The difference makes functional sense, but its physiological basis remains a mystery.

Blood pressure in pulmonary capillaries (average: 10 mm Hg) is lower than that in systemic capillaries. The BCOP (25 mm Hg) is the same as elsewhere in the bloodstream. As a result, reabsorption exceeds filtration in pulmonary capillaries. Fluid moves continuously into the pulmonary capillaries across the alveolar surfaces, thereby preventing a buildup of fluid in the alveoli that could interfere with the diffusion of respiratory gases. If the blood pressure in pulmonary capillaries rises above 25 mm Hg, fluid enters the alveoli, causing *pulmonary edema.*

The Distribution of Blood Vessels: An Overview

The cardiovascular system consists of the *pulmonary circuit* and the *systemic circuit.* The pulmonary circuit is composed of arteries and veins that transport blood between the heart and the lungs. This circuit begins at the right ventricle and ends at the left atrium. From the left ventricle, the arteries of the systemic circuit transport oxygenated blood and nutrients to all organs and tissues, ultimately returning deoxygenated blood to the right atrium. Figure 11.24 summarizes the primary distribution routes within the pulmonary and systemic circuits.

In the pages that follow, we will examine the vessels of the pulmonary and systemic circuits further. Three general functional patterns are worth noting at the outset:

1. The peripheral distributions of arteries and veins on the body's left and right sides are generally identical, except near the heart, where the largest vessels connect to the atria or ventricles. Corresponding arteries and veins usually follow the same path. For example, the distributions of the left and right subclavian *arteries* parallel those of the left and right subclavian *veins.*

2. A single vessel may have several names as it crosses specific anatomical boundaries, making accurate anatomical descriptions possible when the vessel extends far into the periphery. For example, the *external iliac artery* becomes the *femoral artery* as it leaves the trunk and enters the lower limb.

3. Tissues and organs are usually serviced by several arteries and veins. Often, anastomoses between adjacent arteries or veins reduce the impact of a temporary or even permanent occlusion (blockage) of a single blood vessel.

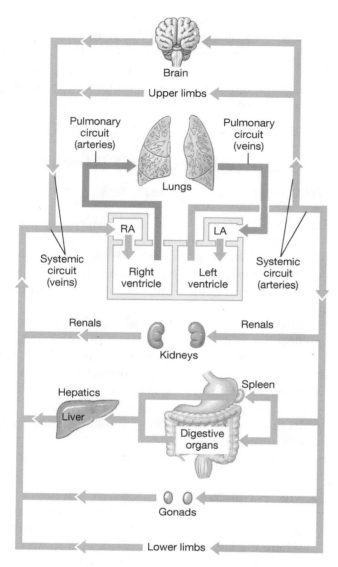

FIGURE 11.24   A schematic overview of the pattern of circulation. *RA* stands for right atrium, *LA* for left atrium.

The Pulmonary Circuit

Blood entering the right atrium has just returned from the peripheral capillary beds, where oxygen was released and carbon dioxide absorbed. After traveling through the right atrium and ventricle, this deoxygenated blood enters the pulmonary trunk, the start of the pulmonary circuit (Figure 11.25). At the lungs, oxygen is replenished, carbon dioxide is released, and the oxygenated blood is returned to the heart for distribution via the systemic circuit. Compared with the systemic circuit, the pulmonary circuit is short: The base of

the pulmonary trunk and the lungs are only about 15 cm (6 in.) apart.

The arteries of the pulmonary circuit differ from those of the systemic circuit in that they carry deoxygenated blood. (For this reason, most color-coded diagrams show the pulmonary arteries in blue, the same color as systemic veins.) As the pulmonary trunk curves over the superior border of the heart, it gives rise to the **left** and **right pulmonary arteries.** These large arteries enter the lungs before branching repeatedly, giving rise to smaller and smaller arteries. The smallest branches, the *pulmonary arterioles,* provide blood to capillary networks that surround *alveoli.* The walls of these small air pockets are thin enough for gas to be exchanged between the capillary blood and inspired air. As it leaves the alveolar capillaries, oxygenated blood enters venules that in turn unite to form larger vessels carrying blood toward the **pulmonary veins.** These four veins, two from each lung, empty into the left atrium, completing the pulmonary circuit.

The Hypophyseal Portal System

By secreting specific regulatory hormones, the hypothalamus controls the production of hormones in the anterior lobe of the pituitary gland. At the *median eminence,* a swelling near the attachment of the infundibulum, hypothalamic neurons release regulatory factors into the surrounding interstitial fluids. Their secretions enter the bloodstream quite easily, because the endothelial cells lining the capillaries in this region are unusually permeable. These **fenestrated** (FEN-es-trā-ted) **capillaries** (*fenestra,* window) allow relatively large molecules to enter or leave the circulatory system.

The capillary networks in the median eminence are supplied by the *superior hypophyseal artery* (Figure 11.26). Before leaving the hypothalamus, the capillary networks unite to form a series of larger vessels that spiral around the infundibulum to reach the anterior lobe of the pituitary gland. Once within the anterior lobe, these vessels form a second capillary network that branches among the endocrine cells.

This vascular arrangement is unusual: A typical artery conducts blood from the heart to a capillary network, and a typical vein carries blood from a capillary network back to the heart. The vessels

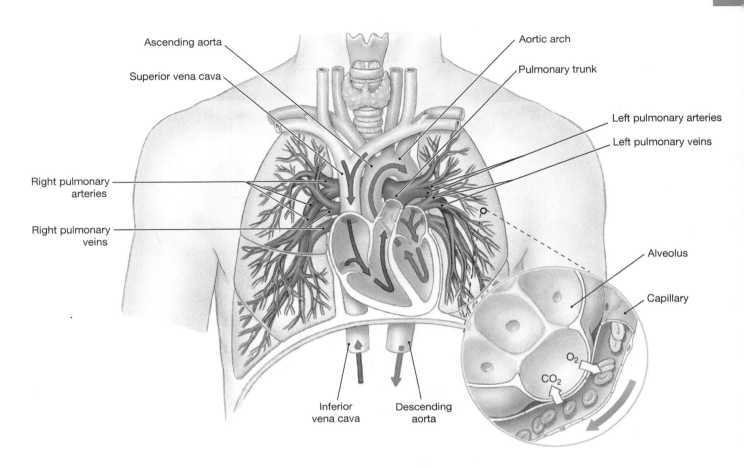

FIGURE 11.25   The pulmonary circuit. The pulmonary circuit consists of pulmonary arteries, which deliver deoxygenated blood from the right ventricle to the lungs; pulmonary capillaries, where gas exchange occurs; and pulmonary veins, which deliver oxygenated blood to the left atrium. As the enlarged view shows, diffusion across the capillary walls at alveoli removes carbon dioxide and provides oxygen to the blood.

between the median eminence and the anterior lobe, however, carry blood from one capillary network to another. Blood vessels that link two capillary networks are called **portal vessels;** in this case, they have the histological structure of veins. The entire complex is a **portal system.** Portal systems are named after their destinations; hence, this particular network is known as the **hypophyseal** (hī-pō-FI-sē-al) **portal system.**

Portal systems provide an efficient means of chemical communication by ensuring that all the hypothalamic hormones entering the portal vessels will reach the target cells in the anterior lobe of the pituitary gland before being diluted through mixing with the general circulation. The communication is strictly one way, however, because any chemicals released by the cells "downstream" must do a complete circuit of the cardiovascular system before they reach the capillaries of the portal system.

Figure 11.23 shows the circulation of the hepatic portal system.

Fetal Circulation   Now let's consider the distribution of blood vessels in a developing fetus. Since the lungs and digestive system are not yet functioning in a fetus, all nutrient, excretory, and gas exchanges occur through the placenta. Nutrients and oxygen move from the mother's blood into the fetal blood, and fetal wastes move in the opposite direction. As shown in Figure 11.27, the *umbilical cord* contains three blood vessels: one large **umbilical vein** and two smaller **umbilical arteries.** The umbilical vein carries blood rich in nutrients and oxygen to the fetus. The umbilical

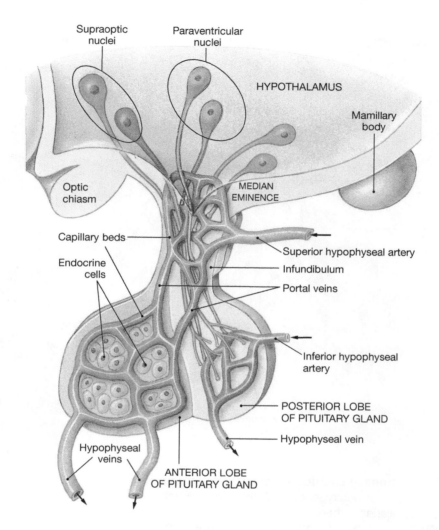

FIGURE 11.26 **The hypophyseal portal system and the blood supply to the pituitary gland.**

arteries carry carbon dioxide and debris-laden blood from the fetus to the placenta. As blood flows superiorly toward the heart of the fetus, most of it bypasses the immature liver through the **ductus venosus** (duk′tus ve-no′sus) and enters the inferior vena cava, which carries the blood to the right atrium of the heart.

Since fetal lungs are nonfunctional and collapsed, two shunts see to it that they are almost entirely bypassed. Some of the blood entering the right atrium is shunted directly into the left atrium through the **foramen ovale** (fo-ra′men o-val′e), a flaplike opening in the interatrial septum. Blood that does manage to enter the right ventricle is pumped out the pulmonary trunk, where it meets a second shunt, the **ductus**

arteriosus (ar-ter″e-o′sus), a short vessel that connects the aorta and the pulmonary trunk. Because the collapsed lungs are a high-pressure area, blood tends to enter the systemic circulation through the ductus arteriosus. The aorta carries blood to the tissues of the fetal body and ultimately back to the placenta through the umbilical arteries.

At birth, or shortly after, the foramen ovale closes, and the ductus arteriosus collapses and is converted to the fibrous **ligamentum arteriosum** (lig″ah-men′tum ar-ter″e-o′sum) (see Figure 11.2a). As blood stops flowing through the umbilical vessels, they become obliterated, and the circulatory pattern converts to that of an adult.

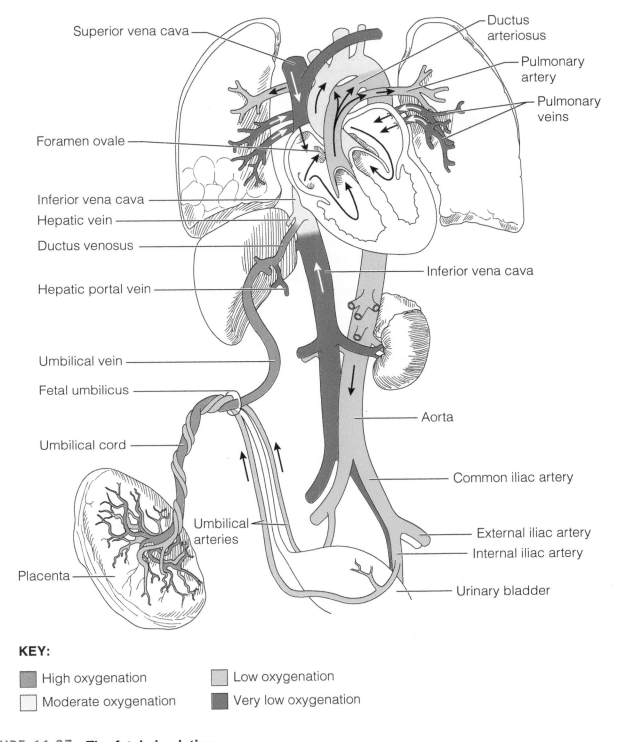

KEY:

- ■ High oxygenation
- □ Moderate oxygenation
- □ Low oxygenation
- ■ Very low oxygenation

FIGURE 11.27 **The fetal circulation.**

Physiology of Circulation

A fairly good indication of the efficiency of a person's circulatory system can be obtained by taking arterial pulse and blood pressure measurements. These measurements, along with those of respiratory rate and body temperature, are referred to collectively as **vital signs** in clinical settings.

Arterial Pulse

The alternating expansion and recoil of an artery that occurs with each beat of the left ventricle creates a pressure wave—a **pulse**—that travels through the entire arterial system. Normally the pulse rate (pressure surges per minute) equals the heart rate (beats per minute). The pulse averages 70 to 76 beats per minute in a normal resting person. It is influenced by activity, postural changes, and emotions.

You can feel a pulse in any artery lying close to the body surface by compressing the artery against firm tissue; this provides an easy way of counting heart rate. Because it is so accessible, the point where the radial artery surfaces at the wrist (the radial pulse) is routinely used to take a pulse measurement, but there are several other clinically important arterial pulse points (Figure 11.28). Because these same points are compressed to stop blood flow into distal tissues during hemorrhage, they are also called **pressure points.** For example, if you seriously cut your hand, you can stop

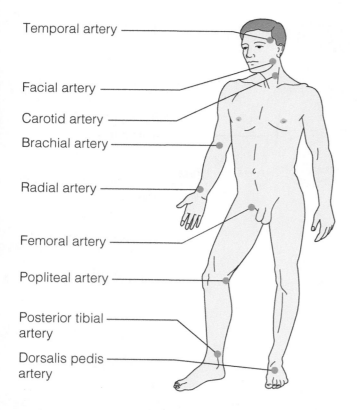

Temporal artery

Facial artery

Carotid artery

Brachial artery

Radial artery

Femoral artery

Popliteal artery

Posterior tibial artery

Dorsalis pedis artery

FIGURE 11.28   Body sites where the pulse is most easily palpated.

the bleeding somewhat by compressing the radial artery or the brachial artery.

Try to palpate each of the pulse points shown in Figure 11.28 by placing the tips of your first two or three fingers of one hand over the artery at the site indicated. It helps to compress the artery firmly as you begin and then immediately ease up on your pressure slightly. In each case, notice the regularity of the pulse and its relative strength.

Blood Pressure

Any system equipped with a pump that forces fluid through a network of closed tubes operates under pressure. The closer you get to the pump, the higher the pressure. **Blood pressure** is the pressure the blood exerts against the inner walls of the blood vessels, and it is the force that keeps blood circulating continuously even between heartbeats. Unless stated otherwise, the term *blood pressure* is understood to mean the pressure within the large systemic arteries near the heart.

Blood Pressure Gradient   When the ventricles contract, they force blood into large, thick-walled elastic arteries that expand as the blood is pushed into them. The high pressure in these arteries forces the blood to continually move into areas where the pressure is lower. The pressure is highest in the large arteries and continues to drop throughout the pathway, reaching zero or negative pressure at the venae cavae (Figure 11.29). Recall that the blood flows into the smaller arteries, then arterioles, capillaries, venules, veins, and finally back to the large venae cavae entering the right atrium of the heart. It flows continually along a pressure gradient (from high to low pressure) as it makes its circuit day in and day out. Notice that if venous return depended entirely on a high blood pressure throughout the system, blood would probably never be able to complete its circuit back to the heart. This is why the valves in the larger veins, the milking activity of the skeletal muscles, and pressure changes in the thorax are so important.

The pressure differences between arteries and veins become very clear when these vessels are cut. If a vein is cut, the blood flows evenly from the wound; a lacerated artery produces rapid spurts of blood.

Continual blood flow absolutely depends on the stretchiness of the larger arteries and their abil-

Q How does the pulsating change in blood pressure on the left side of the graph relate to the structure of the largest arteries?

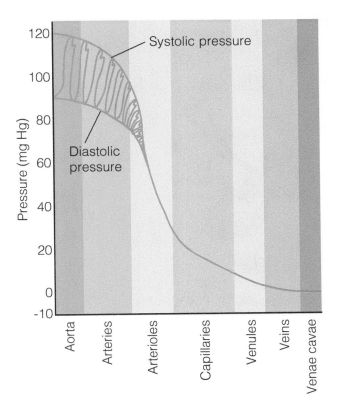

FIGURE 11.29 **Blood pressure in various areas of the cardiovascular system.**

ity to recoil and keep the pressure on the blood as it flows off into the circulation. To illustrate this, think of a garden hose with relatively hard walls. When the water is turned on, the water spurts out under high pressure because the hose walls don't expand. However, when the water faucet is suddenly turned off, the flow of water stops just as abruptly. This is because the walls of the hose cannot recoil to keep pressure on the water; therefore, the pressure drops and the flow of water stops. The importance of the elasticity of the arteries is best appreciated when it is lost, as happens in *arteriosclerosis*. Arteriosclerosis, also called "hardening of the arteries," is discussed in the

A It reveals their elasticity. When the heart contracts and forces blood into the large arteries near the heart, they stretch to accommodate the greater volume of blood (systolic pressure), and then as the blood continues on in the circuit, their walls recoil, keeping pressure on the blood which keeps it moving (diastolic pressure).

"A Closer Look" box on atherosclerosis later in this chapter.

Measuring Blood Pressure   Because the heart alternately contracts and relaxes, the off-and-on flow of blood into the arteries causes the blood pressure to rise and fall during each beat. Thus, two arterial blood pressure measurements are usually made: **systolic** (sis-to′lik) **pressure,** the pressure in the arteries at the peak of ventricular contraction, and **diastolic** (di″us-to′lik) **pressure,** the pressure when the ventricles are relaxing. Blood pressures are reported in millimeters of mercury (mm Hg), with the systolic pressure written first—120/80 (120 over 80) translates to a systolic pressure of 120 mm Hg and a diastolic pressure of 80 mm Hg. Most often, systemic arterial blood pressure is measured indirectly by the **auscultatory** (os-kul′tuh-tor-e) **method.** This procedure, as used to measure blood pressure in the brachial artery of the arm, is illustrated and described in Figure 11.30.

Effects of Various Factors on Blood Pressure   Arterial blood pressure (BP) is directly related to cardiac output (CO; the amount of blood pumped out of the left ventricle per minute) and peripheral resistance (PR). This relationship is expressed by the equation: $BP = CO \times PR$. Since regulation of cardiac output has already been considered, we will concentrate on peripheral resistance here.

Peripheral resistance is the amount of friction encountered by the blood as it flows through the blood vessels. It is increased by many factors, but probably the most important is the constriction, or narrowing, of blood vessels, especially arterioles, as a result of sympathetic nervous system activity or atherosclerosis. Increased blood volume or blood viscosity (thickness) also raises peripheral resistance. Any factor that increases either the cardiac output or peripheral resistance causes an almost immediate reflex rise in blood pressure. Many factors can alter blood pressure—age, weight, time of day, exercise, body position, emotional state, and various drugs, to name a few. The influence of a few of these factors is discussed next.

Cardiovascular Regulation

Homeostatic mechanisms regulate cardiovascular activity to ensure that **tissue perfusion,** or

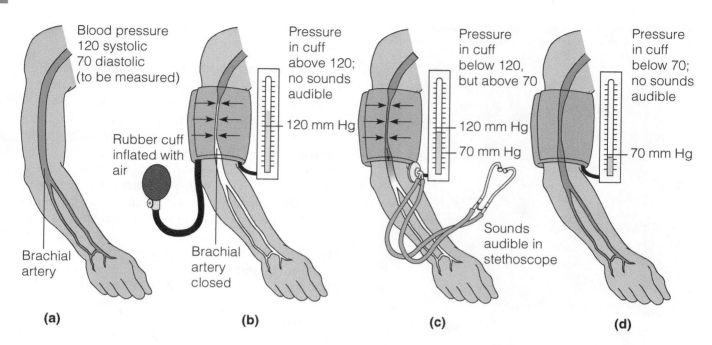

FIGURE 11.30 Measuring blood pressure. (a) The course of the brachial artery of the arm. Assume a blood pressure of 120/70 in a young, healthy person. **(b)** The blood pressure cuff is wrapped snugly around the arm just above the elbow and inflated until the cuff pressure exceeds the systolic blood pressure. At this point, blood flow into the arm is stopped, and a brachial pulse cannot be felt or heard. **(c)** The pressure in the cuff is gradually reduced while the examiner listens (auscultates) carefully for sounds in the brachial artery with a stethoscope. The pressure read as the first soft tapping sounds are heard (the first point at which a small amount of blood is spurting through the constricted artery) is recorded as the systolic pressure. **(d)** As the pressure is reduced still further, the sounds become louder and more distinct; when the artery is no longer constricted and blood flows freely, the sounds can no longer be heard. The pressure at which the sounds disappear is recorded as the diastolic pressure.

blood flow through tissues, meets the demand for oxygen and nutrients. The factors that affect tissue perfusion are (1) cardiac output, (2) peripheral resistance, and (3) blood pressure. We discussed cardiac output and considered peripheral resistance and blood pressure earlier in this chapter.

Most cells are relatively close to capillaries. When a group of cells becomes active, the circulation to that region must increase to deliver the necessary oxygen and nutrients, and to carry away the waste products and carbon dioxide they generate. The purpose of cardiovascular regulation is to ensure that these blood flow changes occur (1) at an appropriate time, (2) in the right area, and (3) without drastically changing blood pressure and blood flow to vital organs.

The regulatory mechanisms focus on controlling cardiac output and blood pressure to restore adequate blood flow after a fall in blood pressure. These mechanisms can be broadly categorized as follows:

- **Autoregulation.** Local factors change the pattern of blood flow within capillary beds in response to chemical changes in interstitial fluids. This is an example of autoregulation at the tissue level. Autoregulation causes immediate, localized homeostatic adjustments. If autoregulation fails to normalize conditions at the tissue level, neural mechanisms and endocrine factors are activated.

- **Neural Mechanisms.** Neural mechanisms respond to changes in arterial pressure or blood gas levels at specific sites. When those changes occur, the cardiovascular centers of the autonomic nervous system adjust cardiac output and peripheral resistance to maintain blood pressure and ensure adequate blood flow.

- **Endocrine Mechanisms.** The endocrine system releases hormones that enhance short-term adjustments and that direct long-term changes in cardiovascular performance.

We will next consider each of these regulatory mechanisms individually by examining regulatory responses to inadequate perfusion of skeletal muscles. The regulatory relationships are diagrammed in Figure 11.31

Autoregulation of Blood Flow within Tissues

Under normal resting conditions, cardiac output remains stable, and peripheral resistance within individual tissues is adjusted to control local blood flow.

Factors that promote the dilation of precapillary sphincters are called **vasodilators. Local vasodilators** act at the tissue level to accelerate blood flow through their tissue of origin. Examples of local vasodilators include the following:

- Decreased tissue oxygen levels or increased CO_2 levels.

- Lactic acid or other acids generated by tissue cells.

- Nitric oxide (NO) released from endothelial cells.

- Rising concentrations of potassium ions or hydrogen ions in the interstitial fluid.

- Chemicals released during local inflammation, including histamine and NO.

- Elevated local temperature.

These factors work by relaxing the smooth muscle cells of the precapillary sphincters. All of them indicate that tissue conditions are in some

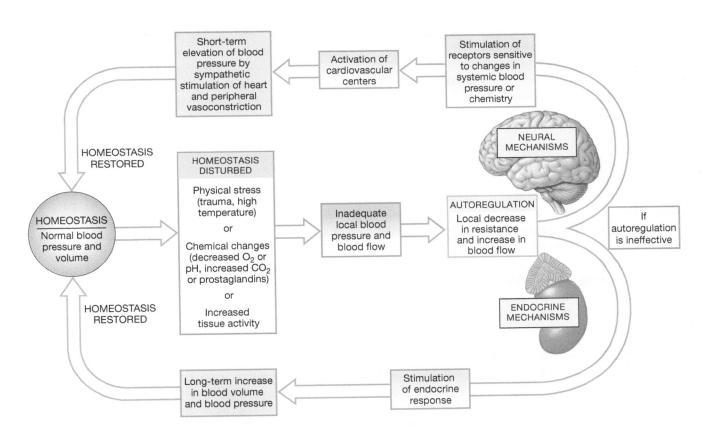

FIGURE 11.31 **Short-term and Long-term cardiovascular responses.** This diagram indicates general mechanisms that compensate for a reduction in blood pressure and blood flow.

way abnormal. An increase in blood flow, which will bring oxygen, nutrients, and buffers, may be sufficient to restore homeostasis.

Aggregating platelets and damaged tissues produce compounds that stimulate the constriction of precapillary sphincters. These compounds are **local vasoconstrictors.** Examples include prostaglandins and thromboxanes released by activated platelets and white blood cells, and the endothelins released by damaged endothelial cells.

Local vasodilators and vasoconstrictors control blood flow within a single capillary bed. In high concentrations, these factors also affect arterioles, increasing or decreasing blood flow to all the capillary beds in a given area.

Neural Mechanisms

The nervous system is responsible for adjusting cardiac output and peripheral resistance in order to maintain adequate blood flow to vital tissues and organs. Centers responsible for these regulatory activities include the *cardiac centers* and the *vasomotor centers* of the medulla oblongata. It is difficult to distinguish the cardiac and vasomotor centers anatomically, and they are often considered to form complex **cardiovascular (CV) centers.** In functional terms, however, the cardiac and vasomotor centers often act independently. As noted earlier, each cardiac center consists of a *cardioacceleratory center,* which increases cardiac output through sympathetic innervation, and a *cardioinhibitory center,* which reduces cardiac output through parasympathetic innervation.

The vasomotor centers contain two populations of neurons: (1) a very large group responsible for widespread vasoconstriction and (2) a smaller group responsible for the vasodilation of arterioles in skeletal muscles and the brain. The vasomotor centers exert their effects by controlling the activity of sympathetic motor neurons:

1. *Control of Vasoconstriction.* The neurons innervating peripheral blood vessels in most tissues are *adrenergic;* that is, they release the neurotransmitter norepinephrine (NE). The response to NE release is the stimulation of smooth muscle in the walls of arterioles, producing vasoconstriction.

2. *Control of Vasodilation.* Vasodilator neurons innervate blood vessels in skeletal muscles and in the brain. The stimulation of these neurons relaxes smooth muscle cells in the walls of arterioles, producing vasodilation. The relaxation of smooth muscle cells is triggered by the appearance of NO in their surroundings. The vasomotor centers may control NO release indirectly or directly. The most common vasodilator synapses are *cholinergic*—their synaptic knobs release ACh. In turn, ACh stimulates endothelial cells in the area to release NO, which causes local vasodilation. Another population of vasodilator synapses is *nitroxidergic*—the synaptic knobs release NO as a neurotransmitter. Nitric oxide has an immediate and direct relaxing effect on the vascular smooth muscle cells in the area.

Vasomotor Tone

We discussed the significance of autonomic tone in setting a background level of neural activity that can increase or decrease on demand. The sympathetic vasoconstrictor nerves are chronically active, producing a significant **vasomotor tone.** Vasoconstrictor activity is normally sufficient to keep the arterioles partially constricted. Under maximal stimulation, arterioles constrict to about half their resting diameter, whereas a fully dilated arteriole increases its resting diameter by roughly 1.5 times. Constriction has a significant effect on resistance, because resistance increases sharply as luminal diameter decreases. The resistance of a maximally constricted arteriole is roughly 80 *times* that of a fully dilated arteriole. Because blood pressure varies directly with peripheral resistance, the vasomotor centers can control arterial blood pressure very effectively by making modest adjustments in vessel diameters. Extreme stimulation of the vasomotor centers also produces venoconstriction and mobilization of the venous reserve.

Reflex Control of Cardiovascular Function

The cardiovascular centers detect changes in tissue demand by monitoring arterial blood, with particular attention to blood pressure, pH, and the concentrations of dissolved gases. The *baroreceptor reflexes* respond to changes in blood pressure, and the *chemoreceptor reflexes* monitor changes in the chemical composition of arterial blood. These reflexes are regulated through a negative feedback loop: The stimulation of a receptor by an abnormal condition leads to a response that counteracts the stimulus and restores normal conditions.

Baroreceptor Reflexes   Baroreceptors are specialized receptors that monitor the degree of stretch in the walls of expandable organs. The baroreceptors involved in cardiovascular regulation are located in the walls of (1) the **carotid sinuses,** expanded chambers near the bases of the *internal carotid arteries* of the neck, (2) the **aortic sinuses,** pockets in the walls of the ascending aorta adjacent to the heart (see Figure 11.9), and (3) the wall of the right atrium. These receptors are components of the **baroreceptor reflexes,** which adjust cardiac output and peripheral resistance to maintain normal arterial pressures.

Aortic baroreceptors monitor blood pressure within the ascending aorta. Any changes trigger the **aortic reflex,** which adjusts blood pressure to maintain adequate blood pressure and blood flow through the systemic circuit. In response to changes in blood pressure at the carotid sinus, carotid sinus baroreceptors trigger reflexes that maintain adequate blood flow to the brain. Because blood flow to the brain must remain constant, the carotid sinus receptors are extremely sensitive. Figure 11.32 presents the basic organization of the baroreceptor reflexes triggered by changes in blood pressure at the carotid and aortic sinuses.

When blood pressure climbs, the increased output from the baroreceptors alters activity in the CV centers and produces two major effects (Figure 11.32a):

1. *A decrease in cardiac output,* due to parasympathetic stimulation and the inhibition of sympathetic activity.

2. *Widespread peripheral vasodilation,* due to the inhibition of excitatory neurons in the vasomotor centers.

The decrease in cardiac output reflects primarily a reduction in heart rate due to the release of acetylcholine at the sinoatrial (SA) node. The widespread vasodilation lowers peripheral resistance, and this effect, combined with a reduction in cardiac output, leads to a decline in blood pressure to normal levels.

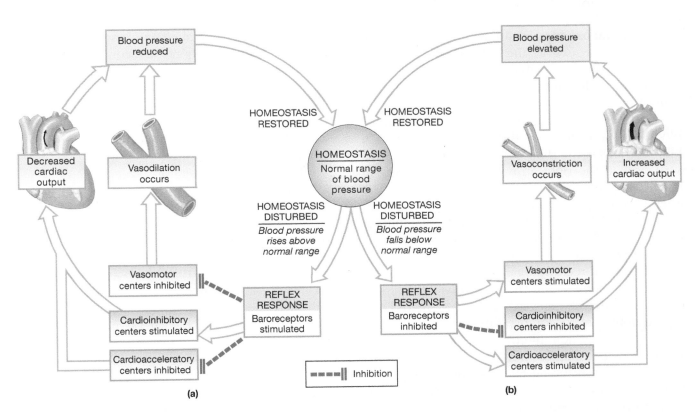

FIGURE 11.32   Baroreceptor reflexes of the carotid and aortic sinuses.

When blood pressure falls below normal, baroreceptor output is reduced accordingly (Figure 11.32b). This change has two major effects:

1. *An increase in cardiac output,* through the stimulation of sympathetic innervation to the heart. This results from the stimulation of the cardioacceleratory centers and is accompanied by an inhibition of the cardioinhibitory centers.

2. *Widespread peripheral vasoconstriction,* caused by the stimulation of sympathetic vasoconstrictor neurons by the vasomotor centers.

The effects on the heart result from the release of NE by sympathetic neurons innervating the SA node, the atrioventricular (AV) node, and the general myocardium. In a crisis, sympathetic activation occurs, and its effects are enhanced by the release of both NE and epinephrine (E) from the adrenal medullae. The net effect is an immediate increase in heart rate and stroke volume, and a corresponding rise in cardiac output. The vasoconstriction, which also results from the release of NE by sympathetic neurons, increases peripheral resistance. These adjustments—increased cardiac output and increased peripheral resistance—work together to elevate blood pressure.

Atrial baroreceptors are receptors that monitor blood pressure at the end of the systemic circuit—at the venae cavae and the right atrium. The **atrial reflex** responds to a stretching of the wall of the right atrium.

Under normal circumstances, the heart pumps blood into the aorta at the same rate at which blood arrives at the right atrium. When blood pressure rises at the right atrium, blood is arriving at the heart faster than it is being pumped out. The atrial baroreceptors correct the situation by stimulating the CV centers and increasing cardiac output until the backlog of venous blood is removed. Atrial pressure then returns to normal.

Exhaling forcefully against a closed glottis, a procedure known as the *Valsalva maneuver,* causes reflexive changes in blood pressure and cardiac output due to compression of the aorta and venae cavae. When internal pressures rise, the venae cavae collapse, and the venous return decreases. The resulting fall in cardiac output and blood pressure stimulates the aortic and carotid baroreceptors, causing reflexive increase in heart rate and peripheral vasoconstriction. When the glottis opens and pressures return to normal, venous return increases suddenly and so does cardiac output. Because vasoconstriction has occurred, blood pressure rises sharply, and this inhibits the baroreceptors. As a result, cardiac output, heart rate, and blood pressure quickly return to normal levels. The Valsalva maneuver is thus a simple way to check for normal cardiovascular responses to changes in arterial pressure and venous return.

Chemoreceptor Reflexes The **chemoreceptor reflexes** respond to changes in carbon dioxide, oxygen, or pH levels in blood and cerebrospinal fluid (CSF) (Figure 11.33). The chemoreceptors involved are sensory neurons located in the **carotid bodies,** situated in the neck near the carotid sinus, and the **aortic bodies,** near the arch of the aorta. These receptors monitor the composition of arterial blood. Additional chemoreceptors located on the ventrolateral surfaces of the medulla oblongata monitor the composition of CSF.

When chemoreceptors in the carotid bodies or aortic bodies detect either a rise in the carbon dioxide content or a fall in the pH of the arterial blood, the cardioacceleratory and vasomotor centers are stimulated, and the cardioinhibitory centers are inhibited. This dual effect causes an increase in cardiac output, peripheral vasoconstriction, and an elevation in arterial blood pressure. A drop in the oxygen level at the aortic bodies has the same effects. Strong stimulation of the carotid or aortic chemoreceptors causes widespread sympathetic activation, with more dramatic increases in heart rate and cardiac output.

The chemoreceptors of the medulla oblongata are involved primarily with the control of respiratory function, and secondarily with regulating blood flow to the brain. For example, a steep rise in CSF carbon dioxide levels will trigger the vasodilation of cerebral vessels, but will produce vasoconstriction in most other organs. The result is increased blood flow—and hence increased oxygen delivery—to the brain.

Arterial CO_2 levels can be reduced and O_2 levels increased most effectively by coordinating cardiovascular and respiratory activities. Chemoreceptor stimulation also stimulates the respiratory centers, and the rise in cardiac output and blood pressure is associated with an increased respiratory rate. Coordination of

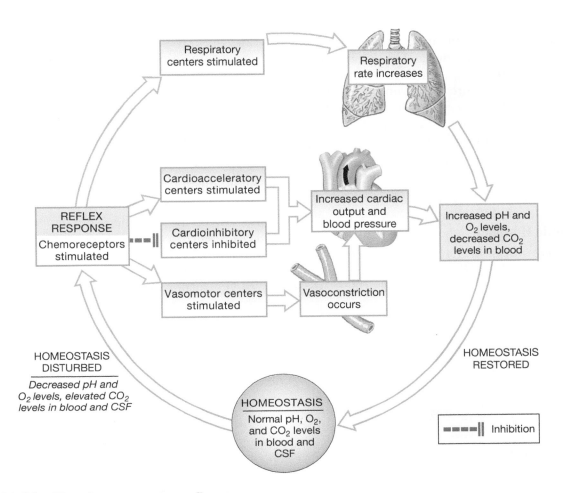

FIGURE 11.33   **The chemoreceptor reflexes.**

cardiovascular and respiratory activities is vital, because accelerating blood flow in the tissues is useful only if the circulating blood contains an adequate amount of oxygen. In addition, a rise in the respiratory rate accelerates venous return through the action of the respiratory pump.

CNS Activities and the Cardiovascular Centers

The output of the cardiovascular centers can also be influenced by activities in other areas of the brain. For example, the activation of either division of the autonomic nervous system will affect output from the cardiovascular centers. The cardioacceleratory and vasomotor centers are stimulated when a general sympathetic activation occurs. The result is an increase in cardiac output and blood pressure. In contrast, when the parasympathetic division is activated, the cardioinhibitory centers are stimulated,

producing a reduction in cardiac output. Parasympathetic activity does not directly affect the vasomotor centers, but vasodilation occurs as sympathetic activity declines.

The activities of higher brain centers can also affect blood pressure. Our thought processes and emotional states can produce significant changes in blood pressure by influencing cardiac output and vasomotor tone. For example, strong emotions of anxiety, fear, and rage are accompanied by an elevation in blood pressure, caused by cardiac stimulation and vasoconstriction.

Hormones and Cardiovascular Regulation

The endocrine system provides both short-term and long-term regulation of cardiovascular performance. As we have seen, E and NE from the adrenal medullae stimulate cardiac output and peripheral vasoconstriction. Other hormones important in regulating cardiovascular function include (1) antidiuretic hormone (ADH), (2) angiotensin II, (3) erythropoietin (EPO), and (4) the natriuretic peptides (ANP and BNP). Although ADH and angiotensin II also affect blood pressure, all four are concerned primarily with the long-term regulation of blood volume (Figure 11.34).

Antidiuretic Hormone

Antidiuretic hormone (ADH) is released at the posterior lobe of the pituitary gland in response to a decrease in blood volume, to an increase in

the osmotic concentration of the plasma, or (secondarily) to circulating angiotensin II. The immediate result is a peripheral vasoconstriction that elevates blood pressure. This hormone also stimulates the conservation of water at the kidneys, thus preventing a reduction in blood volume that would further reduce blood pressure (Figure 11.34a).

Angiotensin II

Angiotensin II appears in the blood after the release of the enzyme renin by *juxtaglomerular cells,* specialized kidney cells, in response to a fall in renal blood pressure (see Figure 11.34a). Once in the bloodstream, renin starts an enzymatic chain reaction. In the first step, renin converts

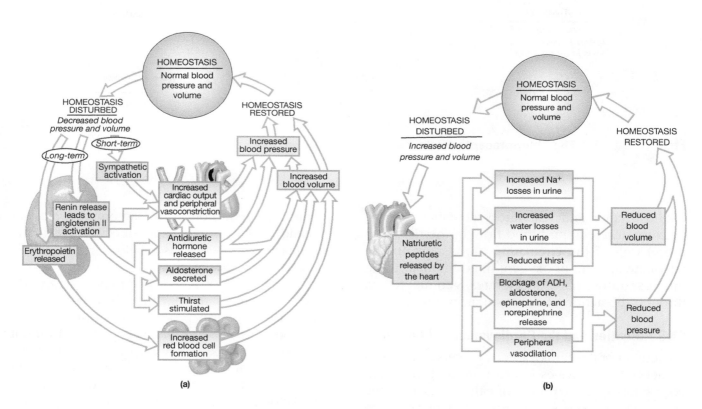

(a)

(b)

FIGURE 11.34 **The hormonal regulation of blood pressure and blood volume.** Shown are factors that compensate for **(a)** decreased blood pressure and volume and for **(b)** increased blood pressure and volume.

angiotensinogen, a plasma protein produced by the liver, to *angiotensin I.* In the capillaries of the lungs, *angiotensin-converting enzyme (ACE)* then modifies angiotensin I to angiotensin II, an active hormone with diverse effects.

Angiotensin II has four important functions: (1) It stimulates the adrenal production of aldosterone, causing Na^+ retention and K^+ loss at the kidneys; (2) it stimulates the secretion of ADH, in turn stimulating water reabsorption at the kidneys and complementing the effects of aldosterone; (3) it stimulates thirst, resulting in increased fluid consumption (the presence of ADH and aldosterone ensures that the additional water consumed will be retained, elevating blood volume); and (4) it stimulates cardiac output and triggers the constriction of arterioles, in turn elevating the systemic blood pressure. The effect of angiotensin II on blood pressure is four to eight times greater than that produced by norepinephrine.

Erythropoietin

Erythropoietin (EPO) is released at the kidneys if blood pressure falls or if the oxygen content of the blood becomes abnormally low (see Figure 11.34a). EPO stimulates the production and maturation of red blood cells, thereby increasing the volume and viscosity of the blood and improving its oxygen-carrying capacity.

Natriuretic Peptides

Atrial natriuretic peptide (nā-trē-ū-RET-ik; *natrium,* sodium + *ouresis,* making water), or *ANP,* is produced by cardiac muscle cells in the wall of the right atrium in response to excessive stretching during diastole. A related hormone called *brain natriuretic peptide,* or *BNP,* is produced by ventricular muscle cells exposed to comparable stimuli. These peptide hormones reduce blood volume and blood pressure by (1) increasing sodium ion excretion at the kidneys, (2) promoting water losses by increasing the volume of urine produced; (3) reducing thirst; (4) blocking the release of ADH, aldosterone, epinephrine, and norepinephrine; and (5) stimulating peripheral vasodilation (Figure 11.34b). As blood volume and blood pressure decline, the stresses on the walls of the heart are removed, and natriuretic peptide production ceases.

100 Keys | Cardiac output cannot increase indefinitely, and blood flow to active versus inactive tissues must be differentially controlled. This control is accomplished by a combination of autoregulation, neural regulation, and hormone release.

Other Factors Causing Change in Blood Pressure

1. **Renal factors: the kidneys.** The kidneys play a major role in regulating arterial blood pressure by altering blood volume. As blood pressure (and/or blood volume) increases beyond normal, the kidneys allow more water to leave the body in the urine. Since the source of this water is the bloodstream, blood volume decreases, which in turn decreases blood pressure. However, when arterial blood pressure falls, the kidneys retain body water, increasing blood volume, and blood pressure rises (see Figure 11.35).

    In addition, when arterial blood pressure is low, certain kidney cells release the enzyme **renin** into the blood. Renin triggers a series of chemical reactions that result in the formation of *angiotensin II,* a potent vasoconstrictor chemical. Angiotensin also stimulates the adrenal cortex to release aldosterone, a hormone that enhances sodium ion reabsorption by the kidneys. As sodium moves into the blood, water follows. Thus, blood volume and blood pressure both rise.

2. **Temperature.** In general, cold has a vasoconstricting effect. This is why your exposed skin feels cold to the touch on a winter day and why cold compresses are recommended to prevent swelling of a bruised area. On the other hand, heat has a **vasodilating** effect, and warm compresses are used to speed the circulation into an inflamed area, relaxing and broading the vessel.

3. **Chemicals.** The effects of chemical substances, many of which are drugs, on blood pressure are widespread and well known in many cases. Just a few examples will be given here. **Epinephrine** increases both heart rate and blood pressure. *Nicotine* increases blood pressure by causing vasoconstriction. Both *alcohol* and *histamine*

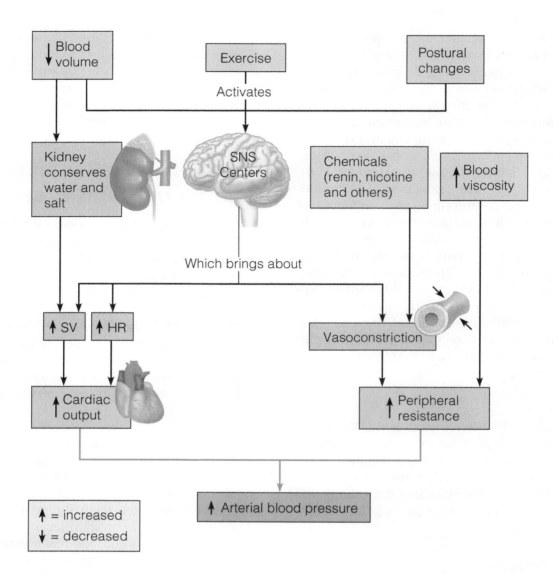

FIGURE 11.35 **Summary of factors causing an increase in arterial blood pressure.** (SV = stroke volume; HR = heart rate)

cause vasodilation and decrease the blood pressure. The reason a person who has "one too many" becomes flushed is that the skin vessels have been dilated by alcohol.

4. **Diet.** Although medical opinions tend to change and are at odds from time to time, it is generally believed that a diet low in salt, saturated fats, and cholesterol helps to prevent *hypertension,* or high blood pressure.

Variations in Blood Pressure In normal adults at rest, systolic blood pressure varies between 110 and 140 mm Hg, and diastolic pressure between 75 and 80 mm Hg—but blood pressure varies considerably from one person to another. What is normal for you may not be normal for your grandfather or your neighbor. Blood pressure varies with age, weight, race, mood, physical activity, and posture. Nearly all these variations can be explained in terms of the factors affecting blood pressure that have already been discussed.

Hypotension, or low blood pressure, is generally considered to be a systolic blood pressure below 100 mm Hg. In many cases, it simply reflects individual differences and is no cause for concern. In fact, low blood pressure is an expected result of physical conditioning and is often associated with long life and an old age free of illness.

Homeostatic Imbalance

Elderly people may experience temporary low blood pressure and dizziness when they rise suddenly from a reclining or sitting position—a condition called *orthostatic hypotension*. Because an aging sympathetic nervous system reacts more slowly to postural changes, blood pools briefly in the lower limbs, reducing blood pressure and, consequently, blood delivery to the brain. Making postural changes more slowly to give the nervous system time to make the necessary adjustments usually prevents this problem. ▲

Chronic hypotension (not explained by physical conditioning) may hint at poor nutrition and inadequate levels of blood proteins. Because blood viscosity is low, blood pressure is also lower than normal. Acute hypotension is one of the most important warnings of *circulatory shock*, a condition in which the blood vessels are inadequately filled and blood cannot circulate normally. The most common cause is blood loss.

A brief elevation in blood pressure is a normal response to fever, physical exertion, and emotional upset, such as anger and fear. Persistent **hypertension, or high blood pressure,** is pathological and is defined as a condition of sustained elevated arterial pressure of 140/90 or higher.

Homeostatic Imbalance

Chronic hypertension is a common and dangerous disease that warns of increased peripheral resistance. Although it progresses without symptoms for the first 10 to 20 years, it slowly and surely strains the heart and damages the arteries. For this reason, hypertension is often called the "silent killer." Because the heart is forced to pump against increased resistance, it must work harder, and in time, the myocardium enlarges. When finally strained beyond its capacity to respond, the heart weakens and its walls become flabby. Hypertension also ravages blood vessels, causing small tears in the endothelium that accelerate the progress of **atherosclerosis.**

Although hypertension and atherosclerosis are often linked, it is difficult to blame hypertension on any distinct anatomical pathology. In fact, about 90 percent of hypertensive people have *primary*, or *essential*, *hypertension*, which cannot be accounted for by any specific organic cause. However, factors such as diet, obesity, heredity, race, and stress appear to be involved. For instance, more women than men and more blacks than whites are hypertensive. Hypertension runs in families. The child of a hypertensive parent is twice as likely to develop high blood pressure as is a child of parents with normal blood pressure. Dietary factors presumed to contribute to hypertension include high cholesterol, saturated fat, and sodium intakes. High blood pressure is common in obese people because the total length of their blood vessels is relatively greater than that in thinner individuals. For each pound of fat, miles of additional blood vessels are required, making the heart work harder to pump blood over longer distances. ▲

Capillary Exchange of Gases and Nutrients

Capillaries form an intricate network among the body's cells such that no substance has to diffuse very far to enter or leave a cell. The substances exchanged first diffuse through an intervening space (Figure 11.36a) filled with **interstitial fluid (tissue fluid).**

Substances tend to move to and from body cells according to their concentration gradients. Thus, oxygen and nutrients leave the blood and move into the tissue cells, and carbon dioxide and other wastes exit the tissue cells and enter the blood. Basically, substances entering or leaving the bloodstream may take one of four routes across the plasma membranes of the single layer of endothelial cells forming the capillary wall (Figure 11.36b).

1. As with all cells, substances can diffuse directly through (cross) their plasma membranes if they are lipid-soluble (like the respiratory gases).

2. Certain lipid-insoluble substances may enter or leave the blood and/or endothelial cells within vesicles, that is, by endocytosis or exocytosis.

Diffusion of substances via the other two routes depends on the specific structural (and permeability) characteristics of the capillary.

3. Limited passage of fluid and small solutes is allowed by **intercellular clefts** (gaps or areas of plasma membrane not joined by tight junctions). It is safe to say that, with the exception of brain capillaries, which are entirely secured together by tight junctions (the basis of the

Q *Assume there is a bacterial infection in the interstitial fluid of (c). How would this affect fluid flows across the capillary walls in the area?*

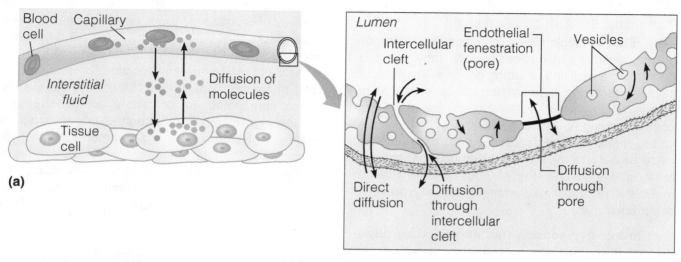

(a)

(b)

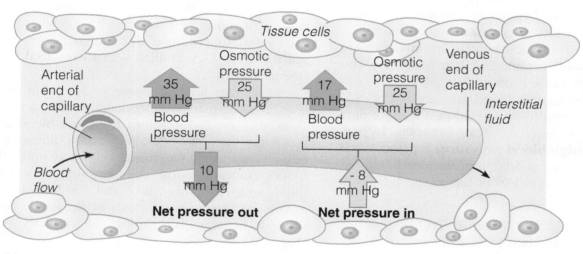

(c)

FIGURE 11.36 Capillary transport mechanisms. (a) Substances exchanged between the blood and the tissue cells must **diffuse** through intervening interstitial fluid. **(b)** The four possible pathways, or routes of transport, across the wall of an endothelial cell. (The endothelial cell is illustrated as if cut in cross section.) **(c)** Bulk fluid flows across capillary walls depend largely on the difference between the **hydrostatic (blood) pressure** and the osmotic pressure at different regions of the capillary bed. Blood pressure, which predominates at the arterial end of the bed (35 mm Hg), provides an outward force. **Osmotic pressure** (25 mm Hg), which predominates at the venous end of the bed where blood pressure is lower (17 mm Hg), produces a negative pressure (−8 mm Hg), which draws the fluid back. Hence, fluid is forced out of a capillary through clefts at the arterial end and returns to the blood at the venous end.

A *It would increase it because the osmotic pressure of the interstitial fluid would rise as inflammatory molecules and debris accumulated in the area.*

A Closer Look

Atherosclerosis? Get Out the Cardiovascular Drāno!

WHEN pipes get clogged, it is usually because something gets stuck in them—a greasy mass of bone bits or a hair ball. But when arteries are narrowed by **atherosclerosis,** the damming-up process occurs from the inside out: the walls of the vessels thicken and then protrude into the vessel lumen. Once this happens, it does not take much to close the vessel completely. A roaming blood clot or arterial spasms can do it.

Although all blood vessels are susceptible to this serious degenerative condition of blood vessel walls, for some unknown reason, the aorta and the coronary arteries serving the heart are most often affected. The disease progresses through many stages before the arterial walls actually become hard and approach the stage of the rigid tube system described in the text, but some of the earlier stages are just as lethal or more so.

Onset and Stages of Atherosclerosis

What triggers this scourge of blood vessels? According to the *response to injury hypothesis*, the initial event is damage to the tunica interna caused by bloodborne chemicals such as carbon monoxide (present in cigarette smoke or auto exhaust); by bacteria or viruses; or by physical factors such as a blow or persistent hypertension. Once a break has occurred, blood platelets cling to the injured site and initiate clotting to prevent blood loss. The injured endothelium sets off the alarm, summoning the immune system and the inflammatory process to repair the damage. If it is a one-time injury, when it's over, it's over. But most plaques grow slowly, through a series of injuries that heal, only to be ruptured again and again. As the plaque grows, the injured endothelial cells release chemotactic agents and chemicals that increase the permeability of the endothelium to fats and cholesterol, allowing them to take up residence just deep to the tunica interna. Monocytes attracted to the area migrate beneath the endothelium, where they become macrophages that gorge themselves on the fat. Soon they are joined by smooth muscle cells migrating from the media of the blood vessel wall. The result is the so-called *fatty streak stage* characterized by thickening of the tunica interna by greasy gray to yellow lesions called *atherosclerotic plaques.* When these small, fatty

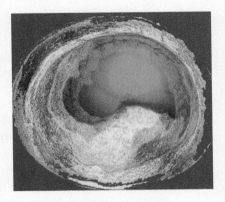

(a) Cross section of an artery that is partially occluded by atherosclerotic plaque.

mounds of muscle begin to protrude into the vessel wall (and ultimately the vessel lumen), the condition is called *atherosclerosis* (see photo a).

Arteriosclerosis is the end stage of the disease. As enlarging plaques hinder diffusion of nutrients from the blood to the deeper tissues of the artery wall, smooth muscle cells in the tunica media die and the elastic fibers deteriorate and are gradually replaced by nonelastic scar tissue. Then, calcium salts are deposited in the lesions. Collectively, these events cause the

Atherosclerosis? Get Out the Cardiovascular Drāno! *(continued)*

arterial wall to fray and ulcerate, conditions that encourage thrombus formation. The increased rigidity of the vessels leads to hypertension. Together, these events increase the risk of myocardial infarctions, strokes, and kidney failure.

However, the popular view that most heart attacks are the consequence of severe vessel narrowing and hardening is now being challenged, particularly since some 70 percent of heart attacks are caused by much smaller obstructions, too small to be seen on an arteriogram or to cause any symptoms in most cases. It now appears that the body's defense system betrays it. The inflammatory process that occurs in the still soft, unstable, cholesterol-rich plaques changes the biology of the vessel wall and makes the plaques susceptible to rupture, exploding off fragments that trigger massive clots that can cause lethal heart attacks. The victim appears perfectly healthy until he drops dead!

Treatment and Prevention

The *vulnerable plaque hypothesis* mentioned above has attracted many medical converts, but the

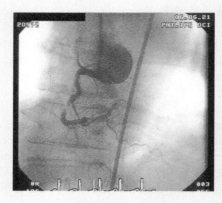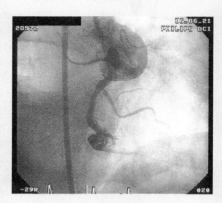

(b) Angiographs of an occluded artery (left) and the same artery after being cleared by balloon angioplasty (right). These views were prepared by a computer imaging technique, digital subtraction angiography (DSA).

question of what to do about it remains. Some medical centers test heart patients for elevated levels of cholesterol and C-reactive protein, a marker of inflammation. Electron beam CT scans may be able to identify those at risk by detecting calcium deposits in their coronary arteries. Antibiotics and anti-inflammatory drugs are being tested as preventative measures. Even the humble aspirin is gaining new respect, and more cardiologists recommend that people at high risk take one baby aspirin daily (81 mg).

So what can help when the damage is done and the heart is at risk because of atherosclerotic coronary vessels? In the past, the only choice has been coronary artery bypass surgery, in which vessels removed from the legs or thoracic cavity are implanted in the heart to restore circulation. More recently, devices threaded through blood vessels to obstructed sites have become part of the ammunition of cardiovascular medicine. *Balloon angioplasty* uses a catheter with a balloon packed into its tip (see the two photos in b).

blood-brain barrier), most of our capillaries have intercellular clefts.

4. Very free passage of small solutes and fluids is allowed by *fenestrated capillaries*. These unique capillaries are found where absorption is a priority (intestinal capillaries or those serving endocrine glands) or where filtration occurs (the kidney). A fenestra is an oval pore (*fenestra =* window) or opening and is usually covered by a delicate membrane (see Figure 11.36b). Even so, a fenestra is much more permeable than other regions of the plasma membrane.

Only substances unable to pass by one of these routes are prevented from leaving (or entering) the capillaries. These include protein molecules (in plasma or interstitial fluid) and blood cells.

Fluid Movements at Capillary Beds

Besides the exchanges made via vesicles, and by passive diffusion through endothelial cell plasma membranes, clefts, or fenestrations, there are active forces operating at capillary beds. Because of their intercellular clefts and fenestrations, some capillaries are leaky and bulk fluid flows occur across their plasma membranes. Hence, blood pressure tends to force fluid (and solutes) outward, and osmotic pressure tends to draw fluid back into the blood stream because blood has a higher solute concentration (due to its plasma proteins) than does interstitial fluid. Whether fluid moves out of or into the capillary depends on the difference between the two pressures. As a rule, blood pressure is higher at the arterial end of the capillary bed, and osmotic pressure is higher at the venous end. Consequently, fluid moves out of the capillaries at the beginning of the bed and is reclaimed at the opposite (venule) end (Figure 11.36c). However, not quite all of the fluid forced out of the blood-stream is reclaimed at the venule end. Returning that lost fluid to the blood is the chore of the lymphatic system.

Developmental Aspects of the Cardiovascular System

The heart begins as a simple tube in the embryo. It is beating and busily pumping blood by the fourth week of pregnancy. During the next three weeks, the heart continues to change and mature, finally becoming a four-chambered structure capable of acting as a double pump—all without missing a beat! During fetal life, the collapsed lungs and non-functional liver are mostly bypassed by the blood, through special vascular shunts. After the seventh week of development, few changes other than growth occur in the fetal circulation until birth. Shortly after birth, the bypass structures become blocked, and the special umbilical vessels stop functioning.

⚠ Homeostatic Imbalance

Congenital heart defects account for about half of infant deaths resulting from all congenital defects. Environmental interferences, such as maternal infection and ingested drugs during the first three months of pregnancy (when the embryonic heart is forming), seem to be the major causes of such problems. Congenital heart defects may include a ductus arteriosus that does not close, septal openings, and other structural abnormalities of the heart. Such problems can usually be corrected surgically. ▲

In the absence of congenital heart problems, the heart usually functions smoothly throughout a long lifetime for most people. Homeostatic mechanisms are so effective that we rarely are aware of when the heart is working harder. The heart will hypertrophy and its cardiac output will increase substantially if we exercise regularly and aerobically (that is, vigorously enough to force it to beat at a higher-than-normal rate for extended periods of time). Not only does the heart become a more powerful pump; it also becomes more efficient: pulse rate and blood pressure decrease. An added benefit of aerobic exercise is that it clears fatty deposits from the blood vessel walls, helping to slow the progress of atherosclerosis. However, let's raise a caution flag here: The once-a-month or once-a-year tennis player or snow shoveler has not built up this type of heart endurance and strength. When such an individual pushes his or her heart too much, it may not be able to cope with the sudden demand. This is why many weekend athletes are myocardial infarction victims.

As we get older, more and more signs of cardiovascular system disturbances start to appear. In some, the venous valves weaken, and purple, snakelike varicose veins appear. Not everyone has varicose veins, but we all have progressive atherosclerosis. Some say the process begins at birth, and there's an old saying that goes, "You are only as old as your arteries," referring to this degenerative process. The gradual loss in elasticity in the blood vessels leads to hypertension and hypertensive heart disease. The insidious filling of the blood vessels with fatty, calcified deposits leads most commonly to **coronary artery disease.** Also, the roughening of the vessel walls encourages thrombus formation. At least 30 percent of the population in the United States has hypertension by the age of 50, and cardiovascular disease causes more than one-half of the deaths in those over age 65. Although the aging process itself contributes to changes in the walls of the blood vessels that can lead to strokes or myocardial infarctions, most researchers feel that diet, not aging, is the single most important contributing factor to cardiovascular diseases. There is some agreement that the risk is lowered if people eat less animal fat, cholesterol, and salt. Other recommendations include avoiding stress, eliminating cigarette smoking, and taking part in a regular, moderate exercise program.

Systems in Sync

Homeostatic Relationships between the Cardiovascular System and Other Body Systems

Endocrine System
- The cardiovascular system delivers oxygen and nutrients; carries away wastes; blood serves as a transport vehicle for hormones
- Several hormones influence blood pressure (epinephrine, ANP, thyroxine, ADH); estrogen maintains vascular health in women

Lymphatic System/Immunity
- The cardiovascular system delivers oxygen and nutrients to lymphatic organs, which house immune cells; transports lymphocytes and antibodies; carries away wastes
- The lymphatic system picks up leaked fluid and plasma proteins and returns them to the cardiovascular system; its immune cells protect cardiovascular organs from specific pathogens

Digestive System
- The cardiovascular system delivers oxygen and nutrients; carries away wastes
- The digestive system provides nutrients to the blood including iron and B vitamins essential for RBC (and hemoglobin) formation

Urinary System
- The cardiovascular system delivers oxygen and nutrients; carries away wastes; blood pressure maintains kidney function
- The urinary system helps regulate blood volume and pressure by altering urine volume and releasing renin

Muscular System
- The cardiovascular system delivers oxygen and nutrients; carries away wastes
- Aerobic exercise enhances cardiovascular efficiency and helps prevent arteriosclerosis; the muscle "pump" aids venous return

Nervous System
- The cardiovascular system delivers oxygen and nutrients; removes wastes
- ANS regulates cardiac rate and force; sympathetic division maintains blood pressure and controls blood distribution according to need

Respiratory System
- The cardiovascular system delivers oxygen and nutrients; carries away wastes
- The respiratory system carries out gas exchange: loads oxygen and unloads carbon dioxide from the blood; respiratory "pump" aids venous return

Cardiovascular System

Reproductive System
- The cardiovascular system delivers oxygen and nutrients; carries away wastes
- Estrogen maintains vascular health in women

Integumentary System
- The cardiovascular system delivers oxygen and nutrients; carries away wastes
- The skin's blood vessels provide an important blood reservoir and a site for heat loss from body

Skeletal System
- The cardiovascular system delivers oxygen and nutrients and carries away wastes
- Bones are the site of hematopoiesis; protect cardiovascular organs by enclosure; provide a calcium depot

12

The Lymphatic System and Body Defenses

PART I: **THE LYMPHATIC SYSTEM**

They can't all be superstars! When we mentally tick off the names of the body's organ systems, the lymphatic (lim-fat'ik) system is probably not the first to come to mind. Yet without this quietly working system, our cardiovascular system would stop working and our immune system would be hopelessly impaired. The **lymphatic system** actually consists of two semi-independent parts: (1) a meandering network of *lymphatic vessels* and (2) various *lymphoid tissues* and *organs* scattered throughout the body. The lymphatic vessels transport fluids that have escaped from the blood vascular system back to the blood. The lymphoid organs house phagocytic cells and lymphocytes, which play essential roles in body defense and resistance to disease.

Lymphatic Vessels

As blood circulates through the body, exchanges of nutrients, wastes, and gases occur between the blood and the interstitial fluid. The hydrostatic and osmotic pressures operating at capillary beds force fluid out of the blood at the arterial ends of capillary beds ("upstream") and cause most of it to be reabsorbed at the venous ends ("downstream"). The fluid that remains behind in the tissue spaces, as much as 3 L daily, becomes part of the interstitial fluid. These leaked fluids, as well as any plasma proteins that escape from the bloodstream, must be carried back to the blood if the vascular system is to have sufficient blood volume to operate properly. If it does not, fluid accumulates in the tissues, producing **edema.** Excessive edema impairs the ability of tissue cells to make exchanges with the interstitial fluid and ultimately the blood. The function of the **lymphatic vessels** is to pick up this excess tissue fluid, now called **lymph fluid** (*lymph* = clear water) and return it to the bloodstream (Figure 12.1).

The lymphatic vessels, also called *lymphatics,* form a one-way system, and lymph flows only toward the heart. The microscopic, blind-ended **lymph capillaries** spiderweb between the tissue cells and blood capillaries in the loose connective tissues of the body (Figures 12.1 and 12.2a) and absorb the leaked fluid (primarily water and a small amount of dissolved proteins). Although similar to blood capillaries, lymphatic capillaries are so remarkably permeable that they were

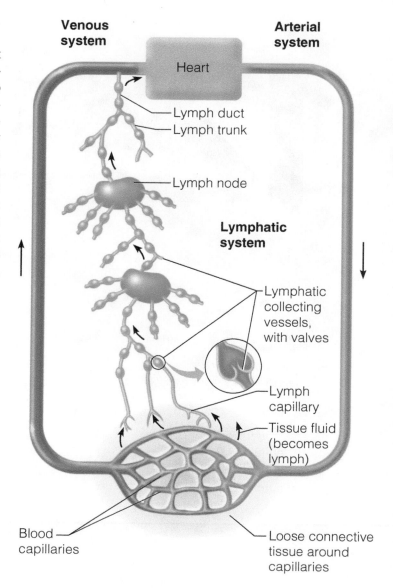

FIGURE 12.1 Relationship of the lymphatic vessels to the blood vessels of the cardiovascular circuit. Beginning at the bottom of this figure, we see that lymph, which begins as tissue fluid derived from blood capillaries, enters the lymph capillaries, travels through the lymphatic vessels and lymph nodes, and enters the bloodstream via the great veins at the root of the neck.

once thought to be open at one end like a straw. Not so—instead, what we find is that the edges of the endothelial cells forming their walls loosely overlap one another, forming flaplike *minivalves* (Figure 12.2b) that act as one-way swinging doors. The flaps, anchored by fine

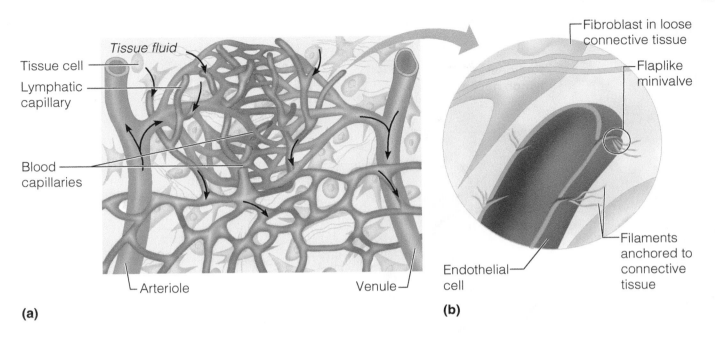

(a)

(b)

FIGURE 12.2   Distribution and special structural features of lymphatic capillaries. (a) Structural relationship between blood capillaries and lymph capillaries. Black arrows indicate direction of fluid movement. **(b)** Lymph capillaries begin as blind-ended tubes. The endothelial cells forming their walls overlap one another, forming flaplike minivalves.

collagen fibers to surrounding structures, gape open when the fluid pressure is higher in the interstitial space, allowing fluid to enter the lymphatic capillary. However, when the pressure is higher inside the lymphatic vessels, the endothelial cell flaps are forced together, preventing the lymph from leaking back out and forcing it along the vessel. Proteins, and even larger particles such as cell debris, bacteria, and viruses, are normally prevented from entering blood capillaries, but they enter the lymphatic capillaries easily, particularly in inflamed areas. But there is a problem here—bacteria and viruses (and cancer cells) that enter the lymphatics can then use them to travel throughout the body. This dilemma is partly resolved by the fact that lymph takes "detours" through the lymph nodes, where it is cleansed of debris and "examined" by cells of the immune system, as explained in more detail shortly.

Lymph is transported from the lymph capillaries through successively larger lymphatic vessels, referred to as *lymphatic collecting vessels,* until it is finally returned to the venous system through one of the two large ducts in the thoracic region.

The **right lymphatic duct** drains the lymph from the right arm and the right side of the head and thorax. The large **thoracic duct** receives lymph from the rest of the body, as shown in Figure 12.3. Both ducts empty the lymph into the subclavian vein on their own side of the body.

Like the veins of the cardiovascular system, the lymphatic vessels are thin-walled, and the larger ones have valves. The lymphatic system is a low-pressure, pumpless system. Lymph is transported by the same mechanisms that aid return of venous blood—the milking action of the skeletal muscles and the pressure changes in the thorax during breathing (that is, the muscular and respiratory "pumps"). In addition, smooth muscle in the walls of the larger lymphatics contracts rhythmically, actually helping to "pump" the lymph along.

Lymph Nodes

More closely related to the immune system, the **lymph nodes** help protect the body by removing foreign material such as bacteria and tumor cells from the lymphatic stream and by producing lymphocytes that function in the immune response.

Q *What would be the consequence of thoracic duct blockage?*

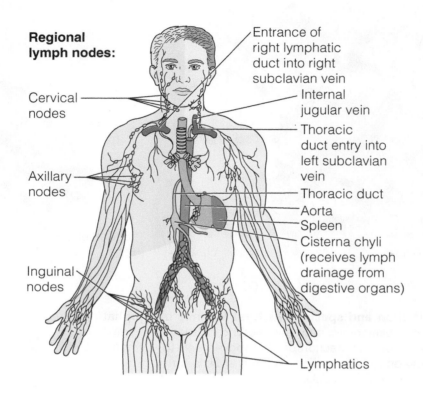

Regional lymph nodes:

Cervical nodes

Axillary nodes

Inguinal nodes

Entrance of right lymphatic duct into right subclavian vein

Internal jugular vein

Thoracic duct entry into left subclavian vein

Thoracic duct

Aorta

Spleen

Cisterna chyli (receives lymph drainage from digestive organs)

Lymphatics

FIGURE 12.3   Distribution of lymphatic vessels and lymph nodes.
Shading shows the body area drained by the right lymphatic duct; the rest of the body is drained by the thoracic duct.

As lymph fluid is transported toward the heart, it is filtered through the thousands of lymph nodes that cluster along the lymphatic vessels (see Figure 12.1). Particularly large clusters are found in the inguinal, axillary, and cervical regions of the body (see Figure 12.3). Within the lymph nodes are **macrophages** (mak′ro-fāj-ez), which engulf and destroy bacteria, viruses, and other foreign substances in the lymph before it is returned to the blood. Collections of **lymphocytes** (a type of white blood cell) are also strategically located in the lymph nodes and respond to foreign substances in the lymphatic stream. Although we are not usually aware of the protective nature of the lymph nodes, most of us have had swollen glands during an active infection. This swelling is a result of the trapping function of the nodes.

Lymph nodes vary in shape and size, but most are kidney-shaped, less than 1 inch (approximately 2.5 centimeters [cm]) long, and "buried" in the connective tissue that surrounds them. Each node is surrounded by a fibrous *capsule* from which strands called *trabeculae* (trah-bek′yu-le) extend inward to divide the node into a number of compartments (Figure 12.4). The internal framework is a network of soft reticular connective tissue that supports a continually changing population of lymphocytes. Lymphocytes arise from the red bone marrow but then migrate to the lymphatic organs, where they proliferate further.)

The outer part of the node, its **cortex,** contains collections of lymphocytes called **follicles.** Many of the follicles have dark-staining centers called **germinal centers.** These centers enlarge when specific lymphocytes (the *B cells*) are generating daughter cells called **plasma cells,** which release antibodies. The rest of the cortical cells are lymphocytes "in transit," the so-called *T cells* that circulate continuously between the blood, lymph

A   *Edema in the areas that drain into the thoracic duct.*

Q *What is the benefit of having fewer efferent than afferent lymphatic vessels?*

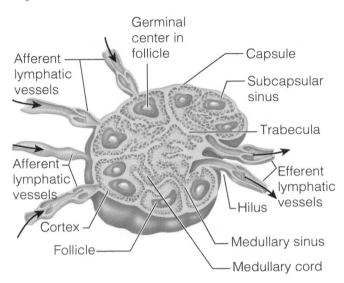

FIGURE 12.4 **Structure of a lymph node.**
Longitudinal view of the internal structure of a lymph node and associated lymphatics. Notice that several afferent lymphatics enter the node, whereas fewer efferent lymphatics exit at its hilus.

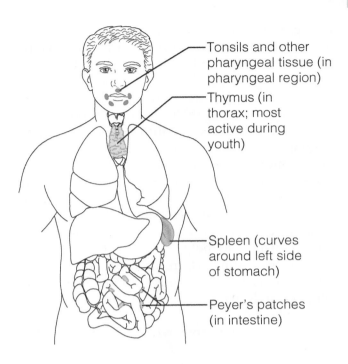

FIGURE 12.5 **Lymphoid organs.** Tonsils, thymus, spleen, and Peyer's patches.

nodes, and lymphatic stream, performing their surveillance role. Phagocytic macrophages are located in the central **medulla** of the lymph node.

Lymph enters the convex side of a lymph node through **afferent lymphatic vessels.** It then flows through a number of **sinuses** that cut through the lymph node and finally exits from the node at its indented region, the **hilus** (hi'lus), via **efferent lymphatic vessels.** Because there are fewer efferent vessels draining the node than afferent vessels feeding it, the flow of lymph through the node is very slow. This allows time for the lymphocytes and macrophages to perform their protective functions. Generally speaking, lymph passes through several nodes before its cleaning process is complete.

◤ Homeostatic Imbalance

Lymph nodes help rid the body of infectious agents and cancer cells, but sometimes they are overwhelmed by the very agents they are trying to destroy. For example, when large numbers of bacteria or viruses are trapped in the nodes, the nodes become inflamed and tender to the touch. The lymph nodes can also become secondary cancer sites, particularly in cancers that use lymphatic vessels to spread throughout the body. The fact that cancer-infiltrated lymph nodes are swollen but not painful helps to distinguish cancerous lymph nodes from those infected by microorganisms. ◤

Other Lymphoid Organs

Lymph nodes are just one example of the many types of **lymphoid organs** in the body. Others are the spleen, thymus gland, tonsils, and Peyer's patches of the intestine (Figure 12.5), as well as bits of lymphatic tissue scattered in the epithelial and connective tissues. The common feature of all these organs is a predominance of reticular connective tissue and lymphocytes. Although all lymphoid organs have roles in protecting the body, only the lymph nodes filter lymph.

The **spleen** is a blood-rich organ that filters blood. It is located in the left side of the abdominal

A *Since the outlet is smaller than the inlet to the lymph node, the lymph fluid stagnates (stops flowing) briefly in the lymph node giving macrophages and lymphocytes time to monitor and process the lymph for pathogens.*

cavity and extends to curl around the anterior aspect of the stomach. Instead of filtering lymph, the spleen filters and cleanses blood of bacteria, viruses, and other debris. Its most important function is to destroy worn-out red blood cells and return some of their breakdown products to the liver. For example, iron is used again for making hemoglobin, and the rest of the hemoglobin molecule is secreted in bile. Other functions of the spleen include storing platelets and acting as a blood reservoir (as does the liver). During hemorrhage, both the spleen and liver contract and empty their contained blood into the circulation to help bring the blood volume back to normal levels. In the fetus, the spleen is an important hematopoietic (blood cell–forming) site, but only lymphocytes are produced by the adult spleen.

The **thymus gland,** which functions at peak levels only during youth, is a lymphatic mass found low in the throat overlying the heart. The thymus produces hormones, *thymosin* and others, that function in the programming of certain lymphocytes so they can carry out their protective roles in the body.

The **tonsils** and **adenoids** are small masses of lymphatic tissue that ring the pharynx (the throat), where they are found in the mucosa. Their job is to trap and remove any bacteria or other foreign pathogens entering the throat. They carry out this function so efficiently that sometimes they become congested with bacteria and become red, swollen, and sore, a condition called *tonsillitis.*

Peyer's patches, which resemble tonsils, are found in the wall of the small intestine. The macrophages of Peyer's patches are in an ideal position to capture and destroy bacteria (always present in tremendous numbers in the intestine), thereby preventing them from penetrating the intestinal wall. Peyer's patches and the tonsils are part of the collection of small lymphoid tissues referred to as **mucosa-associated lymphatic tissue (MALT).** Collectively, MALT acts as a sentinel to protect the upper respiratory and digestive tracts from the never-ending attacks of foreign matter entering those cavities.

Now that we have set the stage on which many of the body's defense mechanisms play their roles, we are ready to consider that topic in more detail.

PART II: BODY DEFENSES

Every second of every day, an army of hostile bacteria, viruses, and fungi swarms on our skin and invades our inner passageways—yet we stay amazingly healthy most of the time. The body seems to have developed a single-minded approach toward such foes—if you're not with us, then you're against us!

The body's defenders against these tiny but mighty enemies are two systems, simply called the *nonspecific* and the *specific defense systems* (Figure 12.6). The **nonspecific defense system** responds immediately to protect the body from all foreign substances, whatever they are. The nonspecific defenses are provided by intact skin and mucous membranes, the inflammatory response, and a number of proteins produced by body cells. This system reduces the workload of the second protective arm, the specific defense system, by preventing entry and spread of microorganisms throughout the body.

Nonspecific defense mechanisms		Specific defense mechanisms (immune system)
First line of defense	Second line of defense	Third line of defense
• Skin • Mucous membranes • Secretions of skin and mucous membranes	• Phagocytic cells • Antimicrobial proteins • The inflammatory response	• Lymphocytes • Antibodies • Macrophages

FIGURE 12.6   **An overview of the body's defenses.**

The **specific defense system,** more commonly called the **immune system,** mounts the attack against *particular* foreign substances. Although certain body organs (lymphatic organs and blood vessels) are intimately involved with the immune response, the immune system is a *functional system* rather than an organ system in an anatomical sense. Its "structures" are a variety of molecules and trillions of immune cells, which inhabit lymphatic tissues and circulate in body fluids. The most important of the immune cells are **lymphocytes** and **macrophages.**

When our immune system is operating effectively, it protects us from most bacteria, viruses, transplanted organs or grafts, and even our own cells that have turned against us. The immune system does this both directly, by cell attack, and indirectly, by releasing mobilizing chemicals and protective antibody molecules. The resulting highly specific resistance to disease is called **immunity** (*immun* = free).

Unlike the nonspecific defenses which are always prepared to defend the body, the immune system must first "meet" or be primed by an initial exposure to a foreign substance (antigen) before it can protect the body against it. Nonetheless, what it lacks in speed it makes up for in the precision of its counterattacks. Although we will consider them separately, keep in mind that specific and nonspecific defenses always work hand-in-hand to protect the body.

Nonspecific Body Defenses

Some nonspecific resistance to disease is inherited. For instance, there are certain diseases that humans never get, such as some forms of tuberculosis that affect birds. Most often, however, the term *nonspecific body defense* refers to the mechanical barriers that cover body surfaces and to cells and chemicals that act on the initial battlefronts to protect the body from invading **pathogens** (harmful or disease-causing microorganisms). Table 12.1 provides a more detailed summary of the most important nonspecific defenses.

Surface Membrane Barriers

The body's *first line of defense* against the invasion of disease-causing microorganisms is the *skin* and *mucous membranes.* As long as the skin is unbroken, its keratinized epidermis is a strong physical barrier to most microorganisms that swarm on the skin. Intact mucous membranes provide similar mechanical barriers within the body. Recall that mucous membranes line all body cavities open to the exterior: the digestive, respiratory, urinary, and reproductive tracts. Besides serving as physical barriers, these membranes produce a variety of protective chemicals:

1. The acid pH of skin secretions inhibits bacterial growth, and sebum contains chemicals that are toxic to bacteria. Vaginal secretions of adult females are also very acidic.

2. The stomach mucosa secretes hydrochloric acid and protein-digesting enzymes. Both kill pathogens.

3. Saliva and lacrimal fluid contain *lysozyme,* an enzyme that destroys bacteria.

4. Sticky mucus traps many microorganisms that enter digestive and respiratory passageways.

Some mucosae also have structural modifications that fend off potential invaders. Mucus-coated hairs inside the nasal cavity trap inhaled particles, and the respiratory tract mucosa is ciliated. The cilia sweep dust- and bacteria-laden mucus superiorly toward the mouth, preventing it from entering the lungs, where the warm, moist environment provides an ideal site for bacterial growth.

Although the surface barriers are very effective, they *are* broken from time to time by small nicks and cuts resulting, for example, from brushing your teeth or shaving. When this happens and microorganisms do invade deeper tissues, other nonspecific mechanisms come into play to defend the body.

Cells and Chemicals

For its *second line of defense,* the body uses an enormous number of cells and chemicals to protect itself. These defenses rely on the destructive powers of *phagocytes* and *natural killer cells,* the inflammatory response, and a variety of chemical substances that kill pathogens and help repair tissue. Fever is also considered to be a nonspecific protective response.

Phagocytes

Pathogens that make it through the mechanical barriers are confronted by **phagocytes** (fa′go-sītz″; *phago*

TABLE 12.1   Summary of Nonspecific Body Defenses

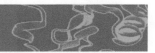

Category and associated elements	Protective mechanism
Surface membrane barriers—First line of defense	
Intact skin (epidermis)	Forms mechanical barrier that prevents entry of pathogens and other harmful substances into body.
• Acid mantle	Skin secretions make epidermal surface acidic, which inhibits bacterial growth; sebum also contains bacteria-killing chemicals.
• Keratin	Provides resistance against acids, alkalis, and bacterial enzymes.
Intact mucous membranes	Form mechanical barrier that prevents entry of pathogens.
• Mucus	Traps microorganisms in respiratory and digestive tracts.
• Nasal hairs	Filter and trap microorganisms in nasal passages.
• Cilia	Propel debris-laden mucus away from lower respiratory passages.
• Gastric juice	Contains concentrated hydrochloric acid and protein-digesting enzymes that destroy pathogens in stomach.
• Acid mantle of vagina	Inhibits growth of bacteria and fungi in female reproductive tract.
• Lacrimal secretion (tears); saliva	Continuously lubricate and cleanse eyes (tears) and oral cavity (saliva); contain lysozyme, an enzyme that destroys microorganisms.
Cellular and chemical defenses—Second line of defense	
Phagocytes	Engulf and destroy pathogens that breach surface membrane barriers; macrophages also contribute to immune response.
Natural killer cells	Promote cell lysis by direct cell attack against virus-infected or cancerous body cells; do not depend on specific antigen recognition.
Inflammatory response	Prevents spread of injurious agents to adjacent tissues, disposes of pathogens and dead tissue cells, and promotes tissue repair; releases chemical mediators that attract phagocytes (and immunocompetent cells) to the area.
Antimicrobial chemicals	
• Complement	Group of plasma proteins that lyses microorganisms, enhances phagocytosis by opsonization, and intensifies inflammatory response.
• Interferons	Proteins released by virus-infected cells that protect uninfected tissue cells from viral takeover; mobilize immune system.
• Urine	Normally acid pH inhibits bacterial growth; cleanses the lower urinary tract as it flushes from the body.
Fever	Systemic response triggered by pyrogens; high body temperature inhibits multiplication of bacteria and enhances body repair processes.

= eat) in nearly every body organ. A phagocyte, such as a *macrophage* or *neutrophil*, engulfs a foreign particle much the way an amoeba ingests a food particle (Figure 12.7). Flowing cytoplasmic extensions bind to the particle and then pull it inside, enclosing it in a vacuole. The vacuole is then fused with the enzymatic contents of a *lysosome*, and its contents are broken down or digested.

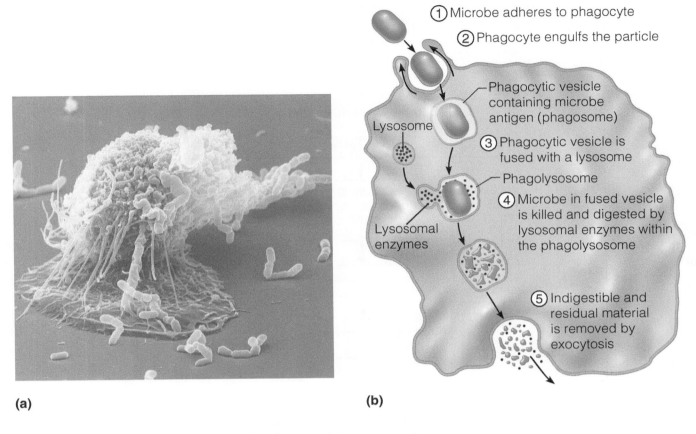

(a)

(b)

FIGURE 12.7   Phagocytosis by a macrophage. (a) This scanning electron micrograph (4300×) in computer-generated color shows a macrophage pulling sausage-shaped *Escherichia coli* bacteria toward it with its long cytoplasmic extensions. Several bacteria on the macrophage's surface are being engulfed. **(b)** Events of phagocytosis.

Natural Killer Cells

Natural killer (NK) cells, which "police" the body in blood and lymph, are a unique group of lymphocytes that can lyse and kill cancer cells and virus-infected body cells well before the immune system is enlisted in the fight. Unlike the lymphocytes of the immune system, which can recognize and react only against *specific* virus-infected or tumor cells, natural killer cells are far less "picky." They can act spontaneously against *any* such target by recognizing certain sugars on the "intruder's" surface. NK cells are not phagocytic. They attack the target cell's membrane and release a lytic chemical called *perforins*. Shortly thereafter, the target cell's membrane and nucleus disintegrate.

Inflammatory Response

The **inflammatory response** is a nonspecific response that is triggered whenever body tissues are injured (Figure 12.8). For example, it occurs in response to physical trauma, intense heat, and irritating chemicals, as well as to infection by viruses and bacteria. The four *cardinal signs* and major symptoms of an acute inflammation are *redness, heat* (*inflamm* = set on fire), *swelling,* and *pain.* It is easy to understand why these symptoms occur, once the events of the inflammatory response are understood.

The inflammatory process begins with a chemical "alarm." When cells are injured, they release inflammatory chemicals, including **histamine** and **kinins** (ki′ninz), that (1) cause blood vessels in

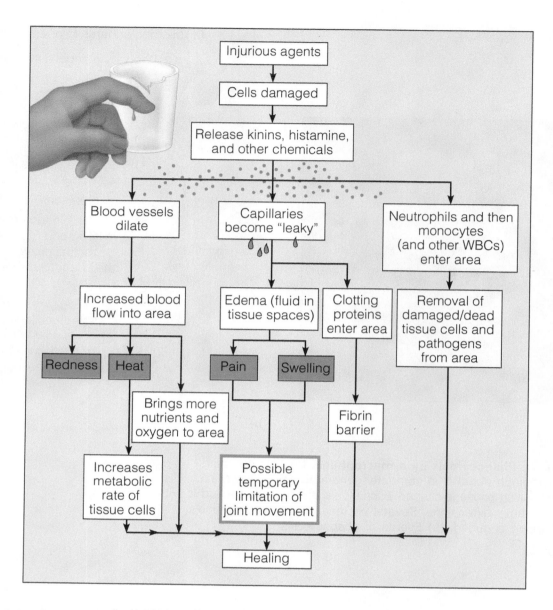

FIGURE 12.8   Flowchart of inflammatory events. The four cardinal signs of acute inflammation are shown in red boxes. Limitation of joint movement (red outlined box) occurs in some cases and is considered to be the fifth cardinal sign of acute inflammation.

the involved area to dilate and capillaries to become leaky, (2) activate pain receptors, and (3) attract phagocytes and white blood cells to the area. (This latter phenomenon is called **chemotaxis** because the cells are following a chemical gradient.) Dilation of the blood vessels increases the blood flow to the area, accounting for the redness and heat observed. Increased permeability of the capillaries allows plasma to leak from the bloodstream into the tissue spaces, causing local edema

(swelling) that also activates pain receptors in the area. If the swollen, painful area is a joint, its function (movement) may be impaired temporarily. This forces the injured part to rest, which aids healing. Some authorities consider limitation of joint movement to be an additional (fifth) cardinal sign of inflammation.

The inflammatory response (1) prevents the spread of damaging agents to nearby tissues, (2) disposes of cell debris and pathogens, and (3) sets the stage for repair. Let's look at how it accomplishes these tasks. Within an hour or so after the inflammatory process has begun, neutrophils are squeezing through the capillary walls, a process called **diapedesis** (Figure 12.9). Drawn to the area by inflammatory chemicals, the neutrophils begin the cleanup detail by engulfing damaged or dead tissue cells and/or pathogens. As the counterattack continues, monocytes begin to leave the bloodstream and follow the neutrophils into the inflamed area. Monocytes are fairly poor phagocytes, but within 8 to 12 hours after entering the tissues they become macrophages with insatiable appetites. The macrophages continue to wage the battle, replacing the short-lived neutrophils on the battlefield. Macrophages are the central actors in the final disposal of cell debris as the inflammation subsides.

Besides phagocytosis, other protective events are also occurring at the inflamed site. Clotting proteins, leaked into the area from the blood, are activated and begin to wall off the damaged area with fibrin to prevent the spread of pathogens or harmful agents to neighboring tissues. The fibrin mesh also forms a scaffolding for permanent repair. The local heat increases the metabolic rate of the tissue cells, speeding up their defensive actions and repair processes.

If the area contains pathogens that have previously invaded the body, the *third line of defense* also comes into play—the immune response mediated by lymphocytes. Both protective antibodies and T cells (T lymphocytes) invade the area to act specifically and directly against the damaging agents. (We will speak more of the immune response shortly.)

Homeostatic Imbalance

In severely infected areas, the battle takes a considerable toll on both sides, and creamy, yellow pus may be formed in the wound. **Pus** is a mixture of dead or dying neutrophils, broken-down tissue cells, and living and dead pathogens. If the inflammatory mechanism fails to fully clear the area of debris, the

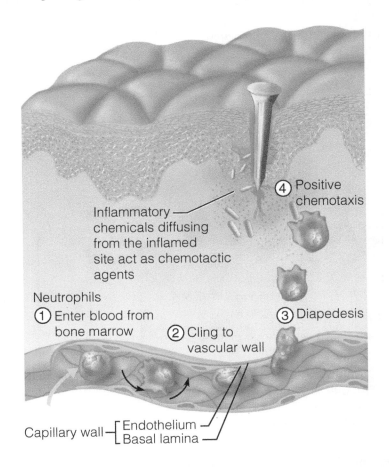

Inflammatory chemicals diffusing from the inflamed site act as chemotactic agents

Neutrophils

(1) Enter blood from bone marrow

(2) Cling to vascular wall

(3) Diapedesis

(4) Positive chemotaxis

Capillary wall — [Endothelium
Basal lamina]

FIGURE 12.9 Phagocyte mobilization.

sac of pus may become walled off, forming an *abscess*. Surgical drainage of abscesses is often necessary before healing can occur. ▲

Antimicrobial Chemicals

The body's most important **antimicrobial chemicals,** apart from those produced in the inflammatory reaction, are *complement proteins* and *interferon*.

Complement   The term ***complement*** refers to a group of at least 20 plasma proteins that circulate in the blood in an inactive state. However, when complement becomes attached, or *fixed*, to foreign cells such as bacteria, fungi, or mismatched red blood cells, it is activated and becomes a major factor in the fight against the foreign cells. This **complement fixation** occurs when complement proteins bind to certain sugars or proteins (such as antibodies) on the foreign cell's surface. One result of complement fixation is the formation of *membrane attack complexes (MAC)* that produce lesions, complete with holes, in the foreign cell's surface (Figure 12.10). These allow water to rush into the cell, causing it to burst. Activated complement also amplifies the inflammatory response. Some of the molecules released during the activation process are *vasodilators,* and some are *chemotaxis chemicals* that attract neutrophils and macrophages into the region. Others cause the cell membranes of the foreign cells to become sticky so they are easier to phagocytize; this effect is called *opsonization*. Although the complement attack is often directed against specific microorganisms that have been "identified" by antibody binding, complement itself is a nonspecific defensive mechanism that "complements," or enhances, the effectiveness of *both* nonspecific and specific defenses.

Interferon   Viruses lack the cellular machinery required to generate ATP or make proteins. They do their "dirty work" or damage in the body by entering tissue cells and taking over the cellular machinery needed to reproduce themselves. Although the virus-infected cells can do little to save themselves, they help defend cells that have not yet been infected by secreting small proteins called **interferons** (in-ter-fer′onz). The interferon molecules diffuse to nearby cells and bind to their membrane receptors. Somehow this binding hinders the ability of viruses to multiply within these cells.

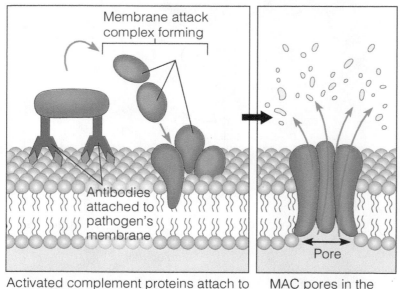

Activated complement proteins attach to pathogen's membrane in step-by-step sequence, forming a membrane attack complex (a MAC attack).

MAC pores in the membrane cause cell lysis.

FIGURE 12.10   Activation of complement, resulting in lysis of a target cell.

Fever

Fever, or abnormally high body temperature, is a systemic response to invading microorganisms. Body temperature is regulated by a part of the hypothalamus, commonly referred to as the body's "thermostat." Normally the thermostat is set at approximately 36.2°C (98.2°F), but it can be reset upward in response to **pyrogens** (*pyro* = fire), chemicals secreted by white blood cells and macrophages exposed to foreign cells or substances in the body.

Although high fevers are dangerous because excess heat "scrambles" enzymes and other body proteins, mild or moderate fever seems to benefit the body. Bacteria require large amounts of iron and zinc to multiply; but, during a fever, the liver and spleen gather up these nutrients, making them less available. Fever also increases the metabolic rate of tissue cells in general, speeding up repair processes.

Specific Body Defenses: The Immune System

Most of us would find it wonderfully convenient if we could walk into a single clothing store and buy a complete wardrobe—hat to shoes—that fit us "to a T" regardless of any special figure problems. We know that such a service would be next to impossible to find—yet we take for granted our *immune system,* our built-in *specific defense system,* which stalks and eliminates with nearly equal precision almost any type of pathogen that intrudes into the body.

The immune system's response to a threat, called the **immune response,** tremendously increases the inflammatory response, and it provides protection that is carefully targeted against *specific* antigens. Furthermore, the initial exposure to an antigen "primes" the body to react more vigorously to later meetings with the same antigen.

Sometimes referred to as the body's *third line of defense,* the immune system is a functional system that recognizes foreign molecules (antigens) and acts to inactivate or destroy them. Normally it protects us from a wide variety of pathogens, as well as from abnormal body cells. When it fails, malfunctions, or is disabled, some of the most devastating diseases—such as cancer, rheumatoid arthritis, and AIDS—may result.

Although *immunology,* the study of immunity, is a fairly new science, the ancient Greeks knew that once someone had suffered through a certain infectious disease, that person was unlikely to have the same disease again. The basis of this immunity was revealed in the late 1800s, when it was shown that animals surviving a serious bacterial infection have "factors" in their blood that protect them from future attacks by the same pathogen. (These factors are now known to be unique proteins, called *antibodies.*) Furthermore, it was demonstrated that if antibody-containing serum from the surviving animals (immune serum) was injected into animals that had not been exposed to the pathogen, those animals would also be protected. These landmark experiments revealed three important aspects of the immune response:

1. **It is antigen specific**—It recognizes and acts against *particular* pathogens or foreign substances.
2. **It is systemic**—Immunity is not restricted to the initial infection site.
3. **It has "memory"**—It recognizes and mounts even stronger attacks on previously encountered pathogens.

This was exciting news. But then, in the mid-1900s, it was discovered that injection of serum containing antibodies did not always protect a recipient from diseases the donor had survived. In such cases, however, injection of the donor's lymphocytes *did* provide immunity.

As the pieces began to fall into place, two separate but overlapping arms of immunity were recognized. **Humoral** (hu′mor-al) **immunity,** also called **antibody-mediated immunity,** is provided by antibodies present in the body's "humors," or fluids. When lymphocytes themselves defend the body, the immunity is called **cellular** or **cell-mediated immunity** because the protective factor is living cells. The cellular arm also has cellular targets—virus-infected tissue cells, cancer cells, and cells of foreign grafts. The lymphocytes act against such targets either *directly,* by lysing the foreign cells, or *indirectly,* by releasing chemicals that enhance the inflammatory response or activate other immune cells. However, before we describe the humoral and cellular responses individually, we will consider the antigens that trigger the activity of the remarkable cells involved in these immune responses.

Antigens

An **antigen** (an'tĭ-jen) **(Ag)** is any substance capable of exciting our immune system and provoking an immune response. Most antigens are large, complex molecules that are not normally present in our bodies. Consequently, as far as our immune system is concerned, they are foreign intruders, or **nonself.** An almost limitless variety of substances can act as antigens, including virtually all foreign proteins, nucleic acids, many large carbohydrates, and some lipids. Of these, proteins are the strongest antigens. Pollen grains and microorganisms such as bacteria, fungi, and virus particles are *antigenic* because their surfaces bear such foreign molecules.

It is also important to remember that our own cells are richly studded with a variety of protein molecules (self-antigens). Somehow, as our immune system develops, it takes an inventory of all these proteins so that, thereafter, they are recognized as self. Although these **self-antigens** do not trigger an immune response in us, they *are* strongly antigenic to other people. This helps explain why our bodies reject cells of transplanted organs or foreign grafts unless special measures (drugs and others) are taken to cripple or stifle the immune response.

As a rule, small molecules are not antigenic. But, when they link up with our own proteins, the immune system may recognize the combination as foreign and mount an attack that is harmful rather than protective. In such cases, the troublesome small molecule is called a *hapten* (*haptein* = to grasp), or *incomplete antigen.* Besides certain drugs, chemicals that act as haptens are found in poison ivy, animal dander, and even in some detergents, hair dyes, cosmetics, and other commonly used household and industrial products.

Homeostatic Imbalance

Perhaps the most dramatic and familiar example of a drug hapten's provoking an immune response involves the binding of penicillin to blood proteins, which causes a *penicillin reaction* in some people. In such cases, the immune system mounts such a vicious attack that the person's life is endangered. ▲

Cells of the Immune System: An Overview

The crucial cells of the immune system are lymphocytes and macrophages. Lymphocytes exist in two major "flavors." The **B lymphocytes,** or **B cells,** produce antibodies and oversee humoral immunity, whereas the **T lymphocytes,** or **T cells,** are non–antibody-producing lymphocytes that constitute the cell-mediated arm of immunity. Unlike the two types of lymphocytes, macrophages do not respond to specific antigens but instead play an essential role in helping the lymphocytes that do.

Lymphocytes

Like all blood cells, lymphocytes originate from hemocytoblasts in red bone marrow (Figure 12.11). The immature lymphocytes released from the marrow are essentially identical. Whether a given lymphocyte matures into a B cell or a T cell depends on where in the body it becomes **immunocompetent,** that is, capable of responding to a specific antigen by binding to it. **T** cells arise from lymphocytes that migrate to the **t**hymus (see Figure 12.11), where they undergo a maturation process of 2 to 3 days, directed by thymic hormones (*thymosin* and others). Within the thymus, the immature lymphocytes divide rapidly and their numbers increase enormously, but only those maturing T cells with the sharpest ability to identify *foreign* antigens survive. Lymphocytes capable of binding strongly with *self-antigens* (and of acting against body cells) are vigorously weeded out and destroyed. Thus, the development of tolerance for self-antigens is an essential part of a lymphocyte's "education." This is true not only for T cells but also for B cells. **B** cells develop immunocompetence in **b**one marrow, but little is known about the factors that regulate B cell maturation.

Once a lymphocyte is immunocompetent, it will be able to react to one distinct antigen and one only, because *all* the antigen receptors on its external surface are the same. For example, the receptors of one lymphocyte can recognize only a part of the hepatitis A virus, those of another lymphocyte can recognize or bind only to pneumococcus bacteria, and so forth.

Although all the details of the maturation process are still beyond our grasp, we know that lymphocytes become immunocompetent *before* meeting the antigens they may later attack. Thus, *it is our genes, not antigens, that determine what specific foreign substances our immune system will be able to recognize and resist.* Only some of the possible antigens our lymphocytes are programmed to

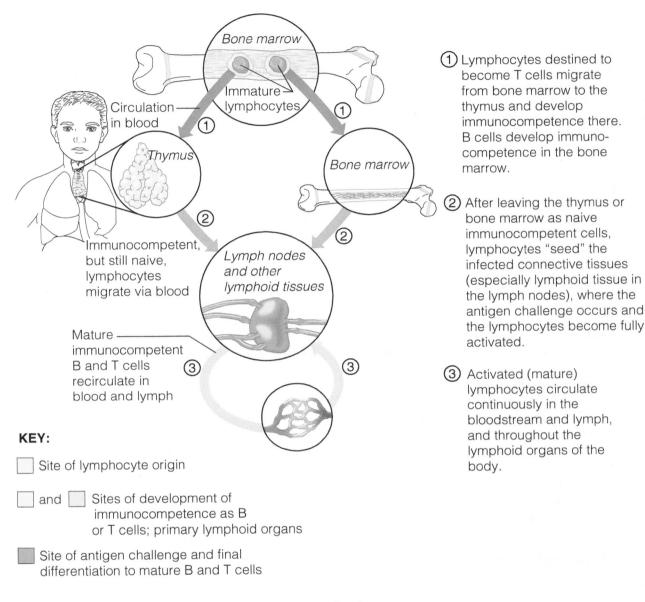

① Lymphocytes destined to become T cells migrate from bone marrow to the thymus and develop immunocompetence there. B cells develop immunocompetence in the bone marrow.

② After leaving the thymus or bone marrow as naive immunocompetent cells, lymphocytes "seed" the infected connective tissues (especially lymphoid tissue in the lymph nodes), where the antigen challenge occurs and the lymphocytes become fully activated.

③ Activated (mature) lymphocytes circulate continuously in the bloodstream and lymph, and throughout the lymphoid organs of the body.

KEY:

☐ Site of lymphocyte origin

☐ and ☐ Sites of development of immunocompetence as B or T cells; primary lymphoid organs

☐ Site of antigen challenge and final differentiation to mature B and T cells

FIGURE 12.11 Lymphocyte differentiation and activation.

resist will ever invade our bodies. Consequently, only some members of our army of immunocompetent cells will be mobilized during our lifetime. The others will be forever idle. As usual, our bodies have done their best to protect us.

After becoming immunocompetent, both T cells and B cells migrate to the lymph nodes and spleen (and loose connective tissues), where their encounters with antigens will occur (see Figure 12.9). Then, when the lymphoctyes bind with recognized antigens, they complete their differentiation into fully mature T cells and B cells.

Macrophages

Macrophages, which also become widely distributed throughout the lymphoid organs and connective tissues, arise from monocytes formed in the bone marrow. As described earlier, a major role of macrophages (literally, "big eaters") in the nonspecific defense system is to engulf foreign particles and rid them from the area. However, their job doesn't stop there. They also present fragments of those antigens, like signal flags, on their own surfaces, where they can be recognized by immunocompetent T cells. Thus, they act as *antigen presenters* in the specific defense system. Macrophages also secrete cytokine proteins, called *monokines,* that are important in the immune response (see Table 12.4). Activated T cells, in turn, release chemicals that cause macrophages to become insatiable phagocytes, or *killer macrophages.* As you will see, interactions between lymphocytes, and between lymphocytes and macrophages, underlie virtually all phases of the immune response.

Macrophages tend to remain fixed in the lymphoid organs (as if waiting for antigens to come to them). But lymphocytes, especially T cells, circulate continuously through the body (see Figure 12.11). This makes sense because it greatly increases a lymphocyte's chance of coming into contact with antigens collected by the lymph capillaries from the tissue spaces, as well as with huge numbers of macrophages and other lymphocytes.

To summarize, the immune system is a two-armed defensive system that uses lymphocytes, macrophages, and specific molecules to identify and destroy all substances—both living and nonliving—that are in the body but are not recognized as being part of the body or as being self. The immune system's ability to respond to such threats depends on the ability of its cells (1) to recognize foreign substances (antigens) in the body by binding to them, and (2) to communicate with one another so that the system as a whole mounts a response specific to those antigens.

Humoral (Antibody-Mediated) Immune Response

An immunocompetent but as yet immature B lymphocyte is stimulated to complete its development into a fully mature B cell when an antigen binds to its surface receptors. This binding event *sensitizes,* or *activates,* the lymphocyte to "switch on" and undergo **clonal selection.** The lymphocyte begins to grow and then multiplies rapidly to form an army of cells all exactly like itself and bearing the same antigen-specific receptors (Figure 12.12). The resulting family of identical cells descended from the *same* ancestor cell is called a **clone,** and clone formation is the **primary humoral response** to that antigen. (As described later, T cells also influence B cell activation.)

Most of the B cell clone members, or descendants, become **plasma cells.** After an initial lag period,

these antibody-producing "factories" swing into action, producing the same highly specific antibodies at an unbelievable rate of about 2000 antibody molecules per second. (The B cells themselves produce only very small amounts of antibodies.) However, this flurry of activity lasts only 4 or 5 days; then the plasma cells begin to die. Antibody levels in the blood during this primary response peak in about 10 days and then slowly decline (Figure 12.13).

B cell clone members that do not become plasma cells become long-lived **memory cells** capable of responding to the same antigen at later meetings with it. Memory cells are responsible for the immunological "memory" mentioned earlier. These later immune responses, called **secondary humoral responses,** are much faster, more prolonged, and more effective because all the preparations for this attack have already been made. Within hours after recognition of the "old-enemy" antigen, a new army of plasma cells is being generated, and antibodies begin to flood into the bloodstream. Within 2 to 3 days, blood antibody levels peak (at much higher levels than seen in the primary response), and their levels remain high for weeks to months. How antibodies protect the body is described shortly.

Active and Passive Humoral Immunity

When your B cells encounter antigens and produce antibodies against them, you are exhibiting **active immunity** (Figure 12.14). Active immunity is (1) *naturally acquired* during bacterial and viral infections, when we may develop the symptoms of the disease and suffer a little (or a lot), and (2) *artificially acquired* when we receive **vaccines.** It makes little difference whether the antigen invades the body under its own power or is introduced in the form of a vaccine. The response of the immune system is pretty much the same. Indeed, once it was recognized that secondary responses are so much more vigorous, the race was on to develop vaccines to "prime" the immune response by providing a first meeting with the antigen. Most vaccines contain dead or *attenuated* (living, but extremely weakened) pathogens.

We receive two benefits from vaccines: (1) we are spared most of the signs and symptoms (and discomfort) of the disease that would otherwise occur during the primary response, and (2) the weakened antigens are still able to stimulate antibody production and promote immunological

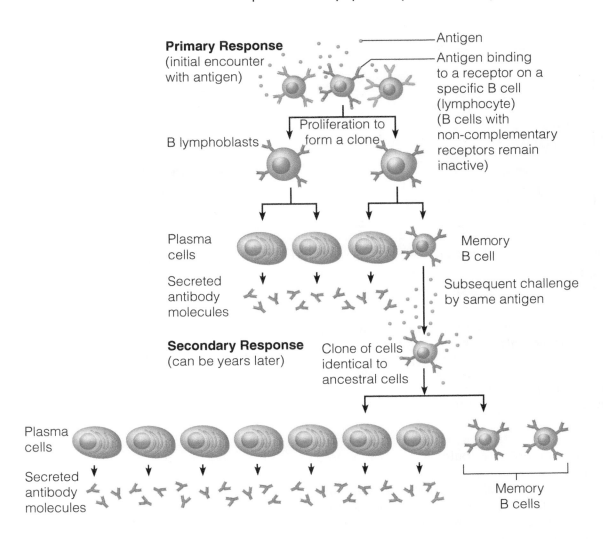

FIGURE 12.12   Clonal selection of a B cell stimulated by antigen binding.
The initial meeting stimulates the primary response in which the B cell proliferates rapidly, forming a clone of like cells (clonal expansion), most of which become antibody-producing plasma cells. Cells that do not differentiate into plasma cells become memory cells, which respond to subsequent exposures to the same antigen. Should such a meeting occur, the memory cells quickly produce more memory cells and larger numbers of effector plasma cells with the same antigen specificity. Responses generated by memory cells are called secondary responses.

memory. So-called booster shots, which may intensify the immune response at later meetings with the same antigen, are also available. Vaccines are currently available against microorganisms that cause pneumonia, smallpox, polio, tetanus, diphtheria, measles, and many other diseases. In the United States, many potentially serious childhood diseases have been virtually wiped out by active immunization programs. A summary of the currently recommended schedule for administering vaccines to U.S. children is provided in Table 12.2.

Passive immunity is quite different from active immunity, both in the antibody source and in the degree of protection it provides (see Figure 12.14). Instead of being made by your plasma cells, the antibodies are obtained from the serum of an immune human or animal donor. As a result, your B cells are *not* challenged by the antigen, immunological memory does *not* occur, and the temporary protection provided by the "borrowed antibodies" ends when they naturally degrade in the body.

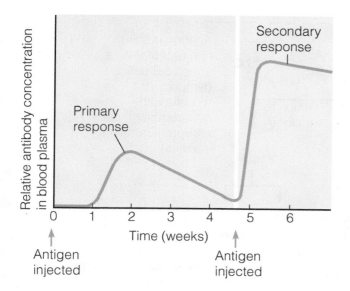

FIGURE 12.13 **Primary and secondary humoral responses to an antigen.** In the primary response, there is a gradual rise and then a rapid decline in the level of antibodies in the blood. The secondary response is both more rapid and more intense. Additionally, antibody levels remain high for a much longer time.

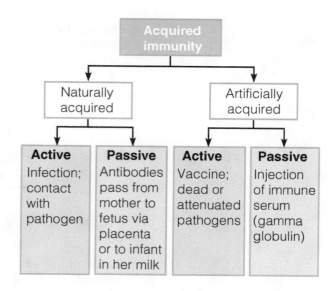

FIGURE 12.14 **Types of acquired immunity.** Orange boxes signify active types of immunity in which immunological memory is established. Gold boxes signify the short-lived passive types of immunity; no immunological memory is established.

Passive immunity is conferred *naturally* on a fetus when the mother's antibodies cross the placenta and enter the fetal circulation, and after birth during breastfeeding. For several months after birth, the baby is protected from all the antigens to which the mother has been exposed.

Passive immunity is *artificially* conferred when one receives immune serum or gamma globulin. Gamma globulin is commonly administered after exposure to hepatitis. Other immune sera are used to treat poisonous snake bites (an antivenom), botulism, rabies, and tetanus (an antitoxin) because these diseases will kill a person before active immunity can be established. The donated antibodies provide immediate protection, but their effect is short-lived (2 to 3 weeks). Meanwhile, however, the body's own defenses take over.

In addition to their use to provide passive immunity, antibodies are prepared commercially for use in research, clinical testing for diagnostic purposes, and treating certain cancers. **Monoclonal antibodies** used for such purposes are produced by descendants of a single cell and are pure antibody preparations that exhibit specificity for one, and only one, antigen. Besides their use in delivering cancer-fighting drugs to cancerous

tissue, monoclonal antibodies are being used for diagnosis of pregnancy, hepatitis, and rabies. They are also used for early diagnosis and to track the extent of cancers hidden deep within the body.

Antibodies

Antibodies, also referred to as **immunoglobulins** (im″mu-no-glob′u-linz), or **Igs,** constitute the *gamma globulin* part of blood proteins. Antibodies are soluble proteins secreted by activated B cells or by their plasma-cell offspring in response to an antigen, and they are capable of binding specifically with that antigen.

Antibodies are formed in response to a huge number of different antigens. Despite their variety, they all have a similar basic anatomy that allows them to be grouped into five Ig classes, each slightly different in structure and function.

Basic Antibody Structure Regardless of its class, every antibody has a basic structure consisting of four amino acid (polypeptide) chains linked together by *disulfide* (sulfur-to-sulfur) *bonds* (Figure 12.15). Two of the four chains are identical and contain approximately 400 amino acids each; these are the *heavy chains*. The other two chains, the *light chains*,

TABLE 12.2	Recommended* Immunization Schedule for Children in the United States
Recommended age	**Immunizing agent in vaccine**
2 months	DPT vaccine (diphtheria toxoid, pertussis [whooping cough] vaccine, and tetanus toxoid); OPV (oral poliomyelitis vaccine)
4 months	DPT vaccine; OPV
6 months	DPT vaccine (OPV optional for areas with high risk of polio exposure)
12–15 months	DPT vaccine; OPV; MMR vaccine (combined mumps vaccine, measles vaccine, and rubella virus vaccine) or individual mumps, measles, and rubella virus vaccines. Completes primary series of DPT and OPV. MMR dose also given one month later.
18 months	HbCV (*Haemophilus* influenza type b); conjugate vaccine preferred over the polysaccharide vaccine (HbPV)
4–6 years	DPT vaccine; OPV (preferably at or before school entry)
11–13 years	MMR (at entrance to middle school or high school); second dose of two.
14–16 years	Td booster (tetanus and diphtheria toxoid); repeat every 10 years throughout life

*Recommended by the American Academy of Pediatrics

are also identical to each other but are only about half as long. When the four chains are combined, the antibody molecule formed has two identical halves, each consisting of a heavy and a light chain, and the molecule as a whole is T- or Y-shaped.

When scientists began investigating antibody structure, they discovered something very peculiar. Each of the four chains forming an antibody had a **variable (V) region** at one end and a much larger **constant (C) region** at the other end. Antibodies responding to different antigens had very different variable regions, but their constant regions were the same or nearly so. This made sense when it was discovered that the variable regions of the heavy and light chains in each arm combine their efforts to form an **antigen-binding site** (Figure 12.15) uniquely shaped to "fit" its specific antigen. Hence, each antibody has two such antigen-binding regions.

The constant regions that form the "stem" of an antibody can be compared to the handle of a key. A key handle has a common function for all keys: it allows you to hold the key and place its tumbler-moving portion into the lock. Similarly, the constant regions of the antibody chains serve common functions in all antibodies: they determine the type of antibody formed (antibody class), as well as how the antibody class will carry out its immune roles in the body, and the cell types or chemicals with which the antibody can bind.

Antibody Classes There are five major immunoglobulin classes—IgM, IgA, IgD, IgG, and IgE. (Remember the woman's name MADGE to recall the five Ig types.) As illustrated in Table 12.3, IgD, IgG, and IgE antibodies have the same basic Y-shaped structure described above and are referred to as *monomers*. IgA antibodies occur in both monomer and *dimer* (two linked monomers) forms. (Only the dimer form is shown in the table.) Compared to the other antibodies, IgM antibodies are huge. Because they are constructed of five linked monomers, IgM antibodies are called *pentamers* (*penta* = five).

The antibodies of each class have slightly different biological roles and locations in the body. For example, IgG is the most abundant antibody in blood plasma and is the only type that can cross the placental barrier. Hence, the passive immunity that a mother transfers to her fetus is "with the compliments" of her IgG antibodies. Only IgM and IgG can fix complement. The IgA dimer, sometimes called

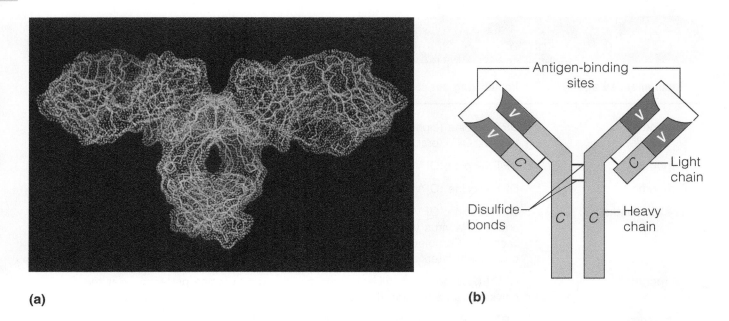

(a)

(b)

FIGURE 12.15   Basic antibody structure. (a) Computer-generated image.
(b) Diagrammed structure. The basic structure (monomer) of each type of
antibody is formed by four polypeptide chains that are joined by disulfide
bonds. Two of the chains are short, light chains; the other two are long, heavy
chains. Each chain has a variable (V) region (different in different antibodies)
and a constant (C) region (essentially identical in different antibodies of the
same class). The variable regions are the antigen-binding sites of the antibody.
Hence, each antibody monomer has two antigen-binding sites.

secretory IgA, is found mainly in mucus and other
secretions that bathe body surfaces. It plays a major
role in preventing pathogens from gaining entry
into the body. IgE antibodies are the "troublemaker"
antibodies involved in allergies. These and other
characteristics unique to each of the immunoglobulin classes are summarized in Table 12.3.

Antibody Function   Antibodies inactivate antigens
in a number of ways—by complement fixation,
neutralization, agglutination, and precipitation
(Figure 12.16). Of these, complement fixation and
neutralization are most important to body protection.

Complement is the chief antibody ammunition
used against cellular antigens, such as bacteria or
mismatched red blood cells. As noted earlier, complement is fixed (activated) during nonspecific body
defenses. It is also activated very efficiently when it
binds to antibodies attached to cellular targets. This
triggers events (described earlier) that result in lysis
of the foreign cell and release of molecules that
tremendously enhance the inflammatory process.

Neutralization occurs when antibodies bind
to specific sites on bacterial *exotoxins* (toxic chemicals secreted by bacteria) or on viruses that can
cause cell injury. In this way, they block the harmful effects of the exotoxin or virus.

Because antibodies have more than one antigen-
binding site, they can bind to more than one antigen at a time; consequently, *antigen-antibody
complexes* can be cross-linked into large lattices.
When the cross-linking involves cell-bound antigens, the process causes clumping of the foreign
cells, a process called **agglutination.** This type of
antigen-antibody reaction occurs when mismatched
blood is transfused (the foreign red blood cells are
clumped) and is the basis of tests used for blood
typing. When the cross-linking process involves
soluble antigenic molecules, the resulting antigen-
antibody complexes are so large that they become
insoluble and settle out of solution. This cross-linking reaction is more precisely called **precipitation.**
There is little question that agglutinated bacteria

TABLE 12.3   Immunoglobin Classes

Class	Generalized structure	Where found	Biological function
IgD		Virtually always attached to B cell.	Believed to be cell surface receptor of immunocompetent B cell; important in activation of B cell.
IgM		Attached to B cell; free in plasma.	When bound to B cell membrane, serves as antigen receptor; first Ig class *released* to plasma by plasma cells during primary response; potent agglutinating agent; fixes complement.
IgG		Most abundant antibody in plasma; represents 75–85% of circulating antibodies.	Main antibody of both primary and secondary responses; crosses placenta and provides passive immunity to fetus; fixes complement.
IgA		Some (monomer) in plasma; dimer in secretions such as saliva, tears, intestinal juice, and milk.	Bathes and protects mucosal surfaces from attachment of pathogens.
IgE		Secreted by plasma cells in skin, mucosae of gastrointestinal and respiratory tracts, and tonsils.	Binds to mast cells and basophils, and triggers release of histamine and other chemicals that mediate inflammation and certain allergic responses.

and immobilized (precipitated) antigen molecules are much more easily captured and engulfed by the body's phagocytes than are freely moving antigens.

Cellular (Cell-Mediated) Immune Response

Like B cells, immunocompetent T cells are activated to form a clone by binding with a "recognized" antigen (see Figure 12.19). However, unlike B cells, the T cells are not able to bind with *free* antigens. Instead, the antigens must be "presented" by macrophages, and a *double recognition* must occur. The macrophages engulf the antigens, process them internally, and then finally display parts of the processed antigens on their external surface in combination with one of their own (self) proteins (Figure 12.17).

Apparently, a T cell must recognize "nonself," the antigen fragment presented by the macrophage, and also "self" by coupling with a specific glycoprotein on the macrophage's surface at the same time. Antigen binding alone is not enough to sensitize T cells. They must be "spoon-fed" the antigens by macrophages, and something like a "double handshake" must occur. Although this idea seemed preposterous when it was first suggested, there is no longer any question that **antigen presentation** is a major role of macrophages and is essential for activation and clonal selection of the T cells. Without macrophage "presenters," the immune response is severely impaired. Cytokine chemicals (monokines, particularly interleukin 1) released by macrophages also play important roles in the immune response, as shown in Table 12.4.

Q   *Complement and agglutination aid phagocytosis, but they assist it in different ways. What is this difference?*

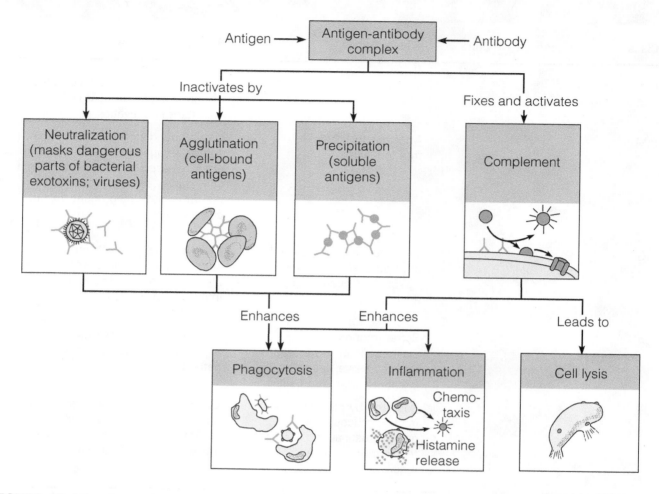

FIGURE 12.16   Mechanisms of antibody action.

The different classes of T cell clones, which provide for cell-mediated immunity, are a diverse lot and produce their deadly effects in a variety of ways (see Table 12.4). Some are **cytotoxic (killer) T cells,** cells that specialize in killing virus-infected, cancer, or foreign graft cells (Figure 12.18). One way they accomplish this is by binding to them and inserting a toxic chemical (*perforin* or others) into the foreign cell's plasma membrane (delivering the so-called kiss of death). Shortly thereafter, the target cell ruptures. By that time, the cytotoxic

T cell is long gone and is seeking other foreign prey to attack.

Helper T cells are the T cells that act as the "directors" or "managers" of the immune system. Once activated, they circulate through the body, recruiting other cells to fight the invaders. For example, helper T cells interact directly with B cells (that have already attached to antigens), prodding them into more rapid division (clone production) and then, like the "boss" of an assembly line, signaling for antibody formation to begin. They also release a variety of cytokine chemicals called - **lymphokines** (see Table 12.4) that act indirectly to rid the body of antigens by (1) stimulating cytotoxic T cells and B cells to grow and divide; (2) attracting other types of protective white blood cells, such as neutrophils, into the area; and (3) enhancing the

A   *Complement fixation provides "knobs" for the phagocyte to attach to, whereas agglutination binds antigens (typically microorganisms) together into large masses that become nonmobile and easier to destroy.*

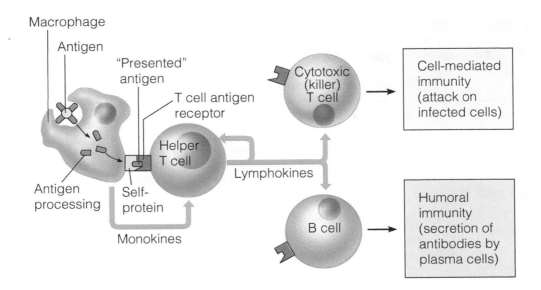

FIGURE 12.17 **T cell activation and interactions with other cells of the immune response.** Macrophages are important both as phagocytes and as antigen presenters. After they have ingested an antigen, they display parts of it on their surface membranes, where it can be recognized by a helper T cell that bears receptors for the same antigen. During the binding process, the T cell binds simultaneously to the antigen and to the macrophage (self) receptor, which leads to T cell activation and cloning (not illustrated). In addition, the macrophage releases monokines, which enhance T cell activation. Activated helper T cells release lymphokines, which stimulate proliferation and activity of other helper T cells and help activate cytotoxic (killer) T cells and B cells.

ability of macrophages to engulf and destroy microorganisms. (Actually, the macrophages are pretty good phagocytes even in the absence of lymphokines, but in their presence, they develop an insatiable appetite.) As the released lymphokines summon more and more cells into the battle, the immune response gains momentum, and the antigens are overwhelmed by the sheer numbers of immune elements acting against them.

Another T cell population, the **suppressor T cells,** releases chemicals that suppress the activity of both T and B cells. Suppressor T cells are vital for winding down and finally stopping the immune response after an antigen has been successfully inactivated or destroyed. This helps prevent uncontrolled or unnecessary immune system activity.

Most of the T cells enlisted to fight in a particular immune response are dead within a few days. However, a few members of each clone are long-lived **memory cells** that remain behind to provide the immunological memory for each antigen

encountered and enable the body to respond quickly to its subsequent invasions.

A summary of the major elements of the immune response appears in Figure 12.19.

Organ Transplants and Rejection

For those suffering with end-stage heart or kidney disease, organ transplants are a desirable treatment option. However, organ transplants have had mixed success because the immune system is ever vigilant, and rejection is a real problem.

Essentially there are four major types of grafts:

1. **Autografts** are tissue grafts transplanted from one site to another in the same person.

2. **Isografts** are tissue grafts donated by a genetically identical person, the only example being an identical twin.

3. **Allografts** are tissue grafts taken from an unrelated person.

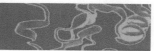

| TABLE 12.4   Functions of Cells and Molecules Involved in Immunity |

Element	Function in the immune response
Cells	
B cell	Lymphocyte that resides in the lymph nodes, spleen, or other lymphoid tissues, where it is induced to replicate by antigen-binding and helper T cell interactions; its progeny (clone members) form plasma cells and memory cells.
Plasma cell	Antibody-producing "machine"; produces huge numbers of the same antibody (immunoglobulin); represents further specialization of B cell clone descendants.
Helper T cell	A *regulatory* T cell that binds with a specific antigen presented by a macrophage; it stimulates the production of other immune cells (cytotoxic T cells and B cells) to help fight the invader; acts both directly and indirectly by releasing lymphokines.
Cytotoxic T cell	Also called a killer T cell; activity enhanced by helper T cells; its specialty is killing virus-invaded body cells, as well as body cells that have become cancerous; involved in graft rejection.
Suppressor T cell	Slows or stops the activity of B and T cells once the infection (or attack by foreign cells) has been conquered.
Memory cell	Descendant of an activated B cell or T cell; generated during the initial immune response (primary response); may exist in the body for years thereafter, enabling it to respond quickly and efficiently to subsequent infections or meetings with the same antigen.
Macrophage	Engulfs and digests antigens that it encounters and presents parts of them on its plasma membrane for recognition by T cells bearing receptors for the same antigen; this function, *antigen presentation,* is essential for normal cell-mediated responses. Also releases chemicals that activate T cells.
Molecules	
Antibody (immunoglobulin)	Protein produced by a B cell or its plasma cell offspring and released into the body fluids (blood, lymph, saliva, mucus, etc.), where it attaches to antigens, causing neutralization, precipitation, or agglutination, which "marks" the antigens for destruction by phagocytes or complement.
Lymphokines	Cytokine chemicals released by sensitized T cells: • Macrophage migration inhibiting factor (MIF)—"inhibits" macrophage migration and keeps them in the local area. • Interleukin 2—stimulates T cells and B cells to proliferate. • Helper factors—enhance antibody formation by plasma cells. • Suppressor factors—suppress antibody formation or T cell–mediated immune responses. • Chemotactic factors—attract leukocytes (neutrophils, eosinophils, and basophils) into inflamed area. • Perforin—a cell toxin; causes cell lysis. • Gamma interferon—helps make tissue cells resistant to viral infection; activates macrophages; activates NK cells; enhances maturation of cytotoxic T cells.

TABLE **12.4** *(continued)*	
Element	**Function in the immune response**
Monokines	Cytokine chemicals released by activated macrophages: • Interleukin 1—stimulates T cells to proliferate and causes fever. • Tumor necrosis factor (TNF)—like perforin, causes cell killing; attracts granulocytes; activates T cells and macrophages.
Complement	Group of bloodborne proteins activated after binding to antibody-covered antigens; when activated, complement causes lysis of the microorganism and enhances inflammatory response.
Antigen	Substance capable of provoking an immune response; typically a large complex molecule not normally present in the body.

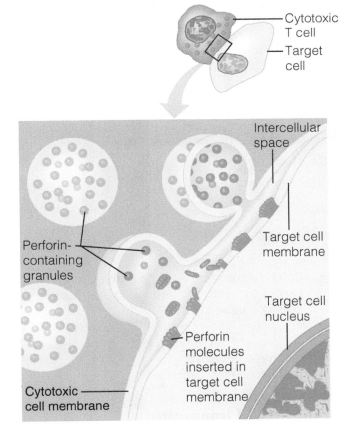

FIGURE 12.18   A proposed mechanism of target cell lysis by cytotoxic T cells.

4. **Xenografts** are tissue grafts harvested from a different animal species, such as transplanting a baboon heart into a human being.

Autografts and isografts are ideal donor organs or tissues and are just about always successful given an adequate blood supply and no infection. Although pig heart valves have been transplanted with success, xenografts of whole organs are never successful. The graft type most used is an allograft taken from a recently deceased person.

Before an allograft is even attempted, the ABO and other blood group antigens of both the donor and recipient must be determined and must match. Then, the cell membrane antigens of their tissue cells are typed to determine how closely they match. At least a 75 percent match is needed to attempt a graft; as you might guess, good tissue matches between unrelated people are hard to find.

After surgery, to prevent rejection, the patient receives **immunosuppressive therapy,** including one or more of the following: corticosteroids to suppress inflammation, cytotoxic drugs, radiation (X-ray) therapy, and immunosuppressor drugs. Many of these drugs kill rapidly dividing cells (such as activated lymphocytes), and all of them have severe side effects. However, the

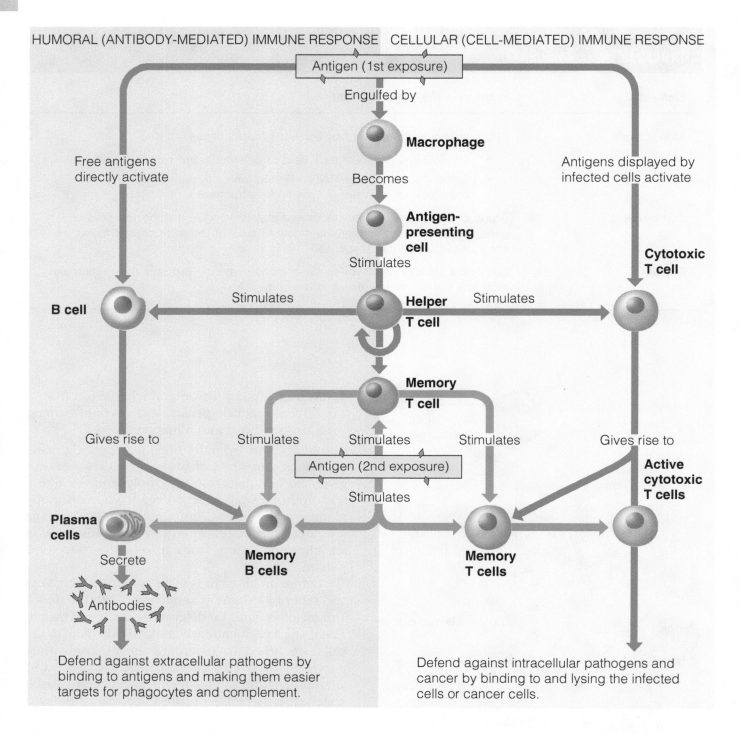

HUMORAL (ANTIBODY-MEDIATED) IMMUNE RESPONSE   CELLULAR (CELL-MEDIATED) IMMUNE RESPONSE

Antigen (1st exposure)

Engulfed by

Macrophage

Free antigens
directly activate

Antigens displayed by
infected cells activate

Becomes

**Antigen-
presenting
cell**

Stimulates

**Cytotoxic
T cell**

B cell   Stimulates   **Helper
T cell**   Stimulates

**Memory
T cell**

Gives rise to   Stimulates   Stimulates   Stimulates   Gives rise to

Antigen (2nd exposure)

**Active
cytotoxic
T cells**

Stimulates

**Plasma
cells**

**Memory
B cells**   **Memory
T cells**

Secrete

Antibodies

Defend against extracellular pathogens by
binding to antigens and making them easier
targets for phagocytes and complement.

Defend against intracellular pathogens and
cancer by binding to and lysing the infected
cells or cancer cells.

FIGURE 12.19   A summary of the immune responses. In this simple flowchart,
green arrows track the primary response, and blue arrows track the secondary response.

major problem with immunosuppressive therapy
is that while the immune system is suppressed, it
cannot protect the body against other foreign
agents. Explosive bacterial and viral infection is
the most frequent cause of death in these
patients.

Disorders of Immunity

Homeostatic Imbalance

The most important disorders of the immune
system are allergies, immunodeficiencies, and autoimmune diseases.

Allergies

At first, the immune response was thought to be purely protective. However, it was not long before its dangerous potentials were discovered. **Allergies** or **hypersensitivities** are abnormally vigorous immune responses in which the immune system causes tissue damage as it fights off a perceived "threat" that would otherwise be harmless to the body. The term *allergen* (*allo* = altered; *erg* = reaction) is used to distinguish this type of antigen from those producing essentially normal responses. People rarely die of allergies; they are just miserable with them.

Although there are several different types of allergies, the most common type is **immediate hypersensitivity** (Figure 12.20). This type of response, also called **acute hypersensitivity,** is triggered by the release of a flood of histamine when IgE antibodies bind to *mast cells*. Histamine causes small blood vessels in the area to become dilated and leaky and is largely to blame for the best-recognized symptoms of allergy: a runny nose, watery eyes, and itching, reddened skin (hives). When the allergen is inhaled, symptoms of asthma appear because smooth muscle in the walls of the bronchioles contracts, constricting the passages and restricting air flow. Over-the-counter (OTC) anti-allergy drugs contain *antihistamines* that counteract these effects. Most of these reactions begin within seconds after contact with the allergen and last about half an hour.

Fortunately, the bodywide or systemic acute allergic response, known as **anaphylactic** (an"ah-fī-lak-tik) **shock,** is fairly rare. Anaphylactic shock occurs when the allergen directly enters the blood and circulates rapidly through the body, as might happen with certain bee stings or spider bites. It may also follow an injection of a foreign substance (such as horse serum, penicillin, or other drugs that act as haptens) into susceptible individuals. The mechanism of anaphylactic shock is essentially the same as that of local responses; but when the entire body is involved, the outcome is life-threatening. For example, it is difficult to breathe when the smooth muscles of lung passages contract, and the sudden vasodilation (and fluid loss) that occurs may cause circulatory collapse and death within minutes. Epinephrine is the drug of choice to reverse these histamine-mediated effects.

Delayed hypersensitivities, mediated mainly by a special subgroup of helper T cells, cytotoxic T cells, and macrophages take much longer to appear (1 to 3 days) than any of the acute reactions produced by antibodies.

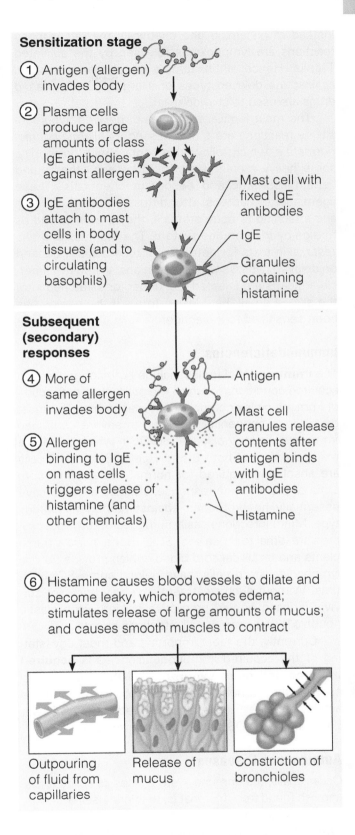

Sensitization stage

① Antigen (allergen) invades body

② Plasma cells produce large amounts of class IgE antibodies against allergen

③ IgE antibodies attach to mast cells in body tissues (and to circulating basophils)

— Mast cell with fixed IgE antibodies
— IgE
— Granules containing histamine

Subsequent (secondary) responses

④ More of same allergen invades body

⑤ Allergen binding to IgE on mast cells triggers release of histamine (and other chemicals)

— Antigen
— Mast cell granules release contents after antigen binds with IgE antibodies
— Histamine

⑥ Histamine causes blood vessels to dilate and become leaky, which promotes edema; stimulates release of large amounts of mucus; and causes smooth muscles to contract

Outpouring of fluid from capillaries

Release of mucus

Constriction of bronchioles

FIGURE 12.20   Mechanism of an immediate (acute) hypersensitivity response.

Instead of histamine, the chemicals mediating these reactions are lymphokines released by the activated T cells. Hence, antihistamine drugs are *not* helpful against the delayed types of allergies. Corticosteroid drugs are used to provide relief.

The most familiar examples of delayed hypersensitivity reactions are those classed as *allergic contact dermatitis,* which follow skin contact with poison ivy, some heavy metals (lead, mercury, and others), and certain cosmetic and deodorant chemicals. These agents act as haptens; after diffusing through the skin and attaching to body proteins, they are perceived as foreign by the immune system. The *Mantoux* and *tine tests,* skin tests for detection of tuberculosis, depend on delayed hypersensitivity reactions. When the tubercle antigens are injected just under (or scratched into) the skin, a small, hard lesion forms if the person has been sensitized to the antigen.

Immunodeficiencies

The **immunodeficiencies** include both congenital and acquired conditions in which the production or function of immune cells or complement is abnormal. The most devastating congenital condition is *severe combined immunodeficiency disease (SCID),* in which there is a marked deficit of both B and T cells. Because T cells are absolutely required for normal operation of *both* arms of the immune response, afflicted children have essentially no protection against pathogens of any type. Minor infections easily shrugged off by most children are lethal to those with SCID. Bone marrow transplants and umbilical cord blood, which provide normal lymphocyte stem cells, have helped some SCID victims. Without such treatment, the only hope for survival is living behind protective barriers (in a plastic "bubble") that keep out all infectious agents.

Currently, the most important and most devastating of the acquired immunodeficiencies is **acquired immune deficiency syndrome (AIDS).** AIDS, which cripples the immune system by interfering with the activity of helper T cells, is highlighted in the "A Closer Look" box on AIDS a little later in this chapter.

Autoimmune Diseases

Occasionally, the immune system loses its ability to distinguish friend from foe, that is, to tolerate self-antigens, while still recognizing and attacking foreign antigens. When this happens, the body produces antibodies (*autoantibodies*) and sensitized T cells that attack and damage its own tissues. This puzzling phenomenon is called **autoimmune disease,** because it is one's own immune system that produces the disorder.

Some 5 percent of adults in North America—two-thirds of them women—are afflicted with autoimmune disease. Most common are:

- *Multiple sclerosis (MS),* which destroys the white matter (myelin sheaths) of the brain and spinal cord
- *Myasthenia gravis,* which impairs communication between nerves and skeletal muscles
- *Graves' disease,* in which the thyroid gland produces excessive amounts of thyroxine
- *Type I diabetes mellitus,* which destroys pancreatic beta cells, resulting in deficient production of insulin
- *Systemic lupus erythematosus (SLE),* a systemic disease that occurs mainly in young females and particularly affects the kidneys, heart, lungs, and skin
- *Glomerulonephritis,* a severe impairment of kidney function
- *Rheumatoid arthritis (RA),* which systematically destroys joints

Current therapies include treatments that depress certain aspects of the immune response.

How does the normal state of self-tolerance break down? It appears that one or more of the following may be triggers:

1. **Inefficient lymphocyte programming.** Instead of being silenced or eliminated, self-reactive B or T lymphocytes escape to the rest of the body. This is believed to occur in MS.

2. **Appearance of self-proteins in the circulation that were not previously exposed to the immune system.** Such "hidden" antigens are found in sperm cells, the eye lens, and certain proteins in the thyroid gland. In addition, "new self-antigens" may appear as a result of gene mutations or alterations in self-proteins by hapten attachment or by bacterial or viral damage.

3. **Cross-reaction of antibodies produced against foreign antigens with self-antigens.** For instance, antibodies produced during an infection caused by streptococcus bacteria are known to cross-react with heart antigens, causing damage to both the heart muscle and its valves, as well as to joints and kidneys. This age-old disease is called *rheumatic fever.* ▲

PART III: DEVELOPMENTAL ASPECTS OF THE LYMPHATIC SYSTEM AND BODY DEFENSES

The lymphatic vessels, which bud from the veins of the blood vascular system, and the main clusters of lymph nodes are obvious by the fifth week of development. Except for the thymus gland and the spleen, the lymphoid organs are poorly developed before birth. However, shortly after birth, they become heavily populated with lymphocytes as the immune system begins to function.

Lymphatic system problems are relatively uncommon, but when they do occur, they are painfully obvious. For example, when the lymphatic vessels are blocked (as in *elephantiasis,* a tropical disease in which the lymphatics become clogged with parasitic worms) or when lymphatics are removed (as in radical breast surgery), severe edema is the result. However, lymphatic vessels removed surgically do grow back in time.

Stem cells of the immune system originate in the spleen and liver during the first month of embryonic development. Later, the bone marrow becomes the predominant source of stem cells (hemocytoblasts), and it persists in this role into adult life. In late fetal life and shortly after birth, the young lymphocytes develop self-tolerance and immunocompetence in their "programming organs" (thymus and bone marrow) and then populate the other lymphoid tissues. Upon meeting "their" antigens, the T and B cells complete their development to fully mature immune cells.

Although the ability of our immune system to recognize foreign substances is determined by our genes, the nervous system may help to control the activity of the immune response. The immune response is definitely impaired in individuals who are under severe stress—for example, in those mourning the death of a beloved family member or friend. Our immune system normally serves us well throughout our lifetime, until old age. But, during the later years, its efficiency begins to wane, as does that of the nonspecific defenses. As a result, the body becomes less able to fight infections and destroy cells that have become cancerous. Additionally, we become more susceptible to both autoimmune and immunodeficiency diseases.

Prove It Yourself

Swollen Lymph Nodes Usually Indicate Infection

The next time you get a bad cold or the flu, you may notice that your lymph nodes become swollen and tender (try feeling the ones in your neck and under your lower jaw). This is a healthy response to the pathogen—it indicates that your lymphatic system is taking the appropriate action to combat an infection. The entry of the pathogen into your lymphatic system has triggered an explosion in the lymphocyte population, and your lymph nodes are swollen with dividing lymphocytes, clumps of virus particles, and pathogens under attack by lymphocytes.

After the infection subsides, check your lymph nodes again. They should have returned to their normal size.

A Closer Look

AIDS: The Modern Day Plague

IN October 1347, several ships made port in Sicily, and within days all the sailors they carried were dead of bubonic plague. By the end of the fourteenth century, approximately 25 percent of the population of Europe had been wiped out by this "black death." In January 1987, the U.S. Secretary of Health and Human Services warned that acquired immune deficiency syndrome, or AIDS, might be the plague of our time. These are strong words. Are they true?

Although AIDS was first identified in this country in 1981 among homosexual men and intravenous drug users of both sexes, it had begun afflicting the heterosexual population of Africa several years earlier. AIDS is characterized by severe weight loss, night sweats, swollen lymph nodes, and increasingly frequent infections, including a rare type of pneumonia called *pneumocystis pneumonia* and the bizarre malignancy *Kaposi's sarcoma,* a cancerlike condition of blood vessels evidenced by purple lesions of the skin. Some AIDS victims develop slurred speech and severe dementia. The course of AIDS is grim, and thus far inescapable, finally ending in complete debilitation and death from cancer or overwhelming infection.

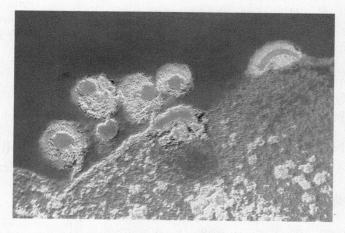

New HIV viruses emerge (yellow and red dots) from an infected human cell.

AIDS is caused by a virus transmitted in blood, semen, vaginal secretions, and saliva. Most commonly, AIDS enters the body via blood transfusions or blood-contaminated needles and during intimate sexual contact in which the mucosa is torn or where open lesions caused by sexually transmitted diseases allow the virus access to the blood.

The virus, named HIV (human immunodeficiency virus), specifically targets and destroys helper T cells, resulting in depression of cell-mediated immunity. Although antibody levels rise and cytotoxic T cells initially mount a vigorous response to viral exposure, in time a profound deficit of normal antibodies develops. Cytotoxic T cells become unresponsive to viral cues, and helper T cells become the prey of the virus. The whole immune system is turned topsy-turvy. It is now clear that the virus multiplies steadily in the lymph nodes throughout most of the chronic asymptomatic period. Symptomatic AIDS appears when the lymph nodes can no longer contain the virus and the immune system collapses. The virus also invades the brain, which accounts for the dementia of some AIDS patients. Although there are exceptions, most AIDS victims have died within a few months to eight years after diagnosis.

AIDS: The Modern Day Plague (continued)

The years since 1981 have witnessed a global AIDS epidemic—worldwide, 16,000 people are infected with the HIV virus daily. As of 2001, more than 40 million people were infected worldwide and almost 90 percent of them live in the developing countries of Asia and southern Africa. In the United States, estimates of Americans infected with HIV topped 700,000 by 2001. Furthermore, because there is a six-month "window" during which antibodies may develop after exposure to HIV, there are probably 100 asymptomatic carriers of the virus for every newly diagnosed case. Moreover, the disease has a long incubation period (from a few months to 10 years) between exposure and the appearance of clinical symptoms.

Not only has the number of identified cases jumped explosively in the at-risk populations, but the "face of AIDS" is changing. Victims have begun to include people who do not belong to the original high-risk group. Before reliable testing of donated blood was available, some people contracted the virus from blood transfusions. Hemophiliacs have been especially vulnerable because the blood factors they need are isolated from pooled blood donations. Although manufacturers began taking measures to kill the virus in 1984, by then an estimated 60 percent of the hemophiliacs in this country were already infected. The virus can also be transmitted from an infected mother to her fetus. Though homosexual men still account for the bulk of cases transmitted by sexual contact, more and more heterosexuals are contracting this disease. Particularly disturbing is the near-epidemic increase in diagnosed cases among teenagers and young adults. AIDS is now the fifth leading killer of all Americans ages 25 to 44.

Large-city hospitals are seeing more AIDS patients daily, and statistics reporting the number of cases in inner-city ghettos, where intravenous drug use is the chief means of AIDS transmission, are alarming. Currently the drug-abusing community accounts for 25 percent of all AIDS cases. Furthermore, 75 percent of AIDS cases in newborns occur where drug abuse abounds.

Diagnostic tests to identify carriers of the AIDS virus are increasingly sophisticated. For example, besides the simple test that scrapes tissue from the oral mucosa, an even easier urine test provides a painless alternative to the standard HIV tests. However, no sure cure has yet been found. Over 100 drugs are now in the U.S. Food and Drug Administration pipeline and more than 20 vaccines are undergoing clinical trials, but it is unlikely that an approved vaccine will be available soon.

Several antiviral drugs (named like alphabet soups) that act by inhibiting the enzymes that the HIV virus needs in order to multiply in the body are now clinically available. The *reverse transcriptase inhibitors*, such as AZT, were early on the scene. AZT has been followed by others, including ddl, ddC, d4T, and 3TC. In late 1995 and early 1996, *protease inhibitors* (saquinavir, ritonavir, and others) were approved. Thus far, it appears that combination therapy using drugs from each class delivers a one-two punch to the HIV virus, at least for a while. Combination therapy postpones drug resistance (a problem with mono-drug therapy using AZT alone) and substantially reduces the amount of HIV virus in the blood while boosting the number of helper T cells. Sadly, the treatments are beginning to fail in about half of those treated. New hope comes from the integrase group of new drugs that block HIV's entry into DNA of the target helper cells.

Given AIDS' poor prognosis, prevention of infection is the way to go. Perhaps, as urged in the media, the best defense is to practice "safer sex" by using condoms and knowing one's sexual partner's history, but the only fool-proof alternative is sexual abstinence.

Homeostatic Relationships between the Lymphatic System and Other Body Systems

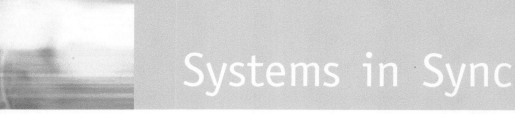

Nervous System
- The lymphatic vessels pick up leaked plasma fluid and proteins in the peripheral nervous system structures; immune cells protect peripheral nervous system structures from specific pathogens
- The nervous system innervates larger lymphatic vessels; the brain helps regulate immune response

Endocrine System
- Lymphatic vessels pick up leaked fluids and proteins; lymph distributes hormones; immune cells protect endocrine organs from pathogens
- The thymus produces hormones that promote development of lymphatic organs and "program" T lymphocytes

Lymphatic System/Immunity

Respiratory System
- Lymphatic vessels pick up leaked fluid and proteins from respiratory organs; immune cells protect respiratory organs from specific pathogens; plasma cells in the respiratory mucosa secrete IgA to prevent pathogen invasion of deeper tissues
- The lungs provide oxygen needed by lymphoid/immune cells and eliminate carbon dioxide; the pharynx houses some lymphoid organs (tonsils); the respiratory "pump" aids lymph flow

Digestive System
- Lymphatic vessels pick up leaked fluids and proteins from digestive organs; lymph transports some products of fat digestion to the blood; lymphoid nodules in the wall of the intestine prevent invasion of pathogens
- The digestive system digests and absorbs nutrients needed by cells of lymphatic organs; gastric acidity inhibits pathogens' entry into blood

Muscular System
- Lymphatic vessels pick up leaked fluid and proteins from skeletal muscle; immune cells protect muscles from specific pathogens
- The skeletal muscle "pump" aids the flow of lymph; muscles protect superficial lymph nodes

Cardiovascular System
- Lymphatic vessels pick up leaked plasma and proteins; spleen destroys aged RBCs, stores iron, and removes debris from blood; immune cells protect cardiovascular organs from specific pathogens
- Blood is the source of lymph; lymphatics develop from veins; blood provides the route for circulation of immune elements

Urinary System
- Lymphatic vessels pick up leaked fluid and proteins from urinary organs; immune cells protect urinary organs from specific pathogens
- Urinary system eliminates wastes and maintains homeostatic water/acid-base/electrolyte balance of the blood for immune cell functioning; urine flushes some pathogens out of the body

Reproductive System
- Lymphatic vessels pick up leaked fluid and proteins from reproductive organs; immune cells protect the organs from specific pathogens
- Acidity of vaginal secretions prevents bacterial multiplication

Integumentary System
- Lymphatic vessels pick up leaked plasma fluid and proteins from the dermis; lymphocytes in lymph enhance the skin's protective role by defending against specific pathogens
- The skin's keratinized epithelium provides a mechanical barrier to pathogens; acid pH of skin secretions inhibits growth of bacteria on skin

Skeletal System
- Lymphatic vessels pick up leaked plasma fluid and proteins from the periostea; immune cells protect bones from specific pathogens
- The bones house hematopoietic tissue (red marrow) which produces the lymphocytes (and macrophages) that populate the lymphoid organs and provide body immunity

13

The Respiratory System

The trillions of cells in the body require an abundant and continuous supply of oxygen to carry out their vital functions. We cannot "do without oxygen" for even a little while, as we can do without food or water. Furthermore, as cells use oxygen, they give off carbon dioxide, a waste product the body must get rid of.

The *cardiovascular* and *respiratory systems* share responsibility for supplying the body with oxygen and disposing of carbon dioxide. The respiratory system organs oversee the gas exchanges that occur between the blood and the external environment. The transportation of respiratory gases between the lungs and the tissue cells is accomplished by the cardiovascular system organs, using blood as the transporting fluid. If either system fails, body cells begin to die from oxygen starvation and accumulation of carbon dioxide.

Functional Anatomy of the Respiratory System

The organs of the **respiratory system** include the nose, pharynx, larynx, trachea, bronchi and their smaller branches, and the lungs, which contain the *alveoli* (al-ve′o-li), or terminal air sacs. Since gas exchanges with the blood happen only in the alveoli, the other respiratory system structures are really just conducting passageways that allow air to reach the lungs. However, these passageways have another, very important job. They purify, humidify, and warm incoming air. Thus, the air finally reaching the lungs has many fewer irritants (such as dust or bacteria) than when it entered the system, and it is warm and damp. As the respiratory system organs are described in detail next, locate each on Figure 13.1.

The Nose

The **nose,** whether "pug" or "ski-jump" in shape, is the only externally visible part of the respiratory system. During breathing, air enters the nose by passing through the **nostrils,** or **external nares.** The interior of the nose consists of the **nasal cavity,** divided by a midline *nasal septum*. The *olfactory receptors* for the sense of smell are located in the mucosa in the slitlike superior part of the nasal cavity, just beneath the ethmoid bone. The rest of the mucosa lining the nasal cavity, called the *respiratory mucosa*, rests on a rich network of thin-walled veins that warms the air as it flows past. (Because of the superficial location of these blood vessels, nosebleeds are common and

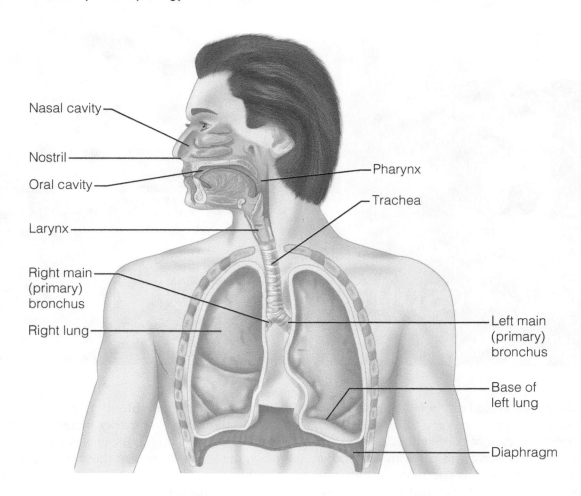

Nasal cavity

Nostril

Oral cavity

Larynx

Right main (primary) bronchus

Right lung

Pharynx

Trachea

Left main (primary) bronchus

Base of left lung

Diaphragm

FIGURE 13.1   The major respiratory organs shown in relation to surrounding structures.

often profuse.) In addition, the sticky mucus produced by the mucosa's glands moistens the air and traps incoming bacteria and other foreign debris. The ciliated cells of the nasal mucosa create a gentle current that moves contaminated mucus posteriorly toward the throat (pharynx), where it is swallowed and digested by stomach juices. We are usually unaware of this important ciliary action, but when the external temperature is extremely cold, these cilia become sluggish, allowing mucus to accumulate in the nasal cavity and to dribble outward through the nostrils. This helps explain why you might have a "runny" nose on a crisp, wintry day.

As shown in Figures 13.1 and 13.2, the lateral walls of the nasal cavity are uneven owing to three mucosa-covered projections or lobes, called **conchae** (kong′ke), which greatly increase

the surface area of the mucosa exposed to the air. The conchae also increase the air turbulence in the nasal cavity. As the air swirls through the twists and turns, inhaled particles are deflected onto the mucus-coated surfaces, where they are trapped and prevented from reaching the lungs.

The nasal cavity is separated from the oral cavity below by a partition, the **palate** (pal′et). Anteriorly, where the palate is supported by bone, is the **hard palate;** the unsupported posterior part is the **soft palate.**

Homeostatic Imbalance

The genetic defect *cleft palate* (failure of the bones forming the palate to fuse medially) results in breathing difficulty as well as problems with oral cavity functions such as chewing and speaking. ▲

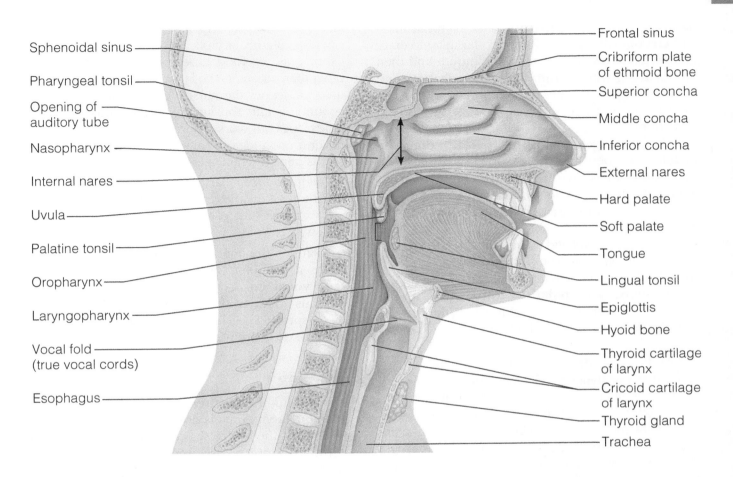

Sphenoidal sinus

Pharyngeal tonsil

Opening of auditory tube

Nasopharynx

Internal nares

Uvula

Palatine tonsil

Oropharynx

Laryngopharynx

Vocal fold (true vocal cords)

Esophagus

Frontal sinus

Cribriform plate of ethmoid bone

Superior concha

Middle concha

Inferior concha

External nares

Hard palate

Soft palate

Tongue

Lingual tonsil

Epiglottis

Hyoid bone

Thyroid cartilage of larynx

Cricoid cartilage of larynx

Thyroid gland

Trachea

FIGURE 13.2   Basic anatomy of the upper respiratory tract, sagittal section.

The nasal cavity is surrounded by a ring of **paranasal sinuses** located in the frontal, sphenoid, ethmoid, and maxillary bones. (See Figure 5.15.) The sinuses lighten the skull, and they act as resonance chambers for speech. They also produce mucus, which drains into the nasal cavities. The suctioning effect created by nose blowing helps to drain the sinuses. The *nasolacrimal ducts,* which drain tears from the eyes, also empty into the nasal cavities.

⚖ Homeostatic Imbalance

Cold viruses and various allergens can cause *rhinitis* (ri-ni′tis), inflammation of the nasal mucosa. The excessive mucus produced results in nasal congestion and postnasal drip. Because the nasal mucosa is continuous throughout the respiratory tract and extends tentacle-like into the nasolacrimal (tear) ducts and paranasal sinuses, nasal cavity infections often spread to those regions as well. *Sinusitis,* or sinus

inflammation, is difficult to treat and can cause marked changes in voice quality. When the passageways connecting the sinuses to the nasal cavity are blocked with mucus or infectious matter, the air in the sinus cavities is absorbed. The result is a partial vacuum and a *sinus headache* localized over the inflamed area. ▲

Pharynx

The **pharynx** (far′inks) is a muscular passageway about 13 cm (5 inches) long that vaguely resembles a short length of red garden hose. Commonly called the *throat,* the pharynx serves as a common passageway for food and air (Figures 13.1 and 13.2). It is continuous with the nasal cavity anteriorly via the **internal nares.**

Air enters the superior portion, the **nasopharynx** (na″zo-far′inks), from the nasal cavity and then descends through the **oropharynx** (o"ro-far'inks) and **laryngopharynx** (lah-ring"go-far'inks) to enter the larynx below. Food enters the mouth and then travels along with air through the oropharynx and laryngopharynx. But instead of entering the larynx, food is directed into the *esophagus* (ĕ-sof'ah-gus) posteriorly.

The pharyngotympanic tubes, which drain the middle ear, open into the nasopharynx. Since the mucosae of these two regions are continuous, ear infections such as *otitis media* (o-ti'tis me'de-ah) may follow a sore throat or other types of pharyngeal infections.

Clusters of lymphatic tissue called *tonsils* are also found in the pharynx. The **pharyngeal** (far-rin'je-al) **tonsil,** often called *adenoid,* is located high in the nasopharynx. The **palatine tonsils** are in the oropharynx at the end of the soft palate; the **lingual tonsils** are at the base of the tongue.

◢ Homeostatic Imbalance

If the pharyngeal tonsil becomes inflamed and swollen (as during a bacterial infection), it obstructs the nasopharynx and forces the person to breathe through the mouth. In mouth breathing, air is not properly moistened, warmed, or filtered before reaching the lungs. Many children seem to have almost continuous *tonsillitis.* Years ago the belief was that the tonsils, though protective, were more trouble than they were worth in such cases, and they were routinely removed. Presently, because of the widespread use of antibiotics, this is no longer necessary (or true). ◢

Larynx

The **larynx** (lar'inks), or *voice box,* routes air and food into the proper channels and plays a role in speech. Located inferior to the pharynx (see Figures 13.1 and 13.2), it is formed by eight rigid hyaline cartilages and a spoon-shaped flap of elastic cartilage, the epiglottis (ep"ĭ-glot'tis). The largest of the hyaline cartilages is the shield-shaped **thyroid cartilage,** which protrudes anteriorly and is commonly called the *Adam's apple.* Sometimes referred to as the "guardian of the airways," the **epiglottis** protects the superior opening of the larynx. When we are not swallowing, the epiglottis does not restrict the passage of air into the lower respiratory passages. When we swallow food or fluids, the situation changes dramatically; the larynx is pulled upward

and the epiglottis tips, forming a lid over the opening of the larynx. This routes food into the esophagus, or food tube, posteriorly. If anything other than air enters the larynx, a *cough reflex* is triggered to expel the substance and prevent it from continuing into the lungs. Because this protective reflex does *not* work when we are unconscious, it is never a good idea to try to give fluids to an unconscious person when attempting to revive him or her.

- Palpate your larynx by placing your hand midway on the anterior surface of your neck. Swallow. Can you feel the larynx rising as you swallow?

Part of the mucous membrane of the larynx forms a pair of folds, called the **vocal folds,** or **true vocal cords,** which vibrate with expelled air. This ability of the vocal folds to vibrate allows us to speak. The slitlike passageway between the vocal folds is the **glottis.**

Trachea

Air entering the **trachea** (tra'ke-ah), or *windpipe,* from the larynx travels down its length (10–12 cm, or about 4 inches) to the level of the fifth thoracic vertebra, which is approximately midchest (Figure 13.1).

The trachea is fairly rigid because its walls are reinforced with C-shaped rings of **hyaline cartilage.** These rings serve a double purpose. The open parts of the rings abut the **esophagus** and allow it to expand anteriorly when we swallow a large piece of food. The solid portions support the trachea walls and keep it *patent,* or open, in spite of the pressure changes that occur during breathing.

◢ Homeostatic Imbalance

Because the trachea is the only way air can enter the lungs, tracheal obstruction is life-threatening. Many people have suffocated after choking on a piece of food that suddenly closed off the trachea (or the glottis of the larynx). The **Heimlich maneuver,** a procedure in which the air in a person's own lungs is used to "pop out," or expel, an obstructing piece of food, has saved many other people from becoming victims of such "café coronaries." The Heimlich maneuver is simple to learn and easy to do. However, it is best learned by demonstration because cracked ribs are a distinct possibility when it is done incorrectly. In some cases of obstructed breathing, an emergency *tracheostomy* (tra'ke-ost'o-me; surgical

Q *In what direction is the power stroke of these cilia directed—superiorly toward the
mouth or inferiorly toward the lungs?*

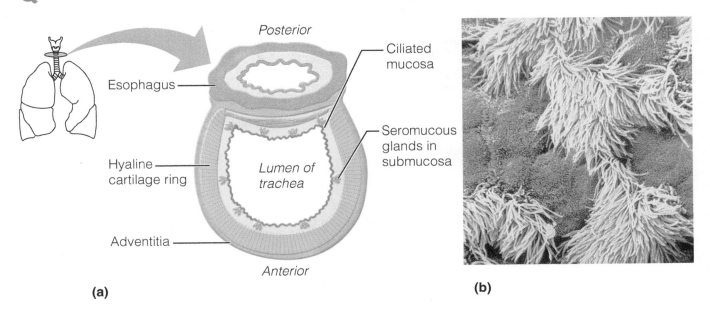

Esophagus

Hyaline
cartilage ring

Adventitia

Posterior

Ciliated
mucosa

Seromucous
glands in
submucosa

*Lumen of
trachea*

Anterior

(a)

(b)

FIGURE 13.3   Structural relationship of the trachea and esophagus.
(a) Cross-sectional view. **(b)** Cilia in the trachea. The cilia are the yellow,
grasslike projections surrounded by the mucus-secreting goblet cells, which
exhibit short microvilli (orange). (Scanning electron micrograph, 221,000×.)

opening of the trachea) is done to provide an alternate
route for air to reach the lungs. Individuals with tracheostomy tubes in place form huge amounts of mucus
the first few days because of irritation to the trachea.
Thus, they must be suctioned frequently during this time
to prevent the mucus from pooling in their lungs. ▲

The trachea is lined with a ciliated mucosa
(Figure 13.3). The cilia beat continuously and in a
direction opposite to that of the incoming air. They
propel mucus, loaded with dust particles and other
debris, away from the lungs to the throat, where it
can be swallowed or spat out.

Homeostatic Imbalance

Smoking inhibits ciliary activity and ultimately
destroys the cilia. Without these cilia, coughing is the
only means of preventing mucus from accumulating in
the lungs. Smokers with respiratory congestion should
avoid medications that inhibit the cough reflex. ▲

Main Bronchi

The right and left **main (primary) bronchi**
(brong′ki) are formed by the division of the trachea. Each main bronchus runs obliquely before
it plunges into the medial depression *(hilus)* of the
lung on its own side (see Figures 13.1 and 13.4).
The right main bronchus is wider, shorter, and
straighter than the left. Consequently, it is the more
common site for an inhaled foreign object to
become lodged. By the time incoming air reaches
the bronchi, it is warm, cleansed of most impurities, and well humidified. The smaller subdivisions
of the main bronchi within the lungs are direct
routes to the air sacs.

Lungs

The paired **lungs** are fairly large organs. They
occupy the entire thoracic cavity except for the
most central area, the **mediastinum** (me″de-
as-ti′num), which houses the heart (in its inferior
pericardial cavity region), the great blood vessels,
bronchi, esophagus, and other organs (Figure 13.4).
The narrow superior portion of each lung, the
apex, is located just deep to the clavicle. The broad

A   *Superiorly toward the mouth to prevent unwanted
substances from entering the lungs.*

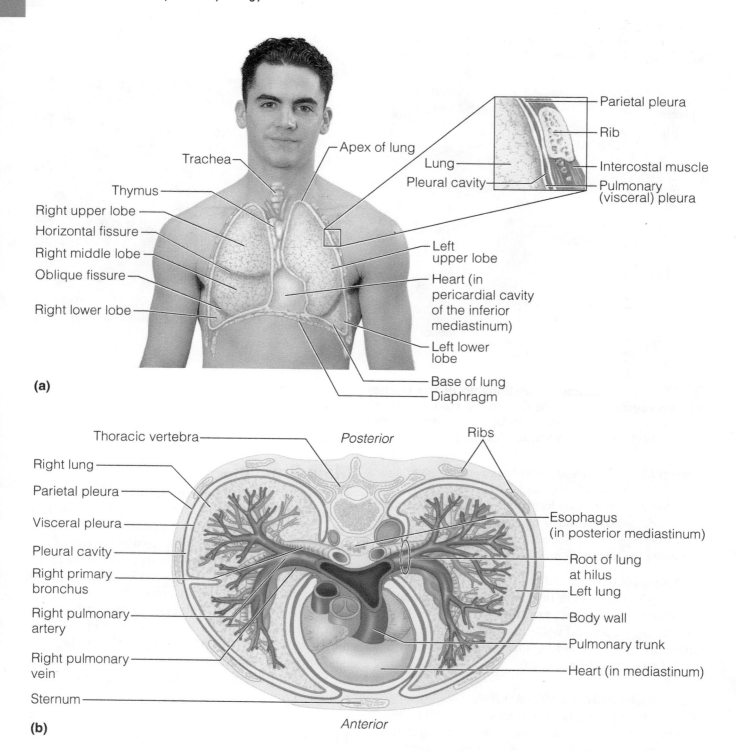

(a)

(b)

FIGURE 13.4   Anatomical relationships of organs in the thoracic cavity. (a) Anterior view of the thoracic cavity organs, showing the position of the lungs, which flank the heart laterally. **(b)** Transverse section through the thorax, showing the relationship of the lungs, the pleural membranes, the major organs present in the mediastinum, and the thorax.

lung area resting on the diaphragm is the **base.** Each lung is divided into lobes by fissures; the left lung has two lobes, and the right lung has three.

The surface of each lung is covered with a visceral serosa called the **pulmonary,** or **visceral, pleura** (ploor'ah), and the walls of the thoracic cavity are lined by the **parietal pleura.** The pleural membranes produce *pleural fluid,* a slippery serous secretion which allows the lungs to glide easily over the thorax wall during breathing movements and causes the two pleural layers to cling together. The pleurae can slide easily from side to side across one another, but they strongly resist being pulled apart. Consequently, the lungs are held tightly to the thorax wall, and the **pleural space** is more of a potential space than an actual one. As described shortly, this condition of tightly adhering pleural membranes is absolutely essential for normal breathing. Figure 13.4 shows the position of the pleura on the lungs and the thorax wall.

◢ Homeostatic Imbalance

Pleurisy (ploo'rĭ-se), inflammation of the pleura, can be caused by decreased secretion of pleural fluid. The pleural surfaces become dry and rough, which results in friction and stabbing pain with each breath. Conversely, the pleurae may produce excessive amounts of fluid, which exerts pressure on the lungs. This type of pleurisy hinders breathing movements, but it is much less painful than the dry rubbing type. ◢

After the primary bronchi enter the lungs, they subdivide into smaller and smaller branches (secondary and tertiary bronchi, and so on), finally ending in the smallest of the conducting passageways, the **bronchioles** (brong'ke-ōlz) (Figure 13.5). Because of this branching and rebranching of the respiratory passageways within the lungs, the network formed is often referred to as the *bronchial* or *respiratory tree.* All but the smallest branches have reinforcing cartilage in their walls.

The *terminal bronchioles* lead into *respiratory zone structures,* even smaller conduits that eventually terminate in **alveoli** (al-ve'o-li; *alveol* = small cavity), or air sacs. The **respiratory zone,** which includes the *respiratory bronchioles, alveolar ducts, alveolar sacs,* and alveoli, is the only site of gas exchange. All other respiratory passages are **conducting zone structures** that serve as conduits to and from the respiratory zone. There are millions of the clustered alveoli, which resemble bunches of grapes, and they make up the bulk of the lungs. Consequently, the lungs are mostly air spaces. The balance of the lung tissue, its *stroma,* is elastic connective tissue. Thus, in spite of their relatively large size, the lungs weigh only about 2½ pounds, and they are soft and spongy.

Histology of the Respiratory Tract

The surface of the respiratory tract is covered in an epithelium, the type of which varies down the tract. There are glands and mucus produced by goblet cells in parts, as well as smooth muscle, elastin, or cartilage.

Most of the epithelium (from the nose to the bronchi) is covered in pseudostratified columnar ciliated epithelial cells, commonly called respiratory epithelium. The cilia beat in one direction, moving mucus toward the throat where it is swallowed. Moving down the bronchioles, the cells get more cuboidal in shape but are still ciliated.

Cartilage is present until the small bronchi. In the trachea they are C-shaped rings, whereas in the bronchi they are interspersed plates.

Glands are abundant in the upper respiratory tract, but there are fewer glands in the lower areas of the tract, and they are absent from the bronchioles onwards. The same is true for goblet cells, although there are a few scattered in the first bronchioles.

Smooth muscle begins in the trachea, where it joins the C-shaped rings of cartilage. It continues down the bronchi and bronchioles, which it completely encircles.

Instead of hard cartilage, the bronchi and bronchioles are mainly composed of elastic tissue.

The Respiratory Membrane

The walls of the alveoli are composed largely of a single, thin layer of squamous epithelial cells. The thinness of their walls is hard to imagine, but a sheet of tissue paper is much thicker. *Alveolar pores* connect neighboring air sacs and provide alternate routes for air to reach alveoli whose feeder bronchioles have been clogged by mucus or otherwise blocked. The external surfaces of the alveoli are covered with a "cobweb" of pulmonary capillaries. Together, the alveolar and capillary walls, their fused basement membranes, and occasional elastic fibers construct the **respiratory membrane (air-blood barrier),** which has gas (air) flowing past on one side and blood flowing past on the other (Figure 13.6). The gas exchanges

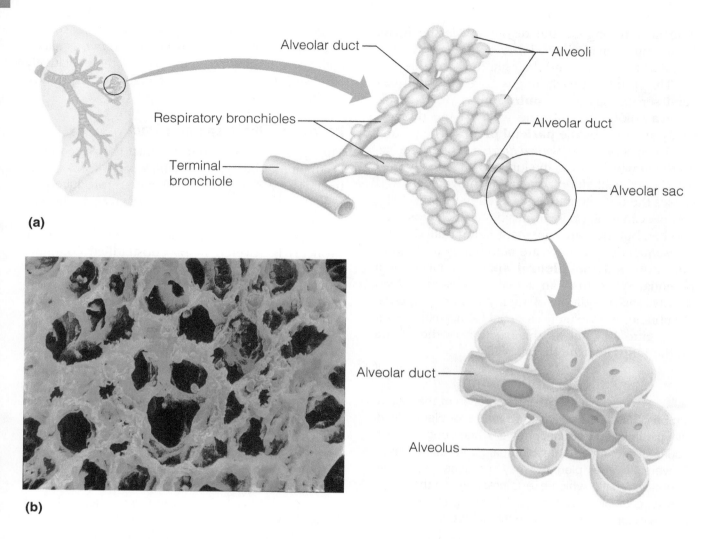

(a)

(b)

FIGURE 13.5 **Respiratory zone structures. (a)** Diagrammatic view of respiratory bronchioles, alveolar ducts, and alveoli. **(b)** Scanning electron micrograph (SEM) of human lung tissue, showing the final divisions of the respiratory tree (475×).

occur by simple diffusion through the respiratory membrane—oxygen passing from the alveolar air into the capillary blood and carbon dioxide leaving the blood to enter the gas-filled alveoli. It has been estimated that the total gas exchange surface provided by the alveolar walls of a healthy man is 50 to 70 square meters, or approximately 40 times greater than the surface area of his skin.

The final line of defense for the respiratory system is in the alveoli. Macrophages, sometimes called "dust cells," wander in and out of the alveoli picking up bacteria, carbon particles, and other debris. Also scattered amid the epithelial cells that form most of the alveolar walls are chunky cuboidal cells, which look very different. The cuboidal cells produce a lipid (fat) molecule called *surfactant,*

which coats the gas-exposed alveolar surfaces and is very important in lung function.

Respiratory Physiology

The major function of the respiratory system is to supply the body with oxygen and to dispose of carbon dioxide. To do this, at least four distinct events, collectively called **respiration,** must occur:

1. **Pulmonary ventilation.** Air must move into and out of the lungs so that the gases in the air sacs (alveoli) of the lungs are continuously changed and refreshed. This process of pulmonary ventilation is commonly called **breathing.**

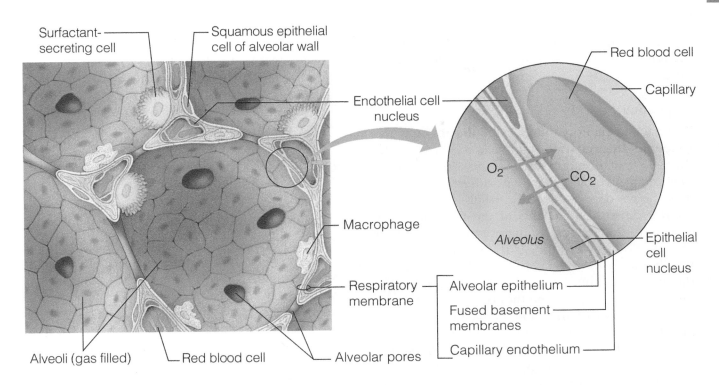

FIGURE 13.6 Anatomy of the respiratory membrane (air-blood barrier). The respiratory membrane is composed of squamous epithelial cells of the alveoli, the capillary endothelium, and the scant basement membranes between. Surfactant-secreting cells are also shown. Oxygen diffuses from the alveolar air into the pulmonary capillary blood; carbon dioxide diffuses from the pulmonary blood into the alveolus. Neighboring alveoli are connected by small pores.

2. **External respiration.** Gas exchange (oxygen loading and carbon dioxide unloading) between the pulmonary blood and alveoli must take place. Remember that in **ex**ternal respiration, gas exchanges are being made between the blood and the body *exterior.*

3. **Respiratory gas transport.** Oxygen and carbon dioxide must be transported to and from the lungs and tissue cells of the body via the bloodstream.

4. **Internal respiration.** At systemic capillaries, gas exchanges must be made between the blood and tissue cells.* In **in**ternal respiration, gas exchanges are occurring between the blood and cells *inside* the body.

Although only the first two processes are the special responsibility of the respiratory system, all four

processes are necessary for it to accomplish its goal of gas exchange. Thus, each process is described in turn next.

Mechanics of Breathing

Breathing, or pulmonary ventilation, is a completely mechanical process that depends on volume changes occurring in the thoracic cavity. Here is a rule to keep in mind about the mechanics of breathing: *Volume changes lead to pressure changes, which lead to the flow of gases to equalize the pressure.*

A gas, like a liquid, always conforms to the shape of its container. However, unlike liquid, a gas *fills* its container. Therefore, in a large volume, the gas molecules will be far apart and the pressure (created by the gas molecules hitting each other and the walls of the container) will be low. If the volume is reduced, the gas molecules will be closer together and the pressure will rise. Let

---

*The actual *use* of oxygen and production of carbon dioxide by tissue cells, that is, **cellular respiration,** is the cornerstone of all energy-producing chemical reactions in the body.

us see how this relates to the two phases of breathing—**inspiration,** when air is flowing into the lungs, and **expiration,** when air is leaving the lungs.

Inspiration

When the inspiratory muscles, the **diaphragm** and **external intercostals,** contract, the size of the thoracic cavity increases. As the dome-shaped diaphragm contracts, it moves inferiorly and flattens out (is depressed). As a result, the superior-inferior dimension (height) of the thoracic cavity increases. Contraction of the external intercostals lifts the rib cage and thrusts the sternum forward, which increases the anteroposterior and lateral dimensions of the thorax (Figure 13.7). Since the lungs adhere tightly to the thorax walls (due to the surface tension of the fluid between the pleural membranes), they are stretched to the new, larger size of the thorax. As *intrapulmonary volume* (the volume within the lungs) increases, the gases within the lungs spread out to fill the larger space. The resulting decrease in the gas pressure in the lungs produces a partial vacuum (pressure less than atmospheric pressure), which sucks air into the lungs (Figure 13.8). Air continues to move into the lungs until the intrapulmonary pressure equals atmospheric pressure. This series of events is called *inspiration* (inhalation).

Expiration

Expiration (exhalation) in healthy people is largely a passive process that depends more on the natural elasticity of the lungs than on muscle contraction. As the inspiratory muscles relax and resume their initial resting length, the rib cage descends and the lungs recoil. Thus, both the thoracic and intrapulmonary volumes decrease (Figure 13.7b). As the intrapulmonary volume decreases, the gases inside the lungs are forced more closely together, and the intrapulmonary pressure rises to a point higher than atmospheric pressure (see Figure 13.8). This causes the gases to flow out to equalize the pressure inside and outside the lungs. Under normal circumstances, expiration is effortless, but if the respiratory passageways are narrowed by spasms of the bronchioles (as in *asthma*) or clogged with mucus or fluid (as in *chronic bronchitis* or *pneumonia*), expiration becomes an active process. In such cases of *forced expiration,* the internal intercostal muscles are activated to help depress the rib cage, and the abdominal muscles contract and help to force air from the lungs by squeezing the abdominal organs upward against the diaphragm.

The normal pressure within the pleural space *(intrapleural pressure)* is *always* negative, and this is the major factor preventing collapse of the lungs. If for any reason the intrapleural pressure becomes equal to the atmospheric pressure, the lungs immediately recoil completely and collapse.

◢ Homeostatic Imbalance

During *atelectasis* (a"teh-lek'tuh-sis), or lung collapse, the lung is useless for ventilation. This phenomenon is seen when air enters the pleural space through a chest wound, but it may also result from a rupture of the visceral pleura, which allows air to enter the pleural space from the respiratory tract. The presence of air in the intrapleural space, which disrupts the fluid bond between the pleurae, is referred to as *pneumothorax* (nu"mo-tho'rakz). Pneumothorax is reversed by drawing air out of the intrapleural space with chest tubes, which allows the lung to reinflate and resume its normal function. ◢

Nonrespiratory Air Movements

Many situations other than breathing move air into or out of the lungs and may modify the normal respiratory rhythm. Coughs and sneezes clear the air passages of debris or collected mucus. Laughing and crying reflect our emotions. For the most part, these **nonrespiratory air movements** are a result of reflex activity, but some may be produced voluntarily.

Respiratory Volumes and Capacities

Many factors affect respiratory capacity—for example, a person's size, sex, age, and physical condition. Normal quiet breathing moves approximately 500 ml of air (about a pint) into and out of the lungs with each breath (see Figure 13.8b). This respiratory volume is referred to as the **tidal volume (TV).**

As a rule, a person *can* inhale much more air than is taken in during a normal, or tidal, breath. The amount of air that can be taken in forcibly over the tidal volume is the **inspiratory reserve volume (IRV).** Normally, the inspiratory reserve volume is between 2100 and 3200 ml.

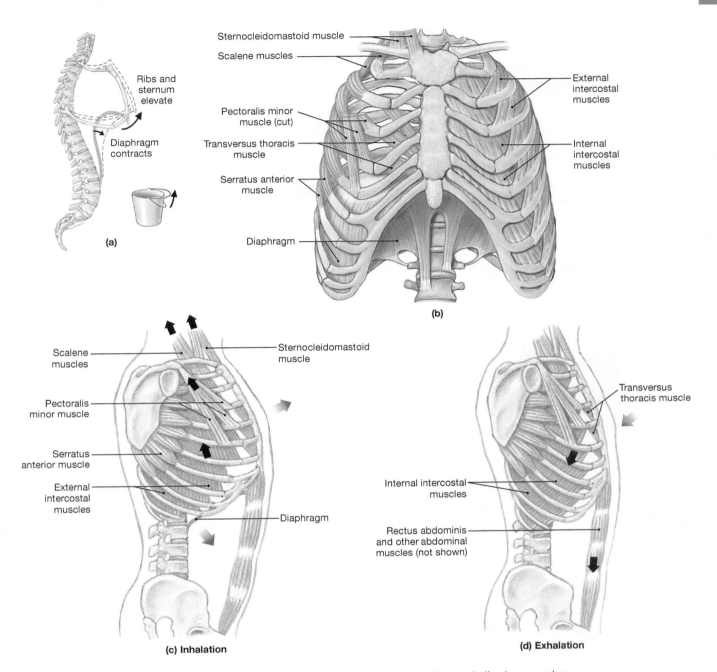

FIGURE 13.7   **The respiratory muscles. (a)** Movements of the ribs and diaphragm that increase the volume of the thoracic cavity. Diaphragmatic movements were also illustrated in *Figure 13.4*. **(b)** An anterior view at rest (with no air movement), showing the primary and accessory respiratory muscles. **(c)** A lateral view during inhalation, showing the muscles that elevate the ribs. **(d)** A lateral view during exhalation, showing the muscles that depress the ribs: The abdominal muscles that assist in exhalation are represented by a single muscle (the rectus abdominis).

Similarly, after a normal expiration, more air can be exhaled. The amount of air that can be forcibly exhaled after a tidal expiration, the **expiratory reserve volume (ERV),** is approximately 1200 ml.

Even after the most strenuous expiration, about 1200 ml of air still remains in the lungs, and it cannot be voluntarily expelled. This is the **residual volume.** Residual volume air is important because it allows gas exchange to go on continuously even

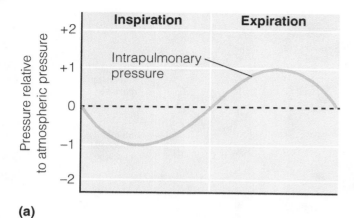

(a)

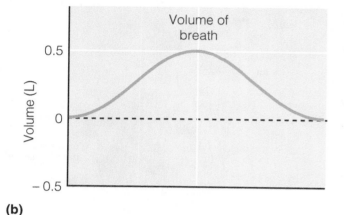

(b)

FIGURE 13.8 Changes in intrapulmonary pressure and air flow during inspiration and expiration.

between breaths and helps to keep the alveoli open (inflated).

The total amount of exchangeable air is typically around 4800 ml in healthy young males, and this respiratory capacity is the **vital capacity (VC).** The vital capacity is the sum of the TV + IRV + ERV. The respiratory volumes are summarized in Figure 13.9.

Obviously, much of the air that enters the respiratory tract remains in the conducting zone passageways and never reaches the alveoli. This is called the **dead space volume,** and during a normal tidal breath, it amounts to about 150 ml. The functional volume—air that actually reaches the respiratory zone and contributes to gas exchange—is about 350 ml.

Respiratory capacities are measured with a *spirometer* (spi-rom'ĕ-ter). As a person breathes, the volumes of air exhaled can be read on an indicator, which shows the changes in air volume

inside the apparatus. Spirometer testing is useful for evaluating losses in respiratory functioning and in following the course of some respiratory diseases. In pneumonia, for example, inspiration is obstructed and the IRV and VC decrease. In emphysema, where expiration is hampered, the ERV is much lower than normal and the residual volume is higher.

Respiratory Sounds

As air flows in and out of the respiratory tree, it produces two recognizable sounds that can be picked up with a stethoscope. **Bronchial sounds** are produced by air rushing through the large respiratory passageways (trachea and bronchi). **Vesicular** (vĕ-sik'u-lar) **breathing sounds** occur as air fills the alveoli. The vesicular sounds are soft and resemble a muffled breeze.

Homeostatic Imbalance

Diseased respiratory tissue, mucus, or pus can produce abnormal sounds such as *crackle* (a bubbling sound) and *wheezing* (a whistling sound). ▲

External Respiration, Gas Transport, and Internal Respiration

As explained earlier, *external respiration* is the actual exchange of gases between the alveoli and the blood (pulmonary gas exchange), and *internal respiration* is the gas exchange process that occurs between the systemic capillaries and the tissue cells. It is important to remember that all gas exchanges are made according to the laws of diffusion; that is, movement occurs *toward* the area of lower concentration of the diffusing substance. The relative amounts of O_2 and CO_2 in the alveolar tissues, and in the arterial and venous blood, are illustrated in Figure 13.10.

External Respiration

During external respiration, dark red blood flowing through the pulmonary circuit is transformed into the scarlet river that is returned to the heart for distribution to the systemic circuit. Although this color change is due to oxygen pickup by hemoglobin in the lungs, carbon dioxide is being unloaded from the blood equally fast. Because body cells continually remove oxygen from blood,

TABLE 13.1   Nonrespiratory Air (Gas) Movements

Movement	Mechanism and result
Cough	Taking a deep breath, closing glottis, and forcing air superiorly from lungs against glottis. Then, the glottis opens suddenly and a blast of air rushes upward. Coughs act to clear the lower respiratory passageways.
Sneeze	Similar to a cough, except that expelled air is directed through nasal cavities instead of through oral cavity. The uvula (u'vu-lah), a tag of tissue hanging from the soft palate, becomes depressed and closes oral cavity off from pharynx, routing the air through nasal cavities. Sneezes clear upper respiratory passages.
Crying	Inspiration followed by release of air in a number of short breaths. Primarily an emotionally induced mechanism.
Laughing	Essentially same as crying in terms of the air movements produced. Also an emotionally induced response.
Hiccups	Sudden inspirations resulting from spasms of diaphragm; initiated by irritation of diaphragm or phrenic nerves, which serve diaphragm. The sound occurs when inspired air hits vocal folds of closed glottis.
Yawn	Very deep inspiration, taken with jaws wide open. Formerly believed to be triggered by need to increase amount of oxygen in blood, but this theory is now being questioned; ventilates all alveoli (this is not the case in normal quiet breathing).

there is always more oxygen in the alveoli than in the blood. Thus, oxygen tends to move from the air of the alveoli through the respiratory membrane into the more oxygen-poor blood of the pulmonary capillaries. On the other hand, as tissue cells remove oxygen from the blood in the systemic circulation, they release carbon dioxide into the blood. Because the concentration of carbon dioxide is much higher in the pulmonary capillaries than it is in the alveolar air, it will move from the blood into the alveoli and be flushed out of the lungs during expiration. Relatively speaking, blood draining from the lungs into the pulmonary veins is oxygen-rich and carbon dioxide-poor and is ready to be pumped to the systemic circulation.

The Movement of Air

To understand the process of respiration, we need to grasp some basic physical principles governing the movement of air. One of the most basic is that our bodies and everything around us are compressed by the weight of Earth's atmosphere.

Although we are seldom aware of it, this **atmospheric pressure** has several important physiological effects. For example, air moves into and out of the respiratory tract as the air pressure in the lungs cycles between below atmospheric pressure and above atmospheric pressure.

Gas Pressure and Volume (Boyle's Law)

The primary differences between liquids and gases reflect the interactions among individual molecules. Although the molecules in a liquid are in constant motion, they are held closely together by weak interactions, such as the hydrogen bonding between adjacent water molecules. Yet because the electrons of adjacent atoms tend to repel one another, liquids tend to resist compression. If you squeeze a balloon filled with water, it will distort into a different shape, but the volumes of the two shapes will be the same.

In a gas, such as air, the molecules bounce around as independent entities. At normal atmospheric pressures, gas molecules are much farther apart than the molecules in a liquid, so the density of

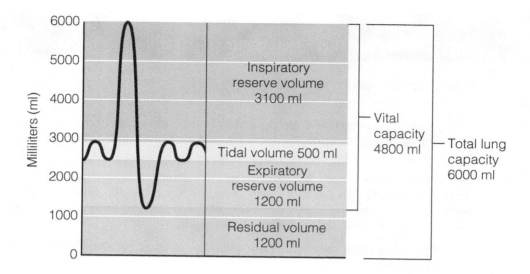

FIGURE 13.9 **Idealized tracing of the various respiratory volumes of a healthy young adult male.**

air is relatively low. The forces acting between gas molecules are minimal (the molecules are too far apart for weak interactions to occur), so an applied pressure can push them closer together. Consider a sealed container of air at atmospheric pressure. The pressure exerted by the enclosed gas results from the collision of gas molecules with the walls of the container. The greater the number of collisions, the higher the pressure.

You can change the gas pressure within a sealed container by changing the volume of the container, thereby giving the gas molecules more or less room in which to bounce around. If you decrease the volume of the container, collisions occur more frequently over a given period, elevating the pressure of the gas (Figure 13.11a). If you increase the volume, fewer collisions occur per unit time, because it takes longer for a gas molecule to travel from one wall to another. As a result, the gas pressure inside the container declines (Figure 13.11b).

For a gas in a closed container and at a constant temperature, pressure (P) is inversely proportional to volume (V). That is, *if you decrease the volume of a gas, its pressure will rise; if you increase the volume of a gas, its pressure will fall.* In particular, the relationship between pressure and volume is reciprocal: If you double the external pressure on a flexible container, its volume will drop by half; if you reduce the external pressure by half, the volume of the container will double. This relationship, $P = 1/V$ first recognized by Robert Boyle in the 1600s, is called **Boyle's law**.

Another law relates temperature and volume of gases. Charles' law states that as the temperature of gases brought into the body increases so will the pressure or volume of the air.

Pressure and Airflow to the Lungs

Air will flow from an area of higher pressure to an area of lower pressure. This tendency for directed airflow, plus the pressure–volume relationship of Boyle's law, provides the basis for pulmonary ventilation. A single respiratory cycle consists of an *inspiration*, or inhalation, and an *expiration*, or exhalation. Inhalation and exhalation involve changes in the volume of the lungs. These volume changes create pressure gradients that move air into or out of the respiratory tract.

Each lung lies within a pleural cavity. The parietal and visceral pleurae are separated by only a thin film of pleural fluid. The two membranes can slide across one another, but they are held together by that fluid film. You encounter the same principle when you set a wet glass on a smooth tabletop. You can slide the glass easily, but when you try to lift it, you experience considerable resistance. As you pull the glass away from the tabletop, you create a powerful suction. The only way to overcome it is to tilt the glass so that air is pulled between the glass and the table, breaking the fluid bond.

A comparable fluid bond exists between the parietal pleura and the visceral pleura covering the lungs. As a result, the surface of each lung sticks to the inner wall of the chest and to the superior surface of the

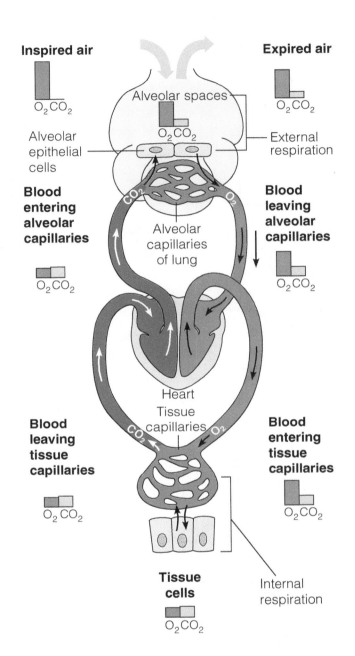

Inspired air

O$_2$ CO$_2$

Alveolar spaces

O$_2$ CO$_2$

Alveolar epithelial cells

Blood entering alveolar capillaries

O$_2$ CO$_2$

Alveolar capillaries of lung

CO$_2$ O$_2$

Expired air

O$_2$ CO$_2$

External respiration

Blood leaving alveolar capillaries

O$_2$ CO$_2$

Heart

Tissue capillaries

CO$_2$ O$_2$

Blood leaving tissue capillaries

O$_2$ CO$_2$

Blood entering tissue capillaries

O$_2$ CO$_2$

Tissue cells

O$_2$ CO$_2$

Internal respiration

FIGURE 13.10 Gas exchanges in the body occur according to the laws of diffusion.

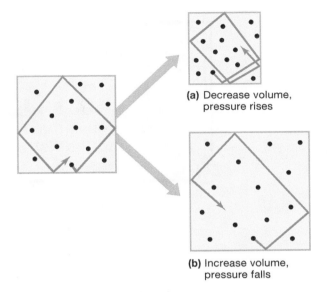

(a) Decrease volume, pressure rises

(b) Increase volume, pressure falls

FIGURE 13.11 Gas pressure and volume relationships. Gas molecules in a sealed container bounce off the walls and off one another, traveling the distance indicated in a given period of time. **(a)** If the volume decreases, each molecule travels the same distance in that same period, but strikes the walls more frequently. The pressure exerted by the gas thus increases. **(b)** If the volume of the container increases, each molecule strikes the walls less often, lowering the pressure in the container.

thoracic cavity. When the diaphragm contracts, it tenses and moves inferiorly. This movement increases the volume of the thoracic cavity, reducing the pressure within it. When the diaphragm relaxes, it returns to its original position, and the volume of the thoracic cavity decreases.

Gas Exchange

Pulmonary ventilation both ensures that your alveoli are supplied with oxygen and removes the carbon dioxide arriving from your bloodstream. The actual process of gas exchange occurs between blood and alveolar air across the respiratory membrane. To understand these events, we will first consider (1) the *partial pressures* of the gases involved and (2) the diffusion of molecules between a gas and a liquid. We can then proceed to discuss the movement of oxygen and carbon dioxide across the respiratory membrane.

diaphragm. As a result, movements of the diaphragm or rib cage that change the volume of the thoracic cavity also change the volume of the lungs.

Changes in the volume of the thoracic cavity result from movements of the diaphragm or rib cage (Figure 13.12a):

- The diaphragm forms the floor of the thoracic cavity. The relaxed diaphragm has the shape of a dome that projects superiorly into the

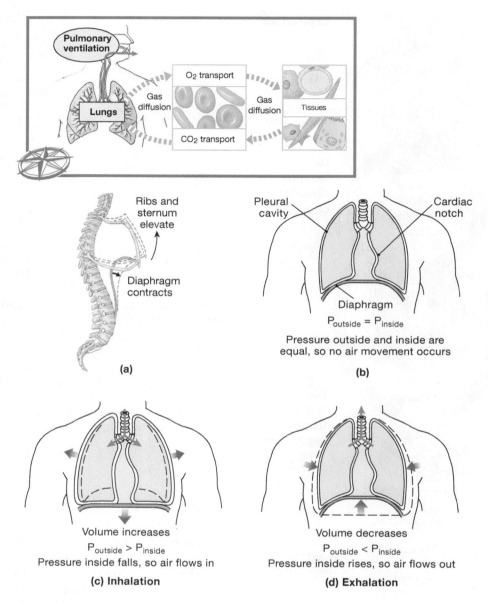

FIGURE 13.12   Mechanisms of pulmonary ventilation. The Navigator icon in the shadow box highlights the topic of the current figure. **(a)** As the rib cage is elevated or the diaphragm is depressed, the volume of the thoracic cavity increases. **(b)** An anterior view with the diaphragm at rest; no air movement occurs. **(c)** *Inhalation*: Elevation of the rib cage and contraction of the diaphragm increase the size of the thoracic cavity. Pressure within the thoracic cavity decreases, and air flows into the lungs. **(d)** *Exhalation*: When the rib cage returns to its original position, the volume of the thoracic cavity decreases. Pressure rises, and air moves out of the lungs.

The Gas Laws

Gases are exchanged between the alveolar air and the blood through diffusion, which occurs in response to concentration gradients. The rate of diffusion varies in response to a variety of factors, including the size of the concentration gradient and the temperature. The principles that govern the movement and diffusion of gas molecules, such as those in the atmosphere, are relatively straightforward. These principles, known as *gas laws*, have been understood for roughly 250 years. You have already heard about Boyle's law, which determines the direction of air movement in pulmonary ventilation. In this section, you will learn about gas laws and other factors that determine the rate of oxygen

TABLE 13.2	Partial Pressures (mm Hg) and Normal Gas Concentrations (%) in Air			
SOURCE OF SAMPLE	Nitrogen (N_2)	Oxygen (O_2)	Carbon Dioxide (CO_2)	Water Vapor (H_2O)
Inhaled air (dry)	597 (78.6%)	159 (20.9%)	0.3 (0.04%)	3.7 (0.5%)
Alveolar air (saturated)	573 (75.4%)	100 (13.2%)	40 (5.2%)	47 (6.2%)
Exhaled air (saturated)	569 (74.8%)	116 (15.3%)	28 (3.7%)	47 (6.2%)

and carbon dioxide diffusion across the respiratory membrane.

Dalton's Law and Partial Pressures

The air we breathe is not a single gas but a mixture of gases. Nitrogen molecules (N_2) are the most abundant, accounting for about 78.6 percent of atmospheric gas molecules. Oxygen molecules (O_2), the second most abundant, make up roughly 20.9 percent of air. Most of the remaining 0.5 percent consists of water molecules, with carbon dioxide (CO_2) contributing a mere 0.04 percent.

Atmospheric pressure, 760 mm Hg, represents the combined effects of collisions involving each type of molecule in air. At any moment, 78.6 percent of those collisions will involve nitrogen molecules, 20.9 percent oxygen molecules, and so on. Thus, each of the gases contributes to the total pressure in proportion to its relative abundance. This relationship is known as **Dalton's law**.

The **partial pressure** of a gas is the pressure contributed by a single gas in a mixture of gases. The partial pressure is abbreviated by the symbol P or p. All the partial pressures added together equal the total pressure exerted by the gas mixture. For the atmosphere, this relationship can be summarized as follows:

$$P_{N_2} + P_{O_2} + P_{H_2O} + P_{CO_2} = 760 \text{ mm Hg}$$

Because we know the individual percentages in air, we can easily calculate the partial pressure of each gas. For example, the partial pressure of oxygen, P_{O_2}, is 20.9 percent of 760 mm Hg, or roughly 159 mm Hg. The partial pressures for other atmospheric gases are included in Table 13.2.

Diffusion between Liquids and Gases (Henry's Law)

Differences in pressure, which move gas molecules from one place to another, also affect the movement of gas molecules into and out of solution. At a given temperature, the amount of a particular gas in solution is directly proportional to the partial pressure of that gas. This principle is known as **Henry's law**.

When a gas under pressure contacts a liquid, the pressure tends to force gas molecules into solution. At a given pressure, the number of dissolved gas molecules will rise until an equilibrium is established. At equilibrium, gas molecules diffuse out of the liquid as quickly as they enter it, so the total number of gas molecules in solution remains constant. If the partial pressure goes up, more gas molecules will go into solution; if the partial pressure goes down, gas molecules will come out of solution.

You see Henry's law in action whenever you open a can of soda. The soda was put into the can under pressure, and the gas (carbon dioxide) is in solution (Figure 13.13a). When you open the can, the pressure falls and the gas molecules begin coming out of solution (Figure 13.13b). Theoretically, the process will continue until an equilibrium develops between the surrounding air and the gas in solution. In fact, the volume of the can is so small, and the volume of the atmosphere so great, that within a half hour or so virtually all the carbon dioxide comes out of solution. You are then left with "flat" soda.

The actual *amount* of a gas in solution at a given partial pressure and temperature depends on the solubility of the gas in that particular liquid. In body fluids, carbon dioxide is highly soluble, oxygen is somewhat less soluble, and nitrogen has very limited solubility. The dissolved gas content is usually reported in milliliters of gas per 100 ml (1 dl) of

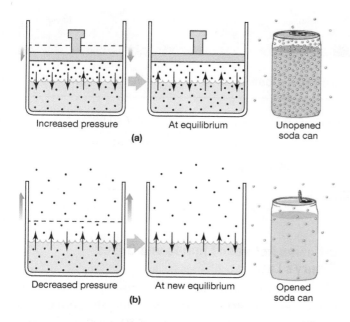

Increased pressure At equilibrium Unopened soda can

(a)

Decreased pressure At new equilibrium Opened soda can

(b)

FIGURE 13.13 **Henry's law and the relationship between solubility and pressure.** **(a)** Increasing the pressure drives gas molecules into solution until an equilibrium is established. A sealed can of carbonated soda is under higher-than-atmospheric pressure. **(b)** When the gas pressure decreases, dissolved gas molecules leave the solution until a new equilibrium is reached. Opening the soda can relieves the pressure, and bubbles form as dissolved gases leave the solution.

Clinical Note

Decompression sickness is a painful condition that develops when a person is exposed to a sudden drop in atmospheric pressure. Nitrogen is the gas responsible for the problems experienced, owing to its high partial pressure in air. When the pressure drops, nitrogen comes out of solution, forming bubbles like those in a shaken can of soda. The bubbles may form in joint cavities, in the bloodstream, and in the cerebrospinal fluid. Individuals with decompression sickness typically curl up from the pain in affected joints; this reaction accounts for the condition's common name: *the bends*. Decompression sickness most commonly affects scuba divers who return to the surface too quickly after breathing air under greater-than-normal pressure while submerged. It can also develop in airline passengers subject to sudden losses of cabin pressure.

solution. To see the differences in relative solubility, we can compare the gas content of blood in the pulmonary veins with the partial pressure of each gas in the alveoli. In a pulmonary vein, plasma generally contains 2.62 ml/dl of dissolved CO_2 (P_{CO_2} = 40 mm Hg), 0.29 ml/dl of dissolved O_2 (P_{O_2} = 100 mm Hg), and 1.25 ml/dl of dissolved N_2 (P_{N_2} = 573 mm Hg).

Gas Transport in the Blood

Oxygen is transported in the blood in two ways. Most attaches to hemoglobin molecules inside the RBCs to form **oxyhemoglobin** (ok″se-he″mo-glo′bin)—HbO_2 in Figure 13.14a. A very small amount of oxygen is carried dissolved in the plasma.

Most carbon dioxide is transported in plasma as the **bicarbonate ion** (HCO_3^-), which plays a very important role in the blood buffer system. (The enzymatic conversion of carbon dioxide to bicarbonate ion actually occurs within the red blood cells, and then the newly formed bicarbonate ions diffuse into the plasma.) A smaller amount (between 20 and 30 percent of the transported CO_2) is carried inside the RBCs bound to hemoglobin. Carbon dioxide carried inside the RBCs binds to hemoglobin at a different site than oxygen does, and so it does not interfere in any way with oxygen transport. Before carbon dioxide can diffuse out of the blood into the alveoli, it must first be released from its bicarbonate ion form. For this to occur, bicarbonate ions must enter the red blood cells where they combine with hydrogen ions (H^+) to form carbonic acid (H_2CO_3). Carbonic acid quickly splits to form water and carbon dioxide, and carbon dioxide then diffuses from the blood and enters the alveoli.

Homeostatic Imbalance

Impaired oxygen transport: Whatever the cause, inadequate oxygen delivery to body tissues is called **hypoxia** (hi-pok′se-ah). This condition is easy to recognize in fair-skinned people because their skin and mucosae take on a bluish cast (become *cyanotic*). In dark-skinned individuals, this color change can be observed only in the mucosae and nailbeds. Hypoxia may be the result of anemia, pulmonary disease, or impaired or blocked blood circulation.

Carbon monoxide poisoning represents a unique type of hypoxia. Carbon monoxide (CO) is an odorless, colorless gas that competes vigorously with

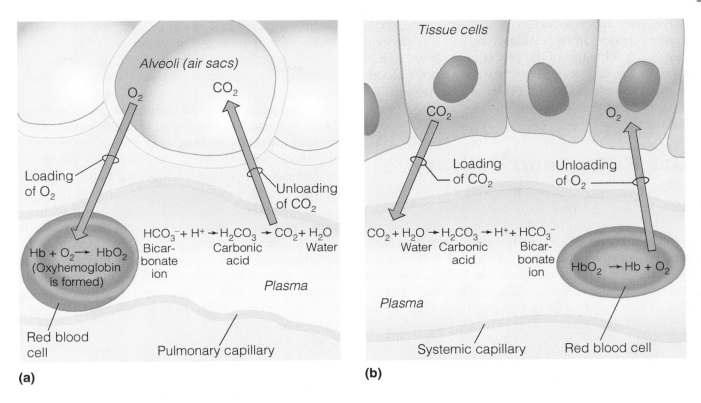

FIGURE 13.14 **Diagrammatic representation of the major means of oxygen (O_2) and carbon dioxide (CO_2) loading and unloading in the body.** **(a)** External respiration in the lungs (pulmonary gas exchange): Oxygen is loaded and carbon dioxide is unloaded. **(b)** Internal respiration in the body tissues (systemic capillary gas exchange): Oxygen is unloaded and carbon dioxide is loaded into the blood. (Note that although the conversion of CO_2 to bicarbonate ion and the reverse reaction are shown occurring in the plasma, most such conversions occur within the red blood cells.) Additionally, though not illustrated, some CO_2 is carried within red blood cells bound to hemoglobin.

oxygen for the same binding sites on hemoglobin. Moreover, since hemoglobin binds to CO more readily than to oxygen, carbon monoxide is a very successful competitor—so much so that it crowds out or displaces oxygen.

Carbon monoxide poisoning is the leading cause of death from fire. It is particularly dangerous because it kills its victims softly and quietly. It does not produce the characteristic signs of hypoxia—cyanosis and respiratory distress. Instead, the victim becomes confused and has a throbbing headache. In rare cases, the skin becomes cherry red (the color of the hemoglobin-CO complex), which is often interpreted as a healthy "blush." Those with CO poisoning are given 100 percent oxygen until the carbon monoxide has been cleared from the body. ▲

Internal Respiration

Internal respiration, the exchange of gases that takes place between the blood and the tissue cells, is opposite to what occurs in the lungs. This process, in which oxygen is unloaded and carbon dioxide is loaded into the blood, is shown in Figure 13.14b. Carbon dioxide diffusing out of tissue cells enters the blood. In the blood, it combines with water to form carbonic acid, which quickly releases the bicarbonate ions. As previously mentioned, most conversion of carbon dioxide to bicarbonate ions actually occurs *inside* the RBCs, where a special enzyme (carbonic anhydrase) is available to speed up this reaction. Then the bicarbonate ions diffuse out into plasma, where they are transported. At the same time, oxygen is released from hemoglobin, and the oxygen diffuses quickly out of the blood to enter the tissue cells. As a result of these exchanges, venous blood in the systemic circulation is much poorer in oxygen and richer in carbon dioxide than that leaving the lungs.

Gas Pickup and Delivery

Let's return to how gas is tranported in the blood and examine this process in more detail.

Oxygen and carbon dioxide have limited solubilities in blood plasma. For example, at the normal Po_2 of alveoli, 100 ml of plasma will absorb only about 0.3 ml of oxygen. The limited solubilities of these gases are a problem, because peripheral tissues need more oxygen and generate more carbon dioxide than the plasma can absorb and transport.

The problem is solved by red blood cells (RBCs), which remove dissolved oxygen and CO_2 molecules from plasma and bind them (in the case of oxygen) or use them to manufacture soluble compounds (in the case of carbon dioxide). Because these reactions remove dissolved gases from blood plasma, gases continue to diffuse into the blood, but never reach equilibrium.

The important thing about these reactions is that they are both temporary and completely reversible. When plasma oxygen or carbon dioxide concentrations are high, the excess molecules are removed by RBCs. When plasma concentrations are falling, the RBCs release their stored reserves.

Oxygen Transport

Each 100 ml of blood leaving the alveolar capillaries carries away roughly 20 ml of oxygen. Of this amount, only about 0.3 ml (1.5 percent) consists of oxygen molecules in solution. The rest of the oxygen molecules are bound to *hemoglobin (Hb) molecules*—specifically, to the iron ions in the center of heme units. Recall that the hemoglobin molecule consists of four globular protein subunits, each containing a heme unit. Thus, each hemoglobin molecule can bind four molecules of oxygen, forming oxyhemoglobin (HbO_2). This is a reversible reaction that can be summarized as

$$Hb + O_2 \rightleftharpoons HbO_2.$$

Each red blood cell has approximately 280 million molecules of hemoglobin. Because a hemoglobin molecule contains four heme units, each RBC potentially can carry more than a billion molecules of oxygen.

The percentage of heme units containing bound oxygen at any given moment is called the **hemoglobin saturation**. If all the Hb molecules in the blood are fully loaded with oxygen, saturation is 100 percent. If, on average, each Hb molecule carries two O_2 molecules, saturation is 50 percent.

In Chapter 2, we saw that the shape and functional properties of a protein change in response to changes in its environment. Hemoglobin is no exception: Any changes in shape that occur can affect oxygen binding. Under normal conditions, the most important environmental factors affecting hemoglobin are (1) the Po_2 of blood, (2) blood pH, (3) temperature, and (4) ongoing metabolic activity within RBCs.

Hemoglobin and Amount of Oxygen in Blood (Po_2)

An **oxygen–hemoglobin saturation curve,** or **oxygen–hemoglobin dissociation curve,** is a graph that relates the saturation of hemoglobin to the partial pressure of oxygen (Figure 13.15). The binding and dissociation of oxygen to hemoglobin is a typical reversible reaction. At equilibrium, oxygen molecules bind to heme at the same rate that other oxygen molecules are being released. If the oxygen concentration (Po_2) increases, the reaction shifts to the right, and more oxygen gets bound to hemoglobin. If the Po_2 decreases, the reaction shifts to the left, and more oxygen is released by hemoglobin. The graph of this relationship is a curve rather than a straight line, because the shape of the Hb molecule changes slightly each time it binds an oxygen molecule, in a way that enhances its ability to bind *another* oxygen molecule. In other words, the attachment of the first oxygen molecule makes it easier to bind the second; binding the second promotes binding of the third; and binding of the third enhances binding of the fourth.

Because each arriving oxygen molecule increases the affinity of hemoglobin for the *next* oxygen molecule, the saturation curve takes the form shown in Figure 13.15. Once the first oxygen molecule binds to the hemoglobin, the slope rises rapidly until reaching a plateau near 100 percent saturation. While the slope is steep, a very small

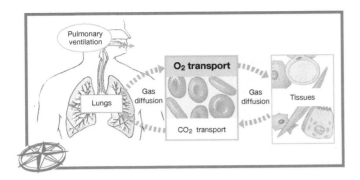

FIGURE 13.15   An oxygen–hemoglobin saturation curve. The saturation characteristics of hemoglobin at various partial pressures of oxygen under normal conditions (body temperature of 37°C and blood pH of 7.4).

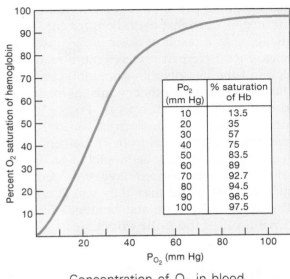

P_{O_2} (mm Hg)	% saturation of Hb
10	13.5
20	35
30	57
40	75
50	83.5
60	89
70	92.7
80	94.5
90	96.5
100	97.5

Concentration of O_2 in blood

change in plasma P_{O_2} will result in a large change in the amount of oxygen bound to Hb or released from HbO_2. Because the curve rises quickly, hemoglobin will be more than 90 percent saturated if exposed to an alveolar P_{O_2} above 60 mm Hg. Thus, near-normal oxygen transport can continue despite a decrease in the oxygen content of alveolar air. Without this ability, you could not survive at high altitudes, and conditions significantly reducing pulmonary ventilation would be immediately fatal.

Note that the relationship between P_{O_2} and hemoglobin saturation remains valid whether the P_{O_2} is rising or falling. If the P_{O_2} increases, the saturation goes up and hemoglobin stores oxygen. If the P_{O_2} decreases, hemoglobin releases oxygen into its surroundings. When oxygenated blood arrives in the peripheral capillaries, the blood P_{O_2} declines rapidly as a result of gas exchange with the interstitial fluid. As the P_{O_2} falls, hemoglobin gives up its oxygen.

The relationship between the P_{O_2} and hemoglobin saturation provides a mechanism for automatic regulation of oxygen delivery. Inactive tissues have little demand for oxygen, and the local P_{O_2} is usually about 40 mm Hg. Under these conditions, hemoglobin will not release much oxygen. As it passes through the capillaries, it will go from 97 percent saturation ($P_{O_2} = 95$ mm Hg) to 75 percent saturation ($P_{O_2} = 40$ mm Hg). Because it still retains three-quarters of its oxygen, venous blood has a relatively large oxygen reserve. This reserve is important, because it can be mobilized if tissue oxygen demands increase.

Active tissues consume oxygen at an accelerated rate, so the P_{O_2} may drop to 15–20 mm Hg. Hemoglobin passing through these capillaries will then go from 97 percent saturation to about 20 percent saturation. In practical terms, this means that as blood circulates through peripheral capillaries, active tissues will receive 3.5 times as much oxygen as will inactive tissues.

The exhaust of automobiles and other petroleum-burning engines, of oil lamps, and of fuel-fired space heaters contains *carbon monoxide* (CO), and each winter entire families die from *carbon monoxide poisoning*. Carbon monoxide competes with oxygen molecules for the binding sites on heme units. Unfortunately, the carbon monoxide usually wins the competition, because at very low partial pressures it has a much stronger affinity for hemoglobin than does oxygen. The bond formed between CO and heme is extremely durable, so the attachment of a CO molecule essentially makes that heme unit inactive for respiratory purposes.

Hemoglobin and pH

The oxygen–hemoglobin saturation curve in Figure 13.15 was determined in normal blood, with a pH of 7.4 and a temperature of 37°C. In addition to consuming oxygen, active tissues generate acids that lower the pH of the interstitial fluid. When the pH drops, the shape of hemoglobin molecules changes. As a result of this change, the molecules release their oxygen reserves more readily, so the slope of the hemoglobin saturation curve changes (Figure 13.16a). In other words, as pH drops, the saturation declines. At a tissue P_{O_2} of 40 mm Hg, for example, a pH drop from 7.4 to 7.2 changes hemoglobin saturation from 75 percent to 60 percent. This means that hemoglobin molecules will release 20 percent more oxygen in peripheral tissues at a pH of 7.2 than they will at a pH of 7.4. This effect of pH on the hemoglobin saturation curve is called the **Bohr effect**.

Control of Respiration

Neural Regulation: Setting the Basic Rhythm

Although our tidelike breathing seems so beautifully simple, its control is fairly complex. We will cover only the most basic aspects of the respiratory controls. The activity of the respiratory muscles, the diaphragm and external intercostals, is regulated by nerve impulses transmitted to them from the brain by the **phrenic** and **intercostal nerves.**

The neural centers that control respiratory rhythm and depth are located in the *medulla* and *pons* (Figure 13.17). The medulla, which sets the basic rhythm of breathing, contains a **self-exciting inspiratory center,** as well as other respiratory centers. The pons centers appear to smooth out the basic rhythm of inspiration and expiration set by the medulla. Impulses going back and forth between the pons and medulla centers maintain a rate of 12–15 respirations/minute. This normal respiratory rate is referred to as **eupnea** (ūp-neʹah).

In addition, the bronchioles and alveoli have stretch receptors that respond to extreme overinflation (which might damage the lungs) by initiating protective reflexes. In the case of overinflation, impulses are sent from the stretch receptors to the medulla by the vagus nerves; soon therafter inspiration ends and expiration occurs.

During exercise, we breathe more vigorously and deeply because the brain centers send more impulses to the respiratory muscles. This respiratory pattern is called **hyperpnea** (hy-perpʹne-ah). However, the *rate* of breathing may not be significantly increased with exercising. After strenuous exercise, expiration becomes active,

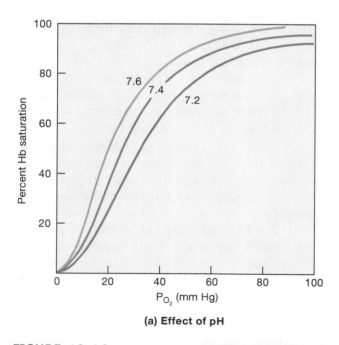

(a) Effect of pH

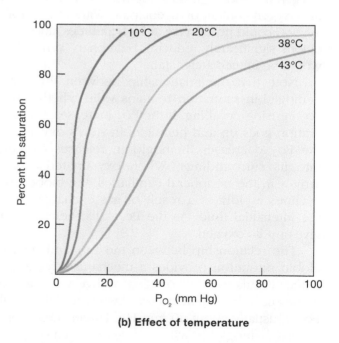

(b) Effect of temperature

FIGURE 13.16   The effects of pH and temperature on hemoglobin saturation. (a) When the pH drops below normal levels, more oxygen is released; the hemoglobin saturation curve shifts to the right. When the pH increases, less oxygen is released; the curve shifts to the left. **(b)** When the temperature rises, the saturation curve shifts to the right.

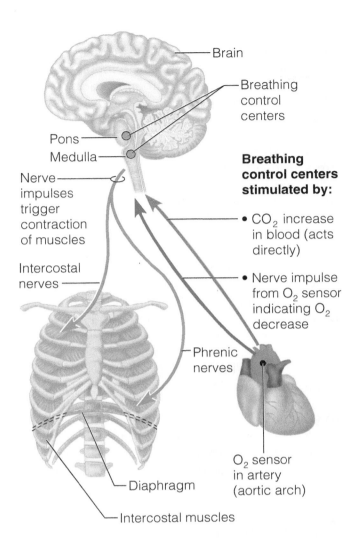

Brain

Breathing control centers

Pons

Medulla

Nerve impulses trigger contraction of muscles

Intercostal nerves

Breathing control centers stimulated by:

- CO_2 increase in blood (acts directly)
- Nerve impulse from O_2 sensor indicating O_2 decrease

Phrenic nerves

O_2 sensor in artery (aortic arch)

Diaphragm

Intercostal muscles

FIGURE 13.17   Breathing control centers, sensory inputs, and effector nerves.

and the abdominal muscles and any other muscles capable of lifting the ribs are used to aid expiration.

Homeostatic Imbalance

If the medullary centers are completely suppressed (as with an overdose of sleeping pills, morphine, or alcohol), respiration stops completely, and death occurs. ▲

Factors Influencing Respiratory Rate and Depth

Physical Factors   Although brain centers set the basic rhythm of breathing, there is no question that physical factors such as talking, coughing, and exercising can modify both the rate and depth of breathing. Some of these factors have

already been examined in the earlier discussion of nonrespiratory air movements. Increased body temperature causes an increase in the rate of breathing.

Volition (Conscious Control)   We all have consciously controlled our breathing pattern at one time or another. During singing and swallowing, breath control is extremely important, and many of us have held our breath for short periods to swim underwater. However, voluntary control of breathing is limited, and the respiratory centers will simply ignore messages from the cortex (our wishes) when the oxygen supply in the blood is getting low or blood pH is falling. All you need do to prove this is to try to talk normally or to hold your breath after running at breakneck speed for a few minutes. It simply cannot be done. Many toddlers try to manipulate their parents by holding their breath "to death." Even though this threat causes many parents to become anxious, they need not worry because the involuntary controls take over and normal respiration begins again.

Emotional Factors   Emotional factors also modify the rate and depth of breathing. Have you ever watched a horror movie with bated (held) breath or been so scared by what you saw that you were nearly panting? Have you ever touched something cold and clammy and gasped? All of these result from reflexes initiated by emotional stimuli acting through centers in the hypothalamus.

Chemical Factors   Although many factors can modify respiratory rate and depth, the most important factors are chemical—the levels of carbon dioxide and oxygen in the blood. Increased levels of carbon dioxide and decreased blood pH are the most important stimuli leading to an increase in the rate and depth of breathing. (Actually, an increase in carbon dioxide levels and decreased blood pH are the same thing in this case because carbon dioxide retention leads to increased levels of carbonic acid, which decrease the blood pH.) Changes in carbon dioxide concentrations in the blood seem to act directly on the medulla centers (see Figure 13.17).

Conversely, changes in oxygen concentration in the blood are detected by chemoreceptor regions in the aorta (aortic arch) and carotid artery (carotid body). These, in turn, send impulses to the medulla when blood oxygen levels are dropping.

Although every cell in the body must have oxygen to live, it is the body's need to rid itself of carbon dioxide (not to take in oxygen) that is the *most* important stimulus for breathing in a healthy person. Decreases in oxygen levels only become important stimuli when they are dangerously low.

Respiratory Control at the Local Level and in the Brain

Peripheral cells continuously absorb oxygen from interstitial fluids and generate carbon dioxide. Under normal conditions, the cellular rates of absorption and generation are matched by the capillary rates of delivery and removal. Both rates are identical to those of oxygen absorption and carbon dioxide excretion at the lungs. If diffusion rates at the peripheral and alveolar capillaries become unbalanced, homeostatic mechanisms intervene to restore equilibrium. Such mechanisms involve (1) changes in blood flow and oxygen delivery that are regulated at the local level and (2) changes in the depth and rate of respiration under the control of the brain's respiratory centers. The activities of the respiratory centers are coordinated with changes in cardiovascular function, such as fluctuations in blood pressure and cardiac output.

Local Regulation of Gas Transport and Alveolar Function

The rate of oxygen delivery in each tissue and the efficiency of oxygen pickup at the lungs are largely regulated at the local level. For example, when a peripheral tissue becomes more active, the interstitial P_{O_2} falls and the P_{CO_2} rises. This change increases the difference between the partial pressures in the tissues and in the arriving blood, so more oxygen is delivered and more carbon dioxide is carried away. In addition, the rising P_{CO_2} levels cause the relaxation of smooth muscles in the walls of arterioles and capillaries in the area, increasing local blood flow.

Local factors also coordinate (1) *lung perfusion*, or blood flow to the alveoli, with (2) *alveolar ventilation*, or airflow, over a wide range of conditions and activity levels. As blood flows toward the alveolar capillaries, it is directed toward lobules in which the P_{O_2} is relatively high. This movement occurs because alveolar capillaries constrict when the local P_{O_2} is low. (This response is the opposite of that seen in peripheral tissues.) Such a shift in blood flow tends to eliminate temporary differences in the oxygen and carbon dioxide contents of alveoli, lobules, or groups of lobules that could otherwise result from minor variations in local blood flow.

Smooth muscles in the walls of bronchioles are sensitive to the P_{CO_2} of the air they contain. When the P_{CO_2} goes up, the bronchioles increase in diameter (bronchodilation). When the P_{CO_2} declines, the bronchioles constrict (bronchoconstriction). Airflow is therefore directed to lobules in which the P_{CO_2} is high. Because these lobules obtain carbon dioxide from blood, they are actively engaged in gas exchange. This response is especially important, because the improvement of airflow to functional alveoli can at least partially compensate for damage to pulmonary lobules.

By directing blood flow to alveoli with low CO_2 levels and increasing airflow to alveoli with high CO_2 levels, local adjustments improve the efficiency of gas transport. When activity levels increase and the demand for oxygen rises, the cardiac output and respiratory rates increase under neural control, but the adjustments in alveolar blood flow and bronchiole diameter occur automatically.

The Respiratory Centers of the Brain

Let's examine how the brain regulates respiration in more detail.

Respiratory control has both involuntary and voluntary components. Your brain's involuntary centers regulate the activities of the respiratory muscles and control the respiratory minute volume by adjusting the frequency and depth of pulmonary ventilation. They do so in response to sensory information arriving from your lungs and other portions of the respiratory tract, as well as from a variety of other sites.

The voluntary control of respiration reflects activity in the cerebral cortex that affects either the output of the respiratory centers in the medulla oblongata and pons or of motor neurons in the spinal cord that control respiratory muscles. The **respiratory centers** are three pairs of nuclei in the reticular formation of the medulla oblongata and pons. The motor neurons in the spinal cord are generally controlled by *respiratory reflexes*, but they can also be controlled voluntarily through commands delivered by the corticospinal pathway.

Respiratory Centers in the Medulla Oblongata

The *respiratory rhythmicity centers* of the medulla oblongata are paired centers that set the pace of respiration. Each center can be subdivided into a **dorsal respiratory group (DRG)** and a **ventral respiratory group (VRG)**. The DRG's *inspiratory center* contains neurons that control lower motor neurons innervating the external intercostal muscles and the diaphragm. The DRG functions in every respiratory cycle, whether quiet or forced. The VRG functions only during forced breathing. It includes neurons that innervate lower motor neurons controlling accessory respiratory muscles involved in active exhalation (an *expiratory center*) and maximal inhalation (an *inspiratory center*).

Reciprocal inhibition occurs between the neurons involved with inhalation and exhalation. When the inspiratory neurons are active, the expiratory neurons are inhibited, and vice versa. The pattern of interaction between these groups differs between quiet breathing and forced breathing. During quiet breathing (Figure 13.18a):

- Activity in the DRG increases over a period of about 2 seconds, providing stimulation to the inspiratory muscles. Over this period, inhalation occurs.

- After 2 seconds, the DRG neurons become inactive. They remain quiet for the next 3 seconds and allow the inspiratory muscles to relax. Over this period, passive exhalation occurs.

During forced breathing (Figure 13.18b):

- Increases in the level of activity in the DRG stimulate neurons of the VRG that activate the accessory muscles involved in inhalation.

- After each inhalation, active exhalation occurs as the neurons of the expiratory center stimulate the appropriate accessory muscles.

The basic pattern of respiration thus reflects a cyclic interaction between the DRG and the VRG. The pace of this interaction is thought to be established by pacemaker cells that spontaneously undergo rhythmic patterns of activity. Attempts to locate the pacemaker, however, have been unsuccessful.

Central nervous system stimulants, such as amphetamines or even caffeine, increase the

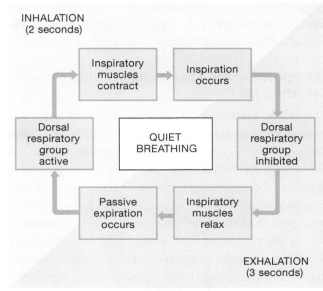

(a) Quiet breathing

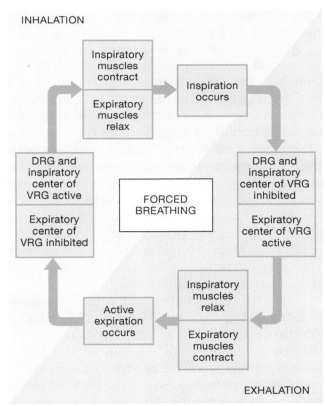

(b) Forced breathing

FIGURE 13.18   Basic regulatory patterns of respiration. (a) Quiet breathing. **(b)** Forced breathing.

respiratory rate by facilitating the respiratory centers. These actions are opposed by CNS depressants, such as barbiturates or opiates.

The Apneustic and Pneumotaxic Centers of the Pons

The **apneustic** (ap-NOO-stik) **centers** and the **pneumotaxic** (noo-mō-TAKS-ik) **centers** of the pons are paired nuclei that adjust the output of the respiratory rhythmicity centers. Their activities regulate the respiratory rate and the depth of respiration in response to sensory stimuli or input from other centers in the brain. Each apneustic center provides continuous stimulation to the DRG on that side of the brain stem. During quiet breathing, stimulation from the apneustic center helps increase the intensity of inhalation over the next 2 seconds. Under normal conditions, after 2 seconds, the apneustic center is inhibited by signals from the pneumotaxic center on that side. During forced breathing, the apneustic centers also respond to sensory input from the vagus nerves regarding the amount of lung inflation.

The pneumotaxic centers inhibit the apneustic centers and promote passive or active exhalation. Centers in the hypothalamus and cerebrum can alter the activity of the pneumotaxic centers, as well as the respiratory rate and depth. However, essentially normal respiratory cycles continue even if the brain stem superior to the pons has been severely damaged. If the inhibitory output of the pneumotaxic centers is cut off by a stroke or other damage to the brain stem, and if sensory innervation from the lungs is eliminated due to damage to the vagus nerves, the person inhales to maximum capacity and maintains that state for 10–20 seconds at a time. Intervening exhalations are brief, and little pulmonary ventilation occurs.

The CNS regions involved with respiratory control are diagrammed in Figure 13.19. Interactions between the DRG and the VRG establish the basic pace and depth of respiration. The pneumotaxic centers modify that pace: An increase in pneumotaxic output quickens the pace of respiration by shortening the duration of each inhalation; a decrease in pneumotaxic output slows the respiratory pace, but increases the depth of respiration, because the apneustic centers are more active.

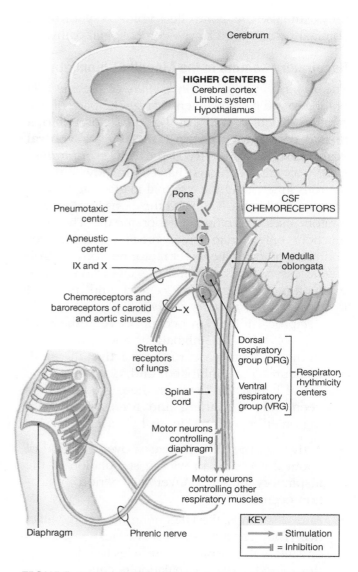

FIGURE 13.19   Respiratory centers and reflex controls. The locations of the major respiratory centers and other structures important to the reflex control of respiration. Pathways for conscious control over respiratory muscles are not shown.

Sudden infant death syndrome (SIDS), also known as *crib death*, kills an estimated 10,000 infants each year in the United States alone. Most crib deaths occur between midnight and 9:00 a.m., in the late fall or winter, and involve infants 2 to 4 months old. Eyewitness accounts indicate that the sleeping infant suddenly stops breathing, turns blue, and relaxes. Genetic factors appear to be involved, but controversy remains as to the relative importance of other factors. The age at the time of death corresponds with a period when the pacemaker complex and respiratory centers are establishing connections with other portions of the brain. It has been suggested that SIDS results from a problem in the interconnection process that disrupts the reflexive respiratory pattern.

Respiratory Reflexes

The activities of the respiratory centers are modified by sensory information from several sources:

- Chemoreceptors sensitive to the P_{CO_2} pH, or P_{O_2} of the blood or cerebrospinal fluid.
- Baroreceptors in the aortic or carotid sinuses sensitive to changes in blood pressure.
- Stretch receptors that respond to changes in the volume of the lungs.
- Irritating physical or chemical stimuli in the nasal cavity, larynx, or bronchial tree.
- Other sensations, including pain, changes in body temperature, and abnormal visceral sensations.

Information from these receptors alters the pattern of respiration. The induced changes have been called *respiratory reflexes.*

The Baroreceptor Reflexes

The output from carotid and aortic baroreceptors affects the respiratory centers. When blood pressure falls, the respiratory rate increases; when blood pressure rises, the respiratory rate declines. This adjustment results from the stimulation or inhibition of the respiratory centers by sensory fibers in the glossopharyngeal (IX) and vagus (X) nerves.

The Hering–Breuer Reflexes

The **Hering–Breuer reflexes** are named after the physiologists who described them in 1865. The sensory information from these reflexes is distributed to the apneustic centers and the ventral respiratory group. The Hering–Breuer reflexes are not involved in normal quiet breathing (eupnea) or in tidal volumes under 1000 ml. There are two such reflexes:

1. The **inflation reflex** prevents overexpansion of the lungs during forced breathing. Stretch receptors located in the smooth muscle tissue around bronchioles are stimulated by lung expansion. Sensory fibers leaving the stretch receptors of each lung reach the respiratory rhythmicity center on the same side via the vagus nerve. As lung volume increases, the dorsal respiratory group is gradually inhibited, and the expiratory center of the VRG is stimulated. Inhalation stops as the lungs near maximum volume, and active exhalation then begins.

2. The **deflation reflex** inhibits the expiratory centers and stimulates the inspiratory centers when the lungs are deflating. These receptors, which are distinct from those of the inflation reflex, are located in the alveolar wall near the alveolar capillary network. The smaller the volume of the lungs, the greater the degree of inhibition, until exhalation stops and inhalation begins. This reflex normally functions only during forced exhalation, when both the inspiratory and expiratory centers are active.

Voluntary Control of Respiration

Activity of the cerebral cortex has an indirect effect on the respiratory centers, as the following examples show:

- Conscious thought processes tied to strong emotions, such as rage or fear, affect the respiratory rate by stimulating centers in the hypothalamus.
- Emotional states can affect respiration through the activation of the sympathetic or parasympathetic division of the autonomic nervous system. Sympathetic activation causes bronchodilation and increases the respiratory rate; parasympathetic stimulation has the opposite effect.
- An anticipation of strenuous exercise can trigger an automatic increase in the respiratory rate, along with increased cardiac output, by sympathetic stimulation.

Conscious control over respiratory activities may bypass the respiratory centers completely, using pyramidal fibers that innervate the same lower motor neurons that are controlled by the DRG and VRG. This control mechanism is an essential part of speaking, singing, and swimming, when respiratory activities must be precisely timed. Higher centers can also have an inhibitory effect on the apneustic centers and on the DRG and VRG; this effect is important when you hold your breath.

Your abilities to override the respiratory centers have limits, however. The chemoreceptor reflexes are extremely powerful respiratory stimulators, and they cannot be consciously suppressed. For example, you cannot kill yourself by holding your breath "till you turn blue." Once the P_{CO_2} rises to critical levels, you will be forced to take a breath.

Developmental Aspects of the Respiratory System

In the fetus, the lungs are filled with fluid, and all respiratory exchanges are made by the placenta. At birth, the fluid-filled pathway is drained, and the respiratory passageways fill with air. The alveoli inflate and begin to function in gas exchange, but the lungs are not fully inflated for two weeks. The success of this change—that is, from nonfunctional to functional respiration—depends on the presence of **surfactant** (sur-fak'tant), a fatty molecule made by the cuboidal alveolar cells (see Figure 13.6). Surfactant lowers the surface tension of the film of water lining each alveolar sac so that the alveoli do not collapse between each breath. Surfactant is not usually present in large enough amounts to accomplish this function until late in pregnancy, that is, between 28 and 30 weeks.

◣ Homeostatic Imbalance

Infants born prematurely (before week 28) or those in which surfactant production is inadequate for other reasons (as in many infants born to diabetic mothers) have *infant respiratory distress syndrome (IRDS)*. These infants have dyspnea within a few hours after birth and use tremendous amounts of energy just to keep reinflating their alveoli, which collapse after each breath. Although IRDS still accounts for over 20,000 newborn deaths a year, many of these babies survive now because of the use of equipment that supplies a positive pressure continuously and keeps the alveoli open and working in gas exchange until adequate amounts of surfactant are produced by the maturing lungs.

Important birth defects of the respiratory system include cleft palate and cystic fibrosis. **Cystic fibrosis (CF),** the most common lethal genetic disease in the United States, strikes 1 out of every 2400 children, and every day 2 children die of it. CF causes oversecretion of a thick mucus that clogs the respiratory passages and puts the child at risk for fatal respiratory infections. It affects other secretory processes as well. Most importantly, it impairs food digestion by clogging ducts that deliver pancreatic enzymes and bile to the small intestine. Also, sweat glands produce an extremely salty perspiration. At the heart of CF is a faulty gene that codes for the CFTR protein, which works as a chloride (Cl^-) channel to control the flow of Cl^- in and out of cells. In those with the mutated gene, CFTR gets "stuck" in the endoplasmic reticulum and is unable to reach the plasma membrane to perform its normal role. Consequently, less Cl^- is secreted and less water follows, resulting in the thick mucus typical of CF. Conventional therapy for CF is mucus-dissolving drugs, "clapping" the chest to loosen the thick mucus, and antibiotics to prevent infection. ◢

The respiratory rate is highest in newborn infants, about 40 to 80 respirations per minute. It continues to drop through life: in the infant it is around 30/minute, at 5 years it is around 25/minute, and in adults it is 12 to 18/minute. However, the rate often increases again in old age. The lungs continue to mature throughout childhood, and more alveoli are formed until young adulthood. But when smoking is begun during the early teens, the lungs never completely mature, and those additional alveoli are lost forever.

Systems in Sync

Homeostatic Relationships between the Respiratory System and Other Body Systems

Endocrine System
- Respiratory system provides oxygen; disposes of carbon dioxide
- Epinephrine dilates the bronchioles; testosterone promotes laryngeal enlargement in pubertal males

Lymphatic System/Immunity
- Respiratory system provides oxygen; disposes of carbon dioxide; tonsils in pharynx house immune cells
- Lymphatic system helps to maintain blood volume required for respiratory gas transport; immune system protects respiratory organs from pathogens and cancer

Digestive System
- Respiratory system provides oxygen; disposes of carbon dioxide
- Digestive system provides nutrients needed by respiratory system

Urinary System
- Respiratory system provides oxygen; disposes of carbon dioxide
- Kidneys dispose of metabolic wastes of respiratory system organs (other than carbon dioxide)

Muscular System
- Respiratory system provides oxygen needed for muscle activity; disposes of carbon dioxide
- The diaphragm and intercostal muscles produce volume changes necessary for breathing; regular exercise increases respiratory efficiency

Nervous System
- Respiratory system provides oxygen needed for normal neural activity; disposes of carbon dioxide
- Medullary and pons centers regulate respiratory rate/depth; stretch receptors in lungs and chemoreceptors in large arteries provide feedback

Respiratory System

Cardiovascular System
- Respiratory system provides oxygen; disposes of carbon dioxide; carbon dioxide present in blood as HCO_3^- and H_2CO_3 contributes to blood buffering
- Blood transports respiratory gases

Reproductive System
- Respiratory system provides oxygen; disposes of carbon dioxide

Integumentary System
- Respiratory system provides oxygen; disposes of carbon dioxide
- Skin protects respiratory system organs by forming surface barriers

Skeletal System
- Respiratory system provides oxygen; disposes of carbon dioxide
- Bones enclose and protect lungs and bronchi

14

The Digestive System and Body Metabolism

KEY TERMS

Children have a special fascination with the workings of the digestive system: They relish crunching a potato chip, delight in making "mustaches" with milk, and giggle when their stomach "growls." As adults, we know that a healthy digestive system is essential for good health because it converts food into the raw materials that build and fuel our body's cells. Specifically, the digestive system takes in food (*ingests* it), breaks it down physically and chemically into nutrient molecules (*digests* it), and *absorbs* the nutrients into the bloodstream. Then it rids the body of the indigestible remains (*defecates*).

PART I: ANATOMY AND PHYSIOLOGY OF THE DIGESTIVE SYSTEM

Anatomy of the Digestive System

The organs of the digestive system can be separated into two main groups: those forming the *alimentary* (al"ĕ-men'tar-e; *aliment* = nourish) *canal,* and the *accessory digestive organs* (see Figure 14.1). The alimentary canal performs the whole menu of digestive functions (ingests, digests, absorbs, and defecates). The accessory organs (teeth, tongue, and several large digestive glands) assist the process of digestive breakdown in various ways.

Organs of the Alimentary Canal

The **alimentary canal,** also called the **gastrointestinal (GI) tract,** is a continuous, coiled, hollow, muscular tube that winds through the ventral body cavity and is open at both ends. Its organs are the *mouth, pharynx, esophagus, stomach, small intestine,* and *large intestine.* The large intestine leads to the terminal opening, or *anus.* In a cadaver, the alimentary canal is approximately 9 m (about 30 feet) long, but in a living person, it is considerably shorter because of its relatively constant muscle tone. Food material within this tube is technically outside the body, because it has contact only with cells lining the tract and the tube is

open to the external environment at both ends. As each organ of the alimentary canal is described next, find it in Figure 14.1.

Mouth

Food enters the digestive tract through the **mouth,** or **oral cavity,** a mucous membrane–lined cavity (Figure 14.2). The **lips (labia)** protect its anterior opening, the **cheeks** form its lateral walls, the **hard palate** forms its anterior roof, and the **soft palate** forms its posterior roof. The **uvula** (u'vu-lah) is a fleshy fingerlike projection of the soft palate, which extends downward from its posterior edge. The space between the lips and cheeks externally and the teeth and gums internally is the **vestibule.** The area contained by the teeth is the **oral cavity proper.** The muscular **tongue** occupies the floor of the mouth. The tongue has several bony attachments—two of these are to the hyoid bone and the styloid processes of the skull. The **lingual frenulum** (ling'gwal fren'u-lum), a fold of mucous membrane, secures the tongue to the floor of the mouth and limits its posterior movements (see Figure 14.2a).

Homeostatic Imbalance

Children born with an extremely short frenulum are often referred to as "tongue-tied" because distorted speech results when tongue movement is restricted. This congenital condition can be corrected surgically by cutting the frenulum. ▲

At the posterior end of the oral cavity are paired masses of lymphatic tissue, the **palatine tonsils.** The **lingual tonsil** covers the base of the tongue just beyond. The tonsils, along with other lymphatic tissues, are part of the body's defense system. When the tonsils become inflamed and enlarge, they partially block the entrance into the throat (pharynx), making swallowing difficult and painful.

As food enters the mouth, it is mixed with saliva and **masticated** (chewed). The cheeks and closed lips hold the food between the teeth during chewing. The nimble tongue continually mixes food with saliva during chewing and initiates swallowing. Thus, the breakdown of food begins before the food has even left the mouth. *Papillae* containing taste buds, or taste receptors, are found on the tongue surface. And so, besides its food-manipulating

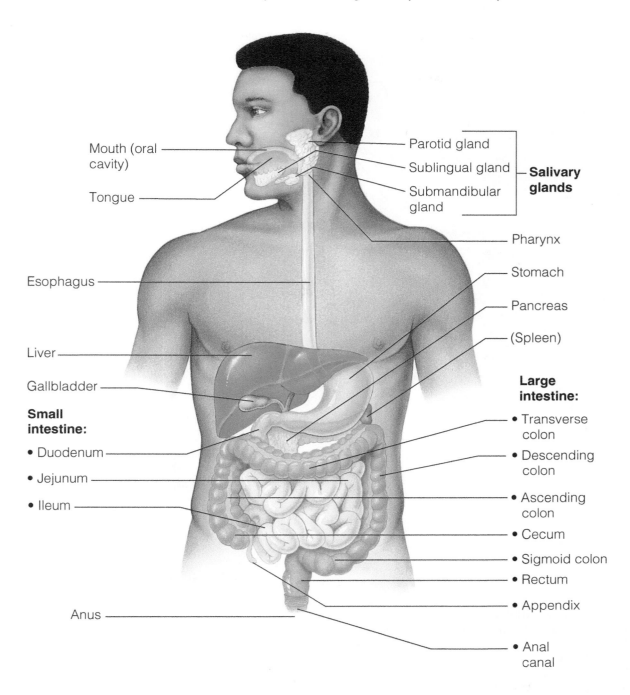

FIGURE 14.1 **The human digestive system: alimentary canal and accessory organs.** (Liver and gallbladder are reflected superiorly and to the right side of the body.)

function, the tongue allows us to enjoy and appreciate the food as it is eaten.

Pharynx

From the mouth, food passes posteriorly into the *oropharynx* and *laryngopharynx,* both of which are common passageways for food, fluids, and air. The pharynx is subdivided into the *nasopharynx,* part of the respiratory passageway; the **oropharynx,** posterior to the oral cavity; and the **laryngopharynx,** which is continuous with the esophagus below.

Q   *What is the protective value of having several sets of tonsils at the oral entrance to the pharynx?*

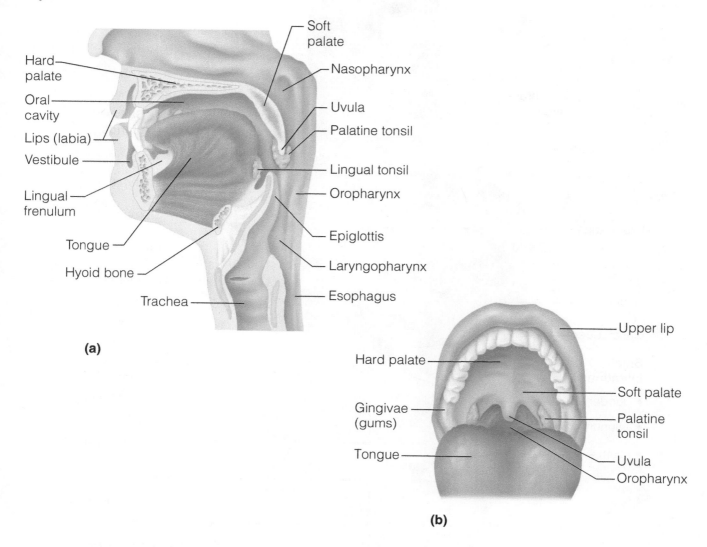

FIGURE 14.2 Anatomy of the mouth (oral cavity). (a) Sagittal view of the oral cavity and pharynx. **(b)** Anterior view of the oral cavity.

The walls of the pharynx contain two skeletal muscle layers. The cells of the inner layer run longitudinally; those of the outer layer (the constrictor muscles) run around the wall in a circular fashion. Alternating contractions of these two muscle layers propel food through the pharynx into the esophagus below. This propelling mechanism, called *peristalsis* (per"i-stal'sis), is described later.

A   *The mouth is a favored site of body entry by bacteria, and the presence of the tonsils (lymphocyte- and macrophage-filled organs) is very effective in preventing many pathogens from getting further into the digestive tract.*

Esophagus

The **esophagus** (ĕ-sof'ah-gus), or *gullet,* runs from the pharynx through the diaphragm to the stomach. About 25 cm (10 inches) long, it is essentially a passageway that conducts food (by peristalsis) to the stomach.

The walls of the alimentary canal organs from the esophagus to the large intestine are made up of the same four basic tissue layers, or tunics (Figure 14.3):

1. The **mucosa** is the innermost layer, a moist membrane that lines the cavity, or **lumen,** of the organ. It consists primarily of a *surface epithelium,* plus a small amount of connective tissue *(lamina propria)* and a scanty *smooth muscle layer.* Beyond the esophagus, which has a friction-resisting stratified squamous epithelium, the epithelium is mostly simple columnar.

2. The **submucosa** is found just beneath the mucosa. It is a soft connective tissue layer containing blood vessels, nerve endings, lymph nodules, and lymphatic vessels.

3. The **muscularis externa** is a muscle layer typically made up of an inner *circular layer* and an outer *longitudinal layer* of smooth muscle cells.

4. The **serosa** is the outermost layer of the wall. It consists of a single layer of flat serous fluid-producing cells, the **visceral peritoneum**

(per"i-to-ne'um). The visceral peritoneum is continuous with the slick, slippery **parietal peritoneum,** which lines the abdominopelvic cavity by way of a membrane extension, the **mesentery** (mes'en-ter"e). These relationships are illustrated in Figure 14.5.

The alimentary canal wall contains two important *intrinsic nerve plexuses*—the **submucosal nerve plexus** and the **myenteric** (mi-en'ter-ik; "intestinal muscle") **nerve plexus.** An additional small *subserous plexus* is associated with the serosa. These networks of nerve fibers are actually part of the autonomic nervous system. They help regulate the mobility and secretory activity of GI tract organs.

Stomach

The C-shaped **stomach** (Figure 14.4) is on the left side of the abdominal cavity, nearly hidden by

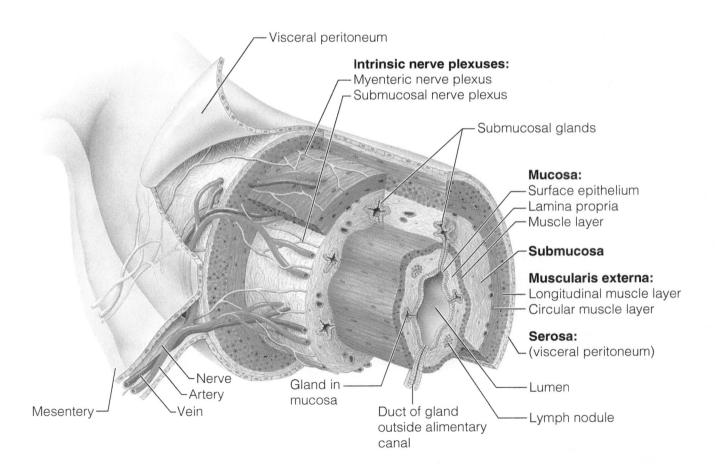

FIGURE 14.3 **Basic structure of the alimentary canal wall.**

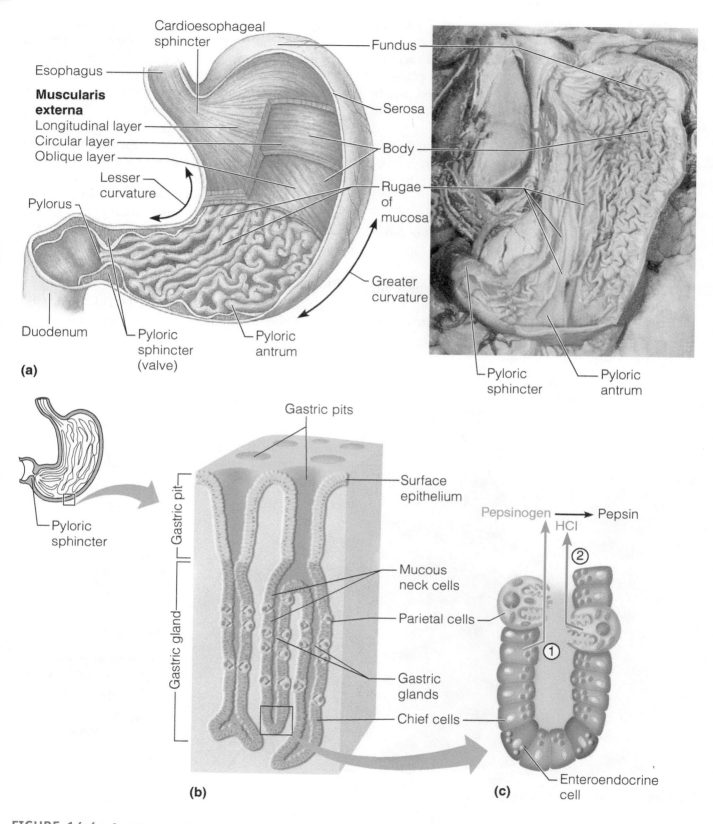

FIGURE 14.4   Anatomy of the stomach. (a) Gross internal anatomy (frontal section). **(b)** Enlarged view of gastric pits and glands (longitudinal section). **(c)** Schematic showing the sequence of events from ① the production of pepsinogen by the chief cells to ② its activation (to pepsin) by HCl secreted by the parietal cells.

the liver and diaphragm. Different regions of the stomach have been named. The *cardiac region* (named for its position near the heart) surrounds the **cardioesophageal** (kar″de-o-ĕ-sof″ah-je′al) **sphincter,** through which food enters the stomach from the esophagus. The *fundus* is the expanded part of the stomach lateral to the cardiac region. The *body* is the midportion, and as it narrows inferiorly, it becomes the *pyloric antrum,* and then the funnel-shaped *pylorus* (pi-lo′rus), the terminal part of the stomach. The pylorus is continuous with the small intestine through the **pyloric sphincter,** or **valve.** The stomach is approximately 25 cm (10 inches) long, but its diameter depends on how much food it contains. When it is full, it can hold about 4 liters (1 gallon) of food. When it is empty, it collapses inward on itself, and its mucosa is thrown into large folds called **rugae** (roo′ge; *ruga* = wrinkle, fold). The convex lateral surface of the stomach is the **greater curvature;** its concave medial surface is the **lesser curvature.**

The **lesser omentum** (o-men′tum), a double layer of peritoneum, extends from the liver to the lesser curvature. The **greater omentum,** another extension of the peritoneum, drapes downward and covers the abdominal organs like a lacy apron before attaching to the posterior body wall (Figure 14.5). The greater omentum is riddled with fat, which helps to insulate, cushion, and protect the abdominal organs, and has large collections of lymph nodules containing macrophages and defensive cells of the immune system.

Homeostatic Imbalance

When the peritoneum is infected, a condition called *peritonitis* (per″i-to-ni′tis), the peritoneal membranes tend to stick together around the infection site. This helps to seal off and localize many intraperitoneal infections (at least initially), providing time for macrophages in the lymphatic tissue to mount an attack. ▲

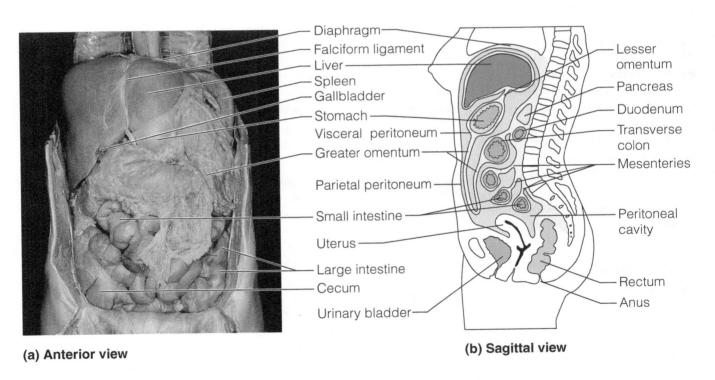

(a) Anterior view

Diaphragm
Falciform ligament
Liver
Spleen
Gallbladder
Stomach
Visceral peritoneum
Greater omentum
Parietal peritoneum
Small intestine
Uterus
Large intestine
Cecum
Urinary bladder

Lesser omentum
Pancreas
Duodenum
Transverse colon
Mesenteries
Peritoneal cavity
Rectum
Anus

(b) Sagittal view

FIGURE 14.5 Peritoneal attachments of the abdominal organs.
(a) Anterior view; the greater omentum is shown in its normal position, covering the abdominal viscera. **(b)** Sagittal view of the abdominopelvic cavity of a female.

The stomach acts as a temporary "storage tank" for food as well as a site for food breakdown. Besides the usual longitudinal and circular muscle layers, its wall contains a third obliquely arranged layer in the *muscularis externa* (see Figure 14.4a). This arrangement allows the stomach not only to move food along the tract, but also to churn, mix, and pummel the food, physically breaking it down to smaller fragments. In addition, chemical breakdown of proteins begins in the stomach. The mucosa of the stomach is a simple columnar epithelium that produces large amounts of mucus. This otherwise smooth lining is dotted with millions of deep *gastric pits,* which lead into *gastric glands* (Figure 14.4b) that secrete the solution called **gastric juice.** For example, some stomach cells produce *intrinsic factor,* a substance needed for the absorption of vitamin B_{12} from the small intestine. The **chief cells** produce protein-digesting enzymes, mostly **pepsinogens,** and the **parietal cells** produce corrosive hydrochloric acid, which makes the stomach contents acidic and activates the enzymes (Figure 14.4c). The *mucous neck cells* produce a sticky alkaline mucus, which clings to the stomach mucosa and protects the stomach wall itself from being damaged by the acid and digested by the enzymes. Still other cells, the **enteroendocrine cells** (*entero* = gut), produce local hormones, such as *gastrin,* that are important to the digestive activities of the stomach (see Table 14.1).

Most digestive activity occurs in the pyloric region of the stomach. After food has been processed in the stomach, it resembles heavy cream and is called **chyme** (kīm). The chyme enters the small intestine through the pyloric sphincter.

Small Intestine

The **small intestine** is the body's major digestive organ. Within its twisted passageways, usable food is finally prepared for its journey into the cells of the body. The small intestine is a muscular tube extending from the pyloric sphincter to the **ileocecal** (il″e-o-se′kal) **valve,** which opens into the large intestine (see Figure 14.10). It is the longest section of the alimentary tube, with an average length of 2.5 to 7 m (8–18 feet) in a living

person. Except for the initial part of the small intestine (the duodenum), which mostly lies in a retroperitoneal position, the small intestine hangs in sausagelike coils in the abdominal cavity, suspended from the posterior abdominal wall by the fan-shaped mesentery (see Figure 14.5). The large intestine encircles and frames it in the abdominal cavity.

The small intestine has three subdivisions: the **duodenum** (du″o-de′num; "twelve finger widths long"), the **jejunum** (je-joo′num: "empty"), and the **ileum** (il′e-um; "twisted intestine"), which contribute 5 percent, nearly 40 percent, and almost 60 percent of the length of the small intestine, respectively (see Figure 14.1). The ileum joins the large intestine at the ileocecal valve.

Chemical digestion of foods begins in earnest in the small intestine. The small intestine is able to process only a small amount of food at one time. The *pyloric sphincter* (literally, "gatekeeper") controls food movement into the small intestine from the stomach and prevents the small intestine from being overwhelmed. Though the C-shaped duodenum is the shortest subdivision of the small intestine, it has the most interesting features. Some enzymes are produced by the intestinal cells. More important are enzymes produced by the pancreas which are ducted into the duodenum through the **pancreatic ducts,** where they complete the chemical breakdown of foods in the small intestine. *Bile* (formed by the liver) also enters the duodenum through the **bile duct** in the same area (Figure 14.6). The main pancreatic and bile ducts join at the duodenum to form the flasklike *hepatopancreatic ampulla* (he-pah″to-pan-kre-a′tik am-pu′lah), literally, the "liver-pancreatic enlargement." From there, the bile and pancreatic juice travel through the *duodenal papilla* and enter the duodenum together.

Nearly all food absorption occurs in the small intestine. The small intestine is well suited for its function. Its wall has three structures that increase the absorptive surface tremendously—microvilli, villi, and circular folds (Figure 14.7). **Microvilli** (mi″kro-vih′lī) are tiny projections of the plasma membrane of the mucosa cells that give the cell surface a fuzzy appearance, sometimes referred to as the **brush border. Villi** are fingerlike projections of the mucosa that give it a velvety appearance and feel, much like the soft nap of a Turkish

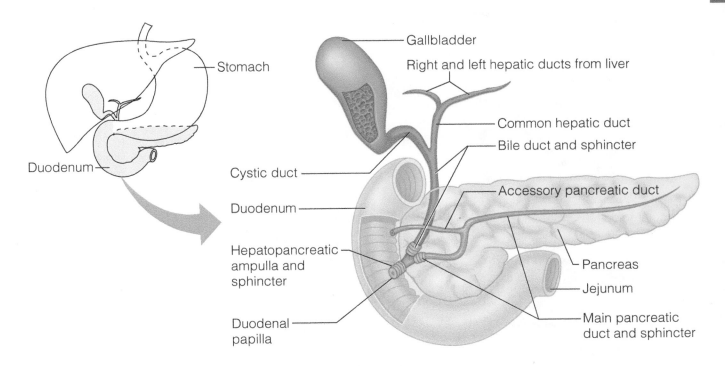

FIGURE 14.6   The duodenum of the small intestine and related organs.

towel. Within each villus is a rich capillary bed and a modified lymphatic capillary called a **lacteal.** The digested foodstuffs are absorbed through the mucosal cells into both the capillaries and the lacteal. **Circular folds,** also called **plicae circulares** (pli′se ser-ku-la′res), are deep folds of both mucosa and submucosa layers. Unlike the rugae of the stomach, the circular folds do not disappear when food fills the small intestine. All these structural modifications, which increase the surface area, decrease in number toward the end of the small intestine. On the other hand, local collections of lymphatic tissue (called **Peyer's patches**) found in the submucosa increase in number toward the end of the small intestine. This reflects the fact that the remaining (undigested) food residue in the intestine contains huge numbers of bacteria, which must be prevented from entering the bloodstream if at all possible.

Histological Organization of the Digestive Tract

The major layers of the digestive tract include (1) the *mucosa,* (2) the *submucosa,* (3) the *muscularis externa,* and (4) the *serosa.* The structure of these layers varies by region; Figure 14.8 is a composite view that most closely resembles the appearance of the small intestine, the longest segment of the digestive tract.

The Mucosa

The inner lining, or **mucosa,** of the digestive tract is a *mucous membrane* consisting of an epithelium, moistened by glandular secretions, and a *lamina propria* of areolar tissue.

The Digestive Epithelium   The mucosal epithelium is either simple or stratified, depending on its location and the stresses to which it is most often subjected. The oral cavity, pharynx, and esophagus (where mechanical stresses are most severe) are lined by a stratified squamous epithelium, whereas the stomach, the small intestine, and almost the entire length of the large intestine (where absorption occurs) have a simple columnar epithelium that contains goblet cells. Scattered among the columnar cells are **enteroendocrine cells,** which secrete hormones that coordinate the activities of the digestive tract and the accessory glands.

Q   *What is the functional value of the microvilli in the absorptive cells of the small intestine?*

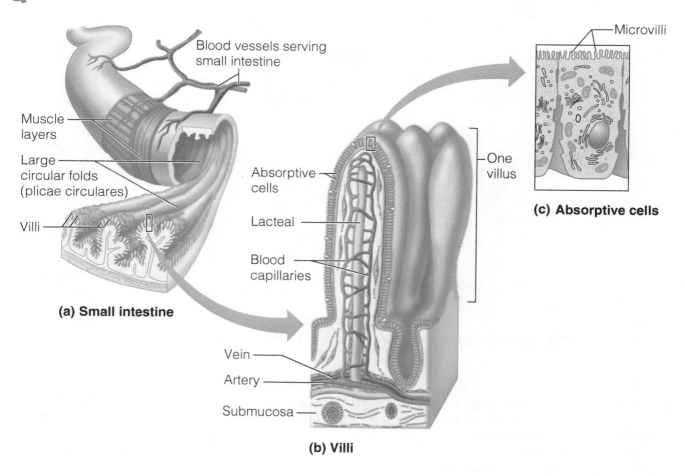

(a) Small intestine

Blood vessels serving small intestine

Muscle layers

Large circular folds (plicae circulares)

Villi

Absorptive cells

Lacteal

Blood capillaries

One villus

Microvilli

(c) Absorptive cells

Vein

Artery

Submucosa

(b) Villi

FIGURE 14.7   Structural modifications of the small intestine.
(a) Several circular folds (plicae circulares), seen on the inner surface of the small intestine. **(b)** Enlargement of one villus extension of the circular fold. **(c)** Enlargement of an absorptive cell to show microvilli (brush border).

The lining of the digestive tract is often thrown into longitudinal folds, which disappear as the tract fills, and permanent transverse folds, or *plicae* (PLĪ-sē; singular, *plica* [PLĪ-ka]) (see Figure 14.8). The folding dramatically increases the surface area available for absorption. The secretions of gland cells located in the mucosa and submucosa—or in accessory glandular organs—are carried to the epithelial surfaces by ducts.

A   *They tremendously increase the surface area available for absorption of digested foodstuffs.*

The Lamina Propria   The lamina propria consists of a layer of areolar tissue that also contains blood vessels, sensory nerve endings, lymphatic vessels, smooth muscle cells, and scattered areas of lymphoid tissue. In the oral cavity, pharynx, esophagus, stomach, and *duodenum* (the proximal portion of the small intestine), the lamina propria also contains the secretory cells of mucous glands.

In most areas of the digestive tract, the lamina propria contains a narrow band of smooth muscle and elastic fibers. This band is called the

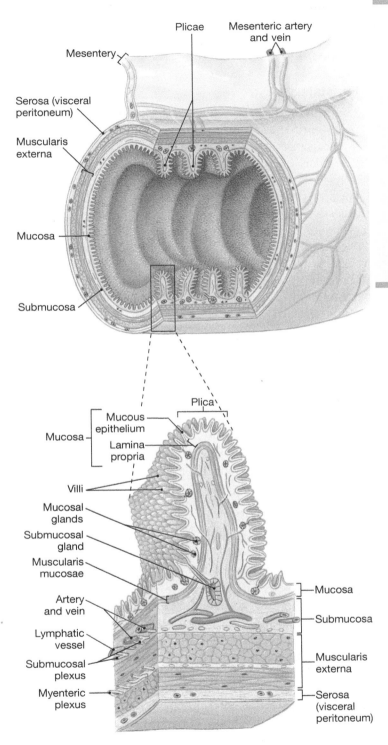

FIGURE 14.8 **The structure of the digestive tract.**
A diagrammatic view of a representative portion of the digestive tract. The features illustrated are typical of those of the small intestine.

Clinical Note

The life span of a typical epithelial cell varies from two to three days in the esophagus to up to six days in the large intestine. The lining of the entire digestive tract is continuously renewed through the divisions of epithelial stem cells, keeping pace with the rates of cell destruction and loss at epithelial surfaces. This high rate of cell division explains why radiation and anticancer drugs that inhibit mitosis have drastic effects on the digestive tract. Lost epithelial cells are no longer replaced, and the cumulative damage to the epithelial lining quickly leads to problems in absorbing nutrients. In addition, the exposure of the lamina propria to digestive enzymes can cause internal bleeding and other serious problems.

muscularis (mus-kū-LA-ris) **mucosae** (mū-KŌ-sē) (see Figure 14.8). The smooth muscle cells in the muscularis mucosae are arranged in two concentric layers. The inner layer encircles the lumen (the *circular muscle*), and the outer layer contains muscle cells oriented parallel to the long axis of the tract (the *longitudinal layer*). Contractions in these layers alter the shape of the lumen and move the epithelial pleats and folds.

The Submucosa

The **submucosa** is a layer of dense irregular connective tissue that surrounds the muscularis mucosae (see Figure 14.8). The submucosa has large blood vessels and lymphatic vessels, and in some regions it also contains exocrine glands that secrete buffers and enzymes into the lumen of the digestive tract. Along its outer margin, the submucosa contains a network of intrinisic nerve fibers and scattered neurons. This **submucosal plexus**, or *plexus of Meissner,* contains sensory neurons, parasympathetic ganglionic neurons, and sympathetic postganglionic fibers that innervate the mucosa and submucosa.

The Muscularis Externa

The submucosal plexus lies along the inner border

of the **muscularis externa,** a region dominated by smooth muscle cells. Like the smooth muscle cells in the muscularis mucosae, those in the muscularis externa are arranged in an inner circular layer and an outer longitudinal layer. These layers play an essential role in mechanical processing and in the movement of materials along the digestive tract. The movements are coordinated primarily by the sensory neurons, interneurons, and motor neurons of the enteric nervous system (ENS). The ENS is innervated primarily by the parasympathetic division of the ANS. Sympathetic postganglionic fibers also synapse here, although many continue onward to innervate the mucosa and the **myent-eric** (mī-en-TER-ik) **plexus** (*mys,* muscle + *enteron,* intestine), or *plexus of Auerbach.* This network of parasympathetic ganglia, sensory neurons, interneurons, and sympathetic postganglionic fibers lies sandwiched between the circular and longitudinal muscle layers. In general, parasympathetic stimulation increases muscle tone and activity; sympathetic stimulation promotes muscular inhibition and relaxation, helping to regulate the activities of the digestive tract.

The Serosa

Along most portions of the digestive tract inside the peritoneal cavity, the muscularis externa is covered by a serous membrane known as the **serosa** (see Figure 14.8). There is no serosa covering the muscularis externa of the oral cavity, pharynx, esophagus, and rectum, where a dense network of collagen fibers firmly attaches the digestive tract to adjacent structures. This fibrous sheath is called an *adventitia* (ad-ven-TISH-ē-uh).

The Movement of Digestive Materials

The muscular layers of the digestive tract consist of *visceral smooth muscle tissue,* a type of smooth muscle. The smooth muscle along the digestive tract has rhythmic cycles of activity due to the presence of *pacesetter cells.* These smooth muscle cells undergo spontaneous depolarization, triggering a wave of contraction that spreads throughout the entire muscular sheet. Pacesetter cells are located in the muscularis mucosae and muscularis externa, the layers of which surround the lumen of the digestive tract. The coordinated contractions of

the muscularis externa play a vital role in the movement of materials along the tract, through *peristalsis,* and in mechanical processing, through *segmentation.*

Peristalsis

The muscularis externa propels materials from one portion of the digestive tract to another by contractions known as **peristalsis** (per-i-STAL-sis). Peristalsis consists of waves of muscular contractions that move a **bolus** (BŌ-lus), or small oval mass of digestive contents, along the length of the digestive tract (Figure 14.9). During a peristaltic movement, the circular muscles contract behind the bolus while circular muscles ahead of the bolus relax. Longitudinal muscles ahead of the bolus then contract, shortening adjacent segments. A wave of contraction in the circular muscles then forces the bolus forward.

Segmentation

Most areas of the small intestine and some portions of the large intestine undergo cycles of contraction that churn and fragment the bolus, mixing the contents with intestinal secretions. This activity, called **segmentation**, does not follow a set pattern, and thus does not push materials along the tract in any one direction.

Large Intestine

The **large intestine** is much larger in diameter than the small intestine (thus its name, the *large* intestine) but shorter in length. About 1.5 m (5 feet) long, it extends from the ileocecal valve to the anus (Figure 14.10). Its major functions are to dry out the indigestible food residue by absorbing water and to eliminate these residues from the body as feces. It frames the small intestine on three sides and has the following subdivisions: **cecum** (se′kum), **appendix, colon, rectum,** and **anal canal.** The saclike cecum is the first part of the large intestine. Hanging from the cecum is the wormlike ("vermiform") appendix, a potential trouble spot. Since it is usually twisted, it is an ideal location for bacteria to accumulate and multiply. Inflammation of the appendix, *appendicitis,* is the usual result. The colon is divided into several distinct regions. The **ascending colon** travels up the right side of the abdominal cavity and

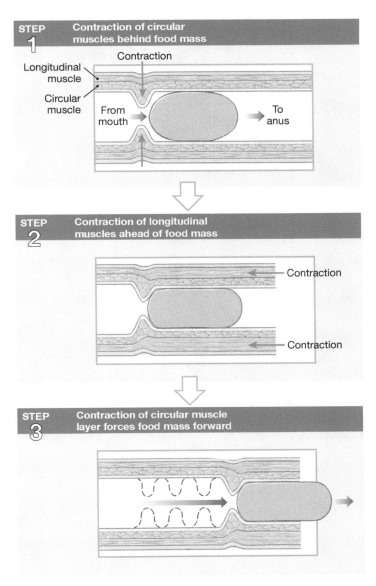

STEP 1 — Contraction of circular muscles behind food mass

Longitudinal muscle
Circular muscle
Contraction
From mouth
To anus

STEP 2 — Contraction of longitudinal muscles ahead of food mass

Contraction
Contraction

STEP 3 — Contraction of circular muscle layer forces food mass forward

FIGURE 14.9 Peristalsis. Peristalsis propels materials along the length of the digestive tract.

makes a turn, the *right colic* (or *hepatic*) *flexure,* to travel across the abdominal cavity as the **transverse colon.** It then turns again at the *left colic* (or *splenic*) *flexure,* and continues down the left side as the **descending colon,** to enter the pelvis, where it becomes the S-shaped **sigmoid** (sig'moid) **colon.** The sigmoid colon, rectum, and anal canal lie in the pelvis. The anal canal ends at the **anus** (a'nus), also called the **rectum,** which

opens to the exterior. The anal canal has an external *voluntary sphincter* (the **external anal sphincter**) composed of skeletal muscle and an internal *involuntary sphincter* formed by smooth muscle. These sphincters, which act rather like purse strings to open and close the anus, are ordinarily closed except during defecation, when feces are eliminated from the body.

Because most nutrient absorption has occurred before the large intestine is reached, no villi are seen in the large intestine, but there are tremendous numbers of *goblet cells* in its mucosa that produce an alkaline (HCO_3^--rich) mucus. The mucus acts as a lubricant to ease the passage of feces to the end of the digestive tract.

In the large intestine, the longitudinal muscle layer of the muscularis externa is reduced to three bands of muscle called *teniae coli* (ten'ne-e ko'li; "ribbons of the colon"). Since these muscle bands usually display some degree of tone (are partially contracted), they cause the wall to pucker into small pocketlike sacs called **haustra** (haws'trah).

Accessory Digestive Organs

Salivary Glands

Three pairs of **salivary glands** empty their secretions into the mouth. The large **parotid** (pah-rot'id) **glands** lie anterior to the ears. *Mumps,* a common childhood disease, is an inflammation of the parotid glands. If you look at the location of the parotid glands in Figure 14.1, you can readily understand why people with mumps complain that it hurts to open their mouth or chew.

The **submandibular glands** and the small **sublingual** (sub-ling'gwal) **glands** empty their secretions into the floor of the mouth through tiny ducts. The product of the salivary glands, **saliva,** is a mixture of mucus and serous fluids. The mucus moistens and helps to bind food together into a mass called a **bolus** (bo'lus), which makes chewing and swallowing easier. The clear serous portion contains an enzyme, **salivary amylase** (am'ĭ-lās), in a bicarbonate-rich (alkaline) juice that begins the process of starch digestion in the mouth. Saliva also contains substances such as lysozyme and antibodies (IgA) that inhibit bacteria; therefore, it has a protective function as well. Last but not least, saliva dissolves food chemicals so they can be tasted.

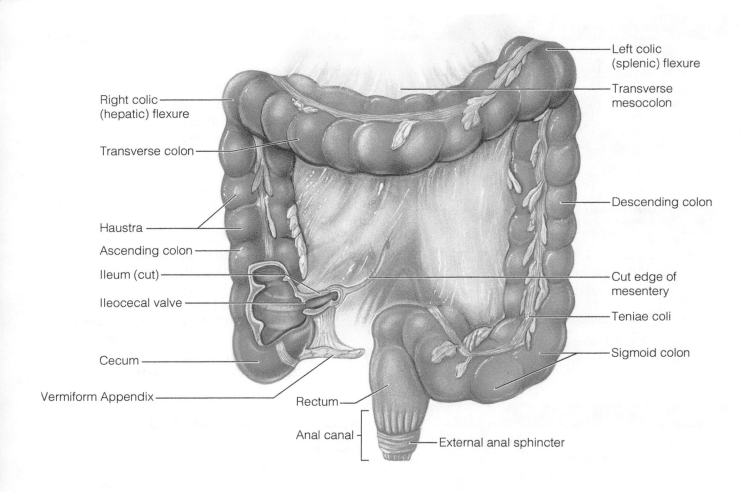

Right colic (hepatic) flexure

Transverse colon

Haustra

Ascending colon

Ileum (cut)

Ileocecal valve

Cecum

Vermiform Appendix

Left colic (splenic) flexure

Transverse mesocolon

Descending colon

Cut edge of mesentery

Teniae coli

Sigmoid colon

Rectum

Anal canal

External anal sphincter

FIGURE 14.10   The large intestine. A section of the cecum is removed to show the ileocecal valve.

Pancreas

The **pancreas** is a soft, pink, triangular gland that extends across the abdomen from the spleen to the duodenum (see Figures 14.1 and 14.6). Most of the pancreas lies posterior to the parietal peritoneum; hence its location is referred to as *retroperitoneal*.

The pancreas produces enzymes (described later) that break down all categories of digestible foods. The pancreatic enzymes are secreted into the duodenum in an alkaline fluid, which neutralizes the acidic chyme coming in from the stomach. The pancreas also has an endocrine function; it produces the hormones insulin and glucagon. Its

enzymes do most of the digestive work in the small intestine, breaking large molecules into small absorbable molecules.

Liver and Gallbladder

The **liver** is the largest gland in the body. It is located under the diaphragm, more to the right side of the body (see Figures 14.1 and 14.5). As described earlier, the liver overlies and almost completely covers the stomach. The liver has four lobes and is suspended from the diaphragm and abdominal wall by a delicate mesentery cord, the **falciform** (fal′si-form) **ligament.**

There is no question that the liver is one of the body's most important organs. It has many metabolic and regulatory roles; however, its digestive function is to produce **bile.** Bile leaves the liver through the **common hepatic duct** and enters the duodenum through the *bile duct* (see Figure 14.6).

Bile is a yellow-to-green, watery solution containing bile salts, bile pigments (chiefly bilirubin, a breakdown product of hemoglobin), cholesterol, phospholipids, and a variety of electrolytes. Of these components, only the bile salts (derived from cholesterol) and phospholipids aid the digestive process. Bile does not contain enzymes, but its bile salts **emulsify** fats by physically breaking large fat globules into smaller ones, thus providing more surface area for the fat-digesting enzymes to work on.

The **gallbladder** is a small, thin-walled green sac that snuggles in a shallow fossa in the inferior surface of the liver (see Figures 14.1 and 14.6). When food digestion is not occurring, bile backs up the **cystic duct** and enters the gallbladder to be stored. While being stored in the gallbladder, bile is concentrated by the removal of water. Later, when fatty food enters the duodenum, a hormonal stimulus prompts the gallbladder to contract and spurt out stored bile, making it available to the duodenum.

Homeostatic Imbalance

If bile is stored in the gallbladder for too long or too much water is removed, the cholesterol it contains may crystallize, forming *gallstones.* Since gallstones tend to be quite sharp, agonizing pain may occur when the gallbladder contracts (the typical *gallbladder attack*).

Blockage of the common hepatic or bile ducts (for example, by wedged gallstones) prevents bile from entering the small intestine, and it begins to accumulate and eventually backs up into the liver. This exerts pressure on the liver cells, and bile salts and bile pigments begin to enter the bloodstream. As the bile pigments circulate through the body, the tissues become yellow, or *jaundiced.* Blockage of the ducts is just one cause of jaundice. More often it results from actual liver problems such as *hepatitis* (an inflammation of the liver) or *cirrhosis* (sir-ro'sis), a chronic inflammatory condition in which the liver is severely damaged and becomes hard and fibrous. Hepatitis is most often due to viral infection resulting from drinking contaminated water or transmitted in blood via transfusion or contaminated needles. Cirrhosis is almost guaranteed when one drinks alcoholic beverages in excess for many years, and it is a common consequence of severe hepatitis. ▲

Functions of the Digestive System

Overview of Gastrointestinal Processes and Controls

The major functions of the digestive tract are usually summarized in two words—*digestion* and *absorption.* However, many of its specific activities (such as smooth muscle activity) and certain regulatory events are not really covered by either term. To describe digestive system processes a little more accurately, we really have to consider a few more functional terms. The essential activities of the GI tract include the following six processes, summarized in Figure 14.11.

1. **Ingestion**—Food must be placed into the mouth before it can be acted on. This is an active, voluntary process called ingestion.

2. **Propulsion**—If foods are to be processed by more than one digestive organ (and indeed they are), they must be propelled from one organ to the next. Swallowing is one example of food movement that depends largely on the propulsive process called **peristalsis.** Peristalsis is involuntary and involves alternating waves of contraction and relaxation of the muscles in the organ wall (Figure 14.12a). The net effect is to squeeze the food along the tract. Although **segmentation** (Figure 14.12b) may help to propel foodstuffs through the small intestine, it normally only moves food back and forth across the internal wall of the organ, serving to mix it with the digestive juices. Thus, segmentation is more an example of mechanical digestion than of propulsion.

3. **Food breakdown: mechanical digestion**— Mixing of food in the mouth by the tongue, churning of food in the stomach, and segmentation in the small intestine are all examples of processes contributing to mechanical digestion. Mechanical digestion prepares food for further

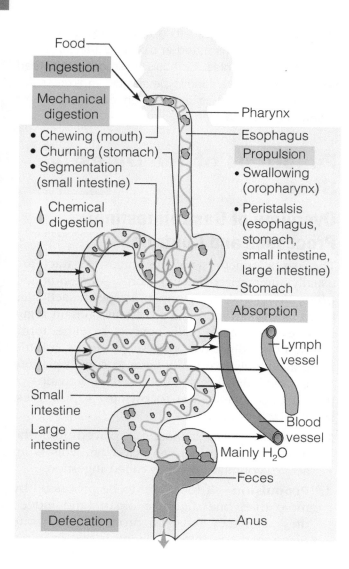

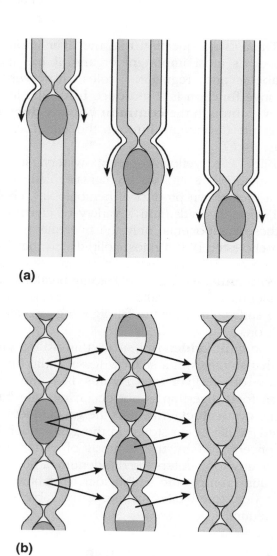

FIGURE 14.11 Schematic summary of gastrointestinal tract activities. Gastrointestinal tract activities include ingestion, mechanical digestion, chemical (enzymatic) digestion, propulsion, absorption, and defecation. Sites of chemical digestion are also sites that produce enzymes or that receive enzymes or other secretions made by accessory organs outside the alimentary canal. The mucosa of virtually the entire GI tract secretes mucus, which protects and lubricates.

FIGURE 14.12 Peristaltic and segmental movements of the digestive tract. (a) In peristalsis, adjacent or neighboring segments of the intestine (or other alimentary canal organs) alternately contract and relax, which moves food distally along the tract. **(b)** In segmentation, single segments of the intestine alternately contract and relax. Because active segments are separated by inactive ones, the food is moved forward and then backward. Thus the food is mixed rather than simply propelled along the tract.

degradation by enzymes by physically fragmenting the foods into smaller particles.

4. **Food breakdown: chemical digestion**—The sequence of steps in which large food molecules are broken down to their building blocks by enzymes (protein molecules that act as catalysts) is called chemical digestion. These

reactions are called **hydrolysis** reactions, because a water molecule is added to each bond to be broken. Water is also necessary as a dissolving medium and a softening agent for food digestion.

Since each of the major food groups has very different building blocks, it is worth taking a little time to review these chemical units. The building blocks, or units, of *carbohydrate* foods are *monosaccharides* (mon"o-sak'ah-rīdz), or simple sugars. We need to remember only three of these that are common in our diet—*glucose, fructose,* and *galactose.* Glucose is by far the most important, and when we talk about blood sugar levels, glucose is the "sugar" being referred to. Fructose is the most abundant sugar in fruits, and galactose is found in milk. Essentially, the only carbohydrates that our digestive system digests, or breaks down to simple sugars, are *sucrose* (table sugar), *lactose* (milk sugar), *maltose* (malt sugar), and *starch.* Sucrose, maltose, and lactose are referred to as *disaccharides,* or double sugars, because each consists of two simple sugars linked together. Starch is a *polysaccharide* (literally, "many sugars") formed of hundreds of glucose units. Although we eat foods containing other polysaccharides, such as *cellulose,* we do not have enzymes capable of breaking them down. The indigestible polysaccharides do not provide us with any nutrients, but they help move the foodstuffs along the gastrointestinal tract by providing bulk, or *fiber,* in our diet.

Proteins are digested to their building blocks, which are amino (ah-me'no) acids. Intermediate products of protein digestion are polypeptides and peptides. When lipids (fats) are digested, they yield two different types of building blocks—fatty acids and an alcohol called glycerol (glis'er-ol). The chemical breakdown of carbohydrates, proteins, and fats is summarized in Figure 14.13.

5. **Absorption**—Transport of digested end products from the lumen of the GI tract to the blood or lymph is absorption. For absorption to occur, the digested foods must first enter the mucosal cells by active or passive transport processes. The small intestine is the major absorptive site.

6. **Defecation**—Defecation is the elimination of indigestible residues from the GI tract via the anus in the form of feces (fe'sēz).

Some of these processes are the job of a single organ. For example, only the mouth ingests, and only the large intestine defecates. But most digestive system activities occur bit by bit as food is moved along the tract. Thus, in one sense, the digestive tract can be viewed as a "disassembly line" in which food is carried from one stage of its processing to the next, and its nutrients are made available to the cells in the body en route.

A point that has been stressed throughout this book has been the drive of the body to maintain a constant internal environment, particularly in terms of homeostasis of the blood, which comes into intimate contact with all body cells. The digestive system, however, creates an optimal environment for itself to function in the lumen (cavity) of the alimentary canal, an area that is actually *outside* the body. Conditions in that lumen are controlled so that digestive processes occur efficiently. Digestive activity is mostly controlled by reflexes via the parasympathetic division of the autonomic nervous system. (This is the "resting-and-digesting" arm.) The sensors (mechanoreceptors, chemoreceptors) involved in these reflexes are located in the walls of the alimentary canal organs and respond to a number of stimuli, the most important being stretch of the organ by food in its lumen, pH of the contents, and presence of certain breakdown products of digestion. When these receptors are activated, they start reflexes that activate or inhibit (1) the glands that secrete digestive juices into the lumen or hormones into the blood, and (2) the smooth muscles of the muscularis that mix and propel the foods along the tract.

Now that we have summarized some points that apply to the function of the digestive organs as a group, we are ready to look at their special capabilities.

Activities Occurring in the Mouth, Pharynx, and Esophagus

Teeth

The role of the teeth in food processing needs little introduction. We **masticate,** or *chew,* by opening and closing our jaws and moving them from side to side while continually using our tongue to move the food between our teeth. In the process, the teeth tear and grind the food, breaking it down into smaller fragments.

Ordinarily, by the age of 21, two sets of teeth have been formed (Figure 14.14). The first set is the **deciduous** (de-sid'u-us) **teeth,** also called **baby teeth** or **milk teeth.** The deciduous teeth begin to erupt around six months, and a baby has a full set (20 teeth) by the age of 2 years. The first

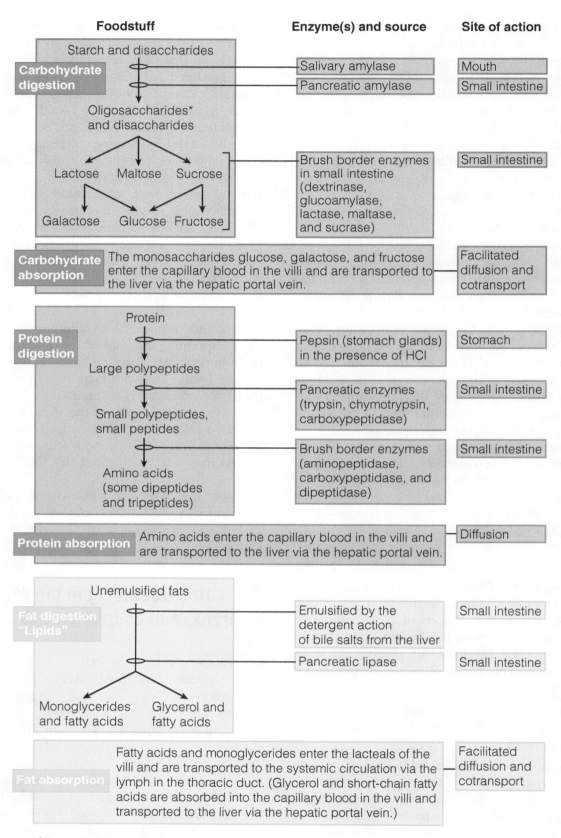

FIGURE 14.13   **Flowchart of chemical digestion and absorption of foodstuffs.**

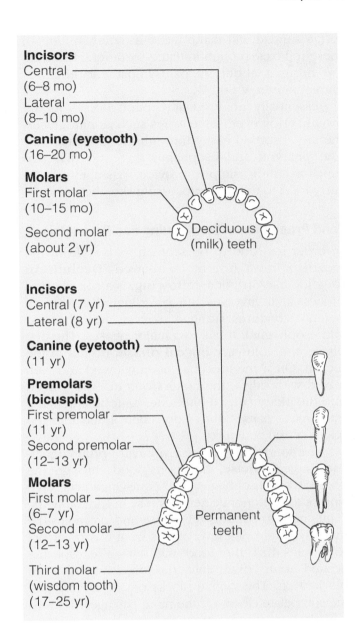

Incisors
Central
(6–8 mo)
Lateral
(8–10 mo)
Canine (eyetooth)
(16–20 mo)
Molars
First molar
(10–15 mo)
Second molar
(about 2 yr)

Deciduous
(milk) teeth

Incisors
Central (7 yr)
Lateral (8 yr)
Canine (eyetooth)
(11 yr)
**Premolars
(bicuspids)**
First premolar
(11 yr)
Second premolar
(12–13 yr)
Molars
First molar
(6–7 yr)
Second molar
(12–13 yr)
Third molar
(wisdom tooth)
(17–25 yr)

Permanent
teeth

FIGURE 14.14   Human deciduous and permanent teeth. Approximate time of tooth eruption is shown in parentheses. Since the same number and arrangement of teeth exist in both upper and lower jaws, only the lower jaw is shown in each case. The shapes of individual teeth are shown on the right.

teeth to appear are the lower central incisors, an event that is usually anxiously awaited by the child's parents.

As the second set of teeth, the deeper **permanent teeth,** enlarge and develop, the roots of

the milk teeth are reabsorbed, and between the ages of 6 and 12 years they loosen and fall out. All of the permanent teeth but the third molars have erupted by the end of adolescence. The third molars, also called *wisdom teeth,* emerge later, between the ages of 17 and 25. Although there are 32 permanent teeth in a full set, the wisdom teeth often fail to erupt; sometimes they are completely absent.

◢ Homeostatic Imbalance

When teeth remain embedded in the jawbone, they are said to be *impacted.* Impacted teeth exert pressure and cause a good deal of pain and must be removed surgically. Wisdom teeth are the most commonly impacted. ◢

The teeth are classified according to shape function as incisors, canines, premolars, and molars (see Figure 14.14). The chisel-shaped **incisors** are adapted for cutting; the fanglike **canines** (eyeteeth) are for tearing or piercing. The **premolars** (bicuspids) and **molars** have broad crowns with rounded cusps (tips) and are best suited for grinding.

A tooth consists of two major regions, the **crown** and the **root,** as shown in Figure 14.15. The enamel-covered crown is the exposed part of the tooth above the **gingiva** (jin-ji'vah), or **gum. Enamel** is the hardest substance in the body and is fairly brittle because it is heavily mineralized with calcium salts. The portion of the tooth embedded in the jawbone is the root; the root and crown are connected by the tooth region called the **neck.** The outer surface of the root is covered by a substance called **cementum,** which attaches the tooth to the **periodontal** (per"e-o-don'tal) **membrane (ligament).** This ligament holds the tooth in place in the bony jaw. **Dentin,** a bonelike material, underlies the enamel and forms the bulk of the tooth. It surrounds a central **pulp cavity,** which contains a number of structures (connective tissue, blood vessels, and nerve fibers) collectively called **pulp.** Pulp supplies nutrients to the tooth tissues and provides for tooth sensations. Where the pulp cavity extends into the root, it becomes the **root canal,** which provides a route for blood vessels, nerves, and other pulp structures to enter the pulp cavity of the tooth.

Q *What substance forms the bulk of the tooth?*

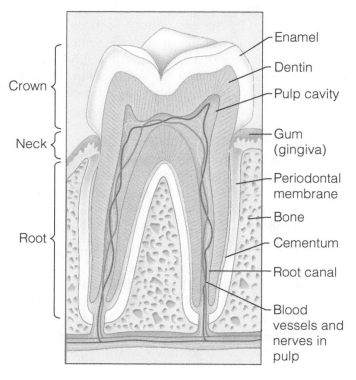

Crown

Neck

Root

— Enamel

— Dentin

— Pulp cavity

— Gum (gingiva)

— Periodontal membrane

— Bone

— Cementum

— Root canal

— Blood vessels and nerves in pulp

FIGURE 14.15 Longitudinal section of a molar.

Food Ingestion and Breakdown

Once food has been placed in the mouth, both mechanical and chemical digestion begin. First the food is *physically* broken down into smaller particles by chewing. Then, as the food is mixed with saliva, salivary amylase begins the *chemical* digestion of starch, breaking it down into maltose (Figure 14.13). The next time you eat a piece of bread, chew it for a few minutes before swallowing it. You will notice that it begins to taste sweet as the sugars are released.

Saliva is normally secreted continuously to keep the mouth moist; but, when food enters the mouth, much larger amounts of saliva pour out. However, the simple pressure of anything put in the mouth and chewed, such as rubber bands or sugarless gum, will also stimulate the release of saliva. Some emotional stimuli can also cause salivation. For example, the mere thought of a hot

A

Dentin.

fudge sundae will make many a mouth water. All these reflexes, though initiated by different stimuli, are brought about by parasympathetic fibers in cranial nerves V and IX.

Essentially no food absorption occurs in the mouth. (However, some drugs such as nitroglycerine are absorbed easily through the oral mucosa.) The pharynx and esophagus have no digestive function; they simply provide passageways to carry food to the next processing site, the stomach.

Food Propulsion—Swallowing and Peristalsis

In order for food to be sent on its way from the mouth, it must first be swallowed. **Deglutition** (deg″loo-tish′un), or **swallowing,** is a complicated process that involves the coordinated activity of several structures (tongue, soft palate, pharynx, and esophagus). It has two major phases. The first phase, the voluntary **buccal phase,** occurs in the mouth. Once the food has been chewed and well mixed with saliva, the bolus (food mass) is forced into the pharynx by the tongue. As food enters the pharynx, it passes out of our control and into the realm of reflex activity.

The second phase, the involuntary **pharyngeal-esophageal phase,** transports food through the pharynx and esophagus. The parasympathetic division of the autonomic nervous system (primarily the vagus nerves) controls this phase and promotes the mobility of the digestive organs from this point on. All routes that the food might take except the desired route distal into the digestive tract are blocked off. The tongue blocks off the mouth, and the soft palate closes off the nasal passages. The larynx rises so that its opening (into the respiratory passageways) is covered by the flaplike epiglottis. Food is moved through the pharynx and then into the esophagus below by wavelike peristaltic contractions of their muscular walls—first the longitudinal muscles contract, and then the circular muscles contract. The events of the swallowing process are illustrated in Figure 14.16.

If we try to talk while swallowing, our routing mechanisms may be "short-circuited," and food may manage to enter the respiratory passages. This triggers still another protective reflex—coughing—during which air rushes upward from the lungs in an attempt to expel the food.

Once food reaches the distal end of the esophagus, it presses against the cardioesophageal

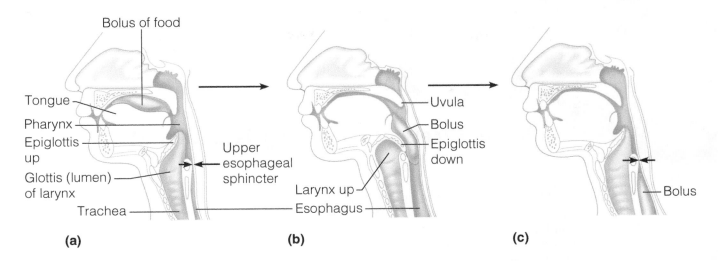

Bolus of food

Tongue
Pharynx
Epiglottis up
Glottis (lumen) of larynx
Trachea

Upper esophageal sphincter

Uvula
Bolus
Epiglottis down
Larynx up
Esophagus

Bolus

(a)   **(b)**   **(c)**

FIGURE 14.16   Swallowing. (a) The tongue pushes the food bolus posteriorly and against the soft palate. **(b)** The soft palate rises to close off the nasal passages as the bolus enters the pharynx. The larynx rises so that the epiglottis covers its opening as peristalsis carries the food through the pharynx and into the esophagus. The upper esophageal sphincter relaxes to allow food entry. **(c)** The upper esophageal sphincter contracts again as the larynx and epiglottis return to their former positions and the food bolus moves inferiorly to the stomach.

sphincter, causing it to open, and the food enters the stomach. The movement of food through the pharynx and esophagus is so automatic that a person can swallow and food will reach the stomach even if he is standing on his head. Gravity plays no part in the transport of food once it has left the mouth, which explains why astronauts (in the zero gravity of outer space) can still swallow and get nourishment.

Regulation of Gastric Activities

Food Breakdown

Secretion of **gastric juice** is regulated by both neural and hormonal factors. The sight, smell, and taste of food stimulate parasympathetic nervous system reflexes (the vagas nerve and synapse in the sub-mucosal plexus), which increase the secretion of gastric juice by the stomach glands. In addition, the presence of food and a falling pH in the stomach stimulate the stomach cells to release the hormone **gastrin.** Gastrin prods the stomach glands to produce still more of the protein-digesting enzymes (pepsinogens), mucus, and hydrochloric acid. Under normal conditions, 2 to 3 liters of gastric juice are produced every day.

Hydrochloric acid makes the stomach contents very acidic. This is (somewhat) dangerous since both hydrochloric acid and the protein-digesting enzymes have the ability to digest the stomach itself, causing *ulcers* (see the "A Closer Look" box a little later in this chapter). However, as long as enough mucus is made, the stomach is "safe" and will remain unharmed.

Homeostatic Imbalance

Occasionally, the cardioesophageal sphincter fails to close tightly and gastric juice backs up into the esophagus, which has little mucus protection. This results in a characteristic pain known as *heartburn,* which, if uncorrected, leads to inflammation of the esophagus (*esophagitis* [ĕ-sof'ah-ji'tis]) and perhaps even to ulceration of the esophagus. A common cause is a *hiatal hernia*, a structural abnormality in which the superior part of the stomach protrudes slightly above the diaphragm. Since the diaphragm no longer reinforces the cardioesophageal sphincter, which is a weak sphincter to begin with, gastric juice flows into the unprotected esophagus. Conservative treatment involves restricting food intake after the evening meal, taking antacids, and sleeping with the head elevated. ▲

A Closer Look

Peptic Ulcers: "Something Is Eating at Me"

ARCHIE, a 53-year-old factory worker, began to experience a gnawing pain in his upper abdomen an hour or two after each meal. At first, he blamed the quality of his home cooking, but he experienced the same symptoms after eating at the factory cafeteria or at restaurants. Archie always responded to stress by drinking and smoking heavily, and his abdominal pain became markedly worse during a hectic week when he worked 15 hours of overtime on the assembly line. Finally, after two months of increasingly severe pain, Archie consulted a physician and was told that he had a peptic ulcer.

Peptic ulcers affect one of every eight Americans. A peptic ulcer is a craterlike erosion in the mucosa of any part of the GI tract that is exposed to the secretions of the stomach. Hydrochloric acid and pepsin cause this damage; people whose stomachs fail to secrete these substances never develop peptic ulcers. A few peptic ulcers occur in the lower esophagus, following the regurgitation of stomach contents, but most (98 percent) occur in the pyloric part of the stomach (gastric ulcers) or the first part of the duodenum (duodenal ulcers). Duodenal ulcers are about three times more common than gastric ulcers. Peptic ulcers may appear at any age, but they develop most frequently between the ages of 50 and 70 years. After developing, they tend to recur—healing, then flaring up periodically—for the rest of one's life if not treated.

Gastric and duodenal ulcers may produce a gnawing or burning pain in the epigastric region of the abdomen. This pain often appears one to three hours after a meal (or causes one to awaken at night) and is relieved by eating. Other potential symptoms include loss of appetite, burping, nausea, and vomiting. Not all people with ulcers experience the above symptoms, however, and many exhibit no symptoms at all.

Despite years of intensive study, the cause of peptic ulcers remains incompletely understood. For over a century, it has been "common knowledge" that stress causes ulcers, and the stereotypical ulcer patient has been the overworked business executive. Recent studies have not been able to demonstrate such a link between stress and ulcers, however, and many researchers now doubt the validity of this claim. Nonetheless, a stressful lifestyle does seem to *aggravate* existing ulcers. Recent studies indicate that many ulcers are actually caused by a strain of acid-resistant bacteria *(Helicobacter pylori)* that inhabit the stomachs of 40 percent of healthy people and 70 to 90 percent of those with ulcers.

The anatomy of a peptic ulcer is shown in the figure in this box. It is a round, sharply defined crater in the mucosa. Typical ulcers are 1 to 4 cm in diameter. The base of the ulcer contains dead tissue cells, granulation tissue, and scar tissue. Eroded blood vessels may sometimes be seen there as well.

Peptic ulcers can produce serious complications. In about 20 percent of cases, eroded blood vessels bleed into the GI tract, causing vomiting of blood and blood in the feces. In such cases, anemia may result from a severe loss of blood. In 5 to 10 percent of ulcer patients, scarring within the stomach obstructs the pyloric opening, blocking digestion. About 5 percent of peptic ulcers *perforate*, allowing the contents of

Peptic Ulcers: "Something Is Eating at Me" *(continued)*

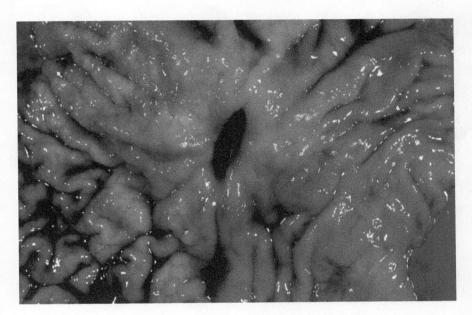

A peptic ulcer.

the stomach or duodenum to leak into the peritoneal cavity. This can cause either peritonitis or digestion and destruction of the nearby pancreas. A perforated ulcer is a life-threatening condition.

In spite of these potential complications, most peptic ulcers heal readily and respond well to treatment. The first steps in treatment are to avoid smoking, alcohol, ibuprofen, and aspirin, all of which aggravate ulcers. Antacid drugs are often suggested to neutralize the stomach acids. In ulcers found to be colonized by *H. pylori,* the goal is to kill the embedded bacteria. Triple drug therapy (a combination of the antibiotics tetracycline and metronidazole, and bismuth subsalicylate, the active ingredient in Pepto-Bismol) effectively promotes healing and prevents recurrence, even in resistant strains. In other cases *H. pylori* is not the cause, such as in esophageal ulcers, which are caused by gastric reflux. Then the therapy of choice is drugs that inhibit HCl secretion (H_2 blockers) such as ranitidine (Zantac). These drugs cure the ulcer by decreasing the production of acid and pepsin.

Recent animal trials using a newly developed vaccine against *H. pylori* have been successful. It is hoped that preventative vaccination, coupled with antibiotic cures, will eradicate peptic ulcers within the next 25 years.

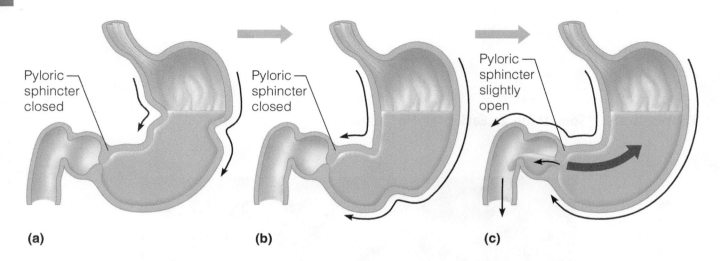

Pyloric sphincter closed

Pyloric sphincter closed

Pyloric sphincter slightly open

(a)   (b)   (c)

FIGURE 14.17   Peristaltic waves act primarily in the inferior portion of the stomach to mix and move chyme through the pyloric valve.
(a) Peristaltic waves move toward the pylorus. **(b)** The most vigorous peristalsis and mixing action occurs close to the pylorus. **(c)** The pyloric end of the stomach acts as a pump that delivers small amounts of chyme into the duodenum while forcing most of the contained material backward into the stomach, where it undergoes further mixing.

The extremely acidic environment that hydrochloric acid provides *is* necessary, because it activates *pepsinogen* to *pepsin,* the active protein-digesting enzyme. *Rennin,* the second protein-digesting enzyme produced by the stomach, works primarily on milk protein and converts it to a substance that looks like sour milk. Many mothers mistakenly think that when their infants spit up a curdy substance after having their bottle that the milk has soured in their stomach. Rennin is produced in large amounts in infants, but it is not believed to be produced in adults.

Other than the beginning of protein digestion, little chemical digestion occurs in the stomach. With the exception of aspirin and alcohol (which seem somehow to have a "special pass"), virtually no absorption occurs through the stomach walls.

As food enters and fills the stomach, its wall begins to stretch (at the same time the gastric juices are being secreted, as just described). Then the three muscle layers of the stomach wall become active. They compress and pummel the food, breaking it apart physically, all the while continually mixing the food with the enzyme-containing gastric juice so that the semifluid chyme is formed. The process looks something like the preparation of a cake mix, in which the floury mixture is

continually folded on itself and mixed with the liquid until it reaches uniform texture.

Food Propulsion

Once the food has been well mixed, a rippling peristalsis begins in the lower half of the stomach, and the contractions increase in force as the pyloric valve is approached. The pylorus of the stomach, which holds about 30 ml of chyme, acts like a meter that allows only liquids and very small particles to pass through the pyloric sphincter (Figure 14.17). Because the pyloric sphincter barely opens, each contraction of the stomach muscle squirts 3 ml or less of chyme into the small intestine. Since the contraction also *closes* the valve, the rest (about 27 ml) is propelled backward into the stomach for more mixing. When the duodenum is filled with chyme and its wall is stretched, a nervous reflex, the *enterogastric* (en"ter-o-gas'trik) *reflex,* occurs. This reflex "puts the brakes on" gastric activity and slows the emptying of the stomach by inhibiting the vagus nerves and tightening the pyloric sphincter, thus allowing time for intestinal processing to catch up. Generally, it takes about 4 hours for the stomach to empty completely after eating a well-balanced meal and 6 hours or more if the meal has a high fat content.

Homeostatic Imbalance

Local irritation of the stomach, such as occurs with bacterial food poisoning, may activate the *emetic* (ē-met′ik) *center* in the brain (medulla). The emetic center, in turn, causes **vomiting (emesis).** Vomiting is essentially a reverse peristalsis occurring in the stomach (and perhaps the small intestine), accompanied by contraction of the abdominal muscles and the diaphragm, which increases the pressure on the abdominal organs. The emetic center may also be activated through other pathways; disturbance of the equilibrium apparatus of the inner ear during a boat ride on rough water is one example. ▲

Activities of the Small Intestine

Food Breakdown and Absorption

Food reaching the small intestine is only partially digested. Carbohydrate and protein digestion have been started, but virtually no fats have been digested up to this point. Here the process of chemical food digestion is accelerated as the food now takes a rather wild 3- to 6-hour journey through the looping coils and twists of the small intestine. By the time the food reaches the end of the small intestine, digestion is complete and nearly all food absorption has occurred.

The microvilli of small intestine cells bear a few important enzymes, the so-called **brush border enzymes** that break down double sugars into simple sugars and complete protein digestion (see Figure 14.13). *Intestinal juice* itself is relatively enzyme-poor, and protective mucus is probably the most important intestinal gland secretion. However, foods entering the small intestine are literally deluged with enzyme-rich **pancreatic juice** ducted in from the pancreas, as well as bile from the liver.

Pancreatic juice contains enzymes that (1) along with brush border enzymes, complete the digestion of starch *(pancreatic amylase);* (2) carry out about half of protein digestion (via the action of *trypsin, chymotrypsin, carboxypeptidase,* and others); (3) are totally responsible for fat digestion since the pancreas is essentially the only source of *lipases;* and (4) digest nucleic acids *(nucleases).*

In addition to enzymes, pancreatic juice contains a rich supply of bicarbonate, which makes it very basic (about pH 8). When pancreatic juice reaches the small intestine, it neutralizes the acidic chyme coming in from the stomach and provides the proper environment for activation and activity of intestinal and pancreatic digestive enzymes.

Homeostatic Imbalance

Pancreatitis (pan″kre-ah-ti′tis) is a rare but extremely serious inflammation of the pancreas that results from activation of pancreatic enzymes in the pancreatic duct. Since pancreatic enzymes break down all categories of biological molecules, the pancreatic tissue and duct are digested. This painful condition can lead to nutritional deficiencies, because pancreatic enzymes are essential to digestion in the small intestine. ▲

The release of pancreatic juice into the duodenum is stimulated by both the vagus nerves and local hormones. When chyme enters the small intestine, it stimulates the mucosa cells to produce several hormones (Table 14.1). Two of these hormones, **secretin** (se-kre′tin) and **cholecystokinin** (ko″le-sis″to-kin′in) **(CCK),** influence the release of pancreatic juice and bile.

The hormones enter the blood and circulate to their target organs, the pancreas, liver, and gallbladder. Both hormones work together to stimulate the pancreas to release its enzyme- and bicarbonate-rich product (Figure 14.18). In addition, secretin causes the liver to increase its output of bile, and cholecystokinin causes the gallbladder to contract and release stored bile into the bile duct so that bile and pancreatic juice enter the small intestine together. As mentioned before, bile is not an enzyme. Instead, it acts like a detergent to emulsify, or mechanically break down, large fat globules into thousands of tiny ones, providing a much greater surface area for the pancreatic lipases to work on. Bile is also necessary for absorption of fats (and other fat-soluble vitamins [K, D, and A] that are absorbed along with them) from the intestinal tract.

Homeostatic Imbalance

If *either* bile or pancreatic juice is absent, essentially no fat digestion or absorption goes on, and fatty, bulky stools are the result. In such cases, blood-clotting problems also occur because the liver needs vitamin K to make prothrombin, one of the clotting factors. ▲

TABLE 14.1   Hormones and Hormonelike Products That Act in Digestion

Hormone	Source	Stimulus for secretion	Action
Gastrin	Stomach	Food in stomach (chemical stimulus)	• Stimulates release of gastric juice • Stimulates mobility of small intestine • Relaxes ileocecal valve.
Histamine	Stomach	Food in stomach	• Activates parietal cells to secrete hydrochloric acid.
Somatostatin	Stomach	Food in stomach	• Inhibits secretion of gastric juice and pancreatic juice • Inhibits emptying of stomach and gallbladder.
Secretin	Duodenum	Acidic chyme and partially digested foods in duodenum	• Increases output of pancreatic juice rich in bicarbonate ions • Increases bile output by liver • Inhibits gastric mobility and gastric gland secretion.
Cholecystokinin (CCK)	Duodenum	Fatty chyme and partially digested proteins in duodenum	• Increases output of enzyme-rich pancreatic juice • Stimulates gallbladder to expel stored bile • Relaxes sphincter of duodenal papilla to allow bile and pancreatic juice to enter the duodenum.
Gastric inhibitory peptide (GIP) "enterogastrone"	Duodenum	Fatty chyme in duodenum	• Inhibits gastric mobility and secretion of gastric juice.

Absorption of water and of the end products of digestion occurs all along the length of the small intestine. Most substances are absorbed through the intestinal cell plasma membranes by the process of *active transport*. Then they enter the capillary beds in the villi to be transported in the blood to the liver via the hepatic portal vein. The exception seems to be lipids, or fats, which are absorbed passively by the process of *diffusion*. Lipid breakdown products enter both the capillary beds and the lacteals in the villi and are carried to the liver by both blood and lymphatic fluids.

At the end of the ileum, all that remains is some water, indigestible food materials (plant fibers such as cellulose), and large amounts of bacteria. This debris enters the large intestine through the ileocecal valve. The complete process of food digestion and absorption is summarized in Figure 14.13

Food Propulsion

As mentioned previously, **peristalsis** is the major means of propelling food through the digestive tract. It involves waves of contraction that move along the length of the intestine, followed by waves of relaxation. The net effect is that the food is moved through the small intestine in much the same way that toothpaste is squeezed from a tube. Rhythmic segmental movements produce local

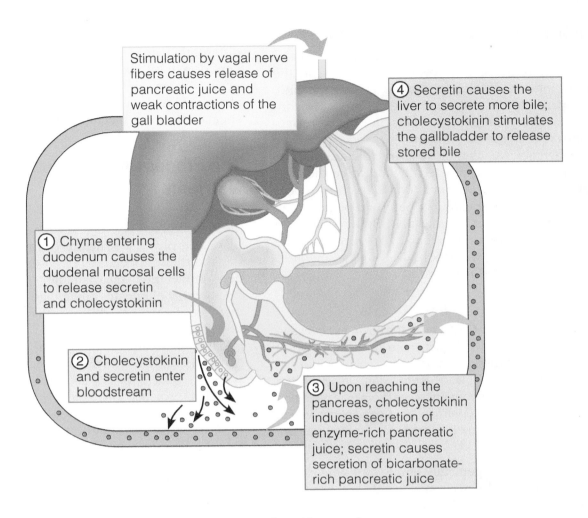

Stimulation by vagal nerve fibers causes release of pancreatic juice and weak contractions of the gall bladder

④ Secretin causes the liver to secrete more bile; cholecystokinin stimulates the gallbladder to release stored bile

① Chyme entering duodenum causes the duodenal mucosal cells to release secretin and cholecystokinin

② Cholecystokinin and secretin enter bloodstream

③ Upon reaching the pancreas, cholecystokinin induces secretion of enzyme-rich pancreatic juice; secretin causes secretion of bicarbonate-rich pancreatic juice

FIGURE 14.18   Regulation of pancreatic juice secretion. Hormonal controls, exerted by secretin and cholecystokinin (steps 1–3), are the main regulatory factors. Neural control is mediated by the vagus nerves.

constrictions of the intestine (see Figure 14.12b) that mix the chyme with the digestive juices, and help to propel food through the intestine. **Pendular movements,** which are longitudinal contractions of the smooth muscle of the small intestine, also assist in the propulsion of food.

Activities of the Large Intestine

Food Breakdown and Absorption

What is finally delivered to the large intestine contains few nutrients, but that residue still has 12 to 24 hours more to spend there. The colon itself produces no digestive enzymes. However, the "resident" bacteria that live within its lumen metabolize some of the remaining nutrients, releasing gases (methane and hydrogen sulfide) that contribute to the odor of feces. About 500 ml of gas (flatus) is produced each day, much more when certain carbohydrate-rich foods (such as beans) are eaten.

Bacteria residing in the large intestine also make some vitamins (vitamin K and some B vitamins). Absorption by the large intestine is limited to the absorption of these vitamins, some ions, and most of the remaining water. **Feces,** the more or less solid product delivered to the rectum, contain undigested food residues, mucus, millions of bacteria, and just enough water to allow their smooth passage.

Propulsion of the Residue and Defecation

Peristalsis and mass movements are the two major types of propulsive movements occurring in the large intestine. Colon peristalsis is sluggish and, compared to the mass movements, probably contributes very little to propulsion. **Mass movements** are long, slow-moving but powerful contractile waves that move over large areas of the colon three or four times daily and force the contents toward the rectum. Typically, they occur during or just after eating, when food begins to fill the stomach and small intestine. Bulk, or fiber, in the diet increases the strength of colon contractions and softens the stool, allowing the colon to act as a well-oiled machine.

Homeostatic Imbalance

When the diet lacks bulk, the colon narrows and its circular muscles contract more powerfully, which increases the pressure on its walls. This encourages formation of *diverticula* (di"ver-tik'u-lah), in which the mucosa protrudes through the colon walls, a condition called *diverticulosis. Diverticulitis,* a condition in which the diverticula become inflamed, can be life-threatening if ruptures occur. ▲

The rectum is generally empty, but when feces are forced into it by mass movements and its wall is stretched, the **defecation reflex** is initiated. The defecation reflex is a spinal (sacral region) reflex that causes the walls of the sigmoid colon and the rectum to contract and the anal sphincters to relax. As the feces are forced through the anal canal, messages reach the brain giving us time to make a decision as to whether the external voluntary sphincter should remain open or be constricted to stop passage of feces. If it is not convenient, defecation (or "moving the bowels") can be delayed temporarily. Within a few seconds, the reflex contractions end and the rectal walls relax. With the next mass movement, the defecation reflex is initiated again.

Digestion and Absorption

Now that we've examined the mechanical process of food ingestion and breakdown, let's take a closer look at how the body digests and absorbs the nutrients it needs.

A typical meal contains carbohydrates, proteins, lipids, water, electrolytes, and vitamins. The digestive system handles each component differently. Large organic molecules must be broken down by digestion before absorption can occur. Water, electrolytes, and vitamins can be absorbed without preliminary processing, but special transport mechanisms may be involved.

The Processing and Absorption of Nutrients

Food contains large organic molecules, many of them insoluble. The digestive system first breaks down the physical structure of the ingested material and then proceeds to disassemble the component molecules into smaller fragments. This disassembly eliminates any antigenic properties, so that the fragments do not trigger an immune response after absorption. The molecules released into the bloodstream are absorbed by cells and either (1) broken down to provide energy for the synthesis of ATP or (2) used to synthesize carbohydrates, proteins, and lipids. This section focuses on the mechanics of digestion and absorption.

Most ingested organic materials are complex chains of simpler molecules. In a typical dietary carbohydrate, the basic molecules are simple sugars; in a protein, the building blocks are amino acids; in lipids, they are generally fatty acids; and in nucleic acids, they are nucleotides. Digestive enzymes break the bonds between the component molecules of carbohydrates, proteins, lipids, and nucleic acids in a process called *hydrolysis.*

The classes of digestive enzymes differ with respect to their targets. *Carbohydrases* break the bonds between simple sugars, *proteases* split the linkages between amino acids, and *lipases* separate fatty acids from glycerides. Some enzymes in each class are even more selective, breaking bonds between specific molecules. For example, a particular carbohydrase might break the bond between two glucose molecules, but not those between glucose and another simple sugar.

Digestive enzymes secreted by the salivary glands, tongue, stomach, and pancreas are mixed into the ingested material as it passes along the digestive tract. These enzymes break down large carbohydrates, proteins, lipids, and nucleic acids into smaller fragments, which in turn must typically be broken down further before absorption can occur. The final enzymatic steps involve brush border enzymes, which are attached to the exposed surfaces of microvilli.

Nucleic acids are broken down into their component nucleotides. Brush border enzymes digest these nucleotides into sugars, phosphates, and nitrogenous bases that are absorbed by active transport. However, nucleic acids represent only a small fraction of all the nutrients absorbed each day. Table 14.2 summarizes the major digestive enzymes and their functions. Next we take a closer look at the digestion and absorption of carbohydrates, lipids, and proteins.

Carbohydrate Digestion and Absorption

The digestion of complex carbohydrates (simple polysaccharides and starches) proceeds in two steps. One step involves carbohydrases produced by the salivary glands and pancreas; the other, brush border enzymes.

The Actions of Salivary and Pancreatic Enzymes

The digestion of complex carbohydrates involves two enzymes—salivary amylase and pancreatic

TABLE 14.2   Digestive Enzymes and Their Functions

Enzyme (proenzyme)	Source	Optimal pH	Target	Products	Remarks
CARBOHYDRASES					
Maltase, sucrase, lactase	Brush border of small intestine	7–8	Maltose, sucrose, lactose	Monosaccharides	Found in membrane surface of microvilli
Pancreatic alpha-amylase	Pancreas	6.7–7.5	Complex carbohydrates	Disaccharides and trisaccharides	Breaks bonds between simple sugars
Salivary amylase	Salivary glands	6.7–7.5	Complex carbohydrates	Disaccharides and trisaccharides	Breaks bonds between simple sugars
PROTEASES					
Carboxypeptidase (procarboxypeptidase)	Pancreas	7–8	Proteins, polypeptides, amino acids	Short-chain peptides	Activated by trypsin
Chymotrypsin (chymotrypsinogen)	Pancreas	7–8	Proteins, polypeptides	Short-chain peptides	Activated by trypsin
Dipeptidases, peptidases	Brush border of small intestine	7–8	Dipeptides, tripeptides	Amino acids	Found in membrane surface of brush border
Elastase (proelastase)	Pancreas	7–8	Elastin	Short-chain peptides	Activated by trypsin
Enterokinase	Brush border and lumen of small intestine	7–8	Trypsinogen	Trypsin	Reaches lumen through disintegration of shed epithelial cells
Pepsin (pepsinogen)	Chief cells of stomach	1.5–2.0	Proteins, polypeptides	Short-chain polypeptides	Secreted as proenzyme pepsinogen; activated by H$^+$ in stomach acid
Rennin	Stomac	3.5–4.0	Milk proteins		Secreted only in infants; causes protein coagulation

TABLE 14.2 *(continued)*

Enzyme (proenzyme)	Source	Optimal pH	Target	Products	Remarks
Trypsin (trypsinogen)	Pancreas	7–8	Proteins, polypeptides	Short-chain peptides	Proenzyme activated by enterokinase; activates other pancreatic proteases
LIPASES					
Lingual lipase	Glands of tongue	3.0–6.0	Triglycerides	Fatty acids and monoglycerides	Begins lipid digestion
Pancreatic lipase	Pancreas	7–8	Triglycerides	Fatty acids and monoglycerides	Bile salts must be present for efficient action
NUCLEASES	Pancreas	7–8	Nucleic acids	Nitrogenous bases and simple sugars	Includes ribonuclease for RNA and deoxy-ribonuclease for DNA

alpha-amylase—that function effectively at a pH of 6.7–7.5. Carbohydrate digestion begins in the mouth during mastication, through the action of salivary amylase from the parotid and sub-mandibular salivary glands. Salivary amylase breaks down starches (complex carbohydrates), producing a mixture composed primarily of *disaccharides* (two simple sugars) and *trisaccharides* (three simple sugars). Salivary amylase continues to digest the starches and glycogen in the food for 1–2 hours before stomach acids render the enzyme inactive. Because the enzymatic content of saliva is not high, only a small amount of digestion occurs over this period.

In the duodenum, the remaining complex carbohydrates are broken down by the action of pancreatic alpha-amylase. Any disaccharides or trisaccharides produced, and any present in the food, are not broken down further by salivary and pancreatic amylases. Additional hydrolysis does not occur until these molecules contact the intestinal mucosa.

Actions of Brush Border Enzymes

Prior to absorption, disaccharides and trisaccharides are fragmented into *monosaccharides* (simple sugars) by brush border enzymes of the intestinal microvilli. The enzyme **maltase** splits bonds between the two glucose molecules of the disaccharide **maltose**. **Sucrase** breaks the disaccharide **sucrose** into glucose and *fructose,* another six-carbon sugar. **Lactase** hydrolyzes the disaccharide **lactose** into a molecule of glucose and one of *galactose.* Lactose is the primary carbohydrate in milk, so by breaking down lactose, lactase provides an essential function throughout infancy and early childhood. If the intestinal mucosa stops producing lactase by the time of adolescence, the individual becomes lactose intolerant. After ingesting milk and other dairy products, lactose-intolerant individuals can experience a variety of unpleasant digestive problems.

Absorption of Monosaccharides

The intestinal epithelium then absorbs the monosaccharides by facilitated diffusion and cotransport mechanisms. Both methods involve a carrier protein. Facilitated diffusion and cotransport differ in three major ways:

1. *Facilitated Diffusion Moves Only One Molecule or Ion through the Cell Membrane, Whereas Cotransport Moves More Than One Molecule or*

Ion through the Membrane at the Same Time. In cotransport, the transported materials move in the same direction: down the concentration gradient for at least one of the transported substances.

2. *Facilitated Diffusion Does Not Require ATP.* Although cotransport by itself does not consume ATP, the cell must often expend ATP to preserve homeostasis. For example, the process may introduce sodium ions that must later be pumped out of the cell.

3. *Facilitated Diffusion Will Not Occur if There Is an Opposing Concentration Gradient for the Particular Molecule or Ion.* By contrast, cotransport can occur despite an opposing concentration gradient for one of the transported substances. For example, cells lining the small intestine will continue to absorb glucose when glucose concentrations inside the cells are much higher than they are in the intestinal contents.

The cotransport system responsible for the uptake of glucose also brings sodium ions into the cell. This passive process resembles facilitated diffusion, except that both a sodium ion and a glucose molecule must bind to the carrier protein before they can move into the cell. Glucose cotransport is an example of sodium-linked cotransport. Comparable cotransport mechanisms exist for other simple sugars and for some amino acids. Although these mechanisms deliver valuable nutrients to the cytoplasm, they also bring in sodium ions that must be ejected by the sodium–potassium exchange pump.

The simple sugars that are transported into the cell at its apical surface diffuse through the cytoplasm and reach the interstitial fluid by facilitated diffusion across the basolateral surfaces. These monosaccharides then diffuse into the capillaries of the villus for eventual transport to the liver in the hepatic portal vein.

Lipid Digestion and Absorption

Lipid digestion involves lingual lipase from glands of the tongue, and pancreatic lipase from the pancreas. The most important and abundant dietary lipids are triglycerides, which consist of three fatty acids attached to a single molecule of glycerol. The lingual and pancreatic lipases break off two of the fatty acids, leaving monoglycerides.

Lipases are water-soluble enzymes, and lipids tend to form large drops that exclude water molecules. As a result, lipases can attack only the exposed surfaces of the lipid drops. Lingual lipase begins breaking down triglycerides in the mouth and continues for a variable time within the stomach, but the lipid drops are so large, and the available time so short, that only about 20 percent of the lipids have been digested by the time the chyme enters the duodenum.

Bile salts improve chemical digestion by emulsifying the lipid drops into tiny emulsion droplets, thereby providing better access for pancreatic lipase. The emulsification occurs only after the chyme has been mixed with bile in the duodenum. Pancreatic lipase then breaks apart the triglycerides to form a mixture of fatty acids and monoglycerides. As these molecules are released, they interact with bile salts in the surrounding chyme to form small lipid-bile salt complexes called **micelles** (mī-SELZ). A micelle is only about 2.5 nm (0.0025 μm) in diameter.

When a micelle contacts the intestinal epithelium, the lipids diffuse across the cell membrane and enter the cytoplasm. The intestinal cells synthesize new triglycerides from the monoglycerides and fatty acids. These triglycerides, in company with absorbed steroids, phospholipids, and fat-soluble vitamins, are then coated with proteins, creating complexes known as **chylomicrons** (kī-lō-MĪ-kronz; *chylos*, milky lymph + *mikros*, small).

The intestinal cells then secrete the chylomicrons into interstitial fluid by exocytosis. The superficial protein coating of the chylomicrons keeps them suspended in the interstitial fluid, but their size generally prevents them from diffusing into capillaries. Most of the chylomicrons released diffuse into the intestinal lacteals, which lack basal laminae and have large gaps between adjacent endothelial cells. From the lacteals, the chylomicrons proceed along the lymphatic vessels and through the thoracic duct, finally entering the bloodstream at the left subclavian vein.

Most of the bile salts within micelles are reabsorbed by sodium-linked cotransport. Only about 5 percent of the bile salts secreted by the liver enters the colon, and only about 1 percent is lost in feces.

Protein Digestion and Absorption

Proteins have very complex structures, so protein digestion is both complex and time-consuming. The first task is to disrupt the three-dimensional organization of the food so that proteolytic enzymes can attack individual proteins. This step involves mechanical processing in the oral cavity, through mastication, and chemical processing in the stomach, through the action of hydrochloric acid. Exposure of the bolus to a strongly acidic environment kills pathogens and breaks down plant cell walls and the connective tissues in animal products.

The acidic contents of the stomach also provide the proper environment for the activity of pepsin, the proteolytic enzyme secreted by chief cells of the stomach. Pepsin, which works effectively at a pH of 1.5–2.0, breaks the peptide bonds within a polypeptide chain. When chyme enters the duodenum, enterokinase produced in the small intestine triggers the conversion of trypsinogen to trypsin, and the pH is adjusted to 7–8. Pancreatic proteases can now begin working. Trypsin, chymotrypsin, and elastase are like pepsin in that they break specific peptide bonds within a polypeptide. For example, trypsin breaks peptide bonds involving the amino acids *arginine* or *lysine*, whereas chymotrypsin targets peptide bonds involving *tyrosine* or *phenylalanine*.

Carboxypeptidase also acts in the small intestine. This enzyme chops off the last amino acid of a polypeptide chain, ignoring the identities of the amino acids involved. Thus, while the other peptidases generate a variety of short peptides, carboxypeptidase produces free amino acids.

Absorption of Amino Acids

The epithelial surfaces of the small intestine contain several peptidases, notably **dipeptidases**—enzymes that break short peptide chains into individual amino acids. (Dipeptidases break apart *dipeptides.*) These amino acids, as well as those produced by the pancreatic enzymes, are absorbed through both facilitated diffusion and cotransport mechanisms.

After diffusing to the basal surface of the cell, the amino acids are released into interstitial fluid by facilitated diffusion and cotransport. Once in the interstitial fluid, the amino acids diffuse into intestinal capillaries for transport to the liver by means of the hepatic portal vein.

Water Absorption

Cells cannot actively absorb or secrete water. All movement of water across the lining of the digestive tract, as well as the production of glandular secretions, involves passive water flow down osmotic gradients. When two fluids are separated by a selectively permeable membrane, water tends to flow into the solution that has the higher concentration of solutes. Osmotic movements are rapid, so interstitial fluid and the fluids in the intestinal lumen always have the same osmolarity (osmotic concentration of solutes).

Intestinal epithelial cells continuously absorb nutrients and ions, and these activities gradually lower the solute concentration in the lumen. As the solute concentration drops, water moves into the surrounding tissues, maintaining osmotic equilibrium.

Each day, roughly 2000 ml of water enters the digestive tract in the form of food or drink. The salivary, gastric, intestinal, pancreatic, and bile secretions provide an additional 7000 ml. Of that total, only about 150 ml is lost in feces. The sites of secretion and absorption of water are indicated in Figure 14.19.

Ion Absorption

Osmosis does not distinguish among solutes; all that matters is the total concentration of solutes. To maintain homeostasis, however, the concentrations of specific ions must be closely regulated. Thus, each ion must be handled individually, and the rate of intestinal absorption of each must be tightly controlled (Table 14.3). Many of the regulatory mechanisms controlling the rates of absorption are poorly understood.

Sodium ions (Na^+), usually the most abundant cations in food, may enter intestinal cells by diffusion, by cotransport with another nutrient, or by active transport. These ions are then pumped into interstitial fluid across the base of the cell. The rate of Na^+ uptake from the lumen is generally proportional to the concentration of Na^+ in the intestinal contents. As a result, eating heavily salted foods leads to increased sodium ion absorption and an associated gain of water through osmosis. The rate of sodium ion absorption by the digestive tract is increased by aldosterone, a steroid hormone from the adrenal cortex.

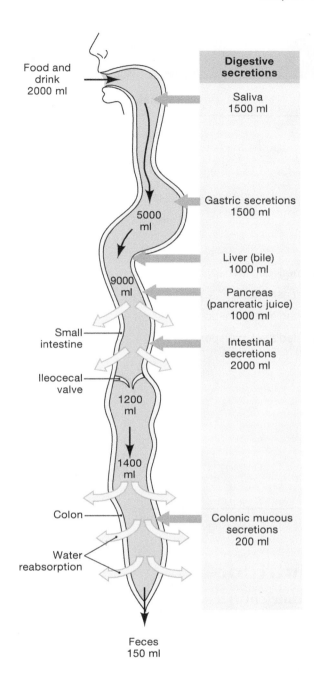

FIGURE 14.19 **Digestive secretion and absorption of water.** The gray arrows indicate secretion, the blue arrows water reabsorption.

along the concentration gradient. The absorption of magnesium (Mg^{2+}), iron (Fe^{2+}), and other cations involves specific carrier proteins; the cell must use ATP to obtain and transport these ions to interstitial fluid. Regulatory factors controlling their absorption are poorly understood.

The anions chloride (Cl^-), iodide (I^-), bicarbonate (HCO_3^-), and nitrate (NO_3^-) are absorbed by diffusion or carrier-mediated transport. Phosphate (PO_4^{3-}) and sulfate ($SO4^{2-}$) ions enter epithelial cells only by active transport.

Vitamin Absorption

Vitamins are organic compounds required in very small quantities. There are two major groups of vitamins: fat-soluble vitamins and water-soluble vitamins. Vitamins A, D, E, and K are **fat-soluble vitamins**; their structure allows them to dissolve in lipids. The nine **water-soluble vitamins** include the B vitamins, common in milk and meats, and vitamin C, found in citrus fruits.

All but one of the water-soluble vitamins are easily absorbed by diffusion across the digestive epithelium. Vitamin B_{12} cannot be absorbed by the intestinal mucosa in normal amounts, unless this vitamin has been bound to *intrinsic factor,* a glycoprotein secreted by the parietal cells of the stomach. The combination is then absorbed through active transport.

Fat-soluble vitamins in the diet enter the duodenum in fat droplets, mixed with triglycerides. The vitamins remain in association with these lipids as they form emulsion droplets and, after further digestion, micelles. The fat-soluble vitamins are then absorbed from the micelles along with the fatty acids and monoglycerides. Vitamin K produced in the colon is absorbed with other lipids released through bacterial action. Taking supplements of fat-soluble vitamins while you have an empty stomach, are fasting, or are on a low-fat diet is relatively ineffective, because proper absorption of these vitamins requires the presence of other lipids.

PART II: NUTRITION AND METABOLISM

Although it seems at times that people can be divided into two camps—those who live to eat and those who eat to live—we all recognize the

Calcium ion (Ca^+) absorption involves active transport at the epithelial surface. The rate of transport is accelerated by parathyroid hormone (PTH) and calcitriol.

As other solutes move out of the lumen, the concentration of potassium ions (K^+) increases. These ions can diffuse into the epithelial cells

TABLE 14.3   The Absorption of Ions and Vitamins

Ion or Vitamin	Transport Mechanism	Regulatory Factors
Na^+	Channel-mediated diffusion, cotransport, or active transport	Increased when sodium-linked cotransport is underway; stimulated by aldosterone
Ca^{2+}	Active transport	Stimulated by calcitriol and PTH
K^+	Channel-mediated diffusion	
Mg^{2+}	Active transport	Follows concentration gradient
Fe^{2+}	Active transport	
Cl^-	Channel-mediated diffusion or carrier-mediated transport	
I^-	Channel-mediated diffusion or active transport	
HCO_3^-	Channel-mediated diffusion or carrier-mediated transport	
NO_3^-	Channel-mediated diffusion or carrier-mediated transport	
PO_4^{3-}	Active transport	
SO_4^{2-}	Active transport	
Water-soluble vitamins (except B_{12})	Channel-mediated diffusion	Follows concentration gradient
Vitamin B_{12}	Active transport	Must be bound to intrinsic factor prior to absorption
Fat-soluble vitamins	Diffusion	Absorbed from micelles along with dietary lipids

vital importance of food for life. It has been said that "you are what you eat," and this is true in that part of the food we eat is converted to our living flesh. In other words, a certain fraction of nutrients is used to build cellular molecules and structures and to replace worn-out parts. However, most foods are used as metabolic fuels. That is, they are oxidized and transformed into **ATP,** the chemical energy form needed by body cells to drive their many activities. The energy value of foods is measured in units called **kilocalories (kcal),** or Calories (with a capital C), the units conscientiously counted by dieters.

We have just considered how foods are digested and absorbed. But what happens to these foods once they enter the blood? Why do we need bread, meat, and fresh vegetables? Why does everything we eat seem to turn to fat? We will try to answer these questions in this section.

Nutrition

A **nutrient** is a substance in food that is used by the body to promote normal growth, maintenance, and repair. The nutrients divide neatly into six categories. The *major nutrients*—carbohydrates, lipids, and proteins—make up the bulk of what we eat. Vitamins and minerals, while equally crucial for health, are required in minute amounts. Water, which accounts for about 60 percent of the volume of the food we eat, is also considered to be a major nutrient. Only the other five classes of nutrients will be considered here.

Most foods offer a combination of nutrients. For example, a bowl of cream of mushroom soup contains all of the major nutrients plus some vitamins and minerals. A diet consisting of foods selected from each of the five food groups (Table 14.5), that is, grains, fruits, vegetables, meats and fish, and milk products, normally guarantees adequate amounts of all of the needed nutrients.

Dietary Sources of the Major Nutrients

Carbohydrates

Except for milk sugar (lactose) and small amounts of glycogen in meats, all the **carbohydrates**—sugars and starches—we ingest are derived from plants. Sugars come mainly from fruits, sugar cane, and milk. The polysaccharide starch is found in grains, legumes, and root vegetables. The polysaccharide cellulose, which is plentiful in most vegetables, is not digested by humans, but it provides roughage, or fiber, which increases the bulk of the stool and aids defecation.

Lipids

Although we also ingest cholesterol and phospholipids, most dietary **lipids** are triglycerides. We eat saturated fats in animal products, such as meat and dairy foods, and in a few plant products, such as coconut. Unsaturated fats are present in seeds, nuts, and most vegetable oils. Major sources of cholesterol are egg yolk, meats, and milk products.

Proteins

Animal products contain the highest-quality **proteins,** molecules that are basically amino acid polymers. Eggs, milk, and most meat proteins are *complete proteins* that meet all of the body's amino acid requirements for tissue maintenance and growth. Legumes (beans and peas), nuts, and cereals are also protein-rich, but their proteins are nutritionally incomplete because they are low in one or more of the essential amino acids.

Metabolic Interactions

The nutrient requirements of each tissue vary with the types and quantities of enzymes present in the cytoplasm of cells. From a metabolic standpoint, we can consider the body to have five distinctive components: the liver, adipose tissue, skeletal muscle, neural tissue, and other peripheral tissues:

1. *The Liver.* The liver is the focal point of metabolic regulation and control. Liver cells contain a great diversity of enzymes, so they can break down or synthesize most of the carbohydrates, lipids, and amino acids needed by other body cells. Liver cells have an extensive blood supply, so they are in an excellent position to monitor and adjust the nutrient composition of circulating blood. The liver also contains significant energy reserves in the form of glycogen deposits.

2. *Adipose Tissue.* Adipose tissue stores lipids, primarily as triglycerides. Adipocytes are located in many areas: in areolar tissue, in mesenteries, within red and yellow marrows, in the epicardium, and around the eyes and the kidneys.

3. *Skeletal Muscle.* Skeletal muscle accounts for almost half of a healthy individual's body weight, and skeletal muscle fibers maintain substantial glycogen reserves. In addition, if other nutrients are unavailable, their contractile proteins can be broken down and the amino acids used as an energy source.

4. *Neural Tissue.* Neural tissue has a high demand for energy, but the cells do not maintain reserves of carbohydrates, lipids, or proteins. Neurons must be provided with a reliable supply of glucose, because they are generally unable to metabolize other molecules. If blood glucose levels become too low, neural tissue in the central nervous system cannot continue to function, and the individual falls unconscious.

5. *Other Peripheral Tissues.* Other peripheral tissues do not maintain large metabolic reserves, but they are able to metabolize glucose, fatty acids, or other substrates. Their preferred source of energy varies according to instructions from the endocrine system.

The interrelationships among these five components can best be understood by considering events over a typical 24-hour period. During this time, the body experiences two broad patterns of metabolic activity: the *absorptive state* and the *postabsorptive state.*

The **absorptive state** is the period following a meal, when nutrient absorption is under way. After a typical meal, the absorptive state continues for about 4 hours. If you are fortunate enough to eat three meals a day, you spend 12 out of every 24 hours in the absorptive state. Insulin is the primary hormone of the absorptive state, although various other hormones stimulate amino acid uptake (growth hormone, or GH) and protein synthesis (GH, androgens, and estrogens) (Table 14.4).

The **postabsorptive state** is the period when nutrient absorption is not under way and your body must rely on internal energy reserves to continue meeting its energy demands. You spend roughly 12 hours each day in the postabsorptive state, although a person who is skipping meals can extend that time considerably. Metabolic activity in the postabsorptive state is focused on the mobilization of energy reserves and the maintenance of normal blood glucose levels. These activities are coordinated by several hormones, including glucagon, epinephrine, glucocorticoids, and growth hormone (see Table 14.4).

During the postabsorptive state, liver cells conserve glucose and break down lipids and amino acids. Both lipid catabolism and amino acid catabolism generate acetyl-CoA. As the concentration of acetyl-CoA rises, compounds called **ketone bodies** begin to form. There are three such compounds: (1) **acetoacetate** (as-ē-tō-AS-e-tāt), (2) **acetone** (AS-e-tōn), and (3) **betahydroxybutyrate** (bā-ta-hī-droks-ē-BŪ-te-rāt). Liver cells do not catabolize any of the ketone bodies, and these compounds diffuse through the cytoplasm and into the general circulation. Cells in peripheral tissues then absorb the ketone bodies and reconvert them to acetyl-CoA for introduction into the TCA cycle.

The normal concentration of ketone bodies in the blood is about 30 mg/dl, and very few of these compounds appear in urine. During even a brief period of fasting, the increased production of ketone bodies results in *ketosis* (kē-TŌ-sis), a high concentration of ketone bodies in body fluids. A ketone body is an acid that dissociates in solution, releasing a hydrogen ion. As a result, the appearance of ketone bodies in the bloodstream—*ketonemia*—lowers plasma pH, which must be controlled by buffers. During prolonged starvation, ketone levels continue to rise. Eventually, buffering capacities are exceeded and a dangerous drop in pH occurs. This acidification of the blood is called *ketoacidosis* (kē-tō-as-i-DŌ-sis). In severe ketoacidosis, the circulating concentration of ketone bodies can reach 200 mg/dl, and the pH may fall below 7.05. A pH that low can disrupt tissue activities and cause coma, cardiac arrhythmias, and death.

In summary, during the postabsorptive state, the liver acts to stabilize blood glucose concentrations, first through the breakdown of glycogen reserves

and later by gluconeogenesis. Over the remainder of the postabsorptive state, the combination of lipid and amino acid catabolism provides the necessary ATP and generates large quantities of ketone bodies that diffuse into the bloodstream.

The changes in activity of the liver, adipose tissue, skeletal muscle, and other peripheral tissues ensure that the supply of glucose to the nervous system continues unaffected, despite daily or even weekly changes in nutrient availability. Only after a prolonged period of starvation will neural tissue begin to metabolize ketone bodies and lactic acid molecules, as well as glucose.

100 Keys | In the absorption state that follows a meal, cells absorb nutrients that are used to support growth and maintenance and stored as energy reserves. Hours later, in the postabsorptive state, blood glucose levels are maintained by gluconeogenesis within the liver, but most cells begin conserving energy and shifting from glucose-based to lipid-based metabolism and, if necessary, ketone bodies become the preferred energy source. This metabolic shift reserves the circulating glucose for use by neurons.

As you can see, strict vegetarians must carefully plan their diets to obtain all the essential amino acids and prevent protein malnutrition.

Vitamins

Vitamins are organic nutrients of various forms that the body requires in small amounts. Although vitamins are found in all major food groups, no one food contains all the required vitamins. Thus, a balanced diet is the best way to ensure a full vitamin complement, particularly since certain vitamins (A, C, and E) appear to have anticancer effects. Diets rich in broccoli, cabbage, and brussels sprouts (all good sources of vitamins A and C) appear to reduce cancer risk. However, controversy abounds concerning the ability of vitamins to work wonders.

Most vitamins function as **coenzymes** (or parts of coenzymes); that is, they act with an enzyme to accomplish a particular type of catalysis.

Minerals

The body also requires adequate supplies of seven **minerals** (that is, inorganic substances including

TABLE 14.4   Regulatory Hormones and Their Effects on Peripheral Metabolism

Hormone	Effect on General Peripheral Tissues	Selective Effects on Target Tissues
ABSORPTIVE STATE		
Insulin	Increased glucose uptake and utilization	*Liver*: Glycogenesis *Adipose tissue*: Lipogenesis *Skeletal muscle*: Glycogenesis
Insulin and growth hormone	Increased amino acid uptake and protein synthesis	*Skeletal muscle*: Fatty acid catabolism
Androgens, estrogens	Increased amino acid use in protein synthesis	*Skeletal muscle*: Muscle hypertrophy (especially androgens)
POSTABSORPTIVE STATE		
Glucagon		*Liver*: Glycogenolysis
Epinephrine		*Liver*: Glycogenolysis *Adipose tissue*: Lipolysis
Glucocorticoids	Decreased use of glucose; increased reliance on ketone bodies and fatty acids	*Liver*: Glycogenolysis *Adipose tissue*: Lipolysis, gluconeogenesis *Skeletal muscle*: Glycogenolysis, protein breakdown, amino acid release
Growth hormone	Complements effects of glucocorticoids	Acts with glucocorticoids

calcium, phosphorus, potassium, sulfur, sodium, chloride, and magnesium) and trace amounts of about a dozen others.

Fats and sugars have practically no minerals, and cereals and grains are poor sources. The most mineral-rich foods are vegetables, legumes, milk, and some meats.

The main uses of the major nutrients in the body are discussed in the section on metabolism.

Metabolism

Metabolism (mĕ-tab′o-lizm; *metabol* = change) is a broad term referring to all chemical reactions that are necessary to maintain life. It involves **catabolism** (kah-tab′o-lizm), in which substances are broken down to simpler substances, and **anabolism** (ah-nab′o-lizm), in which larger molecules or structures are built from smaller ones. During catabolism, energy is released and captured to make ATP, the energy-rich molecule used to energize all cellular activities, including catabolic reactions (Figure 14.20).

Not all foodstuffs are treated in the same way by body cells. For example, carbohydrates, particularly glucose, are usually broken down to make ATP. Fats are used to build cell membranes, make myelin sheaths, and insulate the body with a fatty cushion. They are also used as the body's main energy fuel for making ATP when there are inadequate carbohydrates in the diet. Proteins tend to be carefully conserved (even hoarded) by the body cells. This is easy to understand when you recognize that proteins are the major structural materials used for building cell structures.

TABLE 14.5   Five Basic Food Groups and Some of Their Major Nutrients

Group	Example foods	Major nutrients supplied in significant amounts:	
		By all in group	By only some in group
Fruits	Apples, bananas, dates, oranges, tomatoes	Carbohydrate Water	Vitamins: A, C, folic acid Minerals: iron, potassium Fiber
Vegetables	Broccoli, cabbage, green beans, lettuce, potatoes	Carbohydrate Water	Vitamins: A, C, E, K, and B vitamins except B_{12} Minerals: calcium, magnesium, iodine, manganese, phosphorus Fiber
Grain products (preferably whole grain; otherwise, enriched or fortified)	Breads, rolls, bagels; cereals, dry and cooked; pasta; rice, other grains; tortillas, pancakes, waffles; crackers; popcorn	Carbohydrate Protein Vitamins: thiamin (B_1), niacin	Water Fiber Minerals: iron, magnesium, selenium
Milk products	Milk, yogurt; cheese; ice cream, ice milk, frozen yogurt	Protein Fat Vitamins: riboflavin, B_{12} Minerals: calcium, phosphorus Water	Carbohydrate Vitamins: A, D
Meats and meat alternates	Meat, fish, poultry; eggs; seeds; nuts, nut butters; soybeans, tofu; other legumes (peas and beans)	Protein Vitamins: niacin, B_6 Minerals: iron, zinc	Carbohydrate Fat Vitamins: B_{12}, thiamin (B_1) Water Fiber

Source: Christian, Janet, and Janet Greger. *Nutrition for Living,* 3rd ed. San Francisco, CA: Benjamin Cummings, 1991.

Carbohydrate, Fat, and Protein Metabolism in Body Cells

Carbohydrate Metabolism

Just as an oil furnace uses oil (its fuel) to produce heat, the cells of the body use carbohydrates as their preferred fuel to produce cellular energy (ATP). **Glucose,** also known as **blood sugar,** is the major breakdown product of carbohydrate digestion. Glucose is also the major fuel used for making ATP in most body cells. The liver is an exception; it routinely uses fats as well, thus saving glucose for other body cells. Essentially, glucose is broken apart piece by piece, and some of the chemical energy released when its bonds are broken is captured and used to bind phosphate to ADP molecules to make ATP.

The overall reaction is summed up simply in Figure 14.20. Basically, the carbon atoms released leave the cells as carbon dioxide, and the hydrogen atoms removed (which contain energy-rich electrons) are eventually combined with oxygen to form water. These oxygen-using events are referred to collectively as **cellular respiration.** The events of the three main metabolic pathways controlled by many different enzymes that are involved in cellular respiration—*glycolysis,* the

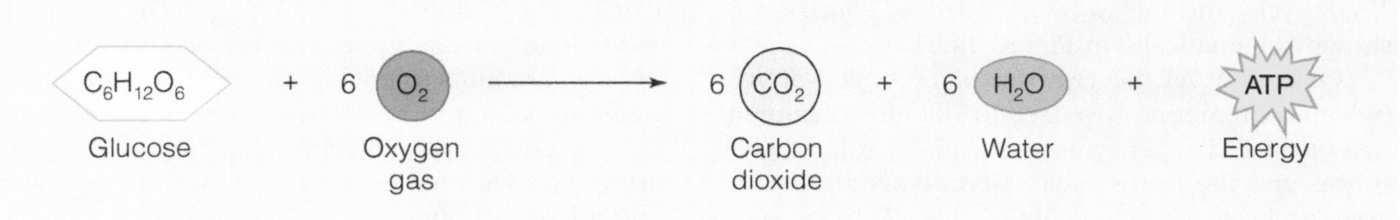

$$C_6H_{12}O_6 \;+\; 6\; O_2 \;\longrightarrow\; 6\; CO_2 \;+\; 6\; H_2O \;+\; ATP$$

| Glucose | Oxygen gas | | Carbon dioxide | Water | Energy |

FIGURE 14.20 Summary equation for cellular respiration. This reaction is **aerobic** because it uses oxygen.

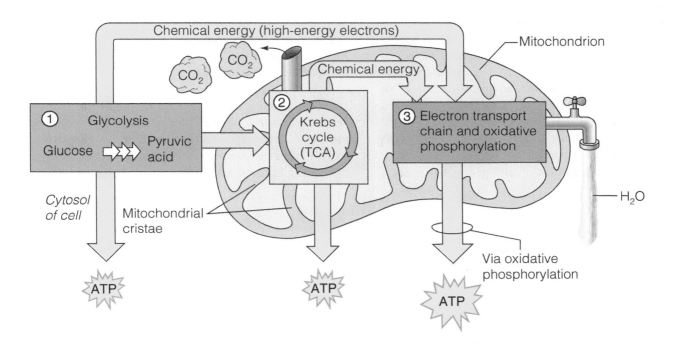

FIGURE 14.21 An overview of sites of ATP formation during cellular respiration. Glycolysis (also called oxidative phosphorylation) occurs outside the mitochondria in the cytosol. The Krebs cycle and the electron transport chain reactions occur within the mitochondria. ① During glycolysis, hydrogen atoms containing high-energy electrons are removed as each glucose molecule is broken down into two molecules of pyruvic acid. ② The pyruvic acid enters the mitochondrion, where Krebs cycle enzymes remove more hydrogen and decompose the pyruvic acid to carbon dioxide. During glycolysis and the Krebs cycle, small amounts of ATP are formed. ③ Chemical energy from glycolysis and the Krebs cycle (also called the TCA cycle), in the form of hydrogen atoms containing energy-rich electrons, is then transferred to the electron transport chain, which is built into the membrane of the cristae. The electron transport chain carries out oxidative phosphorylation, which produces most of the ATP generated by cellular respiration and finally unites the removed hydrogen with oxygen to form water.

Krebs cycle, and the *electron transport chain*—are shown schematically in Figure 14.21.

Oxidation via the removal of hydrogen atoms (which are temporarily passed to vitamin-containing **NAD and FAD** coenzymes) is a major role of glycolysis and the Krebs cycle. **Glycolysis** also energizes each glucose molecule so that it can be split into two pyruvic acid molecules and yield a small amount of ATP in the process (Figure 14.21). The **Krebs cycle** (also called the **TCA cycle**) produces virtually all the carbon dioxide and water that results during cell respiration. Like glycolysis, it yields a small amount of ATP by transferring high energy phosphate groups directly from phosphorylated substances to ADP. Free oxygen is not involved, so it is an **anaerobic reaction.**

The **electron transport chain** is where the action is for ATP production. The hydrogen atoms removed during the first two metabolic phases are loaded with energy. These hydrogens are delivered by the coenzymes to the protein carriers of the electron transport chain, which form part of the mitochondrial cristae membranes (Figure 14.22). There the hydrogen atoms are split into hydrogen ions (H^+) and electrons (e^-). The electrons "fall down an energy hill" going from each

carrier to a carrier of lower energy. They give off their "load" of energy in a series of steps in small enough amounts to enable the cell to attach phosphate to ADP and make ATP. Ultimately free oxygen is reduced (the electrons and hydrogen ions are united with molecular oxygen), forming water and a large amount of ATP. The beauty of this system is that, unlike the explosive reaction that happens when O_2 is combined with hydrogen, relatively small amounts of energy are lost as heat (and light).

Because glucose is the major fuel for making ATP, homeostasis of blood glucose levels is critically important. If there are excessively high levels of glucose in the blood (*hyperglycemia* [hi″per-gli-se′me-ah]), some of the excess is stored in body cells (particularly liver and muscle cells) as glycogen. If blood glucose levels are still too high, excesses are converted to fat. There is no question that eating large amounts of empty-calorie foods such as candy and other sugary sweets causes a rapid deposit of fat in the body's adipose tissues. When blood glucose levels are too low *(hypoglycemia),* the liver breaks down stored glycogen and releases glucose to the blood for cellular use.

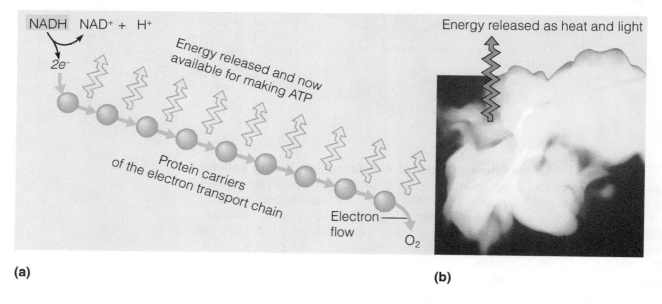

(a)

(b)

FIGURE 14.22   Electron transport chain versus one-step reduction of oxygen. (a) In cellular respiration, cascading electrons release energy in small steps and finally reduce O_2. The energy released is in quantities easily used to form ATP. (NADH is a niacin-containing coenzyme that delivers H^+ to the electron transport chain.) **(b)** When O_2 is reduced (combined with hydrogen) in one step, the result is an explosion of energy. NAD combines with the released hydrogen (H^+).

The complete catabolism of one molecule of glucose provides a typical body cell a net gain of 36 molecules of ATP. Although most ATP production occurs inside mitochondria, the first steps take place in the cytosol. The process of *glycolysis* breaks down glucose in the cytosol and generates smaller molecules that can be absorbed and utilized by mitochondria. Because glycolysis does not require oxygen, the reactions are said to be *anaerobic*. The subsequent reactions, which occur in mitochondria, consume oxygen and are considered *aerobic*. The mitochondrial activity responsible for ATP production is called **aerobic metabolism**, or *cellular respiration*.

Glycolysis

Let's look at the process of glycolysis in more detail. **Glycolysis** (glī-KOL-i-sis; *glykus,* sweet + *lysis,* dissolution) is the breakdown of glucose to **pyruvic acid**. In this process, a series of enzymatic steps breaks the six-carbon glucose molecule ($C_6H_{12}O_6$) into two three-carbon molecules of pyruvic acid (CH_3—CO—COOH). At the normal pH inside cells, each pyruvic acid molecule loses a hydrogen ion and exists as the negatively charged ion CH_3–CO—COO$^-$. This ionized form is usually called *pyruvate,* rather than pyruvic acid.

Glycolysis requires (1) glucose molecules, (2) appropriate cytoplasmic enzymes, (3) ATP and ADP, (4) inorganic phosphates, and (5) **NAD** (***n***icotinamide ***a***denine ***d***inucleotide), a coenzyme that removes hydrogen atoms during one of the enzymatic reactions. If any of these participants is missing, glycolysis cannot occur.

Figure 14.23 provides an overview of the steps in glycolysis. Glycolysis begins when an enzyme *phosphorylates*—that is, attaches a phosphate group—to the last (sixth) carbon atom of a glucose molecule, creating **glucose-6-phosphate**. This step, which "costs" the cell one ATP molecule, has two important results: (1) It traps the glucose molecule within the cell, because phosphorylated glucose cannot cross the cell membrane; and (2) it prepares the glucose molecule for further biochemical reactions.

A second phosphorylation occurs in the cytosol before the six-carbon chain is broken into two three-carbon fragments. Energy benefits begin to appear as these fragments are converted to pyruvic acid. Two of the steps release enough energy to generate ATP from ADP and inorganic phosphate (PO_4^{3-} or P_i). In addition, two molecules of NAD are converted to NADH. The net reaction looks like this:

Glucose + 2 NAD + 2 ADP + 2 P_i $\longrightarrow$

2 Pyruvic acid + 2 NADH + 2 ATP

This anaerobic reaction sequence provides the cell a net gain of two molecules of ATP for each glucose molecule converted to two pyruvic acid molecules. A few highly specialized cells, such as red blood cells, lack mitochondria and derive all their ATP through glycolysis. Skeletal muscle fibers rely on glycolysis for ATP production during periods of active contraction; using the ATP provided by glycolysis alone, most cells can survive for brief periods. However, when oxygen is readily available, mitochondrial activity provides most of the ATP required by cells. This process is called oxidative phosphorylation.

Fat Metabolism

As described shortly, the liver handles most lipid, or fat, metabolism that goes on in the body. The liver cells use some fats to make ATP for their own use; some to synthesize lipoproteins, thromboplastin (a clotting protein), and cholesterol; and then release the rest to the blood in the form of relatively small, fat-breakdown products. Body cells remove the fat products and cholesterol from the blood and build them into their membranes or steroid hormones as needed. Fats are also used to form myelin sheaths of neurons (see Chapter 7) and fatty cushions around body organs. In addition, stored fats are the body's most concentrated source of energy. (Catabolism of 1 gram of fat yields twice as much energy as the breakdown of 1 gram of carbohydrate or protein.)

For fat products to be used for ATP synthesis, they must first be broken down to acetic acid (Figure 14.24d). Within the mitochondria, the acetic acid (like the pyruvic acid product of carbohydrates) is then completely oxidized, and carbon dioxide, water, and ATP are formed. When there is not enough glucose to fuel the needs of the cells for energy, larger amounts of fats are used to produce ATP. Under such conditions, fat oxidation is fast but incomplete, and some of the intermediate products such as acetoacetic acid and acetone begin to accumulate in the blood. These cause the blood to

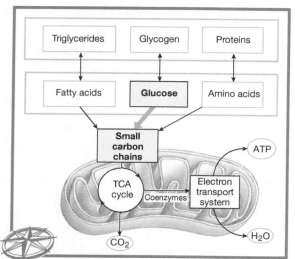

FIGURE 14.23 Glycolysis. The Navigator icon in the shadow box highlights the topic under discussion. Glycolysis breaks down a six-carbon glucose molecule into two three-carbon molecules of pyruvic acid through a series of enzymatic steps. This diagram follows the fate of the carbon chain. There is a net gain of two ATP molecules for each glucose molecule converted to two pyruvic acid molecules. In addition, two molecules of the coenzyme NAD are converted to NADH. Once transferred to mitochondria, both pyruvic acid and NADH can still yield a great deal more energy. The further catabolism of pyruvic acid begins with its entry into a mitochondrion.

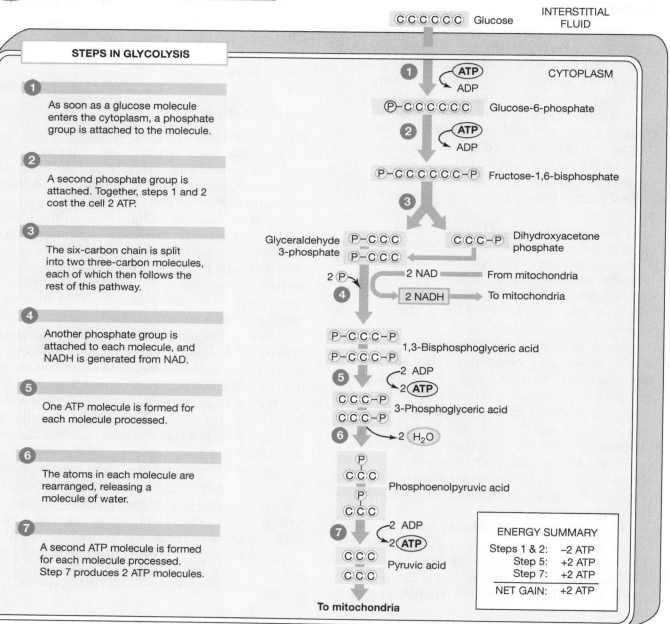

STEPS IN GLYCOLYSIS

1 As soon as a glucose molecule enters the cytoplasm, a phosphate group is attached to the molecule.

2 A second phosphate group is attached. Together, steps 1 and 2 cost the cell 2 ATP.

3 The six-carbon chain is split into two three-carbon molecules, each of which then follows the rest of this pathway.

4 Another phosphate group is attached to each molecule, and NADH is generated from NAD.

5 One ATP molecule is formed for each molecule processed.

6 The atoms in each molecule are rearranged, releasing a molecule of water.

7 A second ATP molecule is formed for each molecule processed. Step 7 produces 2 ATP molecules.

Glucose

INTERSTITIAL FLUID

1 ATP → ADP   CYTOPLASM

Glucose-6-phosphate

2 ATP → ADP

Fructose-1,6-bisphosphate

3

Glyceraldehyde 3-phosphate

Dihydroxyacetone phosphate

2 NAD — From mitochondria
4   2 NADH → To mitochondria

1,3-Bisphosphoglyceric acid

5   2 ADP → 2 ATP

3-Phosphoglyceric acid

6   2 H_2O

Phosphoenolpyruvic acid

7   2 ADP → 2 ATP

Pyruvic acid

ENERGY SUMMARY	
Steps 1 & 2:	−2 ATP
Step 5:	+2 ATP
Step 7:	+2 ATP
NET GAIN:	+2 ATP

To mitochondria

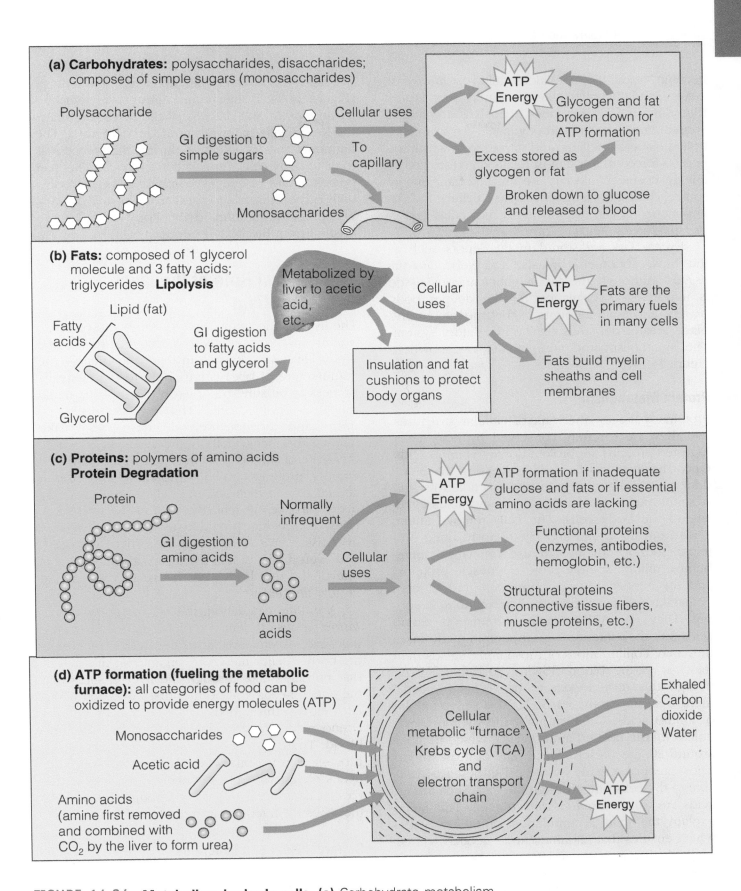

FIGURE 14.24 Metabolism by body cells. (a) Carbohydrate metabolism.
(b) Fat metabolism. **(c)** Protein metabolism. **(d)** ATP formation.

become acidic (a condition called *acidosis,* or *ketosis*), and the breath takes on a fruity odor as acetone diffuses from the lungs. Ketosis is a common consequence of "no-carbohydrate" diets, uncontrolled diabetes mellitus, and starvation in which the body is forced to rely almost totally on fats to fuel its energy needs. While fats are an important energy source, cholesterol is *never* used as a cellular fuel. Its importance lies in the functional molecules and in the structures it helps to form.

Excess fats are stored in fat depots such as the hips, abdomen, breasts, and subcutaneous tissues. Although the fat in subcutaneous tissue is important as insulation for the deeper body organs, excessive amounts restrict movement and place greater demands on the circulatory system. The metabolism and uses of fats are shown in Figure 14.24b.

Protein Metabolism

Proteins make up the bulk of cellular structures, and they are carefully conserved by body cells. Ingested proteins are broken down to amino acids. Once the liver has finished processing the blood draining the digestive tract and has taken its "fill" of amino acids, the remaining amino acids circulate to the body cells. The cells remove amino acids from the blood and use them to build proteins, both for their own use (enzymes, membranes, mitotic spindle proteins, muscle proteins) and for export (mucus, hormones, and others). Cells take few chances with their amino acid supply. They use ATP to actively transport amino acids into their interior even though in many cases they may contain more of those amino acids than there is in the blood flowing past them. Even though this may appear to be "cellular greed," there is an important reason for this active uptake of amino acids. Cells cannot build their proteins unless *all* the needed amino acids, which number around 20, are present. Since nine of these amino acids cannot be made by the cells, they are available to the cells only through the diet. Such amino acids are called *essential amino acids.* This helps explain the avid accumulation of amino acids, which ensures that all amino acids needed will be available for present and (at least some) future protein-building needs of the cells (Figure 14.24c).

Amino acids are used to make ATP only when proteins are overabundant and/or when carbohydrates and fats are not available. When it is

necessary to oxidize amino acids for energy (Figure 14.24d), their amine groups are removed as *ammonia,* and the rest of the molecule enters the Krebs cycle pathways in the mitochondria. The ammonia that is released during this process is toxic to body cells, especially nerve cells. The liver comes to the rescue by combining the ammonia with carbon dioxide to form **urea** (u-re′ah). Urea, which is not harmful to the body cells, is then flushed from the body in urine.

The Central Role of the Liver in Metabolism

The liver is one of the most versatile and complex organs in the body. Without it we would die within 24 hours. Its role in digestion (that is, the manufacture of bile) is important to the digestive process to be sure, but it is only one of the many functions of liver cells. The liver cells detoxify drugs and alcohol, degrade hormones, make many substances vital to the body as a whole (cholesterol, blood proteins such as albumin and clotting proteins, and lipoproteins), and play a central role in metabolism as they process nearly every class of nutrient. Because of the liver's key roles, nature has provided us with a surplus of liver tissue. We have much more than we need, and even if part of it is damaged or removed, it is one of the few body organs that can regenerate rapidly and easily.

A unique circulation, the *hepatic portal circulation,* brings nutrient-rich blood draining from the digestive viscera directly to the liver. The liver is the body's major metabolic organ, and this detour that nutrients take through the liver ensures that the liver's needs will be met first. As blood circulates slowly through the liver, liver cells remove amino acids, fatty acids, and glucose from the blood. These nutrients are stored for later use or processed in various ways. At the same time, the liver's phagocytic cells remove and destroy bacteria that have managed to get through the walls of the digestive tract and into the blood.

General Metabolic Functions

The liver is vitally important in helping to maintain blood glucose levels within normal range (around 100 mg glucose/100 ml of blood). After a carbohydrate-rich meal, thousands of glucose

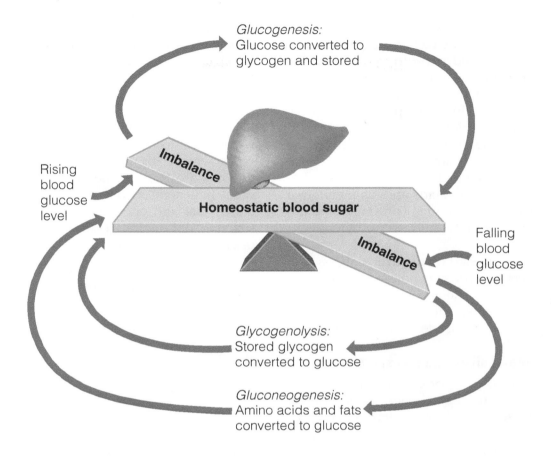

Glucogenesis:
Glucose converted to
glycogen and stored

Rising
blood
glucose
level

Imbalance

Homeostatic blood sugar

Imbalance

Falling
blood
glucose
level

Glycogenolysis:
Stored glycogen
converted to glucose

Gluconeogenesis:
Amino acids and fats
converted to glucose

FIGURE 14.25 Metabolic events occurring in the liver as blood glucose levels rise and fall. When the blood glucose level is rising, the liver removes glucose from the blood and stores it as glycogen (glycogenesis). When the blood glucose level falls, the liver breaks down stored glycogen (glycogenolysis) and makes new glucose from amino acids and fats (gluconeogenesis). The glucose is then released to the blood to restore homeostasis of blood sugar.

molecules are removed from the blood and combined to form the large polysaccharide molecules called **glycogen** (gli′ko-jen), which are then stored in the liver. This process is **glycogenesis** (gli″ko-jen′ĕ-sis), literally, "glycogen formation" (*genesis* = beginning). Later, as body cells continue to remove glucose from the blood to meet their needs, blood glucose levels begin to drop. At this time, liver cells break down the stored glycogen, by a process called **glycogenolysis** (gli″ko-jen-ol′ĭ-sis), which means "glycogen splitting." The liver cells then release glucose bit by bit to the blood to maintain homeostasis of blood glucose levels. If necessary, the liver can also make glucose from noncarbohydrate substances such as fats

and proteins. This process is **gluconeogenesis** (glu″ko-ne″o-jen′ĕ-sis), which means "formation of new sugar" (Figure 14.25). Hormones such as thyroxine, insulin, and glucagon are vitally important in controlling the blood sugar levels and the handling of glucose in all body cells.

Some of the fats and fatty acids picked up by the liver cells are oxidized for energy (to make ATP) for use by the liver cells themselves. The rest are broken down by **lipolysis** to simpler substances such as *acetic acid* and *acetoacetic acid* (two acetic acids linked together) and released into the blood, or stored as fat reserves in the liver. The liver also makes cholesterol and secretes cholesterol's breakdown products in bile.

All blood proteins made by the liver are built from the amino acids its cells pick up from the blood, a process called **protein synthesis.** The completed proteins are then released back into the blood to travel throughout the circulation. *Albumin,* the most abundant protein in blood, holds fluids in the bloodstream. When insufficient albumin is present in blood, fluid leaves the bloodstream and accumulates in the tissue spaces, causing edema. Liver cells also synthesize nonessential amino acids and, as mentioned earlier, detoxify ammonia (produced when amino acids are oxidized for energy) by converting it to urea.

Nutrients not needed by the liver cells, as well as the products of liver metabolism, are released into the blood and drain from the liver in the hepatic vein to enter the systemic circulation, where they become available to other body cells.

Cholesterol Metabolism and Transport

Although it's a very important lipid in the diet, **cholesterol** is not used as an energy fuel. Instead, it serves as the structural basis of steroid hormones and vitamin D and is a major building block of plasma membranes. Because we hear so much about "cutting down our cholesterol intake" in the media, it is always surprising to learn that only about 15 percent of blood cholesterol comes from the diet. The other 85 percent or so is made by the liver. Cholesterol is lost from the body when it is broken down and secreted in bile salts, which eventually leave the body in feces.

Because of the important role they play in fat and cholesterol transport, the lipoproteins, one class of proteins made by the liver and known by the buzzwords *HDLs* and *LDLs,* deserve a bit more attention.

Since fatty acids, fats, and cholesterol are insoluble in water, they cannot circulate freely in the bloodstream. Instead they are transported bound to the small lipid-protein complexes called lipoproteins. Although the entire story is complex, the important thing to know is that the **low-density lipoproteins,** or **LDLs,** transport cholesterol and other lipids *to* body cells, where they are used in various ways. If large amounts of LDLs are circulating, the chance that fatty substances will be deposited on the arterial walls, initiating atherosclerosis, is high. Because of this possibility, the LDLs are unkindly tagged as "bad lipoproteins." By

contrast, the lipoproteins that transport cholesterol *from* the tissue cells (or arteries) to the liver for disposal in bile are **high-density lipoproteins,** or **HDLs.** High HDL levels are considered "good" because the cholesterol is destined to be broken down and eliminated from the body. Obviously both LDLs and HDLs are "good and necessary"; it is just their relative ratio in the blood that determines whether or not potentially lethal cholesterol deposits are likely to be laid down in the artery walls. In general, aerobic exercise, a diet low in saturated fats and cholesterol, and abstaining from smoking and drinking coffee all appear to favor a desirable HDL/LDL ratio.

Body Energy Balance

When any fuel is burned, it consumes oxygen and liberates heat. The "burning" of food fuels by body cells is no exception. Energy cannot be created or destroyed—it can only be converted from one form to another. If we apply this principle to cellular metabolism, it means that a dynamic balance exists between the body's energy intake and its energy output:

Energy intake = total energy output

(heat + work + energy storage)

Energy intake is the energy liberated during food oxidation—that is, during the reactions of glycolysis, the Krebs cycle, and the electron transport chain. **Energy output** includes the energy we immediately lose as heat (about 60 percent of the total), plus that used to do work (driven by ATP), plus energy that is stored in the form of fat or glycogen. Energy storage is important only during periods of growth and during net fat deposit.

Regulation of Food Intake

When energy intake and energy outflow are balanced, body weight remains stable. When they are not, weight is either gained or lost. Since body weight in most people is surprisingly stable, mechanisms that control food intake or heat production or both must exist.

But how is food intake controlled? That is a difficult question, and one that is still not fully answered. Researchers believe that several factors—such as rising or falling blood levels of nutrients (glucose and amino acids), hormones (insulin, glucagon, and leptin), or body temperature

TABLE 14.6   Factors Determining the Basal Metabolic Rate (BMR)

Factor	Variation	Effect on BMR
Surface area	Large surface area in relation to body volume, as in thin, small individuals	Increased
	Small surface area in relation to body volume, as in large, heavy individuals	Decreased
Sex	Male	Increased
	Female	Decreased
Thyroxine production	Increased	Increased
	Decreased	Decreased
Age	Young, rapid growth	Increased
	Aging, elderly	Decreased
Strong emotions (anger or fear) and infections		Increased

(rising temperature is inhibitory), and psychological factors—have an effect on eating behavior through feedback signals to the brain. Indeed, psychological factors are believed to be a very important cause of obesity. However, even when psychological factors *are* the underlying cause of obesity, individuals do *not* continue to gain weight endlessly. It seems that their feeding controls still operate, but they act to maintain total body energy content at higher-than-normal levels.

Metabolic Rate and Body Heat Production

Basal Metabolic Rate   When nutrients are broken down to produce cellular energy (ATP), they yield different amounts of energy. As mentioned earlier, the energy value of foods is measured in a unit called the *kilocalorie (kcal)*. In general, carbohydrates and proteins each yield 4 kcal/gram, and fats yield 9 kcal/gram when they are broken down for energy production. Most meals, and even many individual foods, are mixtures of carbohydrates, fats, and proteins. To determine the caloric value of a meal, we must know how many grams of each type of foodstuff it contains. For most of us, this is a difficult chore indeed, but approximations can easily be made with the help of a simple, calorie-values guide available in most drugstores.

The amount of energy used by the body is also measured in kilocalories. The **basal metabolic rate (BMR)** is the amount of heat produced by the body per unit of time when it is under basal conditions—that is, at rest. It reflects the energy supply a person's body needs just to perform essential life activities such as breathing, maintaining the heartbeat, and kidney function. An average 70-kg (154-pound) adult has a BMR of about 60 to 72 kcal/hour.

Many factors influence BMR, including surface area and gender. As shown in Table 14.6, small, thin males tend to have a higher BMR than large, obese females. Age is also important; children and adolescents require large amounts of energy for growth and have relatively high BMRs. In old age, the BMR decreases dramatically as the muscles begin to atrophy.

The amount of **thyroxine** produced by the thyroid gland is probably the most important factor in determining a person's BMR; hence, thyroxine has been dubbed the "metabolic hormone." The more thyroxine produced, the higher the oxygen consumption and ATP use, and the higher the metabolic rate. In the past, most BMR tests were done to determine whether sufficient thyroxine was being made. Today, thyroid activity is more easily assessed by blood tests.

Homeostatic Imbalance

Hyperthyroidism causes a host of effects due to the excessive metabolic rate it produces. The body catabolizes stored fats and tissue proteins, and despite increased hunger and food intake, the person often loses weight. Bones weaken and body muscles, including the heart, atrophy. In contrast, *hypothyroidism* results in slowed metabolism, obesity, and diminished thought processes. ▲

Total Metabolic Rate   When we are active, more glucose must be oxidized to provide energy for the additional activities. Digesting food and even modest physical activity increase the body's caloric requirements dramatically. These additional fuel requirements are above and beyond the energy required to maintain the body in the basal state. **Total metabolic rate (TMR)** refers to the total amount of kilocalories the body must consume to fuel all ongoing activities. Muscular work is the major body activity that increases the TMR. Even slight increases in skeletal muscle activity cause remarkable leaps in metabolic rate. When a well-trained athlete exercises vigorously for several minutes the TMR may increase to 15 to 20 times normal, and it remains elevated for several hours afterward.

When the total amount of calories consumed is equal to the TMR, homeostasis is maintained, and our weight remains constant. However, if we eat more than we need to sustain our activities, excess calories appear in the form of fat deposits. Conversely, if we are extremely active and do not properly feed the "metabolic furnace," we begin to break down fat reserves and even tissue proteins to satisfy our TMR. This principle is used in every good weight-loss diet. (The total calories needed are calculated on the basis of body size and age. Then, 20 percent or more of the requirements are cut from the daily diet.) If the dieting person exercises regularly, weight drops off even more quickly because the TMR increases above the person's former rate.

Body Temperature Regulation

Although we have been emphasizing that foods are "burned" to produce ATP, remember that ATP is not the only product of cell catabolism. Most of the energy released as foods are oxidized escapes as heat. Less than 40 percent of available food energy is actually captured to form ATP. The heat released warms the tissues and, more importantly, the blood, which circulates to all body tissues, keeping them at homeostatic temperatures, which allows metabolism to occur efficiently.

Body temperature reflects the balance between heat production and heat loss. The body's thermostat is in the *hypothalamus* of the brain. Through autonomic nervous system pathways, the hypothalamus continually regulates body temperature around a set point of 35.6° to 37.8°C (96° to 100°F) by initiating heat-loss or heat-promoting mechanisms (Figure 14.26).

Heat-Promoting Mechanisms   When the environmental temperature is cold (or the temperature of circulating blood falls), body heat must be conserved (increased). Short-term means of accomplishing this are **vasoconstriction** of blood vessels of the skin and **shivering.**

When the skin vasculature constricts, the skin is temporarily bypassed by the blood, and blood is rerouted to the deeper, more vital, body organs. When this happens, the temperature of the exposed skin drops to that of the external environment.

Homeostatic Imbalance

Restriction of blood delivery to the skin is no problem for brief periods of time. But if it is extended, the skin cells, chilled by internal ice crystals and deprived of oxygen and nutrients, begin to die. This condition, called *frostbite,* is extremely serious. ▲

When the *core* body temperature (the temperature of the deep organs) drops to the point beyond which simple constriction of skin capillaries can handle the situation, shivering begins. Shivering, involuntary shudderlike contractions of the voluntary muscles, is very effective in increasing the body temperature, because skeletal muscle activity produces large amounts of heat.

Homeostatic Imbalance

Extremely low body temperature resulting from prolonged exposure to cold is *hypothermia.* In hypothermia, the individual's vital signs (respiratory rate, blood pressure, heart rate) decrease. The person becomes drowsy and oddly comfortable, even though previously he or she felt extremely cold. Uncorrected, the situation progresses to coma and finally death as metabolic processes grind to a stop. ▲

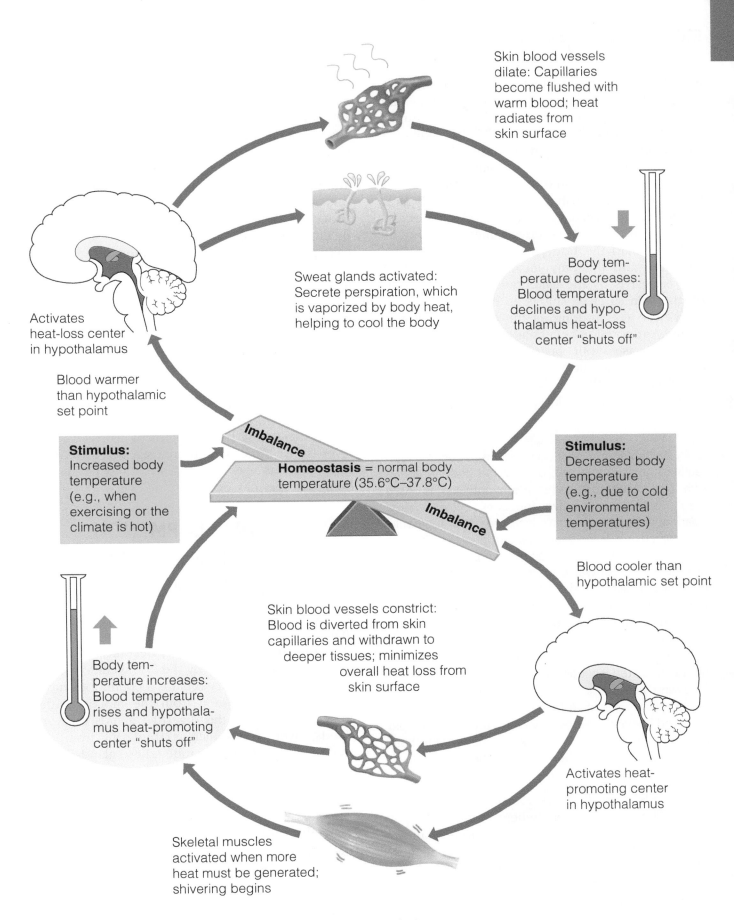

Skin blood vessels dilate: Capillaries become flushed with warm blood; heat radiates from skin surface

Sweat glands activated: Secrete perspiration, which is vaporized by body heat, helping to cool the body

Body temperature decreases: Blood temperature declines and hypothalamus heat-loss center "shuts off"

Activates heat-loss center in hypothalamus

Blood warmer than hypothalamic set point

Stimulus: Increased body temperature (e.g., when exercising or the climate is hot)

Imbalance

Homeostasis = normal body temperature (35.6°C–37.8°C)

Imbalance

Stimulus: Decreased body temperature (e.g., due to cold environmental temperatures)

Blood cooler than hypothalamic set point

Skin blood vessels constrict: Blood is diverted from skin capillaries and withdrawn to deeper tissues; minimizes overall heat loss from skin surface

Body temperature increases: Blood temperature rises and hypothalamus heat-promoting center "shuts off"

Activates heat-promoting center in hypothalamus

Skeletal muscles activated when more heat must be generated; shivering begins

FIGURE 14.26 **Mechanisms of body temperature regulation.**

Heat-Loss Mechanisms   Just as the body must be protected from becoming too cold, it must also be protected from excessively high temperatures. Most heat loss occurs through the skin via **radiation** or **evaporation.** When body temperature increases above what is desirable, the blood vessels serving the skin dilate and capillary beds in the skin become flushed with warm blood. As a result, heat radiates from the skin surface. However, if the external environment is as hot as or hotter than the body, heat cannot be lost by radiation, and the only means of getting rid of excess heat is by the evaporation of perspiration off the skin surface. This is an efficient means of body-heat loss as long as the air is dry. If it is humid, evaporation occurs at a much slower rate. In such cases, our heat-liberating mechanisms don't work well, and we feel miserable and irritable. This is why the hot, humid days of August are often called the "dog days."

Homeostatic Imbalance

When normal heat loss processes become ineffective, the *hyperthermia,* or elevated body temperature, that results depresses the hypothalamus. As a result, a vicious positive feedback cycle occurs: Soaring body temperature increases the metabolic rate, which in turn increases heat production. The skin becomes hot and dry; and, as the temperature continues to spiral upward, permanent brain damage becomes a distinct possibility. This condition, called **heat stroke,** can be fatal unless rapid corrective measures are taken immediately (immersion in cool water and administration of fluids).

Heat exhaustion is the term used to describe the heat-associated collapse of an individual during or following vigorous physical activity. Heat exhaustion results from excessive loss of body fluids (dehydration) and is evidenced by low blood pressure, a rapid heartbeat, and cool, clammy skin. In contrast to heat stroke, heat-loss mechanisms still operate in heat exhaustion. ▲

Fever is *controlled hyperthermia.* Most often, it results from infection somewhere in the body, but it may be caused by other conditions (cancer, allergic reactions, and CNS injuries). Macrophages, white blood cells, and injured tissue cells release chemical substances called *pyrogens* (pi′ro-jenz) that act directly on the hypothalamus, causing its thermostat to be set to a higher temperature (*pyro* = fire). After the thermostat resetting, heat-promoting mechanisms are initiated. Because of vasoconstriction, the skin becomes cool, and shivering begins to generate heat. This situation, called "the chills," is a sure sign that body temperature is rising. Body temperature is allowed to rise until it reaches the new setting. Then, it is maintained at the "fever setting" until natural body defense processes or antibiotics reverse the disease process. At that point, the thermostat is reset again to a lower (or normal) level, causing heat-loss mechanisms to swing into action—the individual begins to sweat, and the skin becomes flushed and warm. Physicians have long recognized that these signs signaled a turn for the better in their patients and said that the patient had "passed the crisis" because body temperature was falling.

Fever, by increasing the metabolic rate, helps speed the various healing processes, and it also appears to inhibit bacterial growth. The danger of fever is that if the body thermostat is set too high, body proteins may be denatured, and permanent brain damage may occur.

PART III: DEVELOPMENTAL ASPECTS OF THE DIGESTIVE SYSTEM AND METABOLISM

The very young embryo is flat and pancake-shaped. However, it soon folds to form a cylindrical body, and its internal cavity becomes the cavity of the alimentary canal. By the fifth week of development, the alimentary canal is a continuous tube-like structure extending from the mouth to the anus. Shortly after, the digestive glands (salivary glands, liver, and pancreas) bud out from the mucosa of the alimentary tube. These glands retain their connections (ducts) and can easily empty their secretions into the alimentary canal to promote its digestive functions.

Homeostatic Imbalance

The digestive system is susceptible to many congenital defects that interfere with feeding. The most common is the *cleft palate/cleft lip* defect. Of the two, cleft palate is more serious because the child is unable to suck properly. Another relatively common congenital defect is a *tracheoesophageal fistula* (tra"ke-o-ĕ-sof'ah-je-al fis'tu-lah). In this condition, there is a connection between the esophagus and the trachea. In addition, the esophagus often (but not always) ends in a blind sac and does not connect to the stomach. The baby chokes, drools, and becomes cyanotic during feedings because food is entering the respiratory passageways. All three defects can be corrected surgically.

There are many types of inborn errors of metabolism (genetically based problems that interfere with metabolism), but perhaps the two most common are *cystic fibrosis (CF)* and *phenylketonuria* (fen"il-ke'to-nu"re-ah) *(PKU)*. CF primarily affects the lungs, but it also significantly impairs the activity of the pancreas. In CF, huge amounts of mucus are produced, which block the passages of involved organs. Blockage of the pancreatic duct prevents pancreatic fluid from reaching the small intestine. As a result, fats and fat-soluble vitamins are not digested or absorbed, and bulky, fat-laden stools result. This condition is usually handled by administering pancreatic enzymes with meals.

PKU involves an inability of tissue cells to use phenylalanine (fen"il-al'ah-nin), an amino acid present in all protein foods. In such cases, brain damage and retardation occur unless a special diet low in phenylalanine is prescribed. ▲

The developing infant receives all its nutrients through the placenta, and at least at this period of life, obtaining and processing nutrients is no problem (assuming the mother is adequately nourished). Obtaining nutrition is the most important activity of the newborn baby, and several reflexes present at this time help in this activity. For example, the *rooting reflex* helps the infant find the nipple (mother's or bottle), and the *sucking reflex* helps him or her to hold on to the nipple and swallow. The stomach of a newborn infant is very small, so feeding must be frequent (every three to four hours). Peristalsis is rather inefficient at this time, and vomiting is not at all unusual.

Teething begins around age 6 months and continues until about the age of 2 years. During this interval, the infant progresses to more and more solid foods and usually is eating an adult diet by toddlerhood. Appetite decreases in the elementary school–aged child and then increases again during the rapid growth of adolescence. (Parents of adolescents usually bewail their high grocery bills!)

All through childhood and into adulthood, the digestive system operates with relatively few problems unless there are abnormal interferences such as contaminated food or extremely spicy or irritating foods (which may cause inflammation of the gastrointestinal tract, or *gastroenteritis* [gas"tro-en-ter-i'tis]). Inflammation of the appendix, *appendicitis*, is particularly common in teenagers for some unknown reason. Between middle age and early old age, the metabolic rate decreases by 5 to 8 percent in every 10-year period. This is the time of life when the weight seems to creep up, and obesity often becomes a fact of life. To maintain desired weight, we must be aware of this gradual change and be

(continued on page 536)

Prove It Yourself

Calculate Your Basal Metabolic Rate

How much energy does your body need just to perform essential life activities? You can calculate your BMR as follows:

1. Calculate your weight in kilograms:
   Divide the number of pounds by 2.2 = _____

2. If you are male:
   Multiply your weight × 1.0 = _____

3. If you are female:
   Multiply your weight × 0.9 = _____

4. This number approximates the number of kilocalories your body consumes per hour. To estimate how many kilocalories you need each day to support basic metabolic functions, multiply this number by 24 = _____

For example, a 200-pound man (91 kg) has a BMR of 91 kcal/hour; his metabolic activities consume approximately 2,184 kilocalories per day. A 130-pound woman (59 kg) has a BMR of 53 kcal/hour, and her metabolic activities consume only 1,272 kilocalories per day. Of course, other factors besides gender and body weight can influence BMR; see Table 14.6.

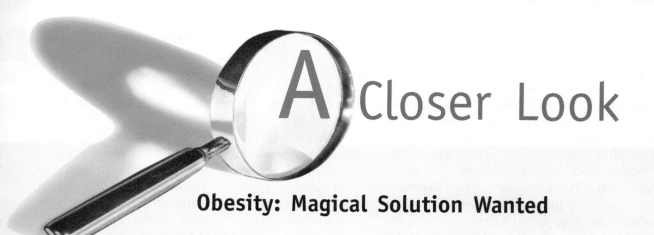

A Closer Look

Obesity: Magical Solution Wanted

HOW fat is too fat? The bathroom scale is an inaccurate guide because body weight tells nothing of body composition. A skilled dancer with dense bones and well-developed muscles may weigh several pounds more than an inactive person of the same relative size.

The most common view of obesity is that it is a condition of excessive triglyceride storage. Although we bewail our inability to rid ourselves of fat, the real problem is that we keep refilling the storehouses by consuming too many calories. A body fat content of 18 to 22 percent of body weight (males and females, respectively) is considered normal for adults. Anything over that is defined as obesity.

The official medical measure of obesity and body fatness is called the *body mass index (BMI)*, an index of a person's weight relative to height. To estimate BMI, multiply weight in pounds by 705 and then divide by your height in inches squared:

$$BMI = \frac{wt\ [lb] \times 705}{(height\ [inches])^2}$$

Overweight is defined by a BMI between 25 and 30; *obese* is a BMI greater than 30.

However it's defined, obesity is a perplexing and poorly understood disease. The term *disease* is appropriate because all forms of obesity involve some imbalance in food intake control mechanisms. Despite its well-known adverse effects on health (the obese have a higher incidence of arteriosclerosis, hypertension, coronary artery disease, and diabetes mellitus), it is the most common health problem in the United States. One out of three of us is obese. Not only are U.S. kids getting fatter, but, because they are opting for home video games and nachos instead of touch football and apples, their general cardiovascular fitness is declining as well.

Besides the health problems mentioned, the obese may store excessive levels of fat-soluble toxic chemicals, such as the insecticide DDT and PCB (a cancer-causing chemical) in their bodies. DDT interferes with the liver's ability to rid the body of other toxins, so these effects may be very far reaching. As if this were not enough, the social stigma and economic disadvantages of obesity are legendary. A fat person pays higher insurance premiums, is discriminated against in the job market, has fewer clothing choices, and is frequently humiliated during both childhood and

adulthood. With all its attendant problems, it's a pretty fair bet that few people choose to be obese. So what causes obesity? Let's look at three of the more recent theories.

Settling Point Theory

Some believe that overeating behaviors develop early in life (the "clean your plate" syndrome) and set the stage for adult obesity by increasing the number of fat cells formed during childhood. During adulthood, increases in adipose tissue mass occur because more fat is deposited in the existing cells. Thus, the more cells there are, the more fat can be stored.

Signals delivered by bloodborne nutrients or so-called satiety chemicals (hormones and others) should prevent massive fat deposit, but it appears that systems controlling hunger and satiety respond too slowly to stop a high-fat intake before the body has had too much. There are also hints that the fat cells themselves may stimulate overeating. Supporting this idea is the observation that when yo-yo dieters lose weight, their metabolic rate falls sharply. But when they subsequently gain weight, their metabolic rate increases like a furnace being stoked. Each successive weight loss occurs more slowly, but lost weight is regained three times as fast. Thus, it appears that people, like laboratory animals subjected to alternating "feasts and fasts," become increasingly food efficient, and their metabolic rates adjust to prevent any deviation from their weight "settling point." The instrument used to solve the problem—dieting (again and again)—becomes self-defeating.

Fuel Efficiency Theory

Obese people are more fuel efficient and more effective "fat storers." Although it is often assumed that obese people eat more than other people, this is not necessarily true—many actually eat less than those of normal weight.

Fat, the nutrient, is the obese person's worst enemy. Fats pack more wallop per calorie (are more fattening) than proteins or carbohydrates because very little energy is used in their processing. For example, when someone ingests 100 excess *fat* calories, only 3 calories are "burned" and the rest (97) are stored.

These facts apply to everyone, but when you are obese, the picture is even bleaker. For example, fat cells of overweight people "sprout" more alpha receptors (the kind that favors fat accumulation), and their lipoprotein lipase enzyme, which unloads fat from the blood (usually to fat cells), is exceptionally efficient.

Genetic Predisposition Theory

Morbid obesity is the fate of those inheriting two obesity genes. However, a true genetic predisposition for "fatness" appears to account for only about 5 percent of obese people in the United States. These people, given excess calories, will always deposit them as fat, as opposed to those who lay down more muscle with some of the excess calories.

False and Risky Cures

Rumors and poor choices for dealing with obesity abound. Some of the most unfortunate strategies used for coping with obesity are listed here.

- *"Water pills."* Diuretics prompt the kidneys to excrete more water. At best, these may cause a few pounds of weight loss for a few hours; they can also cause serious electrolyte imbalance and dehydration.

- *Diet pills.* Some obese people use amphetamines (such as Dexedrine and Benzedrine ["speed"]) to reduce appetite and elevate the metabolic rate. These work, but only temporarily (until tolerance develops) and can cause a dangerous dependency. Furthermore, diet aids that provide fiber to prevent absorption of nutrients can cause serious malnutrition. In the early 1990s, a new combination drug therapy

regimen, the fen-phen program, was conducted with mixed success. Fenfluramine (the "fen") increases levels of serotonin, which causes satiety, and phentermine ("phen") increases metabolic rate. These drugs were shown to promote weight loss of about 10 percent; but in September 1997, spooked by reports of heart valve abnormalities, the makers of these drugs withdrew them from the market. More recently, another diet drug, sibutramine (Merida), has come under fire for suspected cardiovascular side effects.

- *Fad diets.* Many magazines print at least one new diet regimen yearly, and diet products sell well. However, many of these diets are nutritionally unhealthy. For example, some of the liquid high-protein diets contain such poor-quality (incomplete) protein that they are actually dangerous. (The worst are those that contain collagen protein instead of a milk or soybean protein source.)

- *Surgery.* Sometimes sheer desperation prompts surgical solutions, such as having the jaws wired shut or the stomach stapled, intestinal bypass surgery, and biliopancreatic diversion (BPD). BPD "rearranges" the digestive tract: two-thirds of

Obesity: Magical Solution Wanted *(continued)*

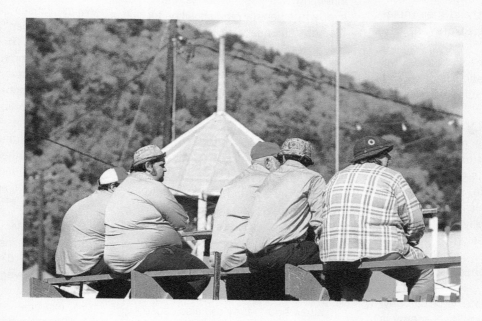

the stomach is removed; the small intestine is cut in half and one 8-foot-long portion is sutured into the stomach opening. Since pancreatic juice and bile are diverted away from this "new intestine," fewer nutrients (and no fats) are digested and absorbed. Although the patients can eat anything they want without gaining weight, BPD is major surgery and carries all of its risks. Liposuction, the removal of adipose tissue by suction to reshape the body, does remove fat, but unless the patient changes his or her eating habits, the remaining fat deposits in other parts of the body overfill.

Unfortunately, there is no magical solution for obesity, and no current explanation of weight regulation leaves much room for voluntary control. Either your genes are helpful and your regulatory peptides are interacting with receptors that are responding as they should—or they're not! Nonetheless, without pharmacological help, the only way for most of us to lose weight is to take in fewer fat calories and increase physical activity. Fidgeting and resistance exercise help to increase muscle mass (muscle consumes more energy at rest than does fat). Low activity levels actually stimulate eating, while physical exercise depresses food intake and increases metabolic rate not only during activity, but also for some time after. The only way to keep the weight off is to make these dietary and exercise changes life-long habits.

Systems in Sync

Homeostatic Relationships between the Digestive System and Other Body Systems

Nervous System
- Digestive system provides nutrients for normal neural functioning
- Neural controls of digestive function; in general, parasympathetic fibers accelerate and sympathetic fibers inhibit digestive activity; reflex and voluntary controls of defecation

Endocrine System
- Liver removes hormones from blood, ending their activity; digestive system provides nutrients needed for energy fuel, growth, and repair; pancreas has hormone-producing cells
- Local hormones help regulate digestive function

Respiratory System
- Digestive system provides nutrients for energy metabolism, growth, and repair
- Respiratory system provides oxygen and carries away carbon dioxide produced by digestive system organs

Lymphatic System/Immunity
- Digestive system provides nutrients for normal functioning; HCl of stomach provides nonspecific protection against bacteria
- Lacteals drain fatty lymph from digestive tract organs and convey it to blood; Peyer's patches and lymphoid tissue in mesentery house macrophages and immune cells that protect digestive tract organs against infection

Cardiovascular System
- Digestive system provides nutrients to heart and blood vessels; absorbs iron needed for hemoglobin synthesis; absorbs water necessary for normal blood volume
- Cardiovascular system transports nutrients absorbed by alimentary canal to all tissues of the body; distributes hormones of the digestive tract

Digestive System

Urinary System
- Digestive system provides nutrients for energy fuel, growth, and repair; excretes some bilirubin produced by the liver
- Kidneys transform vitamin D to its active form, which is needed for calcium absorption

Reproductive System
- Digestive system provides nutrients for energy fuel, growth, and repair and extra nutrition needed to support fetal growth

Integumentary System
- Digestive system provides nutrients for energy fuel, growth, and repair; supplies fats that provide insulation in the dermal and subcutaneous tissues
- The skin synthesizes vitamin D needed for calcium absorption from the intestine; protects by enclosure

Muscular System
- Digestive system provides nutrients for energy fuel, growth, and repair; liver removes lactic acid, resulting from muscle activity, from the blood
- Skeletal muscle activity increases motility of GI tract

Skeletal System
- Digestive system provides nutrients for energy fuel, growth, and repair; absorbs calcium needed for bone salts
- Skeletal system protects some digestive organs by bone; cavities store some nutrients (e.g., calcium, fats)

(continued from page 531)

prepared to reduce caloric intake. Two distinctly middle-age digestive problems are *ulcers* (see the "A Closer Look" box about ulcers earlier in this chapter) and *gallbladder problems* (inflammation of the gallbladder or gallstones).

During old age, activity of the GI tract declines. Fewer digestive juices are produced, and peristalsis slows. Taste and smell become less acute, and periodontal disease often develops. Many elderly individuals live alone or on a reduced income. These factors, along with increasing physical disability, tend to make eating less appealing, and nutrition is inadequate in many of our elderly citizens. Diverticulosis and cancer of the gastrointestinal tract are fairly common problems in the elderly. Cancer of the stomach and colon rarely have early signs and often progress to an inoperable stage (that is, spread to distant parts of the body as well) before the individual seeks medical attention. However, when detected early, both diseases are treatable, and it has been suggested that diets high in plant fiber and low in fat might help to decrease the incidence of colon cancer. Additionally, since most colorectal cancers derive from initially benign mucosal tumors called *polyps*, and the incidence of polyp formation increases with age, a yearly colon examination should be a health priority in everyone over the age of 50.

Unit 6
Urinary System
&
Unit 7
Fluid and Electrolyte Balance

15

The Urinary System

KEY TERMS

The kidneys, which maintain the purity and constancy of our internal fluids, are perfect examples of homeostatic organs. Much like sanitation workers who keep a city's water supply drinkable and dispose of its waste, the kidneys are usually unappreciated until there is a malfunction and "internal garbage" piles up. Every day, the kidneys filter gallons of fluid from the bloodstream. They then process this filtrate, allowing wastes and excess ions to leave the body in urine while returning needed substances to the blood in just the right proportions. Although the lungs and the skin also play roles in excretion, the kidneys bear the major responsibility for eliminating nitrogenous (nitrogen-containing) wastes, toxins, and drugs from the body.

Disposing of wastes and excess ions is only one part of the work of the kidneys. As they perform these excretory functions, they also regulate the blood's volume and chemical makeup so that the proper balance between water and salts and between acids and bases is maintained. Frankly, this would be tricky work for a chemical engineer, but the kidneys do it efficiently most of the time.

The kidneys have other regulatory functions as well: By producing the enzyme *renin* (re'nin), they help regulate blood pressure, and their hormone *erythropoietin* stimulates red blood cell production in bone marrow. Kidney cells also convert vitamin D to its active form.

The kidneys alone perform the functions just described and manufacture urine in the process. The other organs of the **urinary system**—the paired ureters and the single urinary bladder and urethra (Figure 15.1)—provide temporary storage reservoirs for urine or serve as transportation channels to carry it from one body region to another.

Kidneys

Location and Structure

Although many believe that the **kidneys** are located in the lower back, this is *not* their location. Instead, these small, dark red organs with a kidney-bean shape lie against the dorsal body wall in a *retroperitoneal* position (beneath the parietal peritoneum) in the *superior* lumbar region. The kidneys extend from the T_{12} to the L_3 vertebra; thus they receive some protection from the lower part of the rib cage. Because it is crowded by the liver, the right kidney is positioned slightly lower than the left. An adult

kidney is about 12 cm (5 inches) long, 6 cm (2.5 inches) wide, and 3 cm (1 inch) thick, about the size of a large bar of soap. It is convex laterally and has a medial indentation called the *renal hilus*. Several structures, including the ureters, the renal blood vessels, and nerves, enter or exit the kidney at the hilus (see Figures 15.1 and 15.2). Atop each kidney is an *adrenal gland*, which is part of the endocrine system and is a distinctly separate organ functionally.

A fibrous, transparent **renal capsule** encloses each kidney and gives a fresh kidney a glistening appearance. A fatty mass, the *adipose capsule*, surrounds each kidney and helps hold it in place against the muscles of the trunk wall.

▲ Homeostatic Imbalance

The fat surrounding the kidneys is extremely important in holding them in their normal body position. If the amount of fatty tissue dwindles (as with rapid weight loss), the kidneys may drop to a lower position, a condition called *ptosis* (to'sis; "a fall"). Ptosis creates problems if the ureters, which drain urine from the kidneys, become kinked. When this happens, urine that can no longer pass through the ureters backs up and exerts pressure on the kidney tissue. This condition, called *hydronephrosis* (hi"dro-nĕ-fro'sis), can severely damage the kidney. ▲

When a kidney is cut lengthwise, three distinct regions become apparent, as can be seen in Figure 15.2. The outer region, which is light in color, is the **renal cortex.** (The word *cortex* comes from the Latin word meaning "bark.") Deep to the cortex is a darker reddish-brown area, the **renal medulla.** The medulla has many basically triangular regions with a striped appearance, the **medullary** (med'u-lar"e) **pyramids.** The broader *base* of each pyramid faces toward the cortex; its tip, the *apex,* points toward the inner region of the kidney. The pyramids are separated by extensions of cortex-like tissue, the **renal columns.**

Medial to the hilus is a flat, basinlike cavity, the **renal pelvis.** As Figure 15.2b shows, the pelvis is continuous with the ureter leaving the hilus. Extensions of the pelvis, **calyces** (kal'ĭ-sēz; singular *calyx*), form cup-shaped areas that enclose the tips of the pyramids. The calyces collect urine, which continuously drains from the tips of the pyramids into the renal pelvis. Urine then flows from the pelvis into the ureter, which transports it to the bladder for temporary storage.

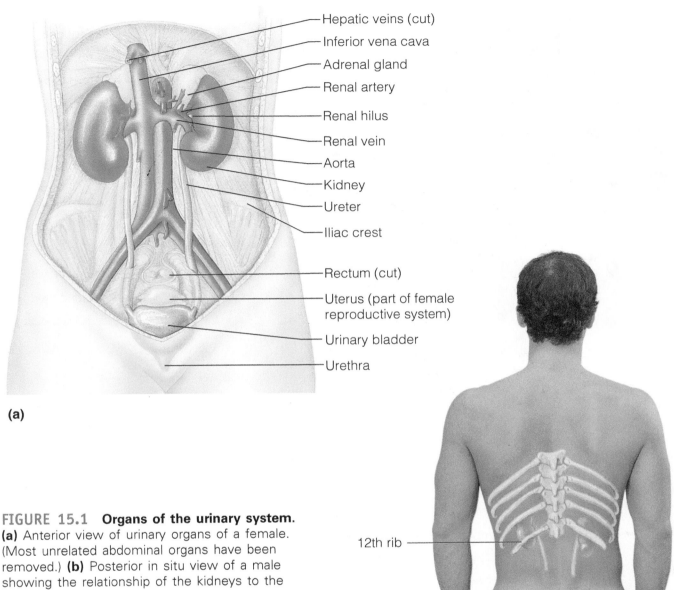

Hepatic veins (cut)
Inferior vena cava
Adrenal gland
Renal artery
Renal hilus
Renal vein
Aorta
Kidney
Ureter
Iliac crest

Rectum (cut)
Uterus (part of female reproductive system)
Urinary bladder
Urethra

(a)

12th rib

FIGURE 15.1   Organs of the urinary system.
(a) Anterior view of urinary organs of a female.
(Most unrelated abdominal organs have been
removed.) **(b)** Posterior in situ view of a male
showing the relationship of the kidneys to the
12th rib pair.

Blood Supply

The kidneys continuously cleanse the blood and
adjust its composition, so it is not surprising that
they have a very rich blood supply (see Figure 15.2b
and c). Approximately one-quarter of the total
blood supply of the body passes through the
kidneys each minute. The arterial supply of each
kidney is the **renal artery.** As the renal artery
approaches the hilus, it divides into **segmental
arteries.** Once inside the pelvis, the segmental
arteries break up into **lobar arteries,** each of
which gives off several branches called **interlobar**

arteries, which travel through the renal columns to
reach the cortex. At the cortex-medulla junction,
interlobar arteries give off the **arcuate** (ar′ku-at)
arteries, which curve over the medullary pyramids.
Small **interlobular arteries** then branch off the arcuate arteries and run outward to supply the cortical
tissue. Venous blood draining from the kidney flows
through veins that trace the pathway of the arterial
supply but in a reverse direction—**interlobular
veins** to **arcuate veins** to **interlobar veins** to the
renal vein, which emerges from the kidney hilus.
(There are no lobar or segmental veins.)

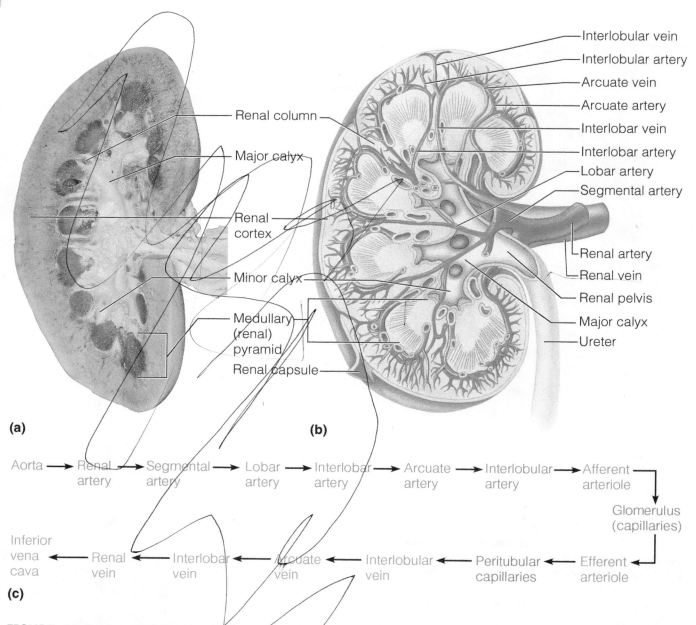

FIGURE 15.2 Internal anatomy of the kidney. (a) Photograph of a coronally sectioned kidney. **(b)** Diagrammatic view of a coronally sectioned kidney, illustrating major blood vessels. **(c)** Summary of the pathway of renal blood vessels.

Nephrons and Urine Formation

Nephrons

Each kidney contains over a million tiny structures called **nephrons** (nef′ronz). Nephrons are the structural and functional units of the kidneys and, as such, are responsible for forming urine. Figure 15.3 shows the anatomy and relative positioning of nephrons in each kidney.

Each nephron consists of two main structures: a **glomerulus** (glo-mer′u-lus), which is a knot of capillaries, and a **renal tubule.** The closed end of the renal tubule is enlarged and cup-shaped and completely surrounds the glomerulus. This portion of the renal tubule is called the **glomerular** (*glom* = little ball), or **Bowman's, capsule.** The inner (visceral) layer of the capsule is made up of highly modified octopus-like cells called **podocytes** (pod′o-sītz).

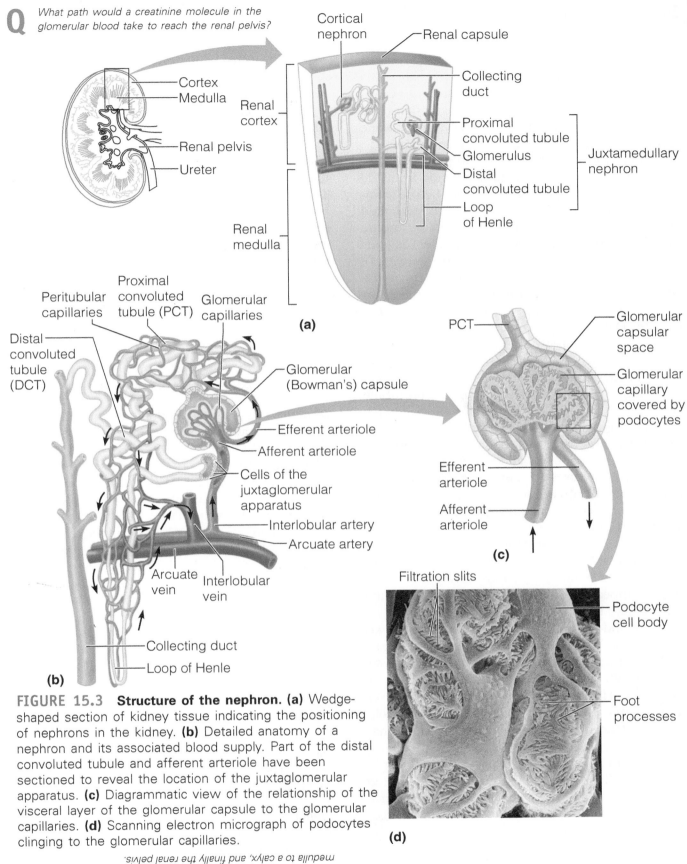

Q What path would a creatinine molecule in the glomerular blood take to reach the renal pelvis?

(a) Cortical nephron · Renal capsule · Cortex · Medulla · Collecting duct · Renal pelvis · Ureter · Renal cortex · Renal medulla · Proximal convoluted tubule · Glomerulus · Distal convoluted tubule · Loop of Henle · Juxtamedullary nephron

(b) Peritubular capillaries · Proximal convoluted tubule (PCT) · Glomerular capillaries · Distal convoluted tubule (DCT) · Glomerular (Bowman's) capsule · Efferent arteriole · Afferent arteriole · Cells of the juxtaglomerular apparatus · Interlobular artery · Arcuate artery · Arcuate vein · Interlobular vein · Collecting duct · Loop of Henle

(c) PCT · Glomerular capsular space · Glomerular capillary covered by podocytes · Efferent arteriole · Afferent arteriole

(d) Filtration slits · Podocyte cell body · Foot processes

FIGURE 15.3 **Structure of the nephron. (a)** Wedge-shaped section of kidney tissue indicating the positioning of nephrons in the kidney. **(b)** Detailed anatomy of a nephron and its associated blood supply. Part of the distal convoluted tubule and afferent arteriole have been sectioned to reveal the location of the juxtaglomerular apparatus. **(c)** Diagrammatic view of the relationship of the visceral layer of the glomerular capsule to the glomerular capillaries. **(d)** Scanning electron micrograph of podocytes clinging to the glomerular capillaries.

A From the glomerular blood into the glomerular capsular space, then the proximal convoluted tubule to the loop of Henle, the distal convoluted tubule, the collecting duct through the renal medulla to a calyx, and finally the renal pelvis.

Podocytes have long branching processes called *foot processes* that intertwine with one another and cling to the glomerulus. Because openings, the so-called *filtration slits,* exist between their extensions, the podocytes form a porous, or "holey," membrane around the glomerulus (Figure 15.3c and d).

The rest of the tubule is about 3 cm (approximately 1.25 inches) long. As it extends from the glomerular capsule, it coils and twists before forming a hairpin loop and then again becomes coiled and twisted before entering a collecting tubule called the **collecting duct.** These different regions of the tubule have specific names (see Figure 15.3); in order from the glomerular capsule they are the **proximal convoluted tubule (PCT), the loop of Henle** (hen′le), and the **distal convoluted tubule (DCT).** The lumen surfaces (surface exposed to the filtrate) of the tubule cells in the proximal convoluted tubules are covered with dense microvilli, which increases their surface area tremendously. Microvilli also occur on the tubule cells in other parts of the tubule but in much reduced numbers.

Most nephrons are called **cortical nephrons** because they are located almost entirely within the cortex. In a few cases, the nephrons are called **juxtamedullary nephrons** because they are situated close to the cortex-medulla junction, and their loops of Henle dip deep into the medulla (see Figure 15.3a). The **collecting ducts,** each of which receives urine from many nephrons, run downward through the medullary pyramids, giving them their striped appearance. They deliver the final urine product into the calyces and renal pelvis.

Each and every nephron is associated with two capillary beds—the glomerulus (mentioned earlier) and the *peritubular* (per″ĭ-tu′bu-lar) *capillary bed.* The glomerulus is both fed and drained by *arterioles.* The **afferent arteriole,** which arises from an *interlobular artery,* is the "feeder vessel," and the **efferent arteriole** receives blood that has passed through the glomerulus. The glomerulus, specialized for filtration, is unlike any other capillary bed in the entire body. Because it is both fed *and* drained by arterioles, which are high-resistance vessels, and the afferent arteriole has a larger diameter than the efferent, blood pressure in the glomerular capillaries is much higher than in other capillary beds. This extremely high pressure forces fluid and solutes (smaller than proteins) out of the blood into the glomerular capsule. Most of this filtrate (99 percent) is eventually reclaimed by the renal tubule cells and returned to the blood in the peritubular capillary beds.

The second capillary bed, the **peritubular capillaries,** arises from the efferent arteriole that drains the glomerulus. Unlike the high-pressure glomerulus, these capillaries are low-pressure, porous vessels that are adapted for absorption instead of filtration. They cling closely to the whole length of the renal tubule, where they are in an ideal position to receive solutes and water from the tubule cells as these substances are reabsorbed from the filtrate percolating through the tubule. The peritubular capillaries drain into interlobular veins leaving the cortex.

Urine Formation

Urine formation is a result of three processes—*filtration, tubular reabsorption,* and *tubular secretion.* Each of these processes is illustrated in Figure 15.4 and described in more detail next.

Filtration   As just described, the glomerulus acts as a filter. **Glomerular filtration** is a nonselective, passive process. The filtrate that is formed is essentially blood plasma without blood proteins. Both proteins and blood cells are normally too large to pass through the filtration membrane, and when either of these appear in the urine, it is a pretty fair bet that there is some problem with the glomerular filters. As long as the systemic blood pressure is normal, filtrate will be formed. If arterial blood pressure drops too low, the glomerular pressure becomes inadequate to force substances out of the blood into the tubules, and filtrate formation stops.

▲ Homeostatic Imbalance

An abnormally low urinary output is called *oliguria* (ol″i-gu′re-ah) if it is between 100 and 400 ml/day, and *anuria* (ah-nu′re-ah) if it is less than 100 ml/day. Low urinary output usually indicates that glomerular blood pressure is too low to cause filtration, but anuria may also result from transfusion reactions and acute inflammation or from crush injuries of the kidneys. ▲

Tubular Reabsorption   Besides wastes and excess ions that must be removed from the blood, the filtrate contains many useful substances (including water, glucose, amino acids, and ions), which must be reclaimed from the filtrate and returned to the blood. **Tubular reabsorption** begins as soon as

Q How would liver disease, in which the liver is unable to make many of the blood proteins, affect process a? (Reviewing Chapter 10 might help.)

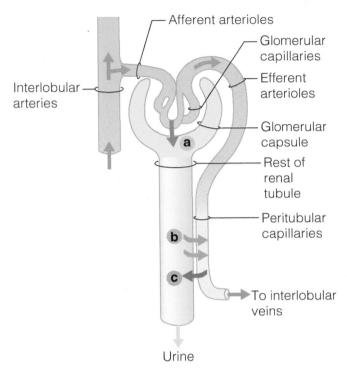

KEY:

a **Filtration:** Water and solutes smaller than proteins are forced through the capillary walls and pores of the glomerular capsule into the renal tubule.

b **Tubular Reabsorption:** Water, glucose, amino acids, and needed ions are transported out of the filtrate into the tubule cells and then enter the capillary blood.

c **Tubular Secretion:** H+, K+, creatinine, and drugs are removed from the peritubular blood and secreted by the tubule cells into the filtrate.

FIGURE 15.4 The kidney depicted schematically as a single large, uncoiled nephron. A kidney actually has millions of nephrons acting in parallel. The three processes by which the kidneys adjust the composition of plasma are **(a)** filtration, **(b)** tubular reabsorption, and **(c)** tubular secretion.

A The amount of renal filtrate formed is a function of filtration (blood) pressure and blood osmotic pressure (exerted largely by blood proteins). Normally the osmotic pressure is a constant; but, in the situation described, more filtrate than normal will be formed because the blood pressure is opposed to a lesser extent by osmotic pressure of the blood.

the filtrate enters the proximal convoluted tubule (Figure 15.5). The tubule cells are "transporters," taking up needed substances from the filtrate and then passing them out their posterior aspect into the extracellular space, from which they are absorbed into peritubular capillary blood. Some reabsorption is done passively (for example, water passes by osmosis), but the reabsorption of most substances depends on active transport processes, which use membrane carriers and are very selective. There is an abundance of carriers for substances that need to be retained, and few or no carriers for substances of no use to the body. Needed substances (for example, glucose and amino acids) are usually entirely removed from the filtrate. **Nitrogenous waste products** are poorly reabsorbed, if at all. These include **urea** (u-re′ah), formed by the liver as an end product of protein breakdown when amino acids are used to produce energy; **uric acid,** released when nucleic acids are metabolized; and **creatinine** (kre-at′ĭ-nin), associated with creatine (kre′ah-tin) metabolism in muscle tissue. Because tubule cells have few membrane carriers to reabsorb these substances, they tend to remain in the filtrate and are found in high concentrations in urine excreted from the body. Various ions are reabsorbed or allowed to go out in the urine, according to what is needed at a particular time to maintain the proper pH and electrolyte composition of the blood. Most reabsorption occurs in the proximal convoluted tubules, but the distal convoluted tubule and the collecting duct are also active.

Tubular Secretion   **Tubular secretion** is essentially reabsorption in reverse. Some substances, such as hydrogen and potassium ions and creatinine, also move from the blood of the peritubular capillaries through the tubule cells or from the tubule cells themselves into the filtrate to be eliminated in urine. This process seems to be important for getting rid of substances not already in the filtrate, such as certain drugs, or as an additional means for controlling blood pH (Figure 15.5).

Filtration at the Glomerulus

Let's look at the processes of urine formation in more detail, starting with filtration. Filtration occurs in the renal corpuscle as fluids move across the wall of the glomerulus and into the capsular space.

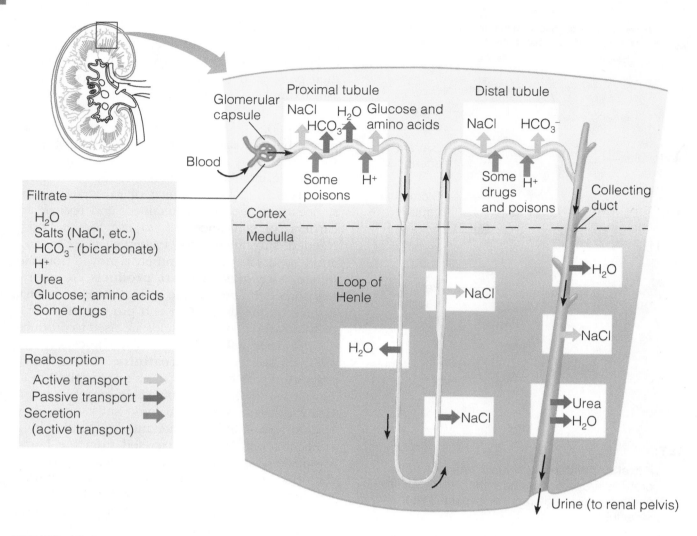

FIGURE 15.5   Sites of filtration, reabsorption, and secretion in a nephron.

The process of glomerular filtration involves passage across a filtration membrane, which has three components: (1) the capillary endothelium, (2) the lamina densa, and (3) the filtration slits (see Figures 15.6).

Glomerular capillaries are fenestrated capillaries with pores ranging from 60 to 100 nm (0.06 to 0.1 μm) in diameter. These openings are small enough to prevent the passage of blood cells, but they are too large to restrict the diffusion of solutes, even those the size of plasma proteins. The lamina densa is more selective: Only small plasma proteins, nutrients, and ions can cross it. The filtration slits are the finest filters of all. Their gaps are only 6–9 nm wide, which is small enough to prevent the passage of most small plasma proteins. As a result, under normal circumstances

no plasma proteins (except a few albumin molecules, with an average diameter of 7 nm) can cross the filtration membrane and enter the capsular space. However, plasma proteins are all that stay behind, so the filtrate contains dissolved ions and small organic molecules in roughly the same concentrations as in plasma.

Filtration Pressures

The primary factor involved in glomerular filtration is basically the same as that governing fluid and solute movement across capillaries throughout the body: the balance between hydrostatic pressure (fluid pressure) and colloid osmotic pressure (pressure due to materials in solution) on either side of the capillary walls.

A Closer Look

Renal Failure and the Artificial Kidney

IKE master chemists, the kidneys continually maintain the purity of our internal environment. Without their continual efforts, body fluids quickly become contaminated with nitrogen-containing wastes, blood pH tumbles into the acidic range, and *uremia* sets in, totally disrupting life processes. Signs and symptoms of uncontrolled uremia include diarrhea, vomiting, labored breathing, irregular heartbeat, convulsions, coma, and finally death.

Although not common, renal failure may occur when the number of functioning units (nephrons) becomes too low to carry out the normal kidney functions. The leading cause of renal failure is diabetes mellitus (approximately 33 percent of new cases each year) with hypertension a close second. (Notice that hypertension is both a cause and a symptom.) Other possible causes of renal failure include:

- Repeated damaging infections of the kidneys
- Physical trauma to the kidneys (crush injury and others)
- Chemical poisoning of the tubule cells by heavy metals (mercury or lead) or organic solvents (dry-cleaning fluids, paint thinner)

- Inadequate blood delivery to the tubule cells (as sometimes happens with arteriosclerosis)
- Prolonged pressure on skeletal muscles (causes release of myoglobin, a muscle pigment that can clog renal tubules)
- Chronic hypertension or immune system problems

In renal failure, filtrate formation decreases or stops completely.

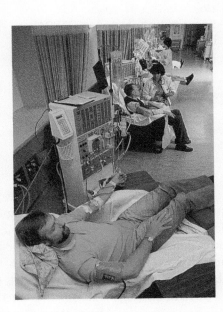

A renal patient undergoing hemodialysis.

Because toxic wastes accumulate quickly in the blood when the kidney tubule cells are not working, *dialysis* (*dialys* = separate) is necessary to cleanse the blood while the kidneys are shut down. In *hemodialysis*, which uses an "artificial kidney" apparatus (see illustration), the patient's blood is passed through a membrane tubing that is permeable only to selected substances, and the tubing is immersed in a bathing solution that differs slightly from normal "cleansed" plasma. As blood circulates through the tubing, substances such as nitrogenous wastes and potassium ions (K^+) present in the blood (but not in the bath) diffuse out of the blood through the tubing into the surrounding solution, and substances to be added to the blood (mainly buffers for hydrogen ions [H^+] and glucose for malnourished patients) move from the bathing solution into the blood. In this way, needed substances are retained in the blood or added to it, while wastes and ion excesses are removed. Hemodialysis is routinely done three times weekly, and each session takes four to eight hours. Serious problems occasionally encountered by hemodialysis patients are

Renal Failure and the Artificial Kidney *(continued)*

thrombosis, infection, and ischemia at the shunt site. Hemorrhage is an added risk, because the blood must be heparinized to prevent clotting during hemodialysis. (*Heparin* is an anticoagulant.)

A less efficient but more convenient procedure for patients who are not hospitalized is *continuous ambulatory peritoneal dialysis (CAPD)*. CAPD uses the patient's own peritoneal membrane as the dialyzing membrane. Fluid that is equal in chemical content to normal plasma and interstitial fluid is introduced into the patient's peritoneal cavity with a catheter and left to equilibrate there for 15 to 60 minutes. Then the dialysis fluid is retrieved from the peritoneal cavity and replaced with fresh dialysis fluid. The procedure is repeated until the patient's blood chemistry reaches normal. Because some ambulatory patients may be inattentive to cloudy or bloody dialysis fluid, infection is more common in CAPD than in hemodialysis.

When renal damage is nonreversible, as in chronic, slowly progressing renal failure, the kidneys become totally unable to process plasma or concentrate urine, and a kidney transplant is the only answer. Unhappily, the signs and symptoms of this life-threatening problem become obvious only after about 75 percent of renal function has been lost. The end-stage of renal failure, *uremia,* occurs when about 90 percent of the nephrons have been lost.

Hydrostatic Pressure

The **glomerular hydrostatic pressure (GHP)** is the blood pressure in the glomerular capillaries. This pressure tends to push water and solute molecules out of the plasma and into the filtrate. The GHP is significantly higher than capillary pressures elsewhere in the systemic circuit, due to the arrangement of vessels at the glomerulus.

Blood pressure is low in typical systemic capillaries because capillary blood flows into the venous system, where resistance is relatively low. However, at the glomerulus, blood leaving the glomerular capillaries flows into an efferent arteriole, whose diameter is *smaller* than that of the afferent arteriole. The efferent arteriole thus offers considerable resistance, so relatively high pressures are needed to force blood into it. As a result, glomerular pressures are similar to those of small arteries, averaging about 50 mm Hg instead of the 35 mm Hg typical of peripheral capillaries.

Glomerular hydrostatic pressure is opposed by the **capsular hydrostatic pressure (CsHP),** which tends to push water and solutes out of the filtrate and into the plasma. This pressure results from the resistance to flow along the nephron and the conducting system. (Before additional filtrate can enter the capsule, some of the filtrate already present must be forced into the PCT.) The CsHP averages about 15 mm Hg.

The *net hydrostatic pressure (NHP)* is the difference between the glomerular hydrostatic pressure, which tends to push water and solutes out of the bloodstream, and the capsular hydrostatic pressure, which tends to push water and solutes into

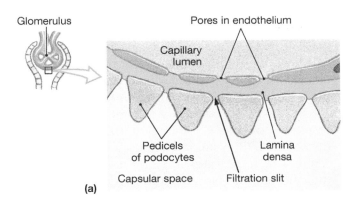

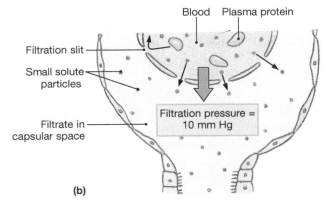

FIGURE 15.6   Glomerular filtration. (a) The filtration membrane. **(b)** Filtration pressure.

the bloodstream. Net hydrostatic pressure can be calculated as follows:

$$NHP = GHP - CsHP = 50 \text{ mm Hg} - 15 \text{ mm Hg} = 35 \text{ mm Hg}$$

Colloid Osmotic Pressure

The colloid osmotic pressure of a solution is the osmotic pressure resulting from the presence of suspended proteins. The **blood colloid osmotic pressure (BCOP)** tends to draw water out of the filtrate and into the plasma; it thus opposes filtration. Over the entire length of the glomerular capillary bed, the BCOP averages about 25 mm Hg. Under normal conditions, very few plasma proteins enter the capsular space, so no opposing colloid osmotic pressure exists within the capsule. However, if the glomeruli are damaged by disease or injury, and plasma proteins begin passing into the capsular space, a *capsular colloid osmotic pressure* is created that promotes filtration and increases fluid losses in urine.

Filtration Pressure

The **filtration pressure (FP)** at the glomerulus is the difference between the hydrostatic pressure and the colloid osmotic pressure acting across the glomerular capillaries. Under normal circumstances, this relationship can be summarized as

$$FP = NHP - BCOP$$

or

$$FP = 35 \text{ mm Hg} - 25 \text{ mm Hg } 10 \text{ mm Hg.}$$

This is the average pressure forcing water and dissolved materials out of the glomerular capillaries and into the capsular spaces (Figure 15.6b). Problems that affect filtration pressure can seriously disrupt kidney function and cause a variety of clinical signs and symptoms.

The Glomerular Filtration Rate

The **glomerular filtration rate (GFR)** is the amount of filtrate the kidneys produce each minute. Each kidney contains about 6 m^2—some 64 square feet—of filtration surface, and the GFR averages an astounding *125 ml per minute*. This means that roughly 10 percent of the fluid delivered to the kidneys by the renal arteries leaves the bloodstream and enters the capsular spaces.

A *creatinine clearance test* is often used to estimate the GFR. Creatinine, which results from the breakdown of creatine phosphate in muscle tissue, is normally eliminated in urine. Creatinine enters the filtrate at the glomerulus and is not reabsorbed in significant amounts. By monitoring the creatinine concentrations in blood and the amount excreted in urine in a 24-hour period, a clinician can easily estimate the GFR. Consider, for example, a person who eliminates 84 mg of creatinine each hour and has a plasma creatinine concentration of 1.4 mg/dl. Because the GFR is equal to the amount secreted, divided by the plasma concentration, this person's GFR is

$$\frac{84 \text{ mg/h}}{1.4 \text{ mg/dl}} = 60 \text{ dl/h} = 100 \text{ ml/min.}$$

The GFR is usually reported in milliliters per minute.

Control of the GFR

Glomerular filtration is the vital first step essential to all other kidney functions. If filtration does not occur, waste products are not excreted, pH control is jeopardized, and an important mechanism for regulating blood volume is lost. It should be no surprise that a variety of regulatory mechanisms ensure that GFR remains within normal limits.

Filtration depends on adequate blood flow to the glomerulus and on the maintenance of normal filtration pressures. Three interacting levels of control stabilize GFR: (1) *autoregulation,* at the local level, (2) *hormonal regulation,* initiated by the kidneys, and (3) *autonomic regulation,* primarily by the sympathetic division of the autonomic nervous system.

Autoregulation of the GFR

Autoregulation maintains an adequate GFR despite changes in local blood pressure and blood flow. Maintenance of the GFR is accomplished by changing the diameters of afferent arterioles, efferent arterioles, and glomerular capillaries. The most important regulatory mechanisms stabilize the GFR when systemic blood pressure declines. A reduction in blood flow and a decline in glomerular blood pressure trigger (1) dilation of the afferent arteriole, (2) relaxation of supporting cells and dilation of the glomerular capillaries, and (3) constriction of the efferent arteriole. This combination increases blood flow and elevates glomerular blood pressure to normal levels. As a result, filtration rates remain relatively constant. The GFR also remains relatively constant when systemic blood pressure rises. A rise in renal blood pressure stretches the walls of afferent arterioles, and the smooth muscle cells respond by contracting. The reduction in the diameter of afferent arterioles decreases glomerular blood flow and keeps the GFR within normal limits.

Hormonal Regulation of the GFR

The GFR is regulated by the hormones of the renin-angiotensin system and the natriuretic peptides (ANP and BNP). There are three triggers for the release of renin by the juxtaglomerular apparatus (JGA): (1) a decline in blood pressure at the glomerulus as the result of a decrease in blood volume, a fall in systemic pressures, or a blockage in the renal artery or its tributaries; (2) stimulation of juxtaglomerular cells by sympathetic innervation; or (3) a decline in the osmotic concentration of the tubular fluid at the macula densa. These stimuli are often interrelated. For example, a decline in systemic blood pressure reduces the glomerular filtration rate while baroreceptor reflexes cause sympathetic activation. Meanwhile,

a reduction in the GFR slows the movement of tubular fluid along the nephron. Because the tubular fluid is then in the ascending limb of the loop of Henle longer, the concentration of sodium and chloride ions in the tubular fluid reaching the macula densa and DCT becomes abnormally low.

Figure 15.7a provides a general overview of the response of the renin-angiotensin system to a decline in GFR. A fall in GFR leads to the release of renin, which activates angiotensin. Angiotensin II then elevates the blood volume and blood pressure, increasing the GFR. Figure 15.7b presents a more detailed view of the mechanisms involved. Once released into the bloodstream by the juxtaglomerular apparatus, renin converts the inactive protein angiotensinogen to angiotensin I. Angiotensin I, which is also inactive, is then converted to angiotensin II by **angiotensin-converting enzyme (ACE),** primarily in the capillaries of the lungs. Angiotensin II is an active hormone whose primary effects include the following:

- *At the nephron,* angiotensin II causes the constriction of the efferent arteriole, further elevating glomerular pressures and filtration rates. Angiotensin II also directly stimulates the reabsorption of sodium ions and water at the PCT.

- *At the adrenal glands,* angiotensin II stimulates the secretion of aldosterone by the adrenal cortex. The aldosterone then accelerates sodium reabsorption in the DCT and cortical portion of the collecting system.

- *In the CNS,* angiotensin II (1) causes the sensation of thirst; (2) triggers the release of antidiuretic hormone (ADH), stimulating the reabsorption of water in the distal portion of the DCT and the collecting system; and (3) increases sympathetic motor tone, mobilizing the venous reserve, increasing cardiac output, and stimulating peripheral vasoconstriction.

- *In peripheral capillary beds,* angiotensin II causes a brief but powerful vasoconstriction of arterioles and precapillary sphincters, elevating arterial pressures throughout the body.

The combined effect is an increase in systemic blood volume and blood pressure and the restoration of normal GFR.

Autonomic Regulation of the GFR

Most of the autonomic innervation of the kidneys consists of sympathetic postganglionic fibers. (The

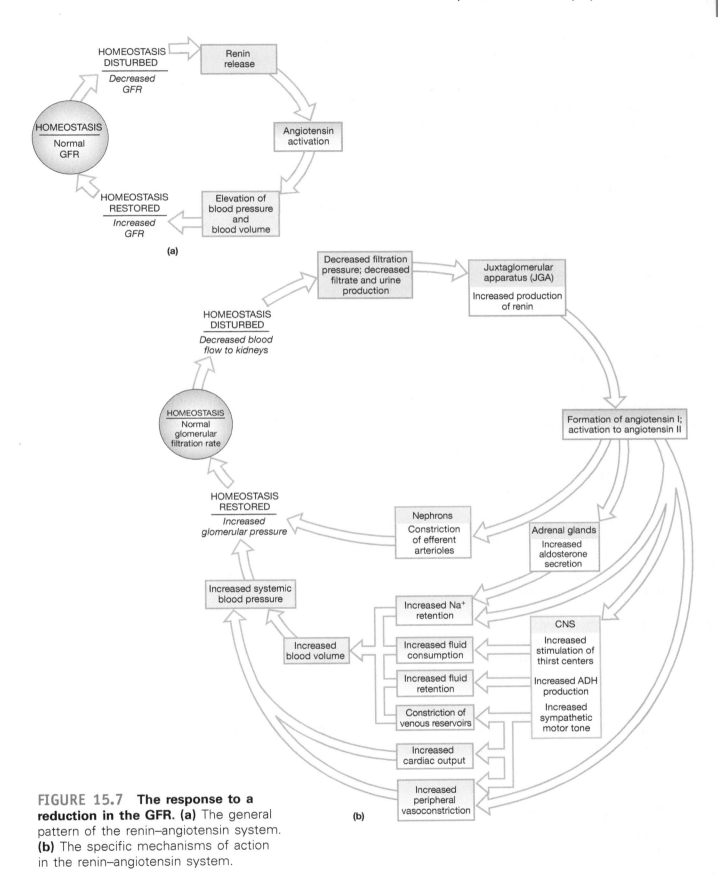

FIGURE 15.7 **The response to a reduction in the GFR. (a)** The general pattern of the renin–angiotensin system. **(b)** The specific mechanisms of action in the renin–angiotensin system.

role of the few parasympathetic fibers in regulating kidney function is not known.) Sympathetic activation has one direct effect on the GFR: It produces a powerful vasoconstriction of afferent arterioles, decreasing the GFR and slowing the production of filtrate. Thus the sympathetic activation triggered by an acute fall in blood pressure or a heart attack overrides the local regulatory mechanisms that act to stabilize the GFR. As the crisis passes and sympathetic tone decreases, the filtration rate gradually returns to normal levels.

When the sympathetic division alters regional patterns of blood circulation, blood flow to the kidneys is often affected. For example, the dilation of superficial vessels in warm weather shunts blood away from the kidneys, so glomerular filtration declines temporarily. The effect becomes especially pronounced during periods of strenuous exercise. As the blood flow to your skin and skeletal muscles increases, kidney perfusion gradually decreases. These changes may be opposed, with variable success, by autoregulation at the local level.

At maximal levels of exertion, renal blood flow may be less than 25 percent of normal resting levels. This reduction can create problems for endurance athletes, because metabolic wastes build up over the course of a long event. *Proteinuria* (protein in the urine) commonly occurs after such events because the glomerular cells have been injured by prolonged hypoxia (low oxygen levels). If the damage is substantial, *hematuria* (blood in the urine) occurs. Hematuria develops in roughly 18 percent of marathon runners. Proteinuria and hematuria generally disappear within 48 hours as the glomerular tissues are repaired. However, a small number of marathon and ultramarathon runners experience *acute renal failure*, with permanent impairment of kidney function.

100 Keys | Roughly 180 L of filtrate is produced at the glomeruli each day, and that represents 70 times the total plasma volume. Almost all of that fluid volume must be reabsorbed to avoid fatal dehydration.

Renal Physiology: Reabsorption and Secretion

Reabsorption recovers useful materials that have entered the filtrate, and secretion ejects waste products, toxins, or other undesirable solutes that did not leave the bloodstream at the glomerulus. Both processes occur in every segment of the nephron except the renal corpuscle, but their relative importance changes from segment to segment.

Reabsorption and Secretion at the PCT

The cells of the proximal convoluted tubule normally reabsorb 60–70 percent of the volume of the filtrate produced in the renal corpuscle. The reabsorbed materials enter the peritubular fluid and diffuse into peritubular capillaries.

The PCT has five major functions:

1. *Reabsorption of Organic Nutrients.* Under normal circumstances, before the tubular fluid enters the loop of Henle, the PCT reabsorbs more than 99 percent of the glucose, amino acids, and other organic nutrients in the fluid. This reabsorption involves a combination of facilitated transport and cotransport.

2. *Active Reabsorption of Ions.* The PCT actively transports several ions, including sodium, potassium, and bicarbonate ions (Figure 15.8), plus magnesium, phosphate, and sulfate ions. The ion pumps involved are individually regulated and may be influenced by circulating ion or hormone levels. For example, angiotensin II stimulates Na^+ reabsorption along the PCT. By absorbing carbon dioxide, the PCT indirectly recaptures roughly 90 percent of the bicarbonate ions from tubular fluid. Bicarbonate is important in stabilizing blood pH.

3. *Reabsorption of Water.* The reabsorptive processes have a direct effect on the solute concentrations inside and outside the tubules. The filtrate entering the PCT has the same osmotic concentration as that of the surrounding peritubular fluid. As transport activities proceed, the solute concentration of tubular fluid decreases, and that of peritubular fluid and adjacent capillaries increases. Osmosis then pulls water out of the tubular fluid and into the peritubular fluid. Along the PCT, this mechanism results in the reabsorption of roughly 108 liters of water each day.

4. *Passive Reabsorption of Ions.* As active reabsorption of ions occurs and water leaves tubular fluid by osmosis, the concentration of

other solutes in tubular fluid increases above that in peritubular fluid. If the tubular cells are permeable to them, those solutes will move across the tubular cells and into the peritubular fluid by passive diffusion. Urea, chloride ions, and lipid-soluble materials may diffuse out of the PCT in this way. Such diffusion further reduces the solute concentration of the tubular fluid and promotes additional water reabsorption by osmosis.

5. *Secretion.* Active secretion also occurs along the PCT. Because the DCT performs comparatively little reabsorption, we will consider secretory mechanisms when we discuss the DCT.

Sodium ion reabsorption plays an important role in all of the foregoing processes. Sodium ions may enter tubular cells by diffusion through Na^+ leak channels; by the sodium-linked cotransport of glucose, amino acids, or other organic solutes; or by countertransport for hydrogen ions (see Figure 15.8). In tubular cells, sodium ions diffuse toward the basal lamina. The cell membrane in this area contains sodium-potassium exchange pumps that eject sodium ions in exchange for extracellular potassium ions. Reabsorbed sodium ions then diffuse into the adjacent peritubular capillaries.

The reabsorption of ions and compounds along the PCT involves many different carrier proteins. Some people have an inherited inability to manufacture one or more of these carrier proteins and are therefore unable to recover specific solutes from tubular fluid. In *renal glycosuria* (glī-kō-SOO-rē-uh), for example, a defective carrier protein makes it impossible for the PCT to reabsorb glucose from tubular fluid.

The Loop of Henle and Countercurrent Multiplication

Roughly 60–70 percent of the volume of filtrate produced at the glomerulus has been reabsorbed before the tubular fluid reaches the loop of Henle. In the process, useful organic substrates and many mineral ions have been reclaimed. The loop of Henle reabsorbs roughly half of the water, and two-thirds of the sodium and chloride ions, remaining in the tubular fluid. This reabsorption is performed efficiently according to the principle of countercurrent exchange, in our discussion of heat conservation mechanisms.

The thin descending limb and the thick ascending limb of the loop of Henle are very close together, separated only by peritubular fluid. The exchange that occurs between these segments is called **countercurrent multiplication.** *Countercurrent* refers to the fact that the exchange occurs between fluids moving in opposite directions: Tubular fluid in the descending limb flows toward the renal pelvis, whereas tubular fluid in the ascending limb flows toward the cortex. *Multiplication* refers to the fact that the effect of the exchange increases as movement of the fluid continues.

The two parallel segments of the loop of Henle have very different permeability characteristics. The thin descending limb is permeable to water but relatively impermeable to solutes. The thick ascending limb, which is relatively impermeable to both water and solutes, contains active transport mechanisms that pump sodium and chloride ions from the tubular fluid into the peritubular fluid of the medulla.

A quick overview of countercurrent multiplication will help you make sense of the details:

- Sodium and chloride are pumped out of the thick ascending limb and into the peritubular fluid.

- This pumping action elevates the osmotic concentration in the peritubular fluid around the thin descending limb.

- The result is an osmotic flow of water out of the thin descending limb and into the peritubular fluid, increasing the solute concentration in the thin descending limb.

- The arrival of the highly concentrated solution in the thick ascending limb accelerates the transport of sodium and chloride ions into the peritubular fluid of the medulla.

Notice that this arrangement is a simple positive feedback loop: Solute pumping at the ascending limb leads to higher solute concentrations in the descending limb, which then result in accelerated solute pumping in the ascending limb.

We can now take a closer look at the mechanics of the process. Figure 15.9a diagrams ion transport across the epithelium of the thick ascending limb. Active transport at the apical surface moves sodium, potassium, and chloride ions out of the tubular fluid. The carrier is called a **$Na^+-N^+/2\ Cl^-$ transporter,** because each cycle of the pump carries a sodium ion, a potassium ion, and two

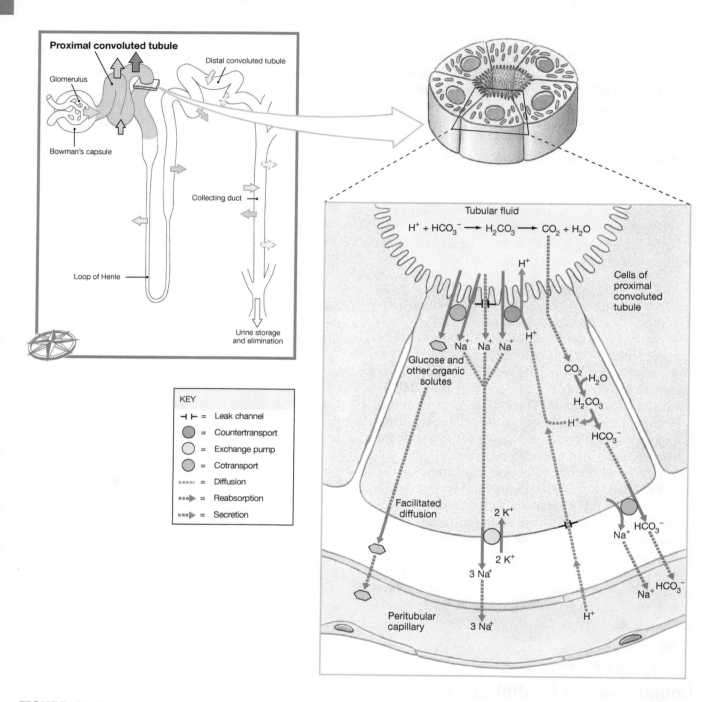

FIGURE 15.8 Transport activities at the PCT. Sodium ions may enter a tubular cell from the filtrate by diffusion, cotransport, or countertransport. The sodium ions are then pumped into the peritubular fluid by the sodium-potassium exchange pump. Other reabsorbed solutes may be ejected into the peritubular fluid by separate active transport mechanisms; the absorption of bicarbonate is indirectly associated with the reabsorption of sodium ions and the secretion of hydrogen ions (a process considered further in *Figure 15-10c*).

chloride ions into the tubular cell. Potassium and chloride ions are pumped into the peritubular fluid by cotransport carriers. However, potassium ions are removed from the peritubular fluid as the sodium-potassium exchange pump pumps sodium ions out of the tubular cell. The potassium ions then diffuse back into the lumen of the tubule through potassium leak channels. The net result is that Na^+ and Cl^- enter the peritubular fluid of the renal medulla.

The removal of sodium and chloride ions from the tubular fluid in the ascending limb elevates the osmotic concentration of the peritubular fluid around the thin descending limb (see Figure 15.9b). Because the thin descending limb is permeable to water but impermeable to solutes, as tubular fluid travels deeper into the medulla along the thin descending limb, osmosis moves water into the peritubular fluid. Solutes remain behind, so the tubular fluid reaching the turn of the loop of Henle has a higher osmotic concentration than it did at the start.

The pumping mechanism of the thick ascending limb is highly effective: Almost two-thirds of the sodium and chloride ions that enter it are pumped out of the tubular fluid before that fluid reaches the DCT. In other tissues, differences in solute concentration are quickly resolved by osmosis. However, osmosis cannot occur across the wall of the thick ascending limb, because the tubular epithelium there is impermeable to water. Thus, as Na^+ and Cl^- are removed, the solute concentration in the tubular fluid declines. Tubular fluid arrives at the DCT with an osmotic concentration of only about 100 mOsm/L, one-third the concentration of the peritubular fluid of the renal cortex.

The rate of ion transport across the thick ascending limb is proportional to an ion's concentration in tubular fluid. As a result, more sodium and chloride ions are pumped into the medulla at the start of the thick ascending limb, where NaCl concentrations are highest, than near the cortex. This regional difference in the rate of ion transport is the basis of the concentration gradient within the medulla.

The Concentration Gradient of the Medulla

Normally, the maximum solute concentration of the peritubular fluid near the turn of the loop of Henle is about 1200 mOsm/L (see Figure 15.9b). Sodium and chloride ions pumped out of the loop's ascending limb account for roughly two-thirds of that gradient (750 mOsm/L). The rest of the concentration gradient results from the presence of urea. To understand how urea arrived in the medulla, we must look ahead to events in the last segments of the collecting system (Figure 15.9c). The thick ascending limb of the loop of Henle, the DCT, and the collecting ducts are impermeable to urea. As water is reabsorbed, the concentration of urea gradually rises. The tubular fluid reaching the papillary duct typically contains urea at a concentration of about 450 mOsm/L. Because the papillary ducts are permeable to urea, the urea concentration in the deepest parts of the medulla also averages 450 mOsm/L.

Benefits of Countercurrent Multiplication

The countercurrent mechanism performs two functions:

1. It efficiently reabsorbs solutes and water before the tubular fluid reaches the DCT and collecting system.

2. It establishes a concentration gradient that permits the passive reabsorption of water from the tubular fluid in the collecting system. This reabsorption is regulated by circulating levels of antidiuretic hormone (ADH).

The tubular fluid arriving at the descending limb of the loop of Henle has an osmotic concentration of roughly 300 mOsm/L, due primarily to the presence of ions such as Na^+ and Cl^-. The concentration of organic wastes, such as urea, is low. Roughly half of the tubular fluid entering the loop of Henle is reabsorbed along the thin descending limb, and two-thirds of the Na^+ and Cl^- is reabsorbed along the thick ascending limb. As a result, the DCT receives a reduced volume of tubular fluid with an osmotic concentration of about 100 mOsm/L. Urea and other organic wastes, which were not pumped out of the thick ascending limb, now represent a significant proportion of the dissolved solutes.

Reabsorption and Secretion at the DCT

The composition and volume of tubular fluid change dramatically as it flows from the capsular space to the distal convoluted tubule. Only 15–20 percent of the

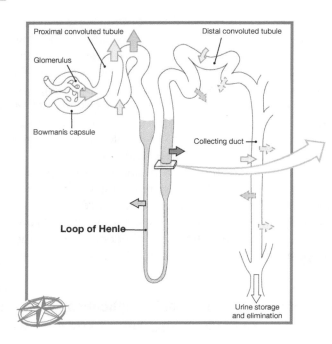

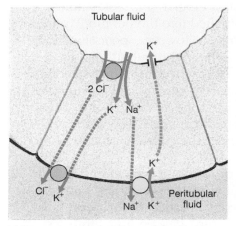

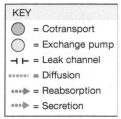

(a) The mechanism of sodium and chloride ion transport involves the Na^+–K^+/2 Cl^- carrier at the apical surface and two carriers at the basal surface of the tubular cell: a potassium-chloride cotransport pump and a sodium-potassium exchange pump. The net result is the transport of sodium and chloride ions into the peritubular fluid.

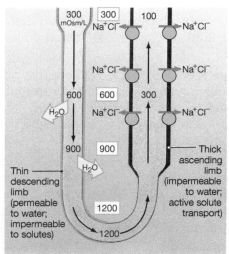

(b) Active transport of NaCl along the ascending thick limb results in the movement of water from the descending limb.

(c) The permeability characteristics of both the loop and the collecting duct tend to concentrate urea in the tubular fluid and in the medulla. The loop of Henle, DCT, and collecting duct are impermeable to urea. As water reabsorption occurs, the urea concentration rises. The papillary ducts' permeability to urea accounts for roughly one-third of the solutes in the deepest portions of the medulla.

FIGURE 15.9 Countercurrent multiplication and concentration of urine.

initial filtrate volume reaches the DCT, and the concentrations of electrolytes and organic wastes in the arriving tubular fluid no longer resemble the concentrations in blood plasma. Selective reabsorption or secretion, primarily along the DCT, makes the final adjustments in the solute composition and volume of the tubular fluid.

Reabsorption at the DCT

Throughout most of the DCT, the tubular cells actively transport Na^+ and Cl^- out of the tubular fluid (Figure 15.10a). Tubular cells along the distal portions of the DCT also contain ion pumps that reabsorb tubular Na^+ in exchange for another cation (usually K^+) (Figure 15.10b). The ion pump and the Na^+ channels involved are controlled by the hormone *aldosterone,* produced by the adrenal cortex. Aldosterone stimulates the synthesis and incorporation of sodium ion pumps and sodium channels in cell membranes along the DCT and collecting duct. The net result is a reduction in the number of sodium ions lost in urine. However, sodium ion conservation is associated with potassium ion loss. Prolonged

aldosterone stimulation can therefore produce *hypokalemia,* a dangerous reduction in the plasma K^+ concentration. The secretion of aldosterone and its actions on the DCT and collecting system are opposed by the natriuretic peptides (ANP and BNP).

The DCT is also the primary site of Ca^{2+} reabsorption, a process regulated by circulating levels of parathyroid hormone and calcitriol.

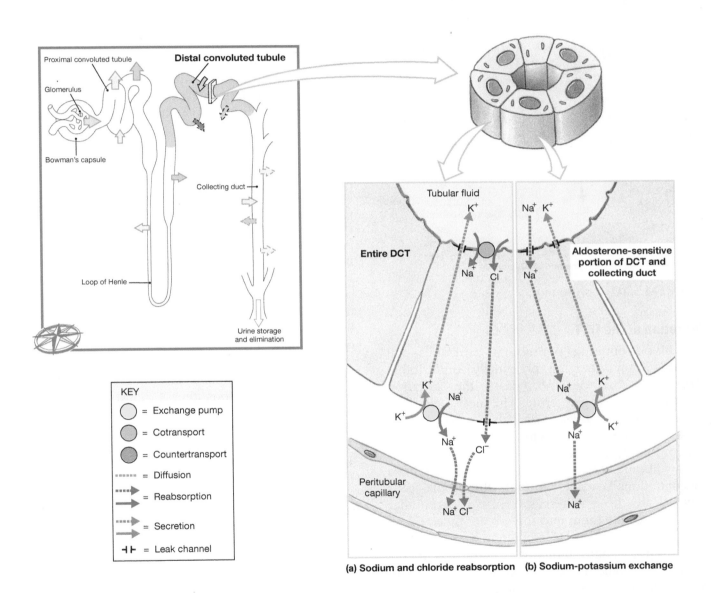

(a) Sodium and chloride reabsorption   (b) Sodium-potassium exchange

FIGURE 15.10   **Tubular secretion and solute reabsorption at the DCT. (a)** The basic pattern of the absorption of sodium and chloride ions and the secretion of potassium ions. **(b)** Aldosterone-regulated absorption of sodium ions, linked to the passive loss of potassium ions. **(c)** Hydrogen ion secretion and the acidification of urine occur by two routes. The central theme is the exchange of hydrogen ions in the cytoplasm for sodium ions in the tubular fluid, and the reabsorption of the bicarbonate ions generated in the process.

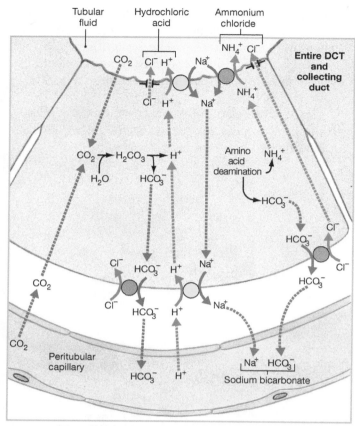

(c) H⁺ secretion and HCO₃⁻ reabsorption

FIGURE 15.10 continued.

Secretion at the DCT

The blood entering peritubular capillaries still contains a number of potentially undesirable substances that did not cross the filtration membrane at the glomerulus. In most cases, the concentrations of these materials are too low to cause physiological problems. However, any ions or compounds that are present in peritubular capillaries will diffuse into the peritubular fluid. If those concentrations become too high, the tubular cells may absorb these materials from the peritubular fluid and secrete them into the tubular fluid.

The rate of K^+ and H^+ secretion rises or falls in response to changes in their concentrations in peritubular fluid. The higher their concentration in the peritubular fluid, the higher the rate of secretion. Potassium and hydrogen ions merit special attention, because their concentrations in body fluids must be maintained within relatively narrow limits.

Potassium Ion Secretion Figure 15.10b diagrams the mechanism of K^+ secretion. Potassium ions are removed from the peritubular fluid in exchange for sodium ions obtained from the tubular fluid. These potassium ions diffuse into the lumen through potassium channels at the apical surfaces of the tubular cells. In effect, tubular cells trade sodium ions in the tubular fluid for excess potassium ions in body fluids.

Hydrogen Ion Secretion Hydrogen ion secretion is also associated with the reabsorption of sodium. Figure 15.10c depicts two routes of secretion. Both involve the generation of carbonic acid by the enzyme *carbonic anhydrase*. Hydrogen ions generated by the dissociation of the carbonic acid are secreted by sodium-linked countertransport in exchange for Na^+ in the tubular fluid. The bicarbonate ions diffuse into the peritubular fluid and then into the bloodstream, where they help prevent changes in plasma pH.

Hydrogen ion secretion acidifies the tubular fluid while elevating the pH of the blood. Hydrogen ion secretion accelerates when the pH of the blood falls—as in *lactic acidosis,* which can develop after exhaustive muscle activity, or *ketoacidosis,* which can develop in starvation or diabetes mellitus. The combination of H^+ removal and HCO_3^- production at the kidneys plays an important role in the control of blood pH. Because one of the secretory pathways is aldosterone sensitive, aldosterone stimulates H^+ secretion. Prolonged aldosterone stimulation can cause *alkalosis,* or abnormally high blood pH.

The production of lactic acid and ketone bodies during the postabsorptive state can cause acidosis. Under these conditions, the PCT and DCT deaminate amino acids in reactions that strip off the amino groups ($-NH_2$). The reaction sequence ties up H^+ and yields both **ammonium ions** (NH_4^+) and HCO_3^-. As indicated in Figure 15.10c, the ammonium ions are then pumped into the tubular fluid by sodium-linked countertransport, and the bicarbonate ions enter the bloodstream by way of the peritubular fluid.

Tubular deamination thus has two major benefits: It provides carbon chains suitable for catabolism, and it generates bicarbonate ions that add to the buffering capabilities of plasma.

Reabsorption and Secretion along the Collecting System

The collecting ducts receive tubular fluid from many nephrons and carry it toward the renal sinus, through the concentration gradient in the medulla. The normal amount of water and solute loss in the collecting system is regulated in two ways:

- By aldosterone, which controls sodium ion pumps along most of the DCT and the proximal portion of the collecting system. As noted above, these actions are opposed by the natriuretic peptides.

- By ADH, which controls the permeability of the DCT and collecting system to water. The secretion of ADH is suppressed by the natriuretic peptides, and this—combined with its effects on aldosterone secretion and action—can dramatically increase urinary water losses.

The collecting system also has other reabsorptive and secretory functions, many of which are important to the control of body fluid pH.

Reabsorption in the Collecting System

Important examples of solute reabsorption in the collecting system include the following:

- **Sodium Ion Reabsorption.** The collecting system contains aldosterone-sensitive ion pumps that exchange Na^+ in tubular fluid for K^+ in peritubular fluid (see Figure 15.10b).

- **Bicarbonate Reabsorption.** Bicarbonate ions are reabsorbed in exchange for chloride ions in the peritubular fluid (see Figure 15.10c).

- **Urea Reabsorption.** The concentration of urea in the tubular fluid entering the collecting duct is relatively high. The fluid entering the papillary duct generally has the same osmotic concentration as that of interstitial fluid of the medulla—about 1200 mOsm/L—but contains a much higher concentration of urea. As a result, urea tends to diffuse out of the tubular fluid and into the peritubular fluid in the deepest portion of the medulla.

Secretion in the Collecting System

The collecting system is an important site for the control of body fluid pH by means of the secretion of hydrogen or bicarbonate ions. If the pH of the peritubular fluid declines, carrier proteins pump hydrogen ions into the tubular fluid and reabsorb bicarbonate ions that help restore normal pH. If the pH of the peritubular fluid rises (a much less common event), the collecting system secretes bicarbonate ions and pumps

hydrogen ions into the peritubular fluid. The net result is that the body eliminates a buffer and gains hydrogen ions that lower the pH.

100 Keys | Reabsorption involves a combination of diffusion, osmosis, channel-mediated diffusion, and active transport. Many of these processes are independently regulated by local or hormonal mechanisms. The primary mechanism governing water reabsorption can be described as "water follows salt." Secretion is a selective, carrier-mediated process.

Characteristics of Urine

In 24 hours, the marvelously complex kidneys filter some 150 to 180 liters of blood plasma through their glomeruli into the tubules, which process the filtrate by taking substances out of it (reabsorption) and adding substances to it (secretion). In the same 24 hours, only about 1.0 to 1.8 liters of urine are produced. Obviously, urine and filtrate are quite different. Filtrate contains everything that blood plasma does (except proteins), but by the time it reaches the collecting ducts, the filtrate has lost most of its water and just about all of its nutrients and necessary ions. What remains, **urine,** contains nitrogenous wastes and unneeded substances. Assuming we are healthy, our kidneys can keep our blood composition fairly constant despite wide variations in diet and cell activity.

Freshly voided urine is generally clear and pale to deep yellow. The normal yellow color is due to *urochrome* (u'ro-krōm), a pigment that results from the body's destruction of hemoglobin. The more solutes are in the urine, the deeper yellow its color; on the other hand, dilute urine is a pale, straw color. At times, urine may be a color other than yellow. This might be a result of eating certain foods (beets, for example) or the presence of bile or blood in the urine.

When formed, urine is sterile, and its odor is slightly aromatic. If it is allowed to stand, it takes on an ammonia odor caused by the action of bacteria on the urine solutes. Some drugs, vegetables (such as asparagus), and various diseases (such as diabetes mellitus) alter the usual odor of urine.

Urine pH is usually slightly acid (around 6), but changes in body metabolism and certain foods may cause it to be much more acidic or basic. For example, a diet that contains large amounts of protein (eggs and cheese) and whole-wheat products

TABLE 15.1   Abnormal Urinary Constituents

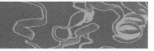

Substance	Name of condition	Possible causes
Glucose	Glycosuria (gli"ko-su're-ah)	Nonpathological: Excessive intake of sugary foods Pathological: Diabetes mellitus
Proteins	Proteinuria (pro"te-ĭ-nu're-ah) (also called albuminuria)	Nonpathological: Physical exertion, pregnancy Pathological: Glomerulonephritis, hypertension
Pus (WBCs and bacteria)	Pyuria (pi-u're-ah)	Urinary tract infection
RBCs	Hematuria (he"mah-tu're-ah)	Bleeding in the urinary tract (due to trauma, kidney stones, infection)
Hemoglobin	Hemoglobinuria (he"mo-glo-bĭ-nu're-ah)	Various: Transfusion reaction, hemolytic anemia
Bile pigment	Bilirubinuria (bil"ĭ-roo-bĭ-nu're-ah)	Liver disease (hepatitis)

causes urine to become quite acidic; thus, such foods are called *acid-ash foods.* Conversely, a vegetarian diet is called an *alkaline-ash diet* because it makes urine quite alkaline as the kidneys excrete the excess bases. Bacterial infection of the urinary tract also may cause the urine to be alkaline.

Since urine is water plus solutes, urine weighs more, or is more dense, than distilled water. The term used to compare how *much* heavier urine is than distilled water is **specific gravity.** Whereas the specific gravity of pure water is 1.0, the specific gravity of urine usually ranges from 1.001 to 1.035 (dilute to concentrated urine, respectively). Urine is generally dilute (that is, it has a low specific gravity) when a person drinks excessive fluids, uses diuretics (drugs that increase urine output), or has chronic renal failure (a condition in which the kidney loses its ability to concentrate urine). Conditions that produce urine with a high specific gravity include inadequate fluid intake, fever, and a kidney inflammation called *pyelonephritis* (pi"ĕ-lo-nĕ-fri'tis).

Solutes normally found in urine include sodium and potassium ions, urea, uric acid, creatinine, ammonia, bicarbonate ions, and various other ions, depending on blood composition. With certain diseases, urine composition can change dramatically, and the presence of abnormal substances in urine is often helpful in diagnosing the problem. This is why a routine urinalysis should always be part of any good physical examination.

Substances *not* normally found in urine are glucose, blood proteins, red blood cells, hemoglobin, white blood cells (pus), and bile. Names and possible causes of conditions in which abnormal urinary constituents and volumes might be seen are given in Table 15.1.

Ureters, Urinary Bladder, and Urethra

Ureters

The **ureters** (u-re'terz) are slender tubes each 25 to 30 cm (10 to 12 inches) long and 6 mm (one-quarter inch) in diameter. Each ureter runs behind the peritoneum from the renal hilus to the posterior aspect of the bladder, which it enters at a slight angle (see Figures 15.1 and 15.11). The superior end of each ureter is continuous with the pelvis of the kidney, and its mucosal lining is continuous with that lining the renal pelvis and the bladder below.

Essentially, the ureters are passageways that carry urine from the kidneys to the bladder. Although it might appear that urine could simply drain to the bladder below by gravity, the ureters *do* play an active role in urine transport. Smooth muscle layers in their walls contract to propel urine into the bladder by peristalsis. Once urine has entered the bladder, it is prevented from flowing

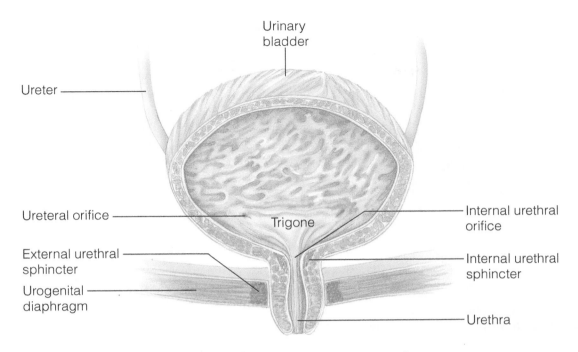

FIGURE 15.11 Basic structure of the urinary bladder and urethra of the female. The urethra of the male, which runs through the length of the penis, is substantially longer than that of the female.

back into the ureters by small valvelike folds of bladder mucosa that flap over the ureter openings.

Homeostatic Imbalance

When urine becomes extremely concentrated, solutes such as uric acid salts form crystals that precipitate in the renal pelvis. These crystals are called **renal calculi** (kal'kyoo-li; *calculus* = little stone), or kidney stones. Excruciating pain that radiates to the flank occurs when the ureter walls close in on the sharp calculi as they are being eased through the ureter by peristalsis or when the calculi become wedged in a ureter. Frequent bacterial infections of the urinary tract, urinary retention, and alkaline urine all favor calculi formation. Surgery has been the treatment of choice, but a newer noninvasive procedure *(lithotripsy)* that uses ultrasound waves to shatter the calculi is becoming more popular. The pulverized, sandlike remnants of the calculi are painlessly eliminated in the urine. ▲

Urinary Bladder

The **urinary bladder** is a smooth, collapsible, muscular sac that stores urine temporarily. It is located retroperitoneally in the pelvis just posterior to the pubic symphysis. If the interior of the bladder is scanned, three openings are seen—the

two ureter openings *(ureteral orifices)* and the single opening of the **urethra** (u-re'thrah) (the *internal urethral orifice*), which drains the bladder (Figure 15.11). The smooth triangular region of the bladder base outlined by these three openings is called the **trigone** (tri'gon). The trigone is important clinically because infections tend to persist in this region. In males, the *prostate gland* (part of the male reproductive system) surrounds the neck of the bladder where it empties into the urethra.

The bladder wall contains three layers of smooth muscle, collectively called the *detrusor muscle,* and its mucosa is a special type of epithelium, *transitional epithelium.* Both of these structural features make the bladder uniquely suited for its function of urine storage. When the bladder is empty, it is collapsed, 5 to 7.5 cm (2 to 3 inches) long at most, and its walls are thick and thrown into folds. As urine accumulates, the bladder expands and rises superiorly in the abdominal cavity (Figure 15.12). Its muscular wall stretches, and the transitional epithelial layer thins, allowing the bladder to store more urine without substantially increasing its internal pressure. A moderately full bladder is about 12.5 cm (5 inches) long and holds about 500 ml (1 pint) of urine, but it is capable of holding more than twice that amount. When the bladder is really distended, or stretched by urine, it

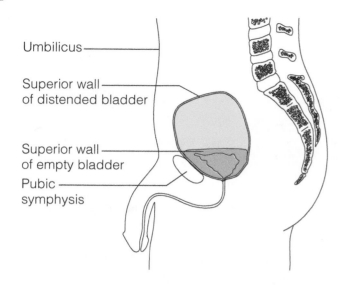

Umbilicus

Superior wall
of distended bladder

Superior wall
of empty bladder

Pubic
symphysis

FIGURE 15.12   Position and shape of a distended and an empty urinary bladder in an adult male.

becomes firm and pear-shaped and may be felt just above the pubic symphysis. Although urine is formed continuously by the kidneys, it is usually stored in the bladder until its release is convenient.

Urethra

The **urethra** is a thin-walled tube that carries urine by peristalsis from the bladder to the outside of the body. At the bladder-urethra junction, a thickening of the smooth muscle forms the **internal urethral sphincter** (see Figure 15.11), an involuntary sphincter that keeps the urethra closed when urine is not being passed. A second sphincter, the **external urethral sphincter,** is fashioned by skeletal muscle as the urethra passes through the pelvic floor. This sphincter is voluntarily controlled.

The length and relative function of the urethra differ in the two sexes. In females, it is about 3 to 4 cm (1½ inches) long, and its external orifice, or opening, lies anteriorly to the vaginal opening (see also Figure16.8a). Its function is to conduct urine to the body exterior.

▲ Homeostatic Imbalance

Since the female urinary orifice is so close to the anal opening, and feces contain a good deal of bacteria, improper toileting habits (that is, wiping from back to front rather than from front to back) can easily carry bacteria into the urethra. Moreover, since the

mucosa of the urethra is continuous with that of the rest of the urinary tract organs, an inflammation of the urethra, or *urethritis* (u"re-thri'tis), can easily ascend the tract to cause bladder inflammation *(cystitis)* or even kidney inflammation *(pyelonephritis,* or *pyelitis).* Symptoms of urinary tract infection include *dysuria* (painful urination), urinary *urgency* and *frequency,* fever, and sometimes cloudy or blood-tinged urine. When the kidneys are involved, back pain and a severe headache are common. ▲

In males, the urethra is approximately 20 cm (8 inches) long and has three named regions (see Figure 16.2), the *prostatic, membranous,* and *spongy* (or *penile*) *urethrae.* It opens at the tip of the penis after traveling down its length. The urethra of the male has a double function. It carries urine out of the body, and it provides the passage-way through which sperm is ejected from the body. Thus, in males, the urethra is part of both the urinary and reproductive systems.

Micturition

Micturition (mik"tu-rish'un), or **voiding,** is the act of emptying the bladder. Two sphincters, or valves, the internal urethral sphincter (more superiorly located) and the external urethral sphincter (more inferiorly located) control the flow of urine from the bladder (see Figure 15.11). Ordinarily, the bladder continues to collect urine until about 200 ml have accumulated. At about this point, stretching of the bladder wall activates stretch receptors. Impulses transmitted to the sacral region of the spinal cord and then back to the bladder via the *pelvic splanchnic nerves* cause the bladder to go into reflex contractions. As the contractions become stronger, stored urine is forced past the internal urethral sphincter (the smooth muscle, involuntary sphincter) into the upper part of the urethra. It is then that a person feels the urge to void. Because the lower external sphincter is skeletal muscle and is voluntarily controlled, we can choose to keep it closed and postpone bladder emptying temporarily. On the other hand, if it is convenient, the external sphincter can be relaxed so that urine is flushed from the body. When one chooses not to void, the reflex contractions of the bladder will stop within a minute or so, and urine will continue to accumulate in the bladder. After 200 to 300 ml more have been collected, the micturition reflex occurs again. Eventually, micturition occurs whether one wills it or not.

Homeostatic Imbalance

Incontinence (in-kon′tĭ-nens) occurs when we are unable to voluntarily control the external sphincter. Incontinence is normal in children 2 years old or younger, because they have not yet gained control over their voluntary sphincter. It may also occur in older children who sleep so soundly that they are not awakened by the stimulus. However, after the toddler years, incontinence is usually a result of emotional problems, pressure (as in pregnancy), or nervous system problems (stroke or spinal cord injury).

Urinary retention is essentially the opposite of incontinence. It is a condition in which the bladder is unable to expel its contained urine. There are various causes for urinary retention. It often occurs after surgery in which general anesthesia has been given because it takes a little time for the smooth muscles to regain their activity. Another cause of urinary retention, occurring primarily in elderly men, is enlargement, or *hyperplasia*, of the prostate gland, which surrounds the neck of the bladder. As it enlarges, it narrows the urethra, making it very difficult to void. When urinary retention is prolonged, a slender flexible drainage tube called a *catheter* (kath′ĭ-ter) must be inserted through the urethra to drain the urine and prevent bladder trauma from excessive stretching. ▲

Fluid, Electrolyte, and Acid-Base Balance

Blood composition depends on three major factors: diet, cellular metabolism, and urine output. In general, the kidneys have four major roles to play, which help keep the blood composition relatively constant. These are (1) excretion of nitrogen-containing wastes, maintaining (2) water and (3) electrolyte balance of the blood, and (4) ensuring proper blood pH. Excretion of nitrogenous wastes has already been considered; roles 2 through 4 are discussed briefly next.

Maintaining Water and Electrolyte Balance of Blood

Body Fluids and Fluid Compartments

If you are a healthy young adult, water probably accounts for half or more of your body weight—50 percent in females and about 60 percent in males. These differences reflect the fact that

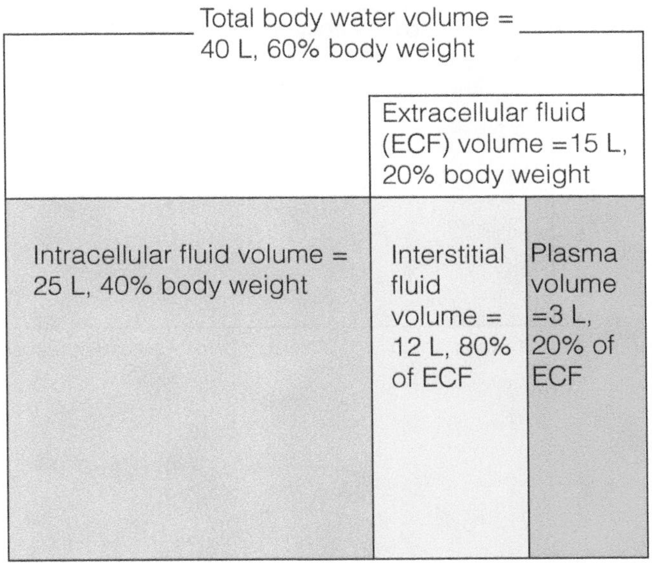

FIGURE 15.13 **The major fluid compartments of the body.** Approximate values are noted for a 70-kg (154-pound) male.

females have relatively less muscle and a larger amount of body fat (and of all body tissues, fat contains the least water). Babies, with little fat and low bone mass, are about 75 percent water, but total body water content declines through life and accounts for only about 45 percent of body weight in old age. Water is the universal body solvent within which all solutes (including the very important electrolytes) are dissolved.

Water occupies three main locations within the body, referred to as *fluid compartments* (Figure 15.13). About two-thirds of body fluid, the so-called **intracellular fluid (ICF),** is contained within the living cells. The remainder, called **extracellular fluid (ECF),** includes all body fluids located outside the cells. Although ECF most importantly includes blood plasma and interstitial (or tissue) fluid, it also accounts for cerebrospinal and serous fluids, the humors of the eye, lymph, and others.

An Introduction to Fluid and Electrolyte Balance

Figure 15.14a presents an overview of the body composition of a 70-kg (154-pound) individual with a minimum of body fat. The distribution was obtained by averaging values for males and females ages

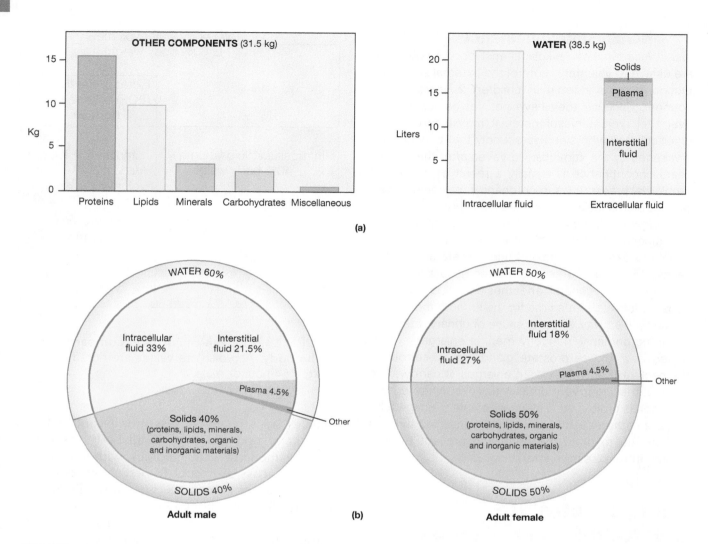

FIGURE 15.14   The composition of the human body. (a) The body composition (by weight, averaged for both sexes) and major body fluid compartments of a 70-kg individual. For technical reasons, it is extremely difficult to determine the precise size of any of these compartments; estimates of their relative sizes vary widely. **(b)** A comparison of the body compositions of adult males and females, ages 18–40 years.

18–40 years. Water accounts for roughly 60 percent of the total body weight of an adult male, and 50 percent of that of an adult female (Figure 15.14b). This difference between the sexes primarily reflects the proportionately larger mass of adipose tissue in adult females, and the greater average muscle mass in adult males. (Adipose tissue is only 10 percent water, whereas skeletal muscle is 75 percent water.) In both sexes, intracellular fluid contains a greater proportion of total body water than does extracellular fluid. Exchange between the ICF and the ECF occurs across cell membranes by osmosis, diffusion, and carrier-mediated transport.

The ECF and the ICF

The largest subdivisions of the ECF are the interstitial fluid of peripheral tissues and the plasma of circulating blood (see Figure 15.14a). Minor components of the ECF include lymph, cerebrospinal fluid (CSF), synovial fluid, serous fluids (pleural, pericardial, and peritoneal fluids), aqueous humor, perilymph, and endolymph. More precise measurements of total body water provide additional information on sex-linked differences in the distribution of body water (see Figure 15.14b). The greatest variation is in the

ICF, as a result of differences in the intracellular water content of fat versus muscle. Less striking differences occur in the ECF values, due to variations in the interstitial fluid volume of various tissues and the larger blood volume in males versus females.

In clinical situations, it is customary to estimate that two-thirds of the total body water is in the ICF and one-third in the ECF. This ratio underestimates the real volume of the ECF, but that underestimation is appropriate because portions of the ECF—including the water in bone, in many dense connective tissues, and in many of the minor ECF components—are relatively isolated. Exchange between these fluid volumes and the rest of the ECF occurs more slowly than does exchange between plasma and other interstitial fluids. As a result, they can be safely ignored in many cases. Clinical attention is usually focused on the rapid fluid and solute movements associated with the administration of blood, plasma, or saline solutions to counteract blood loss or dehydration.

Exchange among the subdivisions of the ECF occurs primarily across the endothelial lining of capillaries. Fluid may also travel from the interstitial spaces to plasma through lymphatic vessels that drain into the venous system. The identities and quantities of dissolved electrolytes, proteins, nutrients, and waste products in the ECF vary regionally. Still, the variations among the segments of the ECF seem minor compared with the major differences between the ECF and the ICF.

The ECF and ICF are called **fluid compartments,** because they commonly behave as distinct entities. The presence of a cell membrane and active transport at the membrane surface enable cells to maintain internal environments with a composition that differs from their surroundings. The principal ions in the ECF are sodium, chloride, and bicarbonate. The ICF contains an abundance of potassium, magnesium, and phosphate ions, plus large numbers of negatively charged proteins. Figure 15.15 compares the ICF with the two major subdivisions of the ECF.

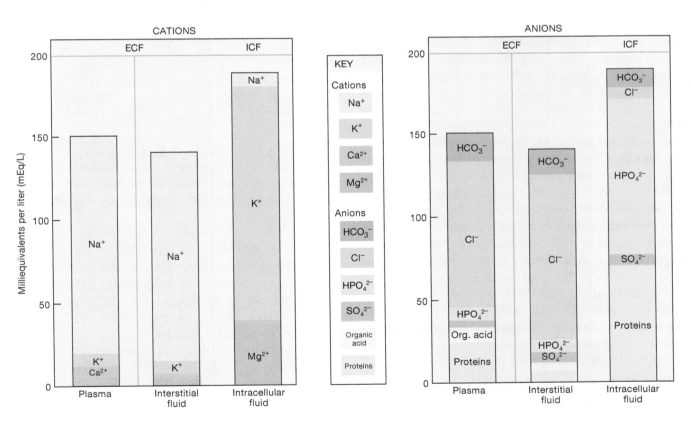

FIGURE 15.15 Cations and anions in body fluids. Notice the differences in cation and anion concentrations in the various body fluid compartments. For information about the composition of other body fluids, see Appendix IV.

If the cell membrane were freely permeable, diffusion would continue until these ions were evenly distributed across the membrane. But it does not, because cell membranes are selectively permeable: Ions can enter or leave the cell only via specific membrane channels. In addition, carrier mechanisms move specific ions into or out of the cell.

Despite the differences in the concentration of specific substances, the osmotic concentrations of the ICF and ECF are identical. Osmosis eliminates minor differences in concentration almost at once, because most cell membranes are freely permeable to water. (The only noteworthy exceptions are the apical surfaces of epithelial cells along the ascending limb of the loop of Henle, the distal convoluted tubule, and the collecting system.) Because changes in solute concentrations lead to immediate changes in water distribution, the regulation of fluid balance and that of electrolyte balance are tightly intertwined.

The Link between Water and Salt in the Compartments

Water certainly accounts for nearly the entire volume of the body fluids, regardless of type, and all body fluids are similar, but there is more to *fluid balance* than just water. The types and amounts of solutes in body fluids, especially electrolytes such as sodium, potassium, and calcium ions, are also vitally important to overall body homeostasis, and water and electrolyte balance are tightly linked as the kidneys continuously process the blood. Electrolytes are charged particles [ions] that conduct an electrical current in an aqueous solution.) Very small changes in **electrolyte balance,** the solute concentrations in the various fluid compartments, cause water to move from one compartment to another. Not only does this alter blood volume and blood pressure, but it can also severely impair the activity of irritable cells like nerve and muscle cells. For example, a deficit of sodium ions (Na^+) in the ECF results in water loss from the bloodstream into the tissue spaces (edema) and muscular weakness.

If the body is to remain properly hydrated, we cannot lose more water than we take in. Most water intake is a result of fluids and foods we ingest in our diet. However, a small amount (about 10 percent) is produced during cellular metabolism, as indicated in Figure 15.16. There are several routes for water to leave the body. Some water vaporizes out of the lungs, some is lost in

Q *How would the values shown here be affected by (1) drinking a six-pack of beer? (2) fasting (only water is ingested)?*

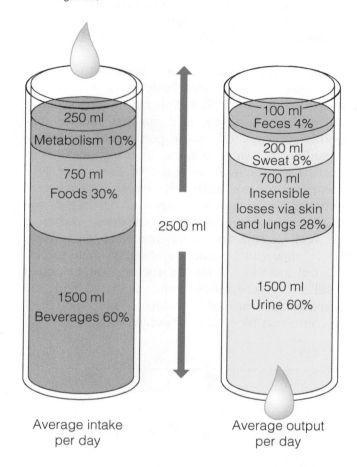

Average intake per day

Average output per day

FIGURE 15.16   Water intake and output. Major sources of body water and routes of water loss from the body are shown. When intake and output are in balance, the body is adequately hydrated.

perspiration, and some leaves the body in the stool. The job of the kidneys is like that of a juggler. If large amounts of water are lost in other ways, they compensate by putting out less urine to conserve body water. On the other hand, when water intake is excessive, the kidneys excrete generous amounts of urine, and the anguish of a too-full bladder becomes very real.

A *In case #1, the fluid ingested would greatly increase as would the amount of urinary output. In case #2, there would be no fluid intake from ingested foods and less fluid resulting from metabolism. Fluid output would be severely curtailed—no output in feces and less in urine to conserve body water. Insensible losses would not change. Loss of water in perspiration would depend on body and ambient temperatures.*

Likewise, the proper concentrations of the various electrolytes must be present in both intracellular and extracellular fluids. Most electrolytes enter the body in foods and "hard" (mineral-rich) water. Although very small amounts are lost in perspiration and in feces, the major factor regulating the electrolyte composition of body fluids is the kidneys. Just how the kidneys accomplish their balancing act is explained in more detail next.

Reabsorption of water and electrolytes by the kidneys is regulated primarily by hormones. When blood volume drops for any reason (for example, due to hemorrhage or excessive water loss through sweating or diarrhea), arterial blood pressure drops, which in turn decreases the amount of filtrate formed by the kidneys. In addition, highly sensitive cells in the hypothalamus called **osmoreceptors** (oz"mo-re-sep'torz) react to the change in blood composition (that is, less water and more solutes) by becoming more active. The result is that nerve impulses are sent to the posterior pituitary (Figure 15.17), which then releases **antidiuretic hormone (ADH) or vasopressin.** (The term *antidiuretic* is derived from *diuresis* [di"u-re'sis], which means "flow of urine from the kidney," and *anti,* which means "against.") As one might guess, this hormone prevents excessive water loss in the urine. ADH travels in the blood to its main target, the kidney's collecting ducts, where it causes the duct cells to reabsorb more water. As more water is returned to the bloodstream, blood volume and blood pressure increase to normal levels, and only a small amount of very concentrated urine is formed. ADH is released more or less continuously unless the solute concentration of the blood drops too low. When this happens, the osmoreceptors become "quiet," and excess water is allowed to leave the body in the urine.

Homeostatic Imbalance

When ADH is *not* released (perhaps because of injury or destruction of the hypothalamus or posterior pituitary gland), huge amounts of very dilute urine (up to 25 liters/day) flush from the body day after day. This condition, *diabetes insipidus* (in-sip'ĭ-dus), can lead to severe dehydration and electrolyte imbalances. Affected individuals are always thirsty and have to drink fluids almost continuously to maintain normal fluid balance. ▲

A second hormone that helps to regulate blood composition and blood volume by acting on the kidney is **aldosterone** (al"dos'ter-on). Aldosterone is the major factor regulating sodium ion content of the ECF and in the process helps regulate the concentration of other ions (Cl^-, K^+, and Mg^{2+} [magnesium]) as well. Sodium ion (Na^+) is the electrolyte most responsible for osmotic water flows. When too little sodium is in the blood, the blood becomes too dilute. Consequently, water leaves the bloodstream and flows out into the tissue spaces, causing edema and possibly a shutdown of the circulatory system. Whether aldosterone is present or not, about 80 percent of the sodium in the filtrate is reabsorbed in the proximal convoluted tubules of the kidneys. When aldosterone concentrations are high, most of the remaining sodium ions are actively reabsorbed in the distal convoluted tubules and the collecting ducts. Generally speaking, for each sodium ion reabsorbed, a chloride ion follows and a potassium ion is secreted into the filtrate. Thus, as the sodium content of the blood increases, potassium concentration decreases, bringing these two ions back to their normal balance in the blood. Still another effect of aldosterone is to increase water reabsorption by the tubule cells, because as sodium is reclaimed, water follows it passively back into the blood. A little rule to keep in mind here is: *water follows salt.*

Recall that aldosterone is produced by the adrenal cortex. Although rising potassium levels or falling sodium levels in the ECF directly stimulate the adrenal cells to release aldosterone, the most important trigger for aldosterone release is the **renin-angiotensin mechanism** (see Figure 15.10) mediated by the *juxtaglomerular (JGA) apparatus* of the renal tubules. The juxtaglomerular apparatus (see Figure 15.3b) consists of a complex of modified smooth muscle cells (JG cells) in the afferent arteriole plus some modified epithelial cells forming part of the distal convoluted tubule. The naming of this cell cluster reflects its location close by (*juxta*) the glomerulus. When the cells of the JGA apparatus are stimulated by low blood pressure in the afferent arteriole or changes in solute content of the filtrate, they respond by releasing the enzyme **renin** into the blood. (Notice the different spelling of this enzyme from *rennin,* an enzyme secreted by stomach glands.) Renin catalyzes the series of reactions that produce angiotensin II, which in turn acts directly on the blood vessels to cause vasoconstriction (and an increase in peripheral resistance) and on the adrenal cortical cells to

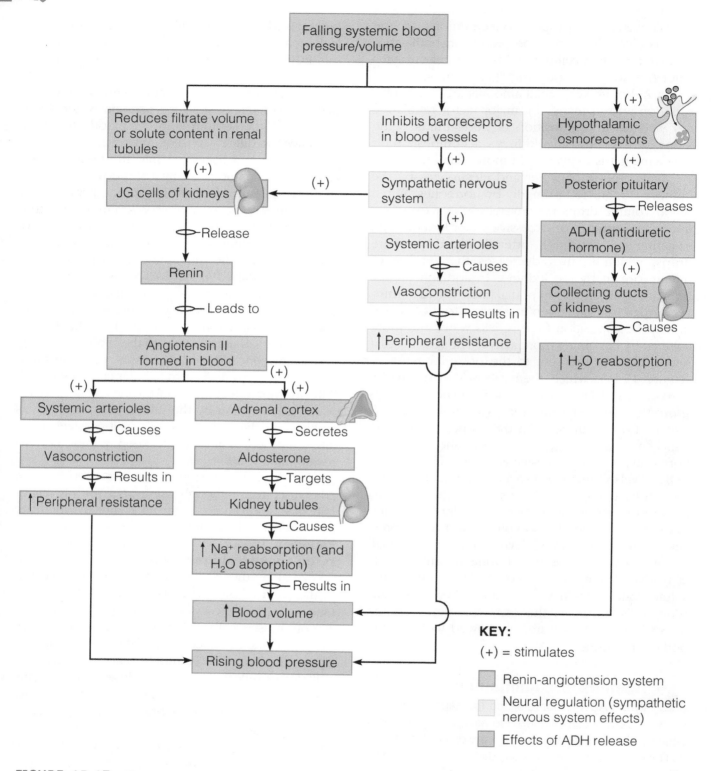

FIGURE 15.17 Flowchart of mechanisms regulating sodium and water balance to help maintain blood pressure homeostasis.

promote aldosterone release. As a result, blood volume and blood pressure increase (see Figure 15.17). The renin-angiotensin mechanism is extremely important for regulating blood pressure.

The pressure drop also excites baroreceptors in the larger blood vessels. These baroreceptors alert sympathetic nervous system centers of the brain to cause vasoconstriction (via release of epinephrine and norepinephrine), which increases the peripheral resistance (see Figure 15.17). However, this neural mechanism's major focus is blood pressure regulation, not water and electrolyte balance.

Homeostatic Imbalance

People with Addison's disease (hypoaldosteronism) have *polyuria* (excrete large volumes of urine) and lose tremendous amounts of salt and water to urine. As long as adequate amounts of salt and fluids are ingested, people with this condition can avoid problems, but they are constantly teetering on the brink of dehydration. ▲

Maintaining Acid-Base Balance of Blood

For the cells of the body to function properly, blood pH must be maintained between 7.35 and 7.45, a very narrow range. Whenever the pH of arterial blood rises above 7.45, a person is said to have **alkalosis** (al″kah-lo′sis). A drop in arterial pH to below 7.35 results in **acidosis** (as″ĭ-do′sis). Because a pH of 7.0 is neutral, 7.35 is not acidic, chemically speaking; however, it represents a higher-than-optimal hydrogen ion concentration for the functioning of most body cells. Therefore, any arterial pH between 7.35 and 7.0 is called **physiological acidosis.**

Although small amounts of acidic substances enter the body in ingested foods, most hydrogen ions originate as by-products of cellular metabolism, which continuously adds substances to the blood that tend to disturb its **acid-base balance.** Many different acids are produced (for example, phosphoric acid, lactic acid, and many types of fatty acids). In addition, carbon dioxide, which is released during energy production, forms carbonic acid. Ammonia and other basic substances are also released to the blood as cells go about their usual "business." Although the chemical buffers in the blood can temporarily "tie up" excess acids and

bases, and the lungs have the chief responsibility for eliminating carbon dioxide from the body, the kidneys assume most of the load for maintaining acid-base balance of the blood. Before describing how the kidneys function in acid-base balance, let's take a look at how each of our other two pH-controlling systems, blood buffers and the respiratory system, works.

Table 15.2 reviews important terms relating to acid-base balance.

Blood Buffers

Chemical buffers are systems of one or two molecules that act to prevent dramatic changes in hydrogen ion (H^+) concentration when acids or bases are added. They do this by binding to hydrogen ions whenever the pH drops and by releasing hydrogen ions when the pH rises. Since the chemical buffers act within a fraction of a second, they are the first line of defense in resisting pH changes.

Prove It Yourself

Demonstrate the Water-retaining Power of Salt

The amount of water your body retains depends more on the amount of salt you consume than on how much water you drink. Here's how to demonstrate this.

On a normal day between meals, empty your bladder. Wait half an hour, and then urinate again. Measure the volume of urine you produced the second time. This is your baseline rate of urine production. Now quickly drink a quart of water and measure your urine output for four more consecutive half-hour periods. Subtract the baseline amount of urine from each time period to find out how much water you excreted in two hours.

Repeat the experiment on another day. This time dissolve 5 grams (approximately ¾ teaspoon) of salt in the water first. You should find that you excrete much less water during the next two hours than you did the first time.

People with certain health conditions, such as hypertension or congestive heart failure, may need to retain less water. Generally, they are advised to restrict their intake of salt, not water. Can you see why?

TABLE 15.2   A Review of Important Terms Relating to Acid–Base Balance

pH	The negative exponent (negative logarithm) of the hydrogen ion concentration [H$^+$]
Neutral	A solution with a pH of 7; the solution contains equal numbers of hydrogen ions and hydroxide ions
Acidic	A solution with a pH below 7; in this solution, hydrogen ions predominate
Basic, or **alkaline**	A solution with a pH above 7; in this solution, hydroxideions [OH$^-$] predominate
Acid	A substance that dissociates to release hydrogen ions, decreasing pH
Base	A substance that dissociates to release hydroxide ions or to tie up hydrogen ions, increasing pH
Salt	An ionic compound consisting of a cation other than hydrogen and an anion other than a hydroxide ion
Buffer	A substance that tends to oppose changes in the pH of a solution by removing or replacing hydrogenions; in body fluids, buffers maintain blood pH within normal limits (7.35–7.45)
Milliequivalents	Electrolytes are measured in milliequivalents per liter, a measure of electrical activity as compared to hydrogen.

To better understand how a chemical buffer system works, let's review the definitions of strong and weak acids and bases. Recall that acids are proton (H$^+$) donors, and that the acidity of a solution reflects only the *free* hydrogen ions, not those still bound to anions. *Strong acids* dissociate completely and liberate all their H$^+$ in water. Consequently they can cause large changes in pH. By contrast, *weak acids* like carbonic acid dissociate only partially and so have a much slighter effect on a solution's pH (Figure 15.18). However, weak acids are very effective at preventing pH changes since they are forced to dissociate and release more H$^+$ when the pH rises over the desirable pH range. This feature allows them to play a very important role in the chemical buffer systems.

Also recall that bases are proton or hydrogen ion acceptors. *Strong bases* like hydroxides dissociate easily in water and quickly tie up H$^+$, but *weak bases* like bicarbonate ion (HCO$_3^-$) and ammonia (NH$_3$) are slower to accept H$^+$. However, as pH drops, the weak bases become "stronger" and begin to tie up more hydrogen ions. Thus, like weak acids, they are valuable members of the chemical buffer systems.

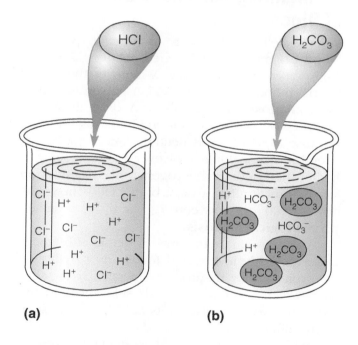

(a)　　　　　　　　**(b)**

FIGURE 15.18   Dissociation of strong and weak acids. (a) When HCl, a strong acid, is added to water it dissociates completely into its ions (H$^+$ and Cl$^-$). **(b)** By contrast, dissociation of H$_2$CO$_3$, a weak acid, is very incomplete, and some molecules of H$_2$CO$_3$ remain undissociated (symbols shown in green ovals) in solution.

The three major chemical buffer systems of the body are the *bicarbonate, phosphate,* and *protein buffer systems,* each of which helps to maintain the pH in one or more of the fluid compartments. They all work together, and anything that causes a shift in H^+ concentration in one compartment also causes changes in the others. Thus, drifts in pH are resisted by the entire buffering system. Since all three systems operate in a similar way, examining just one, the bicarbonate buffer system, which is so important in preventing changes in blood pH, should be sufficient.

The **bicarbonate buffer system** is a mixture of *carbonic acid* (H_2CO_3) and its salt, *sodium bicarbonate* ($NaHCO_3$). Since carbonic acid is a weak acid, it does not dissociate much in neutral or acidic solutions. Thus, when a strong acid, such as hydrochloric acid (HCl) is added, most of the carbonic acid remains intact. However, the *bicarbonate ions* (HCO_3^-) of the salt act as bases to tie up the H^+ released by the stronger acid, forming more carbonic acid:

$$\underset{\substack{\text{strong} \\ \text{acid}}}{HCl} + \underset{\substack{\text{weak} \\ \text{base}}}{NaHCO_3} \longrightarrow \underset{\substack{\text{weak} \\ \text{acid}}}{H_2CO_3} + \underset{\text{salt}}{NaCl}$$

Because the strong acid is (effectively) changed to a weak one, it lowers the pH of the solution only very slightly.

Similarly, if a strong base like sodium hydroxide (NaOH) is added to a solution containing the bicarbonate buffer system, $NaHCO_3$ will not dissociate further under such alkaline conditions. However, carbonic acid will be forced to dissociate further by the presence of the strong base— liberating more H^+ to bind with the OH^- released by NaOH.

$$\underset{\substack{\text{strong} \\ \text{base}}}{NaOH} + \underset{\substack{\text{weak} \\ \text{acid}}}{H_2CO_3} \longrightarrow \underset{\substack{\text{weak} \\ \text{base}}}{NaHCO_3} + \underset{\text{water}}{H_2O}$$

The net result is replacement of a strong base by a weak one, so that the pH of the solution rises very little.

Respiratory System Controls

The respiratory system eliminates carbon dioxide from the blood while it "loads" oxygen into the blood. Remember that when carbon dioxide (CO_2) enters the blood from the tissue cells, most of it enters the red blood cells where it is

converted to bicarbonate ion (HCO_3^-) for transport in the plasma as shown by the equation

$$\underset{\substack{\text{Carbon} \\ \text{dioxide}}}{CO_2} + \underset{\text{water}}{H_2O} \overset{\substack{\text{Carbonic} \\ \text{anhydrase}}}{\rightleftharpoons} \underset{\substack{\text{carbonic} \\ \text{acid}}}{H_2CO_3} \rightleftharpoons \underset{\substack{\text{hydrogen} \\ \text{ion}}}{H^+} + \underset{\substack{\text{bicarbonate} \\ \text{ion}}}{HCO_3^-}$$

The double-headed arrows reveal that an increase in carbon dioxide pushes the reaction to the right, producing more carbonic acid. Likewise, an increase in hydrogen ions pushes the equation to the left, producing more carbonic acid. In healthy people, carbon dioxide is expelled from the lungs at the same rate as it is formed in the tissues. Thus the H^+ released when carbon dioxide is loaded into the blood is not allowed to accumulate because it is tied up in water when CO_2 is unloaded in the lungs. So, under normal conditions, the hydrogen ions produced by carbon dioxide transport have essentially no effect on blood pH. However, when CO_2 accumulates in the blood (for example, during restricted breathing) or more H^+ is released to the blood by metabolic processes, the chemoreceptors in the respiratory control centers of the brain (or in peripheral blood vessels) are activated. As a result, breathing rate and depth increase, and the excess H^+ is "blown off" as more CO_2 is removed from the blood.

On the other hand, when blood pH begins to rise (alkalosis), the respiratory center is depressed. Consequently, the respiratory rate and depth fall, allowing carbon dioxide (hence, H^+) to accumulate in the blood. Again blood pH is restored to the normal range. Generally, these respiratory system corrections of blood pH (via regulation of CO_2 content of the blood) are accomplished within a minute or so.

Renal Mechanisms

Chemical buffers can tie up excess acids or bases temporarily, but they cannot eliminate them from the body. And while the lungs can dispose of carbonic acid by eliminating carbon dioxide, only the kidneys can rid the body of other acids generated during metabolism. Additionally, only the kidneys have the power to regulate blood levels of alkaline substances. Thus, although the kidneys act slowly and require hours or days to bring about changes in blood pH, they are the most potent of the mechanisms for regulating blood pH.

The most important means by which the kidneys maintain acid-base balance of the blood are by (1) excreting bicarbonate ions and (2) conserving (reabsorbing) or generating new bicarbonate ions. Look back again at the equation showing how the carbonic acid–bicarbonate buffer system operates. Notice that losing a HCO_3^- from the body has the same effect as gaining an H^+ because it pushes the equation to the right (that is, it leaves a free hydrogen ion). By the same token, reabsorbing or generating new HCO_3^- is the same as losing H^+ because it tends to combine with a hydrogen ion and pushes the equation to the left. Renal mechanisms undertake these adjustments: As blood pH rises, bicarbonate ions are excreted and hydrogen ions are retained by the tubule cells. Conversely, when blood pH falls, bicarbonate is reabsorbed and hydrogen ions are secreted. Urine pH varies from 4.5 to 8.0, which reflects the ability of the renal tubules to excrete basic or acid ions to maintain blood pH homeostasis. Table 15.3 shows the typical values obtained from standrad urinalysis.

Summary: Renal Function

Table 15.4 lists the functions of each segment of the nephron and collecting system. Figure 15.19 provides a functional overview that summarizes the major steps involved in the reabsorption of water and the production of concentrated urine:

Step 1   The filtrate produced at the renal corpuscle has the same osmotic concentration as does plasma—about 300 mOsm/L. It has the composition of blood plasma, minus the plasma proteins.

Step 2   In the PCT, the active removal of ions and organic substrates produces a continuous osmotic flow of water out of the tubular fluid. This process reduces the volume of filtrate but keeps the solutions inside and outside the tubule isotonic. Between 60 and 70 percent of the filtrate volume has been reabsorbed before the tubular fluid reaches the descending limb of the loop of Henle.

Step 3   In the PCT and descending limb of the loop of Henle, water moves into the surrounding peritubular fluids, leaving a small volume

---

TABLE 15.3   Typical Values Obtained from Standard Urinalysis

Compound	Primary Source	Daily Elimination*	Concentration	Remarks
NITROGENOUS WASTES				
Urea	Deamination of amino acids by liver and kidneys	21 g	1.8 g/dl	Rises if negative nitrogen balance exists
Creatinine	Breakdown of creatine phosphate in skeletal muscle	1.8 g	150 mg/dl	Proportional to muscle mass; decreases during atrophy or muscle disease
Ammonia	Deamination by liver and kidney, absorption from intestinal tract	0.68 g	60 mg/dl	
Uric acid	Breakdown of purines	0.53 g	40 mg/dl	Increases in gout, liver diseases
Hippuric acid	Breakdown of dietary toxins	4.2 mg	350 μg/dl	
Urobilin	Urobilinogens absorbed at colon	1.5 mg	125 μg/dl	Gives urine its yellow color

TABLE 15.3 *(continued)*

Compound	Primary Source	Daily Elimination*	Concentration	Remarks
Bilirubin	Hemoglobin breakdown product	0.3 mg	20 μg/dl	Increase may indicate problem with liver elimination or excess production; causes yellowing of skin and mucous membranes in jaundice
NUTRIENTS AND METABOLITES				
Carbohydrates		0.11 g	9 μg/dl	Primarily glucose; *glycosuria* develops if T_m is exceeded
Ketone bodies		0.21 g	17 μg/dl	Ketonuria may occur during postabsorptive state
Lipids		0.02 g	1.6 μg/dl	May increase in some kidney diseases
Amino acids		2.25 g	287.5 μg/dl	Note relatively high loss compared with other metabolites due to low T_m; excess *(aminoaciduria)* indicates T_m problem
IONS				
Sodium		4.0 g	333 mg/dl	Varies with diet, urine pH, hormones, etc.
Chloride		6.4 g	533 mg/dl	
Potassium		2.0 g	166 mg/dl	Varies with diet, urine pH, hormones, etc.
Calcium		0.2 g	17 mg/dl	Hormonally regulated (PTH/CT)
Magnesium		0.15 g	13 mg/dl	
BLOOD CELLS†				
RBCs		130,000/day	100/ml	Excess *(hematuria)* indicates vascular damage
WBCs		650,000/day	500/ml	Excess *(pyuria)* indicates renal infection or inflammation

*Representative values for a 70-kg male.

†Usually estimated by counting the cells in a sample of sediment after urine centrifugation.

TABLE 15.4   Renal Structures and Their Functions

Segment	General Functions	Specific Functions	Mechanisms
Renal corpuscle	*Filtration* of plasma; generates approximately 180 L/day of filtrate similar in Composition to blood plasma without proteins	*Filtration* of water, inorganic and organic solutes from plasma; retention of plasma proteins and blood cells	Glomerular hydrostatic (blood) pressure working across capillary endothelium, lamina densa, and filtration slits
Proximal convoluted tubule (PCT)	*Reabsorption* of 60–70% of the water (108–116 L/day), 99–100% of the organic substrates, and 60–70% of the sodium and chloride ions in the original filtrate	*Reabsorption:* Active: glucose, other simple sugars, amino acids, vitamins, ions, including (sodium, potassium, calcium, magnesium, phosphate, and bicarbonate) Passive: urea, chloride ions, lipid-solublematerials, water *Secretion:* Hydrogen ions, ammonium ions, creatinine, drugs, and toxins (as at DCT)	Carrier-mediated transport, including facilitated transport (glucose, amino acids), cotransport (glucose, ions), and countertransport (with secretion of H^+) Diffusion (solutes) or osmosis (water) Countertransport with sodium ions
Loop of Henle	*Reabsorption* of 25% of the water (45 L/day) and 20–25% of the sodium and chloride ions present in the original filtrate; creation of the concentration gradient in the medulla	*Reabsorption:* Sodium and chloride ions Water	Active transport via Na^+–K^+/$2Cl^-$ transporter Osmosis
Distal convoluted tubule (DCT)	*Reabsorption* of a variable amount of water (usually 5%, or 9 L/day), under ADH stimulation, and a variable amount of sodium ions, under aldosterone stimulation	*Reabsorption:* Sodium and chloride ions Sodium ions (variable) Calcium ions (variable) Water (variable) *Secretion:* Hydrogen ions, ammonium ions Creatinine, drugs, toxins	Cotransport Countertransport with potassium ions; aldosterone-regulated Carrier-mediated transport stimulated by parathyroid hormone and calcitriol Osmosis; ADH regulated Countertransport with sodium ions Carrier-mediated transport

TABLE 15.4 *(continued)*

Segment	General Functions	Specific Functions	Mechanisms
Collecting system	*Reabsorption* of a variable amount of water (usually 9.3%, or water 16.8 L/day) under ADH stimulation, and a variable amount of sodium ions, under aldosterone stimulation	*Reabsorption:* Sodium ions (variable) Bicarbonate ions (variable) Water (variable) Urea (distal portions only) *Secretion:* Potassium and hydrogen ions (variable)	Countertransport with potassium or hydrogen ions; aldosterone-regulated Diffusion, generated within tubular cells Osmosis; ADH-regulated Diffusion Carrier-mediated transport
Peritubular capillaries	*Redistribution* of water and solutes reabsorbed in the cortex	Return of water and solutes to the general circulation	Osmosis and diffusion
Vasa recta	*Redistribution* of water and solutes reabsorbed in the medulla and stabilization of the concentration gradient of the medulla	Return of water and solutes to the general circulation	Osmosis and diffusion

(15–20 percent of the original filtrate) of highly concentrated tubular fluid. The reduction in volume has occurred by obligatory water reabsorption.

Step 4 The thick ascending limb is impermeable to water and solutes. The tubular cells actively transport Na^+ and Cl^- out of the tubular fluid, thereby lowering the osmotic concentration of tubular fluid without affecting its volume. The tubular fluid reaching the distal convoluted tubule is hypotonic relative to the peritubular fluid, with an osmotic concentration of only about 100 mOsm/L. Because only Na^+ and Cl^- are removed, urea accounts for a significantly higher proportion of the total osmotic concentration at the end of the loop than it did at the start of it.

Step 5 The final adjustments in the composition of the tubular fluid are made in the DCT and the collecting system. Although the DCT and collecting duct are generally impermeable to solutes, the osmotic concentration of tubular fluid can be adjusted through active transport (reabsorption or secretion). Some of these transport activities are hormonally regulated.

Step 6 The final adjustments in the volume and osmotic concentration of the tubular fluid are made by controlling the water permeabilities of the distal portions of the DCT and the collecting system. These segments are relatively impermeable to water unless exposed to ADH. Under maximum ADH stimulation, urine volume is at a minimum, and urine osmotic concentration is equal to that of the peritubular fluid in the deepest portion of the medulla (roughly 1200 mOsm/L).

Step 7 The vasa recta absorbs solutes and water reabsorbed by the loop of Henle and the collecting ducts, thereby maintaining the concentration gradient of the medulla.

Developmental Aspects of the Urinary System

When you trace the development of the kidneys in a young embryo, it almost seems as if they can't "make up their mind" about whether to come or go. The first tubule system forms and then begins to degenerate as a second, lower, set appears. The

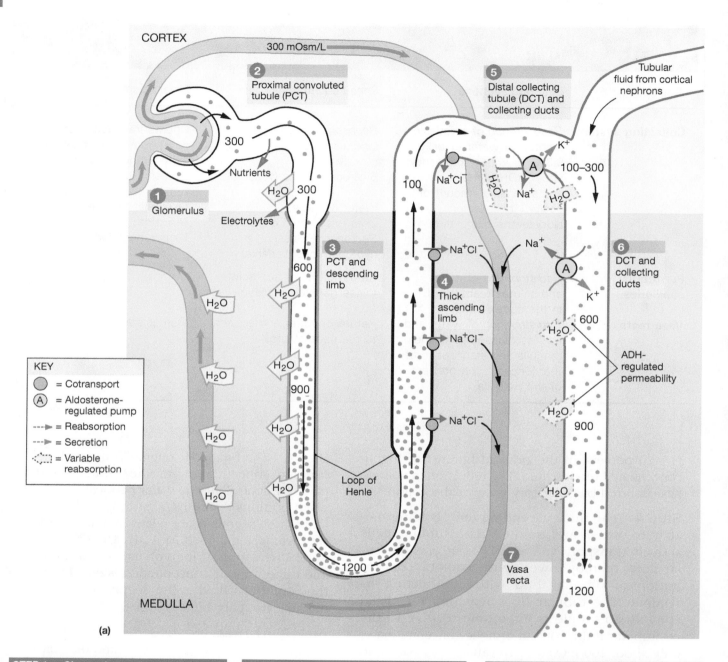

CORTEX

300 mOsm/L

2 Proximal convoluted tubule (PCT)

5 Distal collecting tubule (DCT) and collecting ducts

Tubular fluid from cortical nephrons

300

Nutrients

1 Glomerulus

Electrolytes

H_2O 300

3 PCT and descending limb

600

H_2O

100

Na^+Cl^-

4 Thick ascending limb

Na^+Cl^-

H_2O Na^+

K^+

100–300

Na^+

A

Na^+Cl^-

H_2O

6 DCT and collecting ducts

K^+

600

ADH-regulated permeability

KEY
- = Cotransport
- **A** = Aldosterone-regulated pump
- ---▶ = Reabsorption
- ---▶ = Secretion
- = Variable reabsorption

H_2O

H_2O

900

H_2O

Na^+Cl^-

H_2O

H_2O

900

H_2O

Loop of Henle

H_2O

1200

7 Vasa recta

1200

MEDULLA

(a)

STEP 1:   Glomerulus

The filtrate produced at the renal corpuscle has the same osmotic concentration as plasma—about 300 mOsm/L. It has the same composition as plasma without the plasma proteins.

STEP 2:   Proximal convoluted tubule (PCT)

In the proximal convoluted tubule (PCT), the active removal of ions and organic substrates produces a continuous osmotic flow of water out of the tubular fluid. This reduces the volume of filtrate but keeps the solutions inside and outside the tubule isotonic.

STEP 3:   PCT and descending limb

In the PCT and descending limb of the loop of Henle, water moves into the surrounding peritubular fluids, leaving a small volume of highly concentrated tubular fluid. This reduction occurs by obligatory water reabsorption.

FIGURE 15.19   A summary of renal function. (a) A general overview of steps and events. **(b)** Specific changes in the composition and concentration of the tubular fluid as it flows along the nephron and collecting duct.

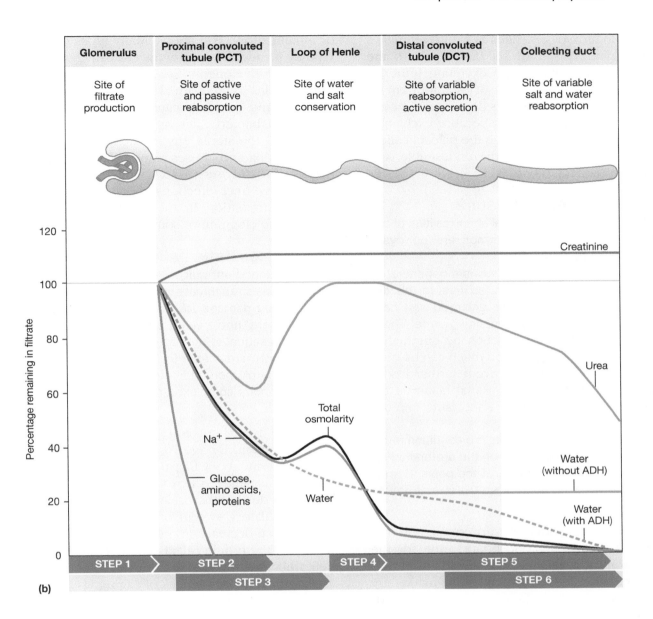

Glomerulus	Proximal convoluted tubule (PCT)	Loop of Henle	Distal convoluted tubule (DCT)	Collecting duct
Site of filtrate production	Site of active and passive reabsorption	Site of water and salt conservation	Site of variable reabsorption, active secretion	Site of variable salt and water reabsorption

(b)

STEP 4: Thick ascending limb

The thick ascending limb is impermeable to water and solutes. The tubular cells actively transport Na^+ and Cl^- out of the tubule, thereby lowering the osmotic concentration of the tubular fluid. Because just Na^+ and Cl^- are removed, urea accounts for a higher proportion of the total osmotic concentration at the end of the loop.

STEP 5: DCT and collecting ducts

The final adjustments in the composition of the tubular fluid occur in the DCT and the collecting system. The osmotic concentration of the tubular fluid can be adjusted through active transport (reabsorption or secretion).

STEP 6: DCT and collecting ducts

The final adjustments in the volume and osmotic concentration of the tubular fluid are made by controlling the water permeabilities of the distal portions of the DCT and the collecting system. The level of exposure to ADH determines the final urine concentration.

STEP 7: Vasa recta

The vasa recta absorbs the solutes and water reabsorbed by the loop of Henle and the collecting ducts. By removing these solutes and water into the main circulatory system, the vasa recta maintains the concentration gradient of the medulla.

second set, in turn, degenerates as a third set makes its appearance. This third set develops into the functional kidneys, which are excreting urine by the third month of fetal life. It is important to remember that the fetal kidneys do not work nearly as hard as they will after birth, because exchanges with the mother's blood through the placenta allow her system to clear many of the undesirable substances from the fetal blood.

⚠ Homeostatic Imbalance

There are many congenital abnormalities of this system. Two of the most common are polycystic kidney and hypospadias.

Polycystic (pol"e-sis'tik) *kidney* is a degenerative condition that appears to run in families. In this disease, one or both kidneys are enlarged and have many blisterlike sacs (cysts) containing urine. These cysts interfere with renal function by obstructing urine drainage. Currently, not too much can be done for this condition except to prevent further kidney damage by avoiding infection. Renal failure is the eventual outcome, but kidney transplants improve chances for survival.

Hypospadias (hi"po-spa'de-as) is a condition found in male babies only. It occurs when the urethral orifice is located on the ventral surface of the penis. Corrective surgery is generally done when the child is around 12 months old. ▲

Because the bladder is very small and the kidneys are unable to concentrate urine for the first two months, a newborn baby voids from 5 to 40 times per day, depending on fluid intake. By 2 months of age, the infant is voiding approximately 400 ml/day, and the amount steadily increases until adolescence, when adult urine output (about 1500 ml/day) is achieved.

Control of the voluntary urethral sphincter goes hand in hand with nervous system development. By 15 months, most toddlers are aware when they have voided. By 18 months they can hold urine in their bladder for about two hours, which is the first sign that toilet training (for voiding) can begin. Daytime control usually occurs well before nighttime control is achieved. It is generally unrealistic to expect that complete nighttime control will occur before the child is 4 years old.

During childhood and through late middle age, most urinary system problems are infectious, or inflammatory, conditions. Many types of bacteria may invade the urinary tract to cause urethritis, cystitis, or pyelonephritis. *Escherichia coli* (esh" er-i'ke-ah ko'li) are normal residents of the digestive tract and generally cause no problems there, but these bacteria act as pathogens (disease-causers) in the sterile environment of the urinary tract. Bacteria and viruses responsible for *sexually transmitted diseases (STDs)*, which are primarily reproductive tract infections, may also invade and cause inflammation in the urinary tract, which leads to the clogging of some of its ducts.

⚠ Homeostatic Imbalance

Childhood streptococcal (strep"to-kok'al) infections, such as strep throat and scarlet fever, may cause inflammatory damage to the kidneys if the original infections are not treated promptly and properly. A common sequel to untreated childhood strep infections is *glomerulonephritis* (glo-mer"u-lo-ne-fri'tis), in which the glomerular filters become clogged with antigen-antibody complexes resulting from the strep infection. ▲

As we age, there is a progressive decline in kidney function. By age 70, the rate of filtrate formation is only about half that of the middle-aged adult. This is believed to result from impaired renal circulation due to atherosclerosis, which affects the entire circulatory system of the aging person. In addition to a decrease in the number of functional nephrons, the tubule cells become less efficient in their ability to concentrate urine.

Another consequence of aging is bladder shrinkage and loss of bladder tone, causing many elderly individuals to experience *urgency* (a feeling that it is necessary to void) and *frequency* (frequent voiding of small amounts of urine). *Nocturia* (nok-tu're-ah), the need to get up during the night to urinate, plagues almost two-thirds of this population. In many, incontinence is the final outcome of the aging process. This loss of control is a tremendous blow to the pride of many aging people. Urinary retention is another common problem; most often it is a result of hypertrophy of the prostate gland in males. Some of the problems of incontinence and retention can be avoided by a regular regimen of activity that keeps the body as a whole in optimum condition and promotes alertness to elimination signals.

Systems in Sync

Homeostatic Relationships between the Urinary System and Other Body Systems

Endocrine System
- Kidneys dispose of nitrogenous wastes; maintain fluid, electrolyte, and acid-base balance of blood; produce the hormone erythropoietin; renal regulation of Na^+ and water balance essential for blood pressure homeostasis and hormone transport in the blood
- ADH, aldosterone, ANP, and other hormones help regulate renal reabsorption of water and electrolytes

Lymphatic System/Immunity
- Kidneys dispose of nitrogenous wastes; maintain fluid, electrolyte, and acid-base balance of blood
- By returning leaked plasma fluid to cardiovascular system, lymphatic vessels help ensure normal systemic blood pressure needed for kidney function; immune cells protect urinary organs from infection, cancer, and other foreign substances

Digestive System
- Kidneys dispose of nitrogenous wastes; maintain fluid, electrolyte, and acid-base balance of blood; also, metabolize vitamin D to the active form needed for calcium absorption
- Digestive organs provide nutrients needed for kidney cell health; liver synthesizes most urea, a nitrogenous waste that must be excreted by the kidneys

Urinary System

Muscular System
- Kidneys dispose of nitrogenous wastes; maintain fluid, electrolyte, and acid-base balance of blood; renal regulation of Na^+, K^+, and Ca^{2+} content in ECF crucial for muscle activity
- Muscles of pelvic diaphragm and external urethral sphincter function in voluntary control of micturition; creatinine is a nitrogenous waste product that must be excreted by the kidneys

Nervous System
- Kidneys dispose of nitrogenous wastes; maintain fluid, electrolyte, and acid-base balance of blood; renal regulation of Na^+, K^+, and Ca^{2+} content in ECF essential for normal neural function
- Neural controls involved in micturition; sympathetic nervous system activity triggers the renin-angiotensin mechanism

Respiratory System
- Kidneys dispose of nitrogenous wastes; maintain fluid, electrolyte, and acid-base balance of blood
- Respiratory system provides oxygen required by kidney cells; disposes of carbon dioxide; cells in the lungs convert angiotensin I to angiotensin II

Cardiovascular System
- Kidneys dispose of nitrogenous wastes; maintain fluid, electrolyte, and acid-base balance of blood; renal regulation of Na^+ and water balance essential for blood pressure homeostasis. Na^+, K^+, and Ca^{2+} regulation help maintain normal heart function
- Systemic arterial blood pressure is the driving force for glomerular filtration; heart secretes atrial natriuretic peptide; blood vessels transport nutrients, oxygen, etc. to urinary organs

Reproductive System
- Kidneys dispose of nitrogenous wastes; maintain fluid, electrolyte, and acid-base balance of blood

Integumentary System
- Kidneys dispose of nitrogenous wastes; maintain fluid, electrolyte, and acid-base balance of blood
- Skin provides external protective barrier; serves as site for water loss (via perspiration); vitamin D synthesis site

Skeletal System
- Kidneys dispose of nitrogenous wastes; maintain fluid, electrolyte, and acid-base balance of blood
- Bones of rib cage provide some protection to kidneys

Unit 8

Reproduction and Development

16

The Reproductive System

Most organ systems of the body function almost continuously to maintain the well-being of the individual. The reproductive system, however, appears to "slumber" until puberty. The **gonads** (go′nadz; "seeds"), or **primary sex organs,** are the *testes* in males and the *ovaries* in females. The gonads produce sex cells, or **gametes** (gam′ēts; "spouses"), and secrete sex hormones. The remaining reproductive system structures are **accessory reproductive organs.** Although male and female **reproductive systems** are quite different, their joint purpose is to produce offspring.

The reproductive role of the male is to manufacture male gametes called **sperm** and deliver them to the female reproductive tract. The female, in turn, produces female gametes, called **ova** (singular, *ovum*), or *eggs*. If the time is suitable, the sperm and egg fuse to produce a fertilized egg, which is the first cell of a new individual. Once fertilization has occurred, the female uterus provides a protective environment in which the *embryo*, later called the *fetus*, develops until birth.

The sex hormones play vital roles both in the development and function of the reproductive organs and in sexual behavior and drives. These gonadal hormones also influence the growth and development of many other organs and tissues of the body.

Anatomy of the Male Reproductive System

As already noted, the primary reproductive organs of the male are the **testes** (tes′tēz), or *male gonads,* which have both an exocrine (sperm-producing) function and an endocrine (testosterone-producing) function. The accessory reproductive structures are ducts or glands that aid in the delivery of sperm to the body exterior or to the female reproductive tract.

Testes

Each olive-sized testis is approximately 4 cm (1½ inches) long and 2.5 cm (1 inch) wide. A fibrous connective tissue capsule, the *tunica albuginea* (tu′nĭ-kah al″bu-jin′e-ah; "white coat") surrounds each testis. Extensions of this capsule *(septa)* plunge into the testis and divide it into a large number of *lobules*. Each lobule contains one to four tightly coiled **seminiferous** (sem″in-if′er-us) **tubules,** the actual "sperm-forming factories"

(Figure 16.1). Seminiferous tubules of each lobe empty sperm into another set of tubules, the *rete* (re′te) *testis,* located at one side of the testis. Sperm travel through the rete testis to enter the first part of the duct system, the *epididymis* (ep″ĭ-did′ĭ-mis), which hugs the external surface of the testis.

Lying in the soft connective tissue surrounding the seminiferous tubules are the *interstitial* (in″ter-stish′al) *cells,* functionally distinct cells that produce androgens—most importantly, *testosterone.* Thus, the sperm-producing and hormone-producing functions of the testes are carried out by completely different cell populations.

Duct System

The accessory organs forming the male duct system, which transports sperm from the body, are the *epididymis, ductus deferens,* and *urethra* (Figure 16.2).

Epididymis

The comma-shaped **epididymis** is a highly coiled tube about 6 m (20 feet) long that caps the superior

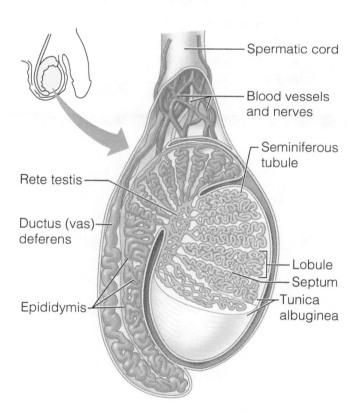

FIGURE 16.1   Sagittal section of the testis and associated epididymis.

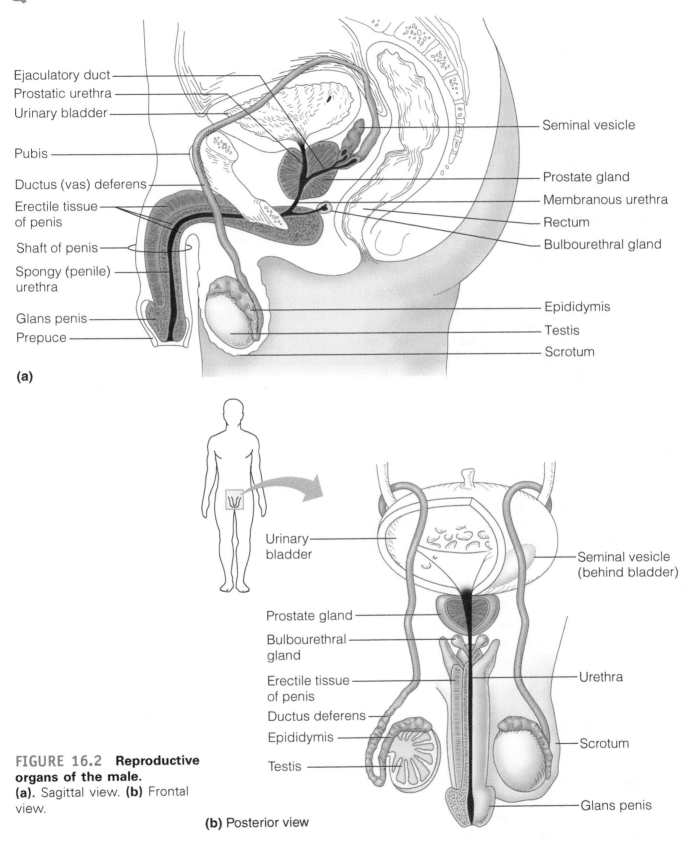

Ejaculatory duct
Prostatic urethra
Urinary bladder

Pubis

Ductus (vas) deferens

Erectile tissue of penis

Shaft of penis

Spongy (penile) urethra

Glans penis
Prepuce

Seminal vesicle

Prostate gland
Membranous urethra
Rectum
Bulbourethral gland

Epididymis
Testis
Scrotum

(a)

Urinary bladder

Prostate gland

Bulbourethral gland

Erectile tissue of penis

Ductus deferens
Epididymis
Testis

Seminal vesicle (behind bladder)

Urethra

Scrotum

Glans penis

FIGURE 16.2 Reproductive organs of the male.
(a). Sagittal view. **(b)** Frontal view.

(b) Posterior view

A Because the prostate gland encircles the superior part of the urethra, prostate hypertrophy would constrict the urethra in that region, impairing urination.

581

part of the testis and then runs down its posterolateral side (see Figure 16.1). The epididymis is the first part of the male duct system and provides a temporary storage site for the immature sperm that enter it from the testis. While the sperm make their way along the snaking course of the epididymis (a trip that takes about 20 days), they mature, gaining the ability to swim. When a male is sexually stimulated, the walls of the epididymis contract to expel the sperm into the next part of the duct system, the ductus deferens.

Ductus Deferens

The **ductus deferens** (duk'tus def'er-enz; "carrying away"), or **vas deferens,** runs upward from the epididymis through the inguinal canal into the pelvic cavity and arches over the superior aspect of the urinary bladder. This tube is enclosed, along with blood vessels and nerves, in a connective tissue sheath called the **spermatic cord** (see Figure 16.1). The end of the ductus deferens empties into the **ejaculatory** (e-jak'u-lah-to"re) **duct,** which passes through the prostate gland to merge with the urethra. The main function of the ductus deferens is to propel live sperm from their storage sites, the epididymis and distal part of the ductus deferens, into the urethra. At the moment of ejaculation (*ejac* = to shoot forth), the thick layers of smooth muscle in its walls create peristaltic waves that rapidly squeeze the sperm forward.

As Figure 16.2 illustrates, part of the ductus deferens lies in the scrotum, which hangs outside the body cavity. Some men voluntarily opt to take full responsibility for birth control by having a ***vasectomy*** (vah-sek'to-me). In this relatively minor operation, the surgeon makes a small incision into the scrotum and then cuts through or cauterizes the ductus deferens. Sperm are still produced, but they can no longer reach the body exterior and eventually they deteriorate and are reabsorbed. A man is sterile after this procedure, but because testosterone is still produced, the sex drive and secondary sex characteristics are retained.

Urethra

The **urethra,** which extends from the base of the urinary bladder to the tip of the penis, is the terminal part of the male duct system. It has three named regions: (1) the **prostatic urethra,** surrounded by the prostate gland; (2) the **membranous urethra,** spanning the distance from the prostatic urethra to the penis; and (3) the **spongy (penile) urethra,**

running within the length of the penis. The male urethra carries both urine and sperm to the body exterior; thus, it serves two masters, the urinary and reproductive systems. However, urine and sperm never pass at the same time. When ejaculation occurs and sperm enter the prostatic urethra from the ejaculatory ducts, the bladder sphincter (internal urethral sphincter) constricts. This event not only prevents the passage of urine into the urethra, but also prevents sperm from entering the urinary bladder.

Accessory Glands and Semen

The accessory glands include the paired *seminal vesicles,* the single *prostate gland,* and the *bulbourethral* (bul-bo-u-re'thral) *glands* (see Figure 16.2). These glands produce the bulk of *semen* (se'men), the sperm-containing fluid that is propelled out of the male's reproductive tract during **ejaculation.**

Seminal Vesicles

The **seminal** (sem'ĭ-nul) **vesicles,** located at the base of the bladder, produce about 60 percent of the fluid volume of semen. Their thick, yellowish secretion is rich in sugar (fructose), vitamin C, prostaglandins, and other substances, which nourish and activate the sperm passing through the tract. The duct of each seminal vesicle joins that of the ductus deferens on the same side to form the ejaculatory duct (see Figure 16.2). Thus, sperm and seminal fluid enter the urethra together during ejaculation.

Prostate Gland

The **prostate gland** is a single gland about the size and shape of a chestnut (see Figure 16.2). It encircles the upper (prostatic) part of the urethra just below the urinary bladder. Prostate gland secretion is a milky fluid that plays a role in activating sperm. During ejaculation, it enters the urethra through several small ducts. Since the prostate is located immediately anterior to the rectum, its size and texture can be palpated (felt) by digital (finger) examination through the anterior rectal wall.

Homeostatic Imbalance

The prostate gland has a reputation as a health destroyer. Hypertrophy of the prostate gland, which affects nearly every elderly male, strangles the urethra. This troublesome condition makes urination difficult and enhances the risk of bladder infections (cystitis) and kidney damage. Traditional treatment has been surgical, but some newer options are becoming more popular. These include:

- Using drugs (finasteride) or microwaves to shrink the prostate,

- Inserting a small inflatable balloon to compress the prostate tissue away from the prostatic urethra,

- Inserting a tiny needle that emits bursts of radio-frequency radiation, which incinerate excess prostate tissue.

Inflammation of the prostate is the single most common reason for a man to consult a urologist, and prostatic cancer is the third most prevalent cancer in men. As a rule, prostatic cancer is a slow-growing, hidden condition, but it can also be a swift and deadly killer. ▲

Bulbourethral Glands

The **bulbourethral glands** (formerly called *Cowper's glands*) are tiny, pea-sized glands inferior to the prostate gland. They produce a thick, clear mucus that drains into the penile urethra. This secretion is the first to pass down the urethra when a man becomes sexually excited. It is believed to cleanse the urethra of traces of acidic urine, and it serves as a lubricant during sexual intercourse.

Semen

Semen is a milky white, somewhat sticky mixture of sperm and accessory gland secretions. The liquid provides a transport medium and nutrients and contains chemicals that protect the sperm and aid their movement. Mature sperm cells are streamlined cellular "missiles" containing little cytoplasm or stored nutrients. The fructose in the seminal vesicle secretion provides essentially all of their energy fuel. The relative alkalinity of semen as a whole (pH 7.2–7.6) helps neutralize the acid environment (pH 3.5–4) of the female's vagina, protecting the delicate sperm. Sperm are very sluggish under acidic conditions (below pH 6). Semen also contains *seminalplasmin* (an antibiotic chemical that inhibits bacterial multiplication), the hormone relaxin, and certain enzymes that enhance sperm motility.

Semen also dilutes sperm; without such dilution, sperm motility is severely impaired. The amount of semen propelled out of the male duct system during ejaculation is relatively small, only 2 to 5 ml (about a teaspoonful), but there are between 50 and 130 million sperm in each milliliter.

Homeostatic Imbalance

Male infertility may be caused by obstructions of the duct system, hormonal imbalances, environmental estrogens, pesticides, excessive alcohol, and many other factors. One of the first series of tests done when a couple has been unable to conceive is *semen analysis*. Factors analyzed include sperm count, motility and morphology (shape and maturity), and semen volume, pH, and fructose content. A sperm count lower than 20 million per milliliter makes impregnation improbable. ▲

External Genitalia

The **external genitalia** (jen"i-tal'e-ah) of the male include the *scrotum* and the *penis* (see Figure 16.2). The **scrotum** (skro'tum; "pouch") is a divided sac of skin that hangs outside the abdominal cavity, between the legs and at the root of the penis. Under normal conditions, the scrotum hangs loosely from its attachments, providing the testes with a temperature that is below body temperature. This is a rather exposed location for a man's testes, which contain his entire genetic heritage, but apparently viable sperm cannot be produced at normal body temperature. The scrotum, which provides a temperature about 3°C (5.4°F) lower, is necessary for the production of healthy sperm. When the external temperature is very cold, the scrotum becomes heavily wrinkled as it pulls the testes closer to the warmth of the body wall. Thus, changes in scrotal surface area can maintain a temperature that favors viable sperm production.

The **penis** (pe'nis; "tail") is designed to deliver sperm into the female reproductive tract. The skin-covered penis consists of a **shaft,** which ends in an enlarged tip, the **glans penis.** The skin covering the penis is loose, and it folds downward to form a cuff of skin, the **prepuce** (pre'pus), or **foreskin,** around the proximal end of the glans. Frequently, the foreskin is surgically removed shortly after birth, by a procedure called *circumcision*.

Internally, the spongy urethra (see Figure 16.2) is surrounded by three elongated areas of *erectile tissue*, a spongy tissue that fills with blood during sexual excitement. This causes the penis to enlarge and become rigid. This event, called **erection,** helps the penis serve as a penetrating organ to deliver the semen into the female's reproductive tract.

Male Reproductive Functions

The chief role of the male in the reproductive process is to produce sperm and the hormone testosterone. These processes are described next.

Spermatogenesis

Sperm production, or **spermatogenesis** (sper″mah-to-jen′ĕ-sis), begins during puberty and continues throughout life. Every day a man makes millions of sperm. Since only one sperm fertilizes an egg, it seems that nature has made sure that the human species will not be endangered for lack of sperm.

Sperm formation occurs in the seminiferous tubules of the testis, as noted earlier. As shown in Figure 16.3, the process is begun by primitive stem cells called **spermatogonia** (sper″mah-to-go′ne-ah), found in the outer edge, or periphery, of each tubule. Spermatogonia go through rapid mitotic divisions to build up the stem cell line. From birth until puberty, all such divisions simply produce more stem cells. During puberty, however, *follicle-stimulating hormone (FSH)* is secreted in increasing amounts by the anterior pituitary gland, and, from this time on, each division of a spermatogonium produces one stem cell (a *type A daughter cell*) and another cell called a *type B daughter cell*. The type A cell remains at the tubule periphery to maintain the stem cell population. The type B cell gets pushed toward the tubule lumen, where it becomes a **primary spermatocyte,** destined to undergo *meiosis* (mi-o′sis) and form four sperm. **Meiosis** is a special type of nuclear division that occurs for the most part only in the gonads (testes and ovaries). It differs from *mitosis* (described in Chapter 3) in two major ways. Meiosis consists of two successive divisions of the nucleus (called meiosis I and II) and results in four (instead of two) daughter cells, or more precisely, four *gametes*. In spermatogenesis, the gametes are called **spermatids** (sper′mah-tidz). Spermatids have only half as much genetic material as other body cells. In humans, this is 23 chromosomes (or the so-called *n* number of chromosomes) rather than the usual 46 (2*n*). Then, when the sperm and the egg (which also has 23 chromosomes) unite, forming the fertilized egg, or zygote, the normal 2*n* number of 46 chromosomes is reestablished and is maintained

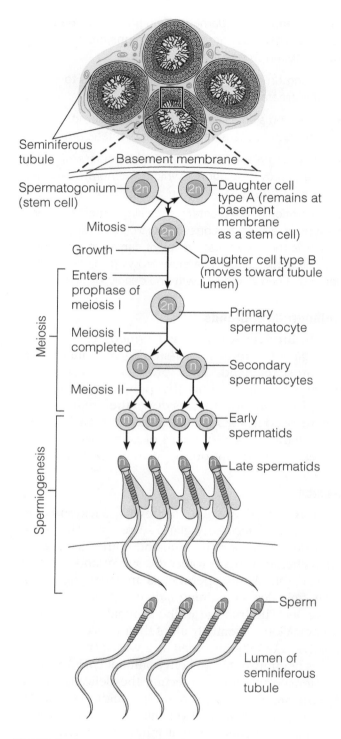

FIGURE 16.3 Spermatogenesis. Flowchart showing the relative position of the spermatogenic cells in the wall of the seminiferous tubule. Although the stem cells and the primary spermatocytes have the same number of chromosomes (46, designated as 2*n*) as other body cells, the products of meiosis (spermatids and sperm) have only half as many (23, designated as *n*).

in subsequent body cells by the process of mitosis (Figure 16.4).

As meiosis occurs, the dividing cells (primary and then secondary spermatocytes) are pushed toward the lumen of the tubule. Thus, the progress of meiosis can be followed from the tubule periphery to the lumen. The spermatids, which are the products of meiosis, are *not* functional sperm. They are nonmotile cells and have too much excess baggage to function well in reproduction. They must undergo further changes, in which their excess cytoplasm is stripped away and a tail is formed (see Figure 16.3). In this last stage of sperm development, called **spermiogenesis** (sper″me-o-gen′ĕ-sis), all the excess cytoplasm is sloughed off, and what remains is compacted into the three regions of the mature sperm—the *head, midpiece,* and *tail* (Figure 16.5). The mature sperm is a greatly streamlined cell equipped with a high rate of metabolism and a means of propelling itself, enabling it to move long distances in a short time to get to the egg. It is a prime example of the fit between form and function.

The sperm head contains DNA, the genetic material. Essentially, it *is* the nucleus of the spermatid. Anterior to the nucleus is the helmetlike

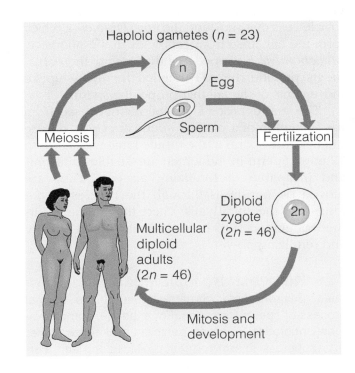

FIGURE 16.4   The human life cycle.

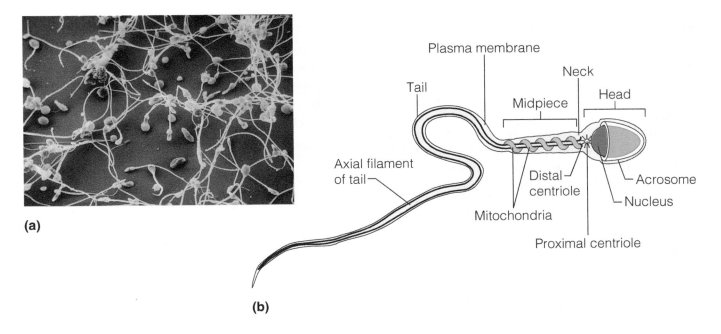

(a)

(b)

FIGURE 16.5   Structure of sperm. (a) Scanning electron micrograph of mature sperm (4303×). **(b)** Diagrammatic view of a sperm.

acrosome (ak'ro-sōm), which is similar to a large lysosome. When a sperm comes into close contact with an egg (or more precisely, an *oocyte*), the acrosomal membrane breaks down and releases enzymes that help the sperm penetrate through the follicle cells that surround the egg. *Filaments,* which form the tail, arise from centrioles in the midpiece. *Mitochondria* wrapped tightly around these filaments provide the ATP needed for the whiplike movements of the tail that propel the sperm.

The entire process of spermatogenesis, from the formation of a primary spermatocyte to release of immature sperm in the tubule lumen, takes 64 to 72 days. Sperm in the lumen are unable to "swim" and incapable of fertilizing an egg. They are moved by peristalsis through the tubules of the testes into the epididymis. There they undergo further maturation, which results in increased motility and fertilizing power.

▲ Homeostatic Imbalance

Environmental threats can alter the normal process of sperm formation. For example, some common antibiotics, such as penicillin and tetracycline, may suppress sperm formation. Radiation, lead, certain pesticides, marijuana, tobacco, and excessive alcohol can cause production of abnormal sperm (two-headed, multiple-tailed, and so on). ▲

Testosterone Production

As noted earlier, the interstitial cells produce **testosterone** (tes-tos'tĕ-rōn), the most important hormonal product of the testes. During puberty, as the seminiferous tubules are being prodded to produce sperm by FSH, the interstitial cells are being activated by **luteinizing hormone (LH),** sometimes called *interstitial cell–stimulating hormone (ICSH),* which is also released by the anterior pituitary gland (Figure 16.6). From this time on, testosterone is produced continuously (more or less) for the rest of a man's life. The rising blood level of testosterone in the young male stimulates the adolescent growth spurt, prods his reproductive organs to develop to their adult size, underlies the sex drive, and causes the secondary male sex characteristics to appear. **Secondary sex characteristics** typical of males include:

- Deepening of the voice due to enlargement of the larynx,

Q *What is the effect of negative feedback of testosterone on anterior pituitary and hypothalamic cells?*

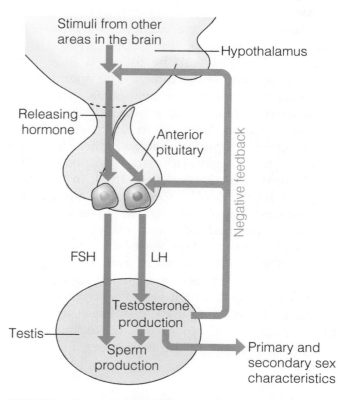

FIGURE 16.6 **Hormonal control of the testis.**

- Increased hair growth all over the body, and particularly in the axillary and pubic regions and the face (the beard and mustache),
- Enlargement of skeletal muscles to produce the heavier muscle mass typical of the male physique,
- Increased heaviness of the skeleton due to thickening of the bones.

Because testosterone is responsible for the appearance of these typical masculine characteristics, it is often referred to as the "masculinizing" hormone.

▲ Homeostatic Imbalance

If testosterone is not produced, the secondary sex characteristics never appear in the young man, and his other reproductive organs remain childlike. This is *sexual infantilism.* Castration of the adult male (or the inability of his interstitial cells to produce testosterone) results in a decrease in the size and function of his

A *It "turns off" the hypothalamic releasing factor that prompts ICSH secretion; hence, ICSH secretion also falls.*

reproductive organs, as well as a decrease in his sex drive. *Sterility* also occurs because testosterone is necessary for the final stages of sperm production. ▲

Anatomy of the Female Reproductive System

The reproductive role of the female is much more complex than that of the male. Not only must she produce the female gametes (ova), but her body must also nurture and protect a developing fetus during nine months of pregnancy. **Ovaries** are the primary reproductive organs of a female. Like the testes of a male, ovaries produce both an exocrine product (eggs, or *ova*) and endocrine products (estrogens and progesterone). The other organs of the female reproductive system serve as accessory structures to transport, nurture, or otherwise serve the needs of the reproductive cells and/or the developing fetus.

Ovaries

The paired *ovaries* (o'vah-rēz) are pretty much the size and shape of almonds. An internal view of an ovary reveals many tiny saclike structures called **ovarian follicles** (Figure 16.7). Each follicle consists of an immature egg, called an **oocyte** (o'o-sīt), surrounded by one or more layers of very different cells called **follicle cells.** As a developing egg within a follicle begins to ripen or mature, the follicle enlarges and develops a fluid-filled central region called an *antrum*. At this stage, the follicle, called a **vesicular,** or **Graafian** (graf'e-an), **follicle,** is mature, and the developing egg is ready to be ejected from the ovary, an event called **ovulation.** After ovulation, the ruptured follicle is transformed into a very different-looking structure called a **corpus luteum** (kor'pus lu'te-um; "yellow body"), which eventually degenerates. Ovulation generally occurs every 28 days, but it can occur more or less frequently in some women. In older women, the surfaces of the ovaries are scarred and pitted, which attests to the fact that many eggs have been released.

The ovaries are secured to the lateral walls of the pelvis by the *suspensory ligaments*. They flank the uterus laterally and anchor to it medially by the *ovarian ligaments* (Figure 16.8). In between, they are enclosed and held in place by a fold of peritoneum, the *broad ligament.*

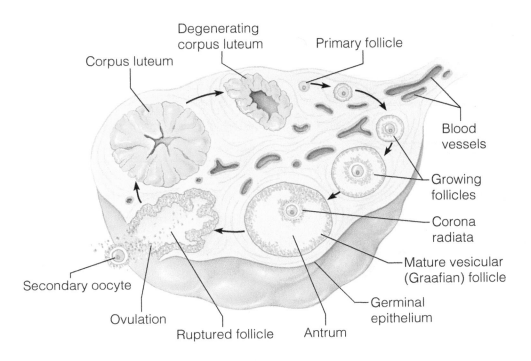

FIGURE 16.7 **Sagittal view of a human ovary showing the developmental stages of an ovarian follicle.**

Duct System

The *uterine tubes, uterus,* and *vagina* form the duct system of the female reproductive tract (Figure 16.8).

Uterine (Fallopian) Tubes

The **uterine** (u'ter-in), or **fallopian** (fal-lo'pe-an), **tubes** form the initial part of the duct system. They receive the ovulated oocyte and provide a site where fertilization can occur. Each of the uterine tubes is about 10 cm (4 inches) long and extends medially from an ovary to empty into the superior region of the uterus. Like the ovaries, the uterine tubes are enclosed and supported by the broad ligament. Unlike in the male duct system, which is continuous with the tubule system of the testes, there is little or no actual contact between the uterine tubes and the ovaries. The distal end of each uterine tube expands as the funnel-shaped *infundibulum,* which has fingerlike projections called **fimbriae** (fim'bre-e) that partially surround the ovary. As an oocyte is expelled from an ovary during ovulation, the waving fimbriae create fluid currents that act to carry the oocyte into the uterine tube, where it begins its journey toward the uterus. (Obviously, however, many potential eggs are lost in the peritoneal cavity.) The oocyte is carried toward the uterus by a combination of peristalsis and the rhythmic beating of *cilia.* Because the journey to the uterus takes 3 to 4 days and the oocyte is viable for up to 24 hours after ovulation, the usual site of fertilization is the uterine tube. To reach the oocyte, the sperm must swim upward through the vagina and uterus to reach the uterine tubes. Because they must swim against the downward current created by the cilia, it is rather like swimming against the tide!

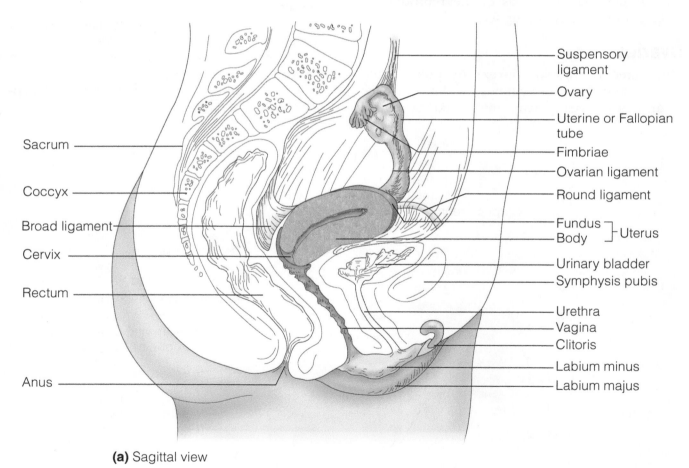

(a) Sagittal view

FIGURE 16.8   The human female reproductive organs. (a) Sagittal section. (The plural of *labium minus* and *majus* is *labia minora* and *majora,* respectively.)

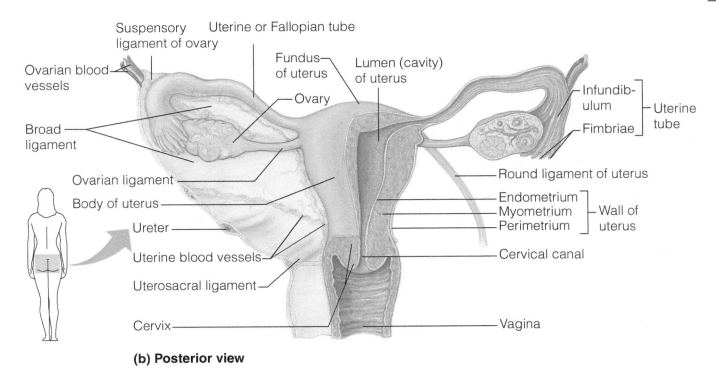

Suspensory ligament of ovary

Uterine or Fallopian tube

Ovarian blood vessels

Fundus of uterus

Lumen (cavity) of uterus

Ovary

Broad ligament

Infundib-ulum

Fimbriae

Uterine tube

Ovarian ligament

Round ligament of uterus

Body of uterus

Endometrium
Myometrium — Wall of
Perimetrium — uterus

Ureter

Uterine blood vessels

Cervical canal

Uterosacral ligament

Cervix

Vagina

(b) Posterior view

FIGURE 16.8   The human female reproductive organs (*continued*)
(b) Posterior view. The posterior organ walls have been removed on the right side to reveal the shape of the lumen of the uterine tube, uterus, and vagina.

Homeostatic Imbalance

The fact that the uterine tubes are not continuous distally with the ovaries places women at risk for infections spreading into the peritoneal cavity from the reproductive tract. *Gonorrhea* (gon"o-re'ah) and other sexually transmitted bacteria sometimes infect the peritoneal cavity in this way, causing an extremely severe inflammation called *pelvic inflammatory disease (PID)*. Unless treated promptly, PID can cause scarring and closure of the narrow uterine tubes, which is one of the major causes of female infertility. ▲

Uterus

The **uterus** (u'ter-us; "womb"), located in the pelvis between the urinary bladder and rectum, is a hollow organ that functions to receive, retain, and nourish a fertilized egg. In a woman who has never been pregnant, it is about the size and shape of a pear. (During pregnancy, the uterus increases tremendously in size and can be felt well above the umbilicus during the latter part of pregnancy.) The uterus is suspended in the pelvis by the broad ligament and anchored anteriorly and posteriorly by the *round* and *uterosacral ligaments,* respectively (see Figure 16.8).

The major portion of the uterus is referred to as the **body.** Its superior rounded region above the entrance of the uterine tubes is the **fundus,** and its narrow outlet, which protrudes into the vagina below, is the **cervix.**

The wall of the uterus is thick and composed of three layers. The inner layer or mucosa is the **endometrium** (en-do-me'tre-um). If fertilization occurs, the fertilized egg (actually the young embryo by the time it reaches the uterus) burrows into the endometrium (this process is called **implantation**) and resides there for the rest of its development. When a woman is not pregnant, the endometrial lining sloughs off periodically, usually about every 28 days, in response to changes in the levels of ovarian hormones in the blood. This process is called menstruation or *menses.*

Homeostatic Imbalance

Cancer of the cervix is common among women between the ages of 30 and 50. Risk factors include frequent cervical inflammation, sexually transmitted diseases, multiple pregnancies, and many sexual partners. A yearly *Pap smear* is the single most important diagnostic test for detecting this slow-growing cancer. ▲

The **myometrium** (mi-o-me′tre-um) is the bulky middle layer of the uterus (see Figure 16.8b). It is composed of interlacing bundles of smooth muscle. The myometrium plays an active role during the delivery of a baby, when it contracts rhythmically to force the baby out of the mother's body. The outermost serous layer of the uterus is the *perimetrium* (per-ĭ-me′tre-um), or the visceral peritoneum.

Vagina

The **vagina** (vah-ji′nah) is a thin-walled tube 8 to 10 cm (3 to 4 inches) long. It lies between the bladder and rectum and extends from the cervix to the body exterior (see Figure 16.8). Often called the *birth canal,* the vagina provides a passageway for the delivery of an infant and for the menstrual flow to leave the body. Since it receives the penis (and semen) during sexual intercourse, it is the female organ of copulation.

The distal end of the vagina is partially closed by a thin fold of the mucosa called the **hymen** (hi′men). The hymen is very vascular and tends to bleed when it is ruptured during the first sexual intercourse. However, its durability varies. In some females, it is torn during a sports activity, tampon insertion, or pelvic examination. Occasionally, it is so tough that it must be ruptured surgically if intercourse is to occur.

External Genitalia

The female reproductive structures that are located external to the vagina are the **external genitalia** (Figure 16.9). The external genitalia, also called the **vulva,** include the *mons pubis, labia, clitoris, urethral* and *vaginal orifices,* and *greater vestibular glands.*

The **mons pubis** ("mountain on the pubis") is a fatty, rounded area overlying the pubic symphysis. After puberty, this area is covered with pubic hair. Running posteriorly from the mons pubis are two elongated hair-covered skin folds, the **labia majora** (la′be-ah ma-jo′ra), which enclose two delicate hair-free folds, the **labia minora.** The labia majora enclose a region called the **vestibule,** which contains the external

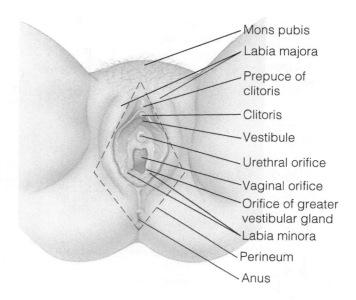

FIGURE 16.9 External genitalia of the human female.

openings of the urethra,* followed posteriorly by that of the vagina. A pair of mucus-producing glands, the **greater vestibular glands** *(Bartholin's glands),* flank the vagina, one on each side. Their secretion lubricates the distal end of the vagina during intercourse.

Just anterior to the vestibule is the **clitoris** (kli′to-ris; "hill"), a small, protruding structure that corresponds to the male penis. Like the penis, it is hooded by a prepuce and is composed of sensitive erectile tissue that becomes swollen with blood during sexual excitement. The clitoris differs from the penis in that it lacks a reproductive duct. The diamond-shaped region between the anterior end of the labial folds, the anus posteriorly, and the ischial tuberosities laterally is the **perineum** (per″ĭ-ne′um).

Female Reproductive Functions and Cycles

Oogenesis and the Ovarian Cycle

As described earlier, sperm production in males begins at puberty and generally continues

---

*The male urethra carries both urine and semen, but the female urethra has no reproductive function—it is strictly a passageway for urine.

throughout life. The situation is quite different in females. The total supply of eggs that a female can release is already determined by the time she is born. In addition, a female's reproductive ability (that is, her ability to release eggs) usually begins during puberty and ends in her fifties or before. The period in which a woman's reproductive capability gradually declines and then finally ends is called *menopause.*

Meiosis, the special kind of cell division that occurs in the male testes to produce sperm, also occurs in the female ovaries. But in this case, female gametes, or sex cells, are produced, and the process is called **oogenesis** (o″o-jen′ĕ-sis; "the beginning of an egg"). This process is shown in Figure 16.10 and described in more detail next.

In the developing female fetus, **oogonia** (o″o-go′ne-ah), the female stem cells, multiply rapidly to increase their number, and then their daughter cells, **primary oocytes,** push into the ovary connective tissue, where they become surrounded by a single layer of cells to form the

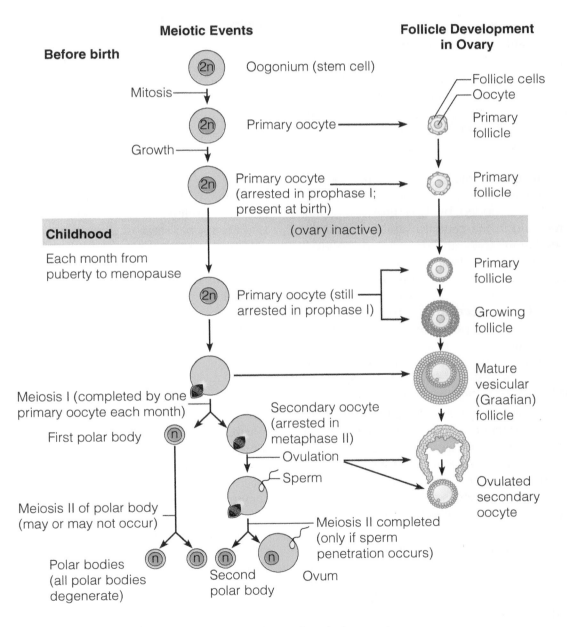

FIGURE 16.10 Events of oogenesis. Left, flowchart of meiotic events. Right, correlation with follicular development and ovulation in the ovary.

primary follicles. By birth, the oogonia no longer exist, and a female's lifetime supply of primary oocytes (approximately 2 million of them) is already in place in the ovarian follicles, awaiting the chance to undergo meiosis to produce functional eggs. Since the primary oocytes remain in this state of suspended animation all through childhood, their wait is a long one—10 to 14 years at the very least.

At puberty, the anterior pituitary gland begins to release **follicle-stimulating hormone (FSH)**, which stimulates a small number of primary follicles to grow and mature each month, and ovulation begins to occur each month. These cyclic changes that occur monthly in the ovary constitute the **ovarian cycle.** At puberty, perhaps 400,000 oocytes remain; and, beginning at this time, a small number of oocytes are activated each month. Since the reproductive life of a female is at best about 40 years (from the age of 11 to approximately 51) and there is typically only one ovulation per month, fewer than 500 ova out of her potential of 400,000 are released during a woman's lifetime. Again, nature has provided us with a generous oversupply of sex cells.

As a follicle prodded by FSH grows larger, it accumulates fluid in the central chamber called the *antrum* (see Figure 16.7), and the primary oocyte it contains replicates its chromosomes and begins meiosis. The first meiotic division produces two cells that are very dissimilar in size (see Figure 16.10). The larger cell is a **secondary oocyte** and the other, very tiny cell is a **polar body.** By the time a follicle has ripened to the mature (*vesicular follicle*) stage, it contains a secondary oocyte and protrudes like an angry boil from the external surface of the ovary. Follicle development to this stage takes about 14 days, and ovulation (of a secondary oocyte) occurs at just about that time in response to the burstlike release of a second anterior pituitary hormone, *luteinizing hormone (LH)*. As shown in Figures 16.7, 16.10, and 16.11, the ovulated secondary oocyte is still surrounded by its follicle-cell capsule, now called the *corona radiata* ("radiating crown"). Some women experience a twinge of abdominal pain in the lower abdomen when ovulation occurs. This phenomenon, called *mittelschmerz* (mit'el-shmārts; German for "middle pain"), is caused by the intense stretching of the ovarian wall during ovulation.

Generally speaking, one of the developing follicles outstrips the others each month to become

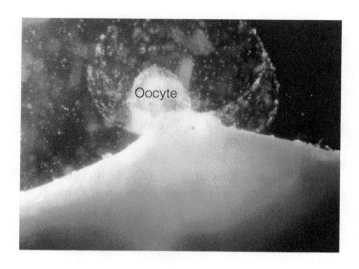

FIGURE 16.11   Ovulation. A secondary oocyte is released from a follicle at the surface of the ovary. The orange mass below the ejected oocyte is part of the ovary. The "halo" of follicle cells around the secondary oocyte is the *corona radiata.*

the dominant follicle. Just how this follicle is selected or selects itself is not understood, but the follicle that is at the proper stage of maturity when the LH stimulus occurs will rupture and release its oocyte into the peritoneal cavity. The mature follicles that are not ovulated soon become overripe and deteriorate. In addition to triggering ovulation, LH also causes the ruptured follicle to change into a very different glandular structure, the *corpus luteum.* (Both the maturing follicles and the corpus luteum produce hormones, as will be described later.)

If the ovulated secondary oocyte is penetrated by a sperm, it undergoes the second meiotic division that produces another polar body and the **ovum.** Once the ovum is formed, its 23 chromosomes are combined with those of the sperm to form the fertilized egg, which is the first cell of the yet-to-be offspring. However, if the secondary oocyte is not penetrated by a sperm, it simply deteriorates without ever completing meiosis to form a functional egg. Although meiosis in males results in four functional sperm, meiosis in females yields only one functional ovum and three tiny polar bodies. Since the polar bodies have essentially no cytoplasm, they deteriorate and die quickly.

Another major difference between males and females concerns the size and structure of their sex cells. Sperm are tiny and equipped with tails for locomotion. They have little nutrient-containing cytoplasm; thus, the nutrients in seminal fluid are vital to their survival. In contrast, the egg is a large, nonmotile cell, well stocked with nutrient reserves that nourish the developing embryo until it can take up residence in the uterus.

Uterine (Menstrual) Cycle

Although the uterus is the receptacle in which the young embryo implants and develops, it is receptive to implantation only for a very short period each month. Not surprisingly, this brief interval coincides exactly with the time when a fertilized egg would begin to implant, approximately seven days after ovulation. The events of the **uterine,** or **menstrual, cycle** are the cyclic changes that the

endometrium, or mucosa of the uterus, goes through month after month as it responds to changes in the levels of ovarian hormones in the blood.

Since the cyclic production of estrogens and progesterone by the ovaries is, in turn, regulated by the anterior pituitary gonadotropic hormones, FSH and LH, it is important to understand how these "hormonal pieces" fit together (see Figure 16.12). Generally speaking, both female cycles are about 28 days long (a period commonly called a *lunar month*), with ovulation typically occurring midway in the cycles, on or about day 14. Figure 16.13 illustrates the events occurring both in the ovary (the ovarian cycle) and in the uterus (menstrual cycle) at the same time. The three stages of the menstrual cycle are described next.

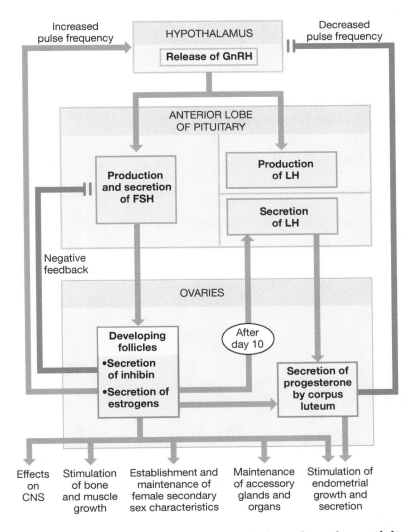
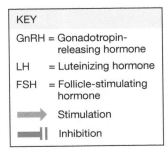

FIGURE 16.12 **The hormonal regulation of ovarian activity.**

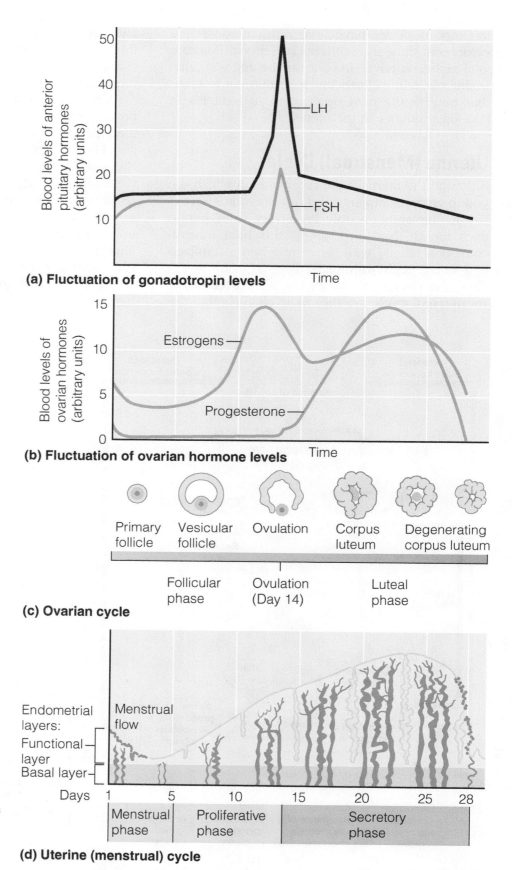

(a) Fluctuation of gonadotropin levels

(b) Fluctuation of ovarian hormone levels

(c) Ovarian cycle

FIGURE 16.13 **Hormonal interactions of the female cycles.** Relative levels of anterior pituitary gonadotropins correlated with hormonal and follicular changes of the ovary and with the menstrual cycle.

(d) Uterine (menstrual) cycle

- **Days 1–5: Menstrual phase.** During this interval, the superficial *functional layer* of the thick endometrial lining of the uterus is sloughing off, or becoming detached, from the uterine wall. This is accompanied by bleeding for three to five days. The detached tissues and blood pass through the vagina as the menstrual flow. The average blood loss during this period is 50 to 150 ml (or about ¼ to ½ cup). By day 5, growing ovarian follicles are beginning to produce more estrogen.

- **Days 6–14: Proliferative phase.** Stimulated by rising estrogen levels produced by the growing follicles of the ovaries, the basal layer of the endometrium regenerates the functional layer, glands are formed in it, and the endometrial blood supply is increased. The endometrium once again becomes velvety, thick, and well vascularized. (Ovulation occurs in the ovary at the end of this stage, in response to the sudden surge of LH in the blood.)

- **Days 15–28: Secretory phase.** Rising levels of progesterone production by the corpus luteum of the ovary act on the estrogen-primed endometrium and increase its blood supply even more. Progesterone also causes the endometrial glands to increase in size and to begin secreting nutrients into the uterine cavity. These nutrients will sustain a developing embryo (if one is present) until it has implanted. If fertilization does occur, the embryo produces a hormone very similar to LH, which causes the corpus luteum to continue producing its hormones. If fertilization does not occur, the corpus luteum begins to degenerate toward the end of this period as LH blood levels decline. Lack of ovarian hormones in the blood causes the blood vessels supplying the functional layer of the endometrium to go into spasms and kink. When deprived of oxygen and nutrients, those endometrial cells begin to die, which sets the stage for menses to begin again on day 28.

Although this explanation assumes a classic 28-day cycle, the length of the menstrual cycle is quite variable. It can be as short as 21 days or as long as 40 days. Only one interval is fairly constant in all females; the time from ovulation to the beginning of menses is almost always 14 or 15 days.

Hormone Production by the Ovaries

As the ovaries become active at puberty and start to produce ova, production of ovarian hormones also begins. The follicle cells of the growing and mature follicles produce **estrogens,*** which cause the appearance of the *secondary sex characteristics* in the young woman. Such changes include:

- Enlargement of the accessory organs of the female reproductive system (uterine tubes, uterus, vagina, external genitals),
- Development of the breasts,
- Appearance of axillary and pubic hair,
- Increased deposits of fat beneath the skin in general, and particularly in the hips and breasts,
- Widening and lightening of the pelvis,
- Onset of menses, or the menstrual cycle.

The second ovarian hormone, **progesterone,** is produced by the glandular *corpus luteum* (see Figure 16.7). As mentioned earlier, after ovulation occurs the ruptured follicle is converted to the corpus luteum, which looks and acts completely different from the growing and mature follicle. Once formed, the corpus luteum produces progesterone (and some estrogen) as long as LH is still present in the blood. Generally speaking, the corpus luteum has stopped producing hormones by 10 to 14 days after ovulation. Except for working with estrogen to establish the menstrual cycle, progesterone does not contribute to the appearance of the secondary sex characteristics. Its other major effects are exerted during pregnancy, when it helps maintain the pregnancy and prepare the breasts for milk production. (However, the source of progesterone during pregnancy is the placenta, not the ovaries.) Table 16.1 summarizes the hormones of the resproductive system.

Mammary Glands

The **mammary glands** are present in both sexes, but they normally function only in females. Since the biological role of the mammary glands is to produce milk to nourish a newborn baby, they are actually important only when reproduction has

---

*Although the ovaries produce several different estrogens, the most important are *estradiol, estrone,* and *estriol.* Of these, estradiol is the most abundant and is most responsible for mediating estrogenic effects.

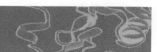

TABLE 16.1 Hormones of the Reproductive System

Hormone	Source	Regulation of Secretion	Primary Effects
Gonadotropin-releasing hormone (GnRH)	Hypothalamus	*Males*: inhibited by testosterone and possibly by inhibin *Females*: GnRH pulse frequency increased by estrogens, decreased by progestins	Stimulates FSH secretion and LH synthesis in males and females
Follicle-stimulating hormone (FSH)	Anterior lobe of pituitary gland	*Males*: stimulated by GnRH, inhibited by inhibin *Females*: stimulated by GnRH, inhibited by inhibin	*Males*: stimulates spermatogenesis and spermiogenesis through effects on sustentacular cells *Females*: stimulates follicle development, estrogen production, and oocyte maturation
Luteinizing hormone (LH)	Anterior lobe of pituitary gland	*Males*: stimulated by GnRH *Females*: production stimulated by GnRH, secretion by the combination of high GnRH pulse frequencies and high estrogen levels	*Males*: stimulates interstitial cells to secrete testosterone *Females*: stimulates ovulation, formation of corpus luteum, and progestin secretion
Androgens (primarily testosterone and dihydrotestosterone)	Interstitial cells of testes	Stimulated by LH	Establish and maintain secondary sex characteristics and sexual behavior; promote maturation of spermatozoa; inhibit GnRH secretion
Estrogens (primarily estradiol)	Granulosa and thecal cells of developing follicles; corpus luteum	Stimulated by FSH	Stimulate LH secretion (at high levels); establish and maintain secondary sex characteristics and sexual behavior; stimulate repair and growth of endometrium; increase frequency of GnRH pulses
Progestins (primarily progesterone)	Granulosa cells from midcycle through functional life of corpus luteum	Stimulated by LH	Stimulate endometrial growth and glandular secretion; reduce frequency of GnRH pulses
Inhibin	Sustentacular cells of testes and granulosa cells of ovaries	Stimulated by factors released by developing spermatozoa (male) and developing follicles (female)	Inhibits secretion of FSH (and possibly of GnRH)

Q *Flat-chested women are perfectly able to nurse their newborn infants; hence, it is not glandular tissue that accounts for the bulk of the breast tissue. So, what does?*

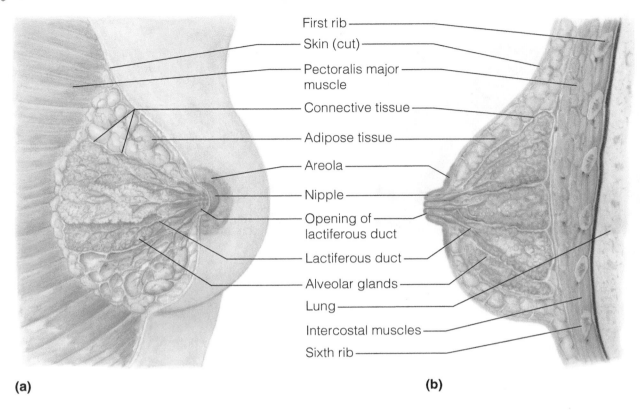

First rib
Skin (cut)
Pectoralis major muscle
Connective tissue
Adipose tissue
Areola
Nipple
Opening of lactiferous duct
Lactiferous duct
Alveolar glands
Lung
Intercostal muscles
Sixth rib

(a)   **(b)**

FIGURE 16.14 Female mammary glands. (a) Anterior view.
(b) Sagittal section.

already been accomplished. Stimulation by female sex hormones, especially estrogens, causes the female mammary glands to increase in size at puberty.

Developmentally, the mammary glands are modified *sweat glands* that are actually part of the skin. Each mammary gland is contained within a rounded skin-covered breast anterior to the pectoral muscles of the thorax. Slightly below the center of each breast is a pigmented area, the **areola** (ah-re′o-lah), which surrounds a central protruding **nipple** (Figure 16.14).

Internally, each mammary gland consists of 15 to 25 *lobes,* which radiate around the nipple. The lobes are padded and separated from each other by connective tissue and fat. Within each lobe are smaller chambers called *lobules,* which contain clusters of **alveolar glands** that produce

the milk when a woman is **lactating** (producing milk). The alveolar glands of each lobule pass the milk into the **lactiferous** (lak-tif′er-us) **ducts,** which open to the outside at the nipple.

Homeostatic Imbalance

Cancer of the breast is the second most common cause of death in American women. One woman in eight will develop this condition. Breast cancer is often signaled by a change in skin texture, puckering, or leakage from the nipple. Early detection by breast self-examination and mammography is unquestionably the best way to increase one's chances of surviving breast cancer. Since most breast lumps are discovered by women themselves in routine monthly breast exams, this simple examination should be a priority in every woman's life. Currently, the American Cancer Society recommends scheduling **mammography**—X-ray examination that detects breast cancers too small to feel (less than 1 cm)—every 2 years for women between 40 and 49 years old and yearly thereafter (Figure 16.15). ▲

A   *Adipose tissue.*

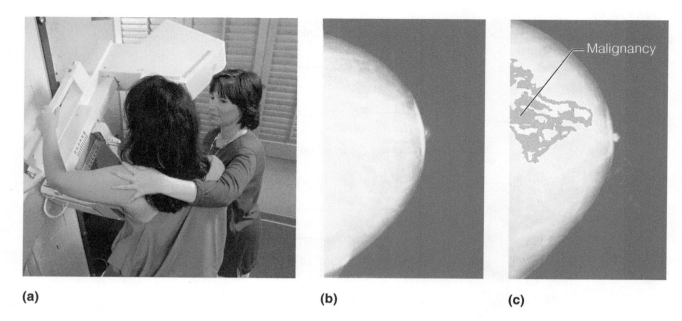

(a)   **(b)**   **(c)**

FIGURE 16.15 **Mammograms. (a)** Photograph of woman undergoing mammography. **(b)** Normal breast. **(c)** Breast with tumor.

Survey of Pregnancy and Embryonic Development

Because the birth of a baby is such a familiar event, we tend to lose sight of the wonder of this accomplishment. In every instance, it begins with a single cell, the fertilized egg, and ends with an extremely complex human being consisting of trillions of cells. The development of an embryo is very complex, and the details of this process can fill a good-sized book. Our intention here is simply to outline the important events of pregnancy and embryonic development.

100 Keys | Cyclic changes in FSH and LH levels are responsible for the maintenance of the ovarian cycle; the hormones produced by the ovaries in turn regulate the uterine cycle. Inadequate hormone levels, inappropriate or inadequate responses to circulating hormones, or poor coordination and timing of hormone production or secondary oocyte release will reduce or eliminate the chances of pregnancy.

The Physiology of Sexual Intercourse

Sexual intercourse, also known as *coitus* (KŌ-i-tus) or *copulation*, introduces semen into the female reproductive tract. We will now consider the process as it affects the reproductive systems of males and females.

Male Sexual Function

Sexual function in males is coordinated by complex neural reflexes that we do not yet understand completely. The reflex pathways utilize the sympathetic and parasympathetic divisions of the autonomic nervous system. During sexual **arousal,** erotic thoughts, the stimulation of sensory nerves in the genital region, or both lead to an *increase in parasympathetic outflow* over the pelvic nerves. This outflow in turn leads to erection of the penis. The integument covering the glans of the penis contains numerous sensory receptors, and **erection** tenses the skin and increases their sensitivity. Subsequent stimulation can initiate the secretion of the bulbourethral glands, lubricating the penile urethra and the surface of the glans.

During intercourse, the sensory receptors of the penis are rhythmically stimulated. This stimulation eventually results in the coordinated processes of emission and ejaculation. **Emission** *occurs under sympathetic stimulation.* The process begins when the peristaltic contractions of the ampulla push fluid and spermatozoa into the prostatic urethra. The seminal vesicles then begin contracting, and the contractions increase in force and duration over the next few seconds. Peristaltic contractions also appear in the walls of the prostate gland. The combination moves the seminal mixture into the membranous and penile portions of the urethra. While the contractions are proceeding, sympathetic commands also cause the contraction of the urinary bladder and the internal urethral sphincter. The combination of elevated pressure inside the bladder and the contraction of the sphincter effectively prevents the passage of semen into the bladder.

Ejaculation occurs as powerful, rhythmic contractions appear in the *ischiocavernosus* and *bulbospongiosus muscles*, two superficial skeletal muscles of the pelvic floor. The ischiocavernosus muscles insert along the sides of the penis; their contractions serve primarily to stiffen that organ. The bulbospongiosus muscle wraps around the base of the penis; the contraction of this muscle pushes semen toward the external urethral opening. The contractions of both muscles are controlled by somatic motor neurons in the inferior lumbar and superior sacral segments of the spinal cord.

Ejaculation is associated with intensely pleasurable sensations, an experience known as male **orgasm** (OR-gazm). Several other noteworthy physiological changes occur at this time, including pronounced but temporary increases in heart rate and blood pressure. After ejaculation, blood begins to leave the erectile tissue, and the erection begins to subside. This subsidence, called **detumescence** (de-tū-MES-ens), is mediated by the sympathetic nervous system.

In sum, arousal, erection, emission, and ejaculation are controlled by a complex interplay between the sympathetic and parasympathetic divisions of the autonomic nervous system. Higher centers, including the cerebral cortex, can facilitate or inhibit many of the important reflexes, thereby modifying the patterns of sexual function. Any physical or psychological factor that affects a single component of the system can result in male sexual dysfunction, also called **impotence.**

Impotence is defined as an inability to achieve or maintain an erection. Various physical causes may be responsible for impotence, because erection involves vascular changes as well as neural commands. For example, low blood pressure in the arteries supplying the penis, due to a circulatory blockage such as a plaque, will reduce the ability to attain an erection. Drugs, alcohol, trauma, or illnesses that affect the autonomic nervous system or the central nervous system can have the same effect. But male sexual performance can also be strongly affected by the psychological state of the individual. Temporary periods of impotence are relatively common in healthy individuals who are experiencing severe stresses or emotional problems. Depression, anxiety, and fear of impotence are examples of emotional factors that can result in sexual dysfunction. The prescription drug Viagra, which enhances and prolongs the effects of nitric oxide on the erectile tissue of the penis, has proven useful in treating many cases of impotence.

Female Sexual Function

The phases of female sexual function are comparable to those of male sexual function. During sexual arousal, parasympathetic activation leads to engorgement of the erectile tissues of the clitoris and increased secretion of cervical mucous glands and the greater vestibular glands. Clitoral erection increases the receptors' sensitivity to stimulation, and the cervical and vestibular glands lubricate the vaginal walls. A network of blood vessels in the vaginal walls becomes filled with blood at this time, and the vaginal surfaces are also moistened by fluid that moves across the epithelium from underlying connective tissues. (This process accelerates during intercourse as the result of mechanical stimulation.) Parasympathetic stimulation also causes contraction of subcutaneous smooth muscle of the nipples, making them more sensitive to touch and pressure.

During sexual intercourse, rhythmic contact of the penis with the clitoris and vaginal walls—reinforced by touch sensations from the breasts and other stimuli (visual, olfactory, and auditory)—provides stimulation that leads to orgasm. Female orgasm is accompanied by peristaltic contractions of the uterine and vaginal walls and, by means of impulses traveling over the pudendal nerves, rhythmic contractions of the bulbospongiosus and ischiocavernosus muscles. The latter contractions give rise to the intensely pleasurable sensations of orgasm.

Accomplishing Fertilization

Before fertilization can occur, the sperm must reach the ovulated secondary oocyte. The oocyte is viable for 12 to 24 hours after it is cast out of the ovary, and sperm generally retain their fertilizing power within the female reproductive tract for 12 to 48 hours after ejaculation. Some "super sperm," however, are viable for 72 hours. Consequently, for fertilization to occur, sexual intercourse must occur no more than 72 hours before ovulation and no later than 24 hours after, at which point the oocyte is approximately one-third of the way down the length of the uterine tube. Remember that sperm are motile cells that can propel themselves by lashing movements of their tails. If sperm are deposited in a female's vagina at the approximate time of ovulation, they are attracted to the oocyte by chemicals that act as "homing devices," allowing them to locate the oocyte. It takes one to two hours for sperm to complete the journey up the female duct system to the end of the uterine tubes, and if an oocyte is en route in the tube, fertilization is a distinct possibility.

When the swarming sperm reach the oocyte, hundreds of their acrosomes rupture, releasing enzymes that break down the "cement" that holds the follicle cells of the corona radiata together around the oocyte. Once a path has been cleared and a single sperm makes contact with the oocyte's membrane receptors, its head (nucleus) is pulled into the oocyte cytoplasm. This is one case that does not bear out the adage, "The early bird catches the worm." A sperm that comes along later, after hundreds of sperm have undergone acrosomal reactions to expose the oocyte membrane, is in the best position to be *the* fertilizing sperm. Once a single sperm has penetrated the oocyte, the oocyte nucleus completes the second meiotic division, forming the ovum and a polar body.

After sperm entry, changes occur in the fertilized egg to prevent other sperm from gaining entry. Of the millions of sperm ejaculated by a male, only *one* can penetrate an oocyte. **Fertilization** occurs at the moment the genetic material of a sperm combines with that of an ovum to form a fertilized egg, or **zygote** (zi'gōt). The zygote represents the first cell of the new individual.

Events of Embryonic and Fetal Development

As the zygote journeys down the uterine tube (propelled by peristalsis and cilia), it begins to undergo rapid mitotic cell divisions—forming first two cells, then four, and so on. This early stage of embryonic development, called **cleavage,** is shown in Figure 16.16. Since there is not much time for cell growth between divisions, the daughter cells become smaller and smaller. Cleavage provides a large number of cells to serve as building blocks for constructing the **embryo** (developmental stage until the ninth week). Consider for a moment how difficult it would be to construct a building from one huge block of granite. If you now consider how much easier your task would be if you could use hundreds of brick-size granite blocks, you will quickly grasp the importance of cleavage. By the time the developing embryo reaches the uterus (about 3 days after ovulation, or on day 17 of the woman's cycle), it is a *morula,* a tiny ball of 16 cells that looks like a microscopic raspberry. The uterine endometrium is still not fully prepared to receive the embryo at this point, so the embryo floats free in the uterine cavity, temporarily using the uterine secretions for nutrition. While still unattached, the embryo continues to develop until it has about 100 cells, and then it hollows out to form a ball-like structure, a **blastocyst** (blas'to-sist) or **chorionic** (ko″re-on'ik) **vesicle.** At the same time, it secretes an LH-like hormone called **human chorionic gonadotropin (hCG),** which prods the corpus luteum of the ovary to continue producing its hormones. (If this were not the case, the functional layer of the endometrium would be sloughing off shortly in menses.) It is hCG that many home pregnancy tests assay for in a woman's urine.

The blastocyst has two important functional areas: the *trophoblast,* which forms the large fluid-filled sphere, and the *inner cell mass,* a small cluster of cells displaced to one side (see Figure 16.16e). By day 7 after ovulation, the blastocyst has attached to the endometrium and has eroded away the lining in a small area, embedding

Q *Why is the multicellular blastocyst only slightly larger than the single-cell zygote?*

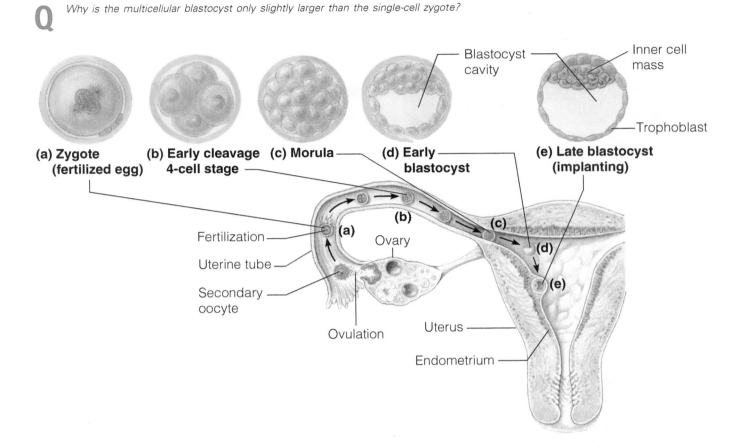

(a) Zygote (fertilized egg)   **(b) Early cleavage 4-cell stage**   **(c) Morula**   **(d) Early blastocyst**   **(e) Late blastocyst (implanting)**

Blastocyst cavity — Inner cell mass — Trophoblast

Fertilization — Uterine tube — Secondary oocyte — Ovary — Ovulation — Uterus — Endometrium

FIGURE 16.16 Cleavage is a rapid series of mitotic divisions that begins with the zygote and ends with the blastocyst. The zygote begins to divide about 24 hours after fertilization and continues to divide rapidly (undergo cleavage) as it travels down the uterine tube. Three to four days after ovulation, the preembryo reaches the uterus and floats freely for two to three days, nourished by secretions of the endometrial glands. At the late blastocyst stage, the embryo is implanting into the endometrium; this begins at about day 7 after ovulation. **(a)** Zygote (fertilized egg). **(b)** Four-cell stage. **(c)** Morula, a solid ball of blastomeres. **(d)** Early blastocyst; the morula hollows out, and fills with fluid. **(e)** Late blastocyst, composed of an outer sphere of trophoblast cells and an off-center cell cluster called the inner cell mass.

itself in the thick velvety mucosa. All of this is occurring even while development is continuing and the three primary germ layers are being formed from the inner cell mass (Figure 16.17). The *primary germ layers* are the **ectoderm** (which gives rise to the nervous system and the epidermis of the skin), the **endoderm** (which forms mucosae and associated glands), and the **mesoderm** (which gives rise to virtually everything else). Implantation has usually been completed and the uterine mucosa has grown over the burrowed-in embryo by day 14 after ovulation—the day the woman would ordinarily be expecting to start menses. After it is securely implanted, the trophoblast part of the blastocyst develops elaborate projections, called **chorionic villi,** which

A Because as the zygote and then its descendents divide, little or no time is provided for growth between subsequent division cycles. As a result, the cells get smaller and smaller and the size of the cell mass stays approximately the same size as the initial zygote.

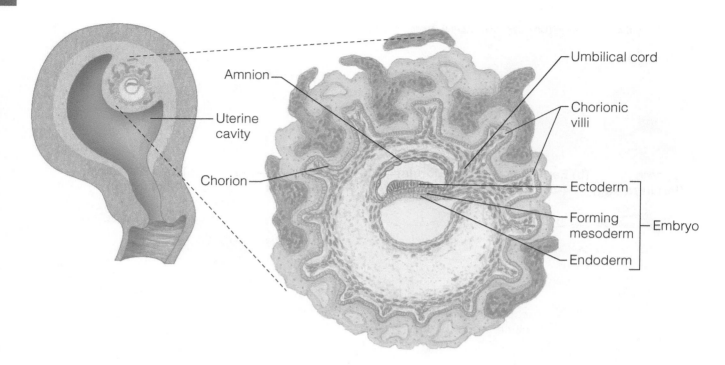

FIGURE 16.17 **Embryo of approximately 22 days.** Embryonic membranes present.

cooperate with the tissues of the mother's uterus to form the **placenta** (plah-sen'tah). Once the placenta has formed, the platelike embryonic body, now surrounded by a fluid-filled sac called the **amnion** (am'ne-on), is attached to the placenta by a blood vessel–containing stalk of tissue, the **umbilical cord** (Figure 16.17). Generally by the third week, the placenta is functioning to deliver nutrients and oxygen to and remove wastes from the embryonic blood. All exchanges are made through the placental barrier. By the end of the second month of pregnancy, the placenta has also become an endocrine organ and is producing estrogen, progesterone, and other hormones that help to maintain the pregnancy. At this time, the corpus luteum of the ovary becomes inactive.

By the eighth week of embryonic development, all the groundwork has been completed. All the organ systems have been laid down, at least in rudimentary form, and the embryo looks distinctly human. Beginning in the ninth week of development, the embryo is referred to as a **fetus.** From this point on, the major activities are growth and organ specialization, accompanied by changes in body proportions. During the fetal period, the developing fetus grows from a crown-to-rump length of about 3 cm (slightly more than 1 inch) and a weight of approximately 1 g (0.03 ounce) to about 36 cm (14 inches) and 2.7 to 4.1 kg (6–10 pounds) or more. (Total body length at birth is about 55 cm, or 22 inches.) As you might expect with such tremendous growth, the changes in fetal appearance are quite dramatic (Figure 16.18). The most significant of these changes are summarized in Table 16.2. By approximately 270 days after fertilization (the end of the tenth lunar month), the fetus is said to be "full-term" and is ready to be born.

Effects of Pregnancy on the Mother

Pregnancy (the period from conception to the birth of her baby) can be a difficult time for the mother. Not only are there obvious anatomical changes, but striking changes occur in her physiology as well.

Anatomical Changes

The ability of the uterus to enlarge during pregnancy is nothing less than remarkable. Starting as a fist-sized organ, the uterus grows to occupy most of the pelvic cavity by 16 weeks. As pregnancy

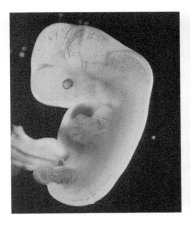 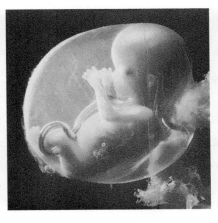 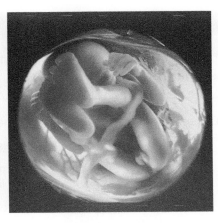

(a) 5 weeks. Limb buds, eyes, the heart, the liver, and rudiments of all other organs have started to develop in the embryo, which is only about 1 cm long.

(b) 14 weeks. Growth and development of the offspring, now called a fetus, continue during the second trimester. This fetus is about 6 cm long.

(c) 20 weeks. By the end of the second trimester (at 24 weeks), the fetus grows to about 30 cm in length.

FIGURE 16.18 **Human fetal development.**

continues, the uterus pushes higher and higher into the abdominal cavity. As birth nears, the uterus reaches the level of the xiphoid process and occupies the bulk of the abdominal cavity. The crowded abdominal organs press superiorly against the diaphragm, which intrudes on the thoracic cavity. As a result, the ribs flare, causing the thorax to widen.

The increasing bulkiness of the abdomen changes the woman's center of gravity, and many women develop an accentuated lumbar curvature (lordosis), often accompanied by backaches, during the last few months of pregnancy. Placental production of the hormone **relaxin** causes pelvic ligaments and the pubic symphysis to relax, widen, and become more flexible. This increased motility eases birth passage, but it may also result in a waddling gait during pregnancy.

Obviously, good maternal nutrition is necessary throughout pregnancy if the developing fetus is to have all the building materials (proteins, calcium, iron, and the like) it needs to form its tissues and organs. The old expression "A pregnant woman is eating for two" has encouraged many women to eat *twice* the amount of food actually needed during pregnancy, which, of course, leads to excessive weight gain. Actually, a pregnant

woman needs only about 300 additional calories daily to sustain proper fetal growth. The emphasis should be on high-quality food, not just more food.

Homeostatic Imbalance

Since many potentially harmful substances can cross through the placental barrier into the fetal blood, the pregnant woman should be very much aware of what she is taking into her body. Substances that may cause life-threatening birth defects (and even fetal death) include alcohol, nicotine, and many types of drugs (anticoagulants, antihypertensives, sedatives, and some antibiotics). Maternal infections, particularly German measles (rubella), may also cause severe fetal damage. Termination of a pregnancy by loss of a fetus during the first 20 weeks of pregnancy is called **abortion.** ▲

Physiological Changes

Gastrointestinal System Many women suffer nausea, commonly called *morning sickness,* during the first few months of pregnancy, until their system adjusts to the elevated levels of progesterone and estrogens. *Heartburn* is common because the esophagus is displaced and the stomach is crowded by the growing uterus,

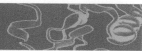

TABLE 16.2   Development of the Human Fetus

Time	Changes/accomplishments
8 weeks (end of embryonic period) 8 weeks	Head nearly as large as body; all major brain regions present Liver disproportionately large and begins to form blood cells Limbs present; though initially webbed, fingers and toes are free by the end of this interval Bone formation begun Heart has been pumping blood since the fourth week All body systems present in at least rudimentary form Approximate crown-to-rump length: 30 mm (3 cm; 1.2 inches); weight: 1 gram (0.03 ounces)
9–12 weeks (third month) 12 weeks	Head still dominant, but body elongating; brain continues to enlarge Facial features present in crude form Walls of hollow visceral organs gaining smooth muscle Blood cell formation begins in bone marrow Bone formation accelerating Sex readily detected from the genitals Approximate crown-to-rump length at end of interval: 90 mm (9 cm)
13–16 weeks (fourth month) 16 weeks	General sensory organs are present; eyes and ears assume characteristic position and shape; blinking of eyes and sucking motions of lips occur Face looks human and body beginning to outgrow head Kidneys attain typical structure Most bones are distinct and joint cavities apparent Approximate crown-to-rump length at end of interval: 140 mm (14 cm)

which favors reflux of stomach acid into the esophagus. Another problem is constipation, because motility of the digestive tract declines during pregnancy.

Urinary System   The kidneys have the additional burden of disposing of fetal metabolic wastes, and they produce more urine during pregnancy. Because the uterus compresses the bladder, urination becomes more frequent, more urgent, and sometimes uncontrollable. (The last condition is called *stress incontinence.*)

Respiratory System   The nasal mucosa responds to estrogen by becoming swollen and congested; thus, nasal stuffiness and occasional nosebleeds may occur. Vital capacity and respiratory rate increase during pregnancy, but residual volume declines, and many women exhibit *dyspnea* (difficult breathing) during the later stages of pregnancy.

Cardiovascular System   Perhaps the most dramatic physiological changes occur in the cardiovascular system. Total body water rises and blood volume

TABLE 16.2	(continued)

Time	Changes/accomplishments
17–20 weeks (fifth month)	Vernix caseosa (fatty secretions of sebaceous glands) covers body; silklike hair (lanugo) covers skin
	Fetal position (body flexed anteriorly) assumed because of space restrictions
	Limbs achieve near-final proportions
	Quickening occurs (mother feels spontaneous muscular activity of fetus)
	Approximate crown-to-rump length at end of interval: 190 mm (19 cm)
21–30 weeks (sixth and seventh months)	Substantial increase in weight (may survive if born prematurely at 27–28 weeks, but hypothalamus still too immature to regulate body temperature, and surfactant production by the lungs is still inadequate)
	Myelination of spinal cord begins; eyes are open
	Skin is wrinkled and red; fingernails and toenails are present
	Body is lean and well proportioned
	Bone marrow becomes sole site of blood cell formation
	Testes enter scrotum in seventh month (in males)
At birth	Approximate crown-to-rump length at end of interval: 280 mm (28 cm)
30–40 weeks (term) (eighth and ninth months)	Skin whitish pink; fat laid down in subcutaneous tissue
	Approximate crown-to-rump length at end of interval: 350–400 mm (35–40 cm; 14–16 inches); weight: 2.7–4.1 kg (6–10 pounds)

increases by 25 to 40 percent to accommodate the additional needs of the fetus. The rise in blood volume also acts as a safeguard against blood loss during birth. Blood pressure and pulse typically rise and increase cardiac output by 20 to 40 percent; this helps propel the greater blood volume around the body. Because the uterus presses on the pelvic blood vessels, venous return from the lower limbs may be impaired somewhat, resulting in varicose veins.

Childbirth

Childbirth, also called **parturition** (par″tu-rish′un; "bringing forth young"), is the culmination of pregnancy. It usually occurs within 15 days of the calculated due date (which is 280 days from the last menstrual period). The series of events that expel the infant from the uterus are referred to collectively as **labor.**

Initiation of Labor

The precise trigger for labor is not clear, but several events appear to be interlocked in this process. During the last few weeks of pregnancy, estrogens reach their highest levels in the mother's blood. This has two important consequences: it causes the myometrium to form abundant *oxytocin* receptors (so that it becomes more sensitive to the hormone oxytocin), and it interferes with progesterone's quieting influence on the uterine muscle. As a result, weak, irregular uterine contractions begin to occur. These contractions, called *Braxton Hicks contractions,* have caused many women to go to the hospital, only to be told that they were in **false labor** and sent home.

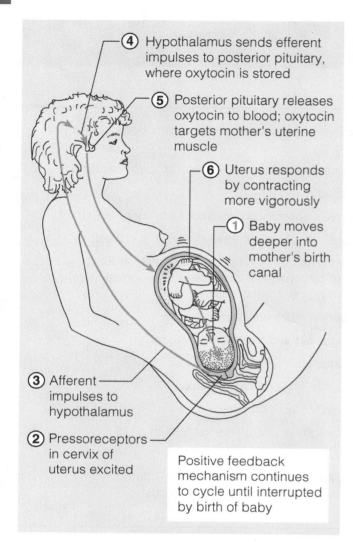

④ Hypothalamus sends efferent impulses to posterior pituitary, where oxytocin is stored

⑤ Posterior pituitary releases oxytocin to blood; oxytocin targets mother's uterine muscle

⑥ Uterus responds by contracting more vigorously

① Baby moves deeper into mother's birth canal

③ Afferent impulses to hypothalamus

② Pressoreceptors in cervix of uterus excited

Positive feedback mechanism continues to cycle until interrupted by birth of baby

FIGURE 16.19   The positive feedback mechanism by which oxytocin promotes labor contractions during birth.

As birth nears, two more chemical signals cooperate to convert these false labor pains into the real thing. Certain cells of the fetus begin to produce oxytocin, which in turn stimulates the placenta to release *prostaglandins*. Both hormones stimulate more frequent and powerful contractions of the uterus. At this point, the increasing emotional and physical stresses activate the mother's hypothalamus, which signals for oxytocin release by the posterior pituitary. The combined effects of rising levels of oxytocin and prostaglandins initiate the rhythmic, expulsive contractions of true labor. Once the hypothalamus is involved, a positive feedback mechanism is propelled into action: Stronger

contractions cause the release of more oxytocin, which causes even more vigorous contractions, forcing the baby ever deeper into the mother's pelvis, and so on (Figure 16.19).

Since both oxytocin and prostaglandins are needed to initiate labor in humans, anything that interferes with production of either of these hormones will hinder the onset of labor. For example, antiprostaglandin drugs such as aspirin and ibuprofen can inhibit labor at the early stages, and such drugs are used occasionally to prevent premature births.

Stages of Labor

The process of labor is commonly divided into three stages (Figure 16.20). These stages are described next.

Stage 1: Dilation Stage   The **dilation stage** is the time from the appearance of true contractions until the cervix is fully dilated by the baby's head (about 10 cm in diameter). As labor starts, regular but weak uterine contractions begin in the upper part of the uterus and move downward toward the vagina. Gradually, the contractions become more vigorous and more rapid, and, as the infant's head is forced against the cervix with each contraction, the cervix begins to soften, becomes thinner *(effaces)*, and dilates. Eventually, the amnion ruptures, releasing the amniotic fluid, an event commonly referred to as "breaking the water." The dilation stage is the longest part of labor and usually lasts for 6 to 12 hours (sometimes considerably more).

Stage 2: Expulsion Stage   The **expulsion stage** is the period from full dilation to delivery of the infant. In this stage, the infant passes through the cervix and vagina to the outside of the body. During this stage, a mother experiencing natural childbirth (that is, undergoing labor without local anesthesia) has an increasing urge to push, or bear down, with the abdominal muscles. Although this phase can take as long as 2 hours, it is typically 50 minutes in a first birth and around 20 minutes in subsequent births.

When the infant is in the usual head-first *(vertex)* position, the skull (its largest diameter) acts as a wedge to dilate the cervix. The head-first presentation also allows the baby to be suctioned free of mucus and to breathe even before it has completely exited from the birth canal. Once the

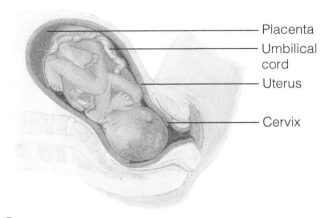

Placenta
Umbilical cord
Uterus
Cervix

① Dilation of the cervix

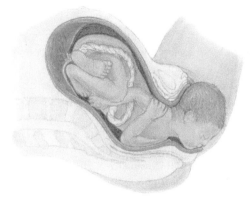

② Expulsion: delivery of the infant

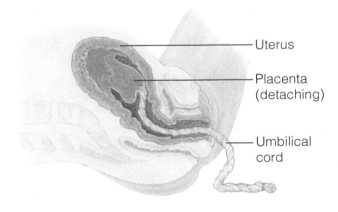

Uterus
Placenta (detaching)
Umbilical cord

FIGURE 16.20 **The three stages of labor.**

head has been delivered, the rest of the baby's body is delivered much more easily. After birth, the umbilical cord is clamped and cut. In *breech* (buttocks-first) presentations and other nonvertex presentations, these advantages are lost and delivery is much more difficult, sometimes requiring the use of forceps or a vacuum extractor.

▲ Homeostatic Imbalance

During an extremely prolonged or difficult stage 2, a condition called *dystocia* (dis-to'se-ah) may occur. In dystocia, oxygen delivery to the infant is inadequate, leading to fetal brain damage (resulting in cerebral palsy or epilepsy) and decreased viability of the infant. To prevent these outcomes, a *cesarean* (se-zayr'e-an) *section,* also called a *C-section*, may be performed. A C-section is delivery of the infant through a surgical incision made through the abdominal and uterine walls. ▲

Stage 3: Placental Stage   The **placental stage,** or the delivery of the placenta, is usually accomplished within 15 minutes after birth of the infant. The strong uterine contractions that continue after birth compress uterine blood vessels, limit bleeding, and cause the placenta to detach from the uterine wall. The placenta and its attached fetal membranes, collectively called the **afterbirth,** are then easily removed by a slight tug on the umbilical cord. It is very important that all placental fragments be removed to prevent continued uterine bleeding after birth *(postpartum bleeding).*

Lactation and the Mammary Glands   By the end of the sixth month of pregnancy, the mammary glands are fully developed, and the gland cells begin to produce a secretion known as **colostrum** (ko-LOS-trum). Ingested by the infant during the first two or three days of life, colostrum contains more proteins and far less fat than breast milk. Many of the proteins are antibodies that may help the infant ward off infections until its own immune system becomes fully functional. In addition, the mucins present in both colostrum and milk can inhibit the replication of a family of viruses *(rotaviruses)* that can cause dangerous forms of gastroenteritis and diarrhea in infants.

As colostrum production drops, the mammary glands convert to milk production. Breast milk consists of water, proteins, amino acids, lipids, sugars, and salts. It also contains large quantities of

A Closer Look

Contraception: To Be or Not To Be

IN a society such as ours, where many women opt for professional careers or must work for economic reasons, **contraception** (*contra* = against; *cept* = taking), or *birth control,* is often seen as a necessity. Thus far, much of the burden for birth control has fallen on women's shoulders, and most birth control products are female-directed.

The key to birth control is dependability. As shown by the red arrows in the accompanying flowchart, the birth control techniques and products currently available have many sites of action for blocking the reproductive process. Let's examine the relative advantages of a few of these current methods more closely.

The most-used contraceptive product in the United States is the *birth control pill,* or simply, "the pill," a preparation taken daily that contains tiny amounts of estrogens and progestins (progesterone-like hormones), except that for the last seven days of the 28-day cycle the tablets are hormone-free. The pill tricks the hypothalamic-pituitary control system and "lulls it to sleep" because the relatively constant blood levels of ovarian hormones make it appear that the woman is pregnant (both estrogen and progesterone are pro-duced throughout pregnancy). Ovarian follicles do not mature, and ovulation ceases. The endometrium does proliferate slightly and is sloughed off when the hormones are discontinued each month, but menstrual flow is much reduced. However, since hormonal balance in the body is precisely controlled, some women simply cannot tolerate the changes caused by the pill—they become nauseated and/or hypertensive.

For a while, the pill was suspected of increasing the incidence of breast and uterine cancer. Its influence on breast cancer is still a question. However, it appears that the new, very low-dose preparations may actually help protect against some forms of cancer (ovarian and endometrial) and may also have reduced the incidence of serious cardiovascular side effects, such as strokes, heart attacks, and blood clots, that occurred (rarely) with earlier forms of the pill.

Presently, the pill is one of the most widely used drugs in the world; well over 50 million women use these drugs to prevent pregnancy. The incidence of failure is less than 6 pregnancies per 100 women per year.

A different hormone pill, the *morning-after pill (MAP),* is widely prescribed on college campuses and the therapy of choice for rape victims and is one of the best-kept secrets in the United States—most teenagers and women in their 30s and 40s have never heard of them. Taken within 72 hours of unprotected intercourse, the concentrated estrogen-progesterone combination pills "mess up" the normal hormonal signals so much that fertilization is prevented altogether or a fertilized egg is prevented from implanting. Planned Parenthood clinics have begun to publicize the availability of MAPs for postcoital contraception, a use now approved by the U.S. Food and Drug Administration (FDA).

Other approaches include a device that is implanted just under the skin and injections of synthetic progesterone. The Norplant implant, six tiny silicone rods that release progestin over a 5-year period (see the photo), was approved late in 1990 and quickly gained users. Its failure rate (0.05 percent) is even lower than that of the pill, but there have been some problems with rod removal. *Depo-Provera,* a synthetic progesterone developed 35 years before, was finally approved for use as an injectable contraceptive in October 1992. Administered in a 150-mg dose once every three

Contraception: To Be or Not To Be *(continued)*

months, Depo-Provera's failure rate is only 0.4 percent.

For several years, the second most used contraceptive method was the *intrauterine device (IUD),* a plastic or metal device inserted into the uterus that prevented implantation of the fertilized egg (see photo). The failure rate of the IUD was nearly as low as that of the pill. For a while, IUDs were taken off the market in the United States because of problems with occasional contraceptive failure, uterine perforation, or pelvic inflammatory disease (PID). New IUD products that deliver sustained doses of synthetic progesterone to the endometrium are currently being recommended for those who have given birth and for those with a lower risk of developing PID in monogamous relationships.

Some methods, such as *tubal ligation* and *vasectomy* (cutting or cauterizing the uterine tubes or ductus deferens, respectively), are nearly foolproof and are the choice of approximately 33 percent of couples of childbearing age in the United States. Both procedures can be done in the physician's office. These changes are usually permanent, however, so they are not for individuals who still plan to have children but want to choose the time.

Coitus interruptus, or withdrawal of the penis just before ejaculation, is simply against nature, and control

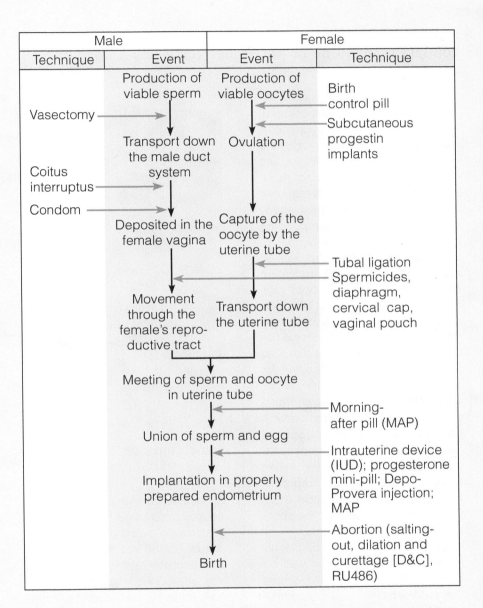

Flowchart of the events that must occur to produce a baby. Techniques or products that interfere with the process are indicated by red arrows at the site of interference; they act to prevent the next step.

Contraception: To Be or Not To Be *(continued)*

of ejaculation is never assured. *Rhythm,* or *fertility awareness, methods* depend on recognizing the period of ovulation or fertility and avoiding intercourse during those intervals. This may be accomplished by (1) recording daily basal body temperatures (body temperature drops slightly immediately prior to ovulation and then rises slightly after ovulation) or (2) recording changes in the consistency of vaginal mucus (the mucus first becomes sticky and then clear and stringy, much like egg white, during the fertile period). Rhythm techniques require accurate record-keeping for several cycles before they can be used with confidence. *Barrier methods,* such as diaphragms, cervical caps, condoms (see photo), spermicidal foams, gels, and sponges, are quite effective, especially when some agent is used by both partners. But many people avoid them because they can reduce the spontaneity of sexual encounters.

RU486, the so-called *abortion pill* developed in France, may well be the next "big seller" in the United States. When taken during the first 7 weeks of pregnancy in conjunction with a tiny amount of prostaglandin

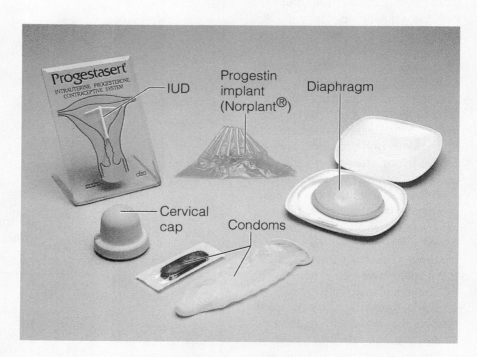

Some contraceptive devices.

to induce uterine contractions, it induces miscarriage by blocking progesterone's quieting effect on the uterus. RU486 has a 96 to 98 percent success rate with virtually no side effects. Now approved by the FDA, it has become a topic of bitter controversy among pro-choice and pro-life groups in the United States.

This summary has barely touched on the large number of experimental birth control drugs now awaiting clinical trials; and other methods are sure to be developed in the near future. In the final analysis, however, the only 100 percent effective means of birth control is the age-old one—*total abstinence.*

lysozymes—enzymes with antibiotic properties. Human milk provides roughly 750 Calories per liter. The secretory rate varies with the demand, but a 5–6-kg (11–13-lb) infant usually requires about 850 ml of milk per day. (The production of milk throughout this period is maintained through the combined actions of several hormones.

Milk becomes available to infants through the **milk let-down reflex** (Figure 16.21). Mammary gland secretion is triggered when the infant sucks on the nipple (STEP 1). The stimulation of tactile receptors there leads to the stimulation of secretory neurons in the paraventricular nucleus of the mother's hypothalamus (STEPS 2 and 3). These neurons release oxytocin at the posterior lobe of the pituitary gland (STEP 4). When circulating oxytocin reaches the mammary gland, this hormone causes the contraction of *myoepithelial cells*, contractile cells in the walls of the lactiferous ducts and sinuses. The result is milk ejection (STEP 5), or *milk let-down.*

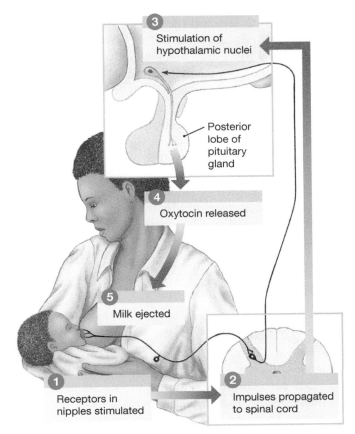

FIGURE 16.21   The milk let-down reflex.

The milk let-down reflex continues to function until *weaning*, typically one to two years after birth. Milk production ceases soon after, and the mammary glands gradually return to a resting state. Earlier weaning is a common practice in the United States, where women take advantage of commercially prepared milk- or soy-based infant formulas that closely approximate the composition of natural breast milk. The major difference between such substitutes and natural milk is that the substitutes lack antibodies and lysozymes, which play important roles in maintaining the health of the infant. Consequently, early weaning is associated with an increased risk of infections and allergies in the infant.

Developmental Aspects of the Reproductive System

Although the sex of an individual is determined at the time of fertilization (males have X and Y sex chromosomes and females have two X sex chromosomes), the gonads do not begin to form until about the eighth week of embryonic development. Prior to this time, the embryonic reproductive structures of males and females are identical and are said to be in the *indifferent stage*. After the gonads have formed, development of the accessory structures and external genitalia begins. Whether male or female structures will form depends entirely on whether testosterone is present or absent. The usual case is that, once formed, the embryonic testes produce testosterone, and the development of the male duct system and external genitalia follows. When testosterone is not produced, as is the case in female embryos that form ovaries, the female ducts and external genitalia result.

Homeostatic Imbalance

Any interference with the normal pattern of sex hormone production in the embryo results in bizarre abnormalities. For example, if the embryonic testes fail to produce testosterone, a genetic male develops the female accessory structures and external genitalia. On the other hand, if a genetic female is exposed to testosterone (as might happen if the mother has an androgen-producing tumor of her adrenal gland), the embryo has ovaries but develops male accessory ducts and glands, as well as a penis and an empty scrotum. Individuals having accessory reproductive structures that do not "match" their gonads are called *pseudo-hermaphrodites* (su"do-her-maf'ro-dītz) to distinguish them from true *hermaphrodites,* rare individuals who possess both ovarian and testicular tissues. In recent years, many pseudohermaphrodites have sought sex change operations to match their outer selves (external genitalia) with their inner selves (gonads). ▲

The male testes, formed in the abdominal cavity at approximately the same location as the female ovaries, descend to enter the scrotum about one month before birth. Failure of the testes to make their normal descent leads to a condition called *cryptorchidism* (krip-tor'kĭ-dizm). Because this condition results in sterility of a male (and also puts him at risk for cancer of the testes), surgery is usually performed during childhood to rectify this problem.

▲ **Homeostatic Imbalance**

Abnormal separation of chromosomes during meiosis can lead to congenital defects of this system. For example, males who have an extra female sex chromosome have the normal male accessory structures, but their testes atrophy, causing them to be sterile. Other abnormalities occur when a child has only one sex chromosome. An XO female appears normal but lacks ovaries; YO males die during development. Other much less serious conditions affect males primarily; these include *phimosis* (fi-mo'sis), which essentially is a narrowing of the foreskin of the penis, and misplaced urethral openings. ▲

Since the reproductive system organs do not function until puberty, there are few problems with this system during childhood. **Puberty** is the period of life, generally between the ages of 10 and 15 years, when the reproductive organs grow to their adult size and become functional under the influence of rising levels of gonadal hormones (testosterone in males and estrogen in females). After this time, reproductive capability continues until old age in males and menopause in females. Since the secondary sex characteristics and major events of puberty were described earlier, these details will not be repeated here. It is important to remember, however, that puberty represents the earliest period of reproductive system activity.

The events of puberty occur in the same sequence in all individuals, but the age at which they occur varies widely. In males, the event that signals puberty's onset is enlargement of the testes and scrotum, around the age of 13 years, followed by the appearance of pubic, axillary, and facial hair. Growth of the penis goes on over the next 2 years, and sexual maturation is indicated by the presence of mature sperm in the semen. In the meantime, the young man has unexpected, and often embarrassing, erections and frequent nocturnal emissions ("wet dreams") as his hormones surge and hormonal controls struggle to achieve a normal balance.

The first sign of puberty in females is budding breasts, often apparent by the age of 11 years. The first menstrual period, called **menarche** (mĕ-nar'ke), usually occurs about two years later. Dependable ovulation and fertility are deferred until the hormonal controls mature, an event that takes nearly two more years.

Prove It Yourself

The Stages of Mitosis and Meiosis Are Similar but Different

Here is a low-tech, but effective, way to compare the stages of mitosis and meiosis.

You'll need two pens of one color and two of another color, each with removable caps. Each pair of pens of a given color can represent the duplicated sister chromatids of a single chromosome (2 sister chromatids = 1 chromosome). Together, the four pens represent the sister chromatids of a pair of corresponding chromosomes (4 sister chromatids = a pair of sister chromosomes).

Now look at Figure 16.3 and move the pens through the stages of meiosis. To represent crossing-over, switch pen caps. How do the events of mitosis and meiosis differ?

▲ **Homeostatic Imbalance**

In adults, the most common reproductive system problems are infections. Vaginal infections are more common in young and elderly women and in those whose resistance is low. Common infections include those caused by *Escherichia coli* (spread from the digestive tract); sexually transmitted microorganisms (such as gonorrhea, syphilis, and herpesvirus);

and yeasts (a type of fungus). Untreated vaginal infections may spread throughout the female reproductive tract, causing pelvic inflammatory disease and sterility. Problems involving painful or abnormal menses may result from infection or hormone imbalance.

The most common inflammatory conditions in males are *urethritis, prostatitis,* and *epididymitis* (ep"ĭ-did-ĭ-mi'tis), all of which may follow sexual contacts in which sexually transmitted disease (STD) microorganisms are transmitted. *Orchiditis* (or"kĭ-di'tis), inflammation of the testes, is rather uncommon but is serious because it can cause sterility. Orchiditis most commonly follows STD or mumps (in an adult male).

As noted earlier, neoplasms represent a major threat to reproductive system organs. Tumors of the breast and cervix are the most common reproductive cancers in adult females, and prostate cancer (a common sequel to prostatic hypertrophy) is a widespread problem in adult males. ▲

Most women reach peak reproductive abilities in their late twenties. After that, a natural decrease in ovarian function occurs. As estrogen production declines, ovulation becomes irregular and menstrual periods become scanty and shorter in length. Eventually, ovulation and menses cease entirely, ending childbearing ability. This event, called **menopause,** is considered to have occurred when a whole year has passed without menstruation.

Although estrogen production continues for a while after menopause, the ovaries finally stop functioning as endocrine organs. When deprived of the stimulatory effects of estrogen, the reproductive organs and breasts begin to atrophy. The vagina becomes dry; intercourse may become painful (particularly if infrequent), and vaginal infections become increasingly common. Other consequences of estrogen deficit include irritability and other mood changes (depression in some); intense vasodilation of the skin's blood vessels, which causes uncomfortable sweat-drenching "hot flashes"; gradual thinning of the skin and loss of bone mass; and slowly rising blood cholesterol levels, which place postmenopausal women at risk for cardiovascular disorders. Some physicians prescribe low-dose estrogen-progestin preparations to help women through this often difficult period and to prevent the skeletal and cardiovascular complications.

There is no equivalent of menopause in males. Although aging men exhibit a steady decline in testosterone secretion, their reproductive capability seems unending. Healthy men well into their eighties and beyond are able to father offspring.

Systems in Sync

Homeostatic Relationships between the Reproductive System and Other Body Systems

Endocrine System
- Gonadal hormones exert feedback effects on hypothalamic-pituitary axis; placental hormones help to maintain pregnancy
- Gonadotropins help regulate function of gonads

Lymphatic System/Immunity
- Developing embryo/fetus escapes immune surveillance (not rejected)
- Lymphatic vessels drain leaked tissue fluids; transport sex hormones; immune cells protect reproductive organs from disease; IgA is present in breast milk

Digestive System
- Digestive organs crowded by developing fetus; heartburn, constipation common during pregnancy
- Digestive system provides nutrients needed for health

Urinary System
- Hypertrophy of the prostate gland inhibits urination; compression of bladder during pregnancy leads to urinary frequency and urgency
- Kidneys dispose of nitrogenous wastes and maintain acid-base balance of blood of mother and fetus; semen exits the body through the urethra of the male

Muscular System
- Androgens promote increased muscle mass
- Abdominal muscles active during childbirth; muscles of the pelvic floor support reproductive organs and aid erection of penis/clitoris

Nervous System
- Sex hormones masculinize or feminize the brain and influence sex drive
- Hypothalamus regulates timing of puberty; neural reflexes regulate sexual response

Respiratory System
- Pregnancy impairs descent of the diaphragm, causing difficult breathing
- Respiratory system provides oxygen; disposes of carbon dioxide; vital capacity and respiratory rate increase during pregnancy

Cardiovascular System
- Estrogens lower blood cholesterol levels and promote cardiovascular health in premenopausal women; pregnancy increases workload of the cardiovascular system
- Cardiovascular system transports needed substances to organs of reproductive system; local vasodilation involved in erection; blood transports sex hormones

Reproductive System

Integumentary System (Skin)
- Male sex hormones (androgens) activate oil glands, which lubricate skin and hair; gonadal hormones stimulate characteristic fat distribution and appearance of pubic and axillary hair; estrogen increases skin hydration; enhances facial skin pigmentation during pregnancy
- Skin protects all body organs by enclosing them externally; mammary gland secretions (milk) nourish the infant

Skeletal System
- Androgens masculinize the skeleton and increase bone density; estrogen feminizes skeleton and maintains bone mass in females
- The bony pelvis encloses some reproductive organs; if narrow, the bony pelvis may hinder vaginal delivery of an infant

Appendices

Appendix I

Summary Table   An Overview of Prenatal Development

Background Material

ATLAS: Embryology Summaries 1–4:
The Development of Tissues
The Development of Epithelia
The Development of
Connective Tissues
The Development of
Organ Systems

Gestational Age (Months)	Size and Weight	Integumentary System	Skeletal System	Muscular System	Nervous System	Special Sense Organs
1	5 mm, 0.02 g		(b) Formation of somites	(b) Formation of somites	(b) Formation of neural tube	(b) Formation of eyes and ears
2	28 mm, 2.7 g	(b) Formation of nail beds, hair follicles, sweat glands	(b) Formation of axial and appendicular cartilages	(c) Rudiments of axial musculature	(b) CNS, PNS organization, growth of cerebrum	(b) Formation of taste buds, olfactory epithelium
3	78 mm, 26 g	(b) Epidermal layers appear	(b) Spreading of ossification centers	(c) Rudiments of appendicular musculature	(c) Basic spinal cord and brain structure	
4	133 mm, 0.15 kg	(b) Formation of hair, sebaceous glands (c) Sweat glands	(b) Articulations (c) Facial and palatal organization	Fetal movements can be felt by the mother	(b) Rapid expansion of cerebrum	(c) Basic eye and ear structure (b) Formation of peripheral receptors
5	185 mm, 0.46 kg	(b) Keratin production, nail production			(b) Myelination of spinal cord	
6	230 mm, 0.64 kg			(c) Perineal muscles	(b) Formation of CNS tract (c) Layering of cortex	

(continued)

SUMMARY TABLE   An Overview of Prenatal Development *(continued)*

Background Material

ATLAS: Embryology Summaries 1–4:
The Development of Tissues
The Development of Epithelia
The Development of
Connective Tissues
The Development of
Organ Systems

Gestational Age (Months)	Size and Weight	Integumentary System	Skeletal System	Muscular System	Nervous System	Special Sense Organs
7	270 mm, 1.492 kg	(b) Keratinization, formation of nails, hair				(c) Eyelids open, retinae sensitive to light
8	310 mm, 2.274 kg		(b) Formation of epiphyseal cartilages			(c) Taste receptors functional
9	346 mm, 3.2 kg					
Early postnatal development		Hair changes in consistency and distribution	Formation and growth of epiphyseal cartilages continue	Muscle mass and control increase	Myelination, layering, CNS tract formation continue	

Note: (b) = beginning; (c) = completion.

SUMMARY TABLE   **An Overview of Prenatal Development** *(continued)*

Gestational Age (Months)	Endocrine System	Cardiovascular and Lymphatic Systems	Respiratory System	Digestive System	Urinary System	Reproductive System
1		(b) Heartbeat	(b) Formation of trachea and lungs	(b) Formation of intestinal tract, liver, pancreas (c) Yolk sac	(c) Allantois	
2	(b) Formation of thymus, thyroid, pituitary, adrenal glands	(c) Basic heart structure, major blood vessels, lymph nodes and ducts (b) Blood formation in liver	(b) Extensive bronchial branching into mediastinum (c) Diaphragm	(b) Formation of intestinal subdivisions, into villi, salivary glands	(b) Formation of kidneys (metanephros)	(b) Formation of mammary glands
3	(c) Thymus, thyroid gland	(b) Tonsils, blood formation in bone marrow		(c) Gallbladder, pancreas		(b) Formation of gonads, ducts, genitalia; oogonia in female
4		(b) Migration of lymphocytes to lymphoid organs; blood formation in spleen			(b) Degeneration of embryonic kidneys (mesonephros)	
5		(c) Tonsils	(c) Nostrils open	(c) Intestinal subdivisions		
6	(c) Adrenal glands	(c) Spleen, liver, bone marrow	(b) Formation of alveoli	(c) Epithelial organization, glands		
7	(c) Pituitary gland			(c) Intestinal plicae	(b) Descent of testes	

(continued)

SUMMARY TABLE   An Overview of Prenatal Development *(continued)*

Gestational Age (Months)	Endocrine System	Cardiovascular and Lymphatic Systems	Respiratory System	Digestive System	Urinary System	Reproductive System
8			Complete pulmonary branching and alveolar structure		(c) Nephron formation	Descent of testes at or near time of birth
9						
Postnatal development		Cardiovascular changes at birth; immune response gradually becomes fully operational				

Note: (b) = beginning; (c) = completion.

Appendix II

Weights and Measures

Accurate descriptions of physical objects would be impossible without a precise method of reporting the pertinent data. Dimensions such as length and width are reported in standardized units of measurement, such as inches or centimeters. These values can be used to calculate the **volume** of an object, a measurement of the amount of space the object fills. Mass is another important physical property. The **mass** of an object is determined by the amount of matter the object contains; on Earth, the mass of an object determines the object's weight.

In the United States, length and width are typically described in inches, feet, or yards; volumes in pints, quarts, or gallons; and weights in ounces, pounds, or tons. These are units of the **U.S. system** of measurement. Table 1 summarizes the terms used in the U.S. system. The U.S. system

TABLE 1	The U.S. System of Measurement	
Physical Property	Unit	Relationship to Other U.S. Units
Length	inch (in.)	1 in. = 0.083 ft
	foot (ft)	1 ft = 12 in.
		= 0.33 yd
	yard (yd)	1 yd = 36 in.
		= 3 ft
	mile (mi)	1 mi = 5280 ft
		= 1760 yd
Volume	fluidram (fl dr)	1 fl dr = 0.125 fl oz
	fluid ounce (fl oz)	1 fl oz = 8 fl dr
		= 0.0625 pt
	pint (pt)	1 pt = 128 fl dr
		= 16 fl oz
		= 0.5 qt
	quart (qt)	1 qt = 256 fl dr
		= 32 fl oz
		= 2 pt
		= 0.25 gal
	gallon (gal)	1 gal = 128 fl oz
		= 8 pt
		= 4 *qt*
Mass	grain (gr)	1 gr = 0.002 oz
	dram (dr)	1 dr = 27.3 gr
		= 0.063 oz
	ounce (oz)	1 oz = 437.5 gr
		= 16 dr
	pound (lb)	1 lb = 7000 gr
		= 256 dr
		= 16 oz
	ton (t)	1 t = 2000 lb

can be very difficult to work with, because there is no logical relationship among the various units. For example, there are 12 inches in a foot, 3 feet in a yard, and 1760 yards in a mile. Without a clear pattern of organization, the conversion of feet to inches or miles to feet can be confusing and time-consuming. The relationships among ounces, pints, quarts, and gallons are no more logical than those among ounces, pounds, and tons.

In contrast, the **metric system** has a logical organization based on powers of 10, as indicated in Table 2. For example, a **meter (m)** is the basic unit for the measurement of size. For measurements of larger objects, data can be reported in **dekameters** (*deka,* ten), **hectometers** (*hekaton,* hundred), or **kilometers** (**km**; *chilioi,* thousand); for smaller objects, data can be reported in **decimeters** (0.1 m; *decem,* ten), **centimeters** (**cm** = 0.01 m; *centum,* hundred), **millimeters** (**mm** = 0.001 m; *mille,* thousand), and so forth. In the metric system, the same prefixes are used to report weights, based on the **gram (g),** and

volumes, based on the **liter (L).** This text reports data in metric units, in most cases with U.S. system equivalents. Use this opportunity to become familiar with the metric system, because most technical sources report data only in metric units; most of the world outside the United States uses the metric system exclusively. Conversion factors are included in Table 2.

The U.S. and metric systems also differ in their methods of reporting temperatures. In the United States, temperatures are usually reported in degrees Fahrenheit (°F), whereas scientific literature and individuals in most other countries report temperatures in degrees centigrade or Celsius (°C). The relationship between temperatures in degrees Fahrenheit and those in degrees centigrade is indicated in Table 2.

The following illustration spans the entire range of measurements that we will consider in this book. Gross anatomy traditionally deals with structural organization as seen with the naked eye or with a simple hand lens. A microscope can

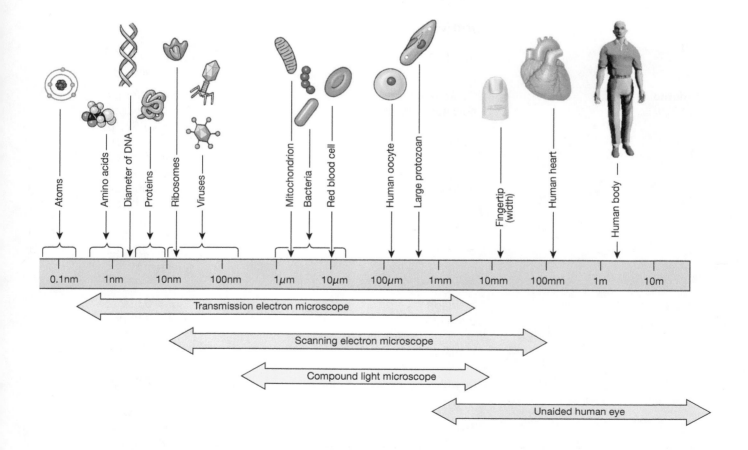

TABLE 2	The U.S. System of Measurement		
Physical Property	Unit	Relationship to Standard Metric Units	Conversion to U.S. Units	
Length	nanometer (nm)	1 nm = 0.000000001 m (10^{-9})	= 3.94×10^{-8} in.	25,400,000 nm = 1 in.
	micrometer (μm)	1 μm = 0.000001 m (10^{-6})	= 3.94×10^{-5} in.	25,400 μm = 1 in.
	millimeter (mm)	1 mm = 0.001 m (10^{-3})	= 0.0394 in.	25.4 mm = 1 in.
	centimeter (cm)	1 cm = 0.01 m (10^{-2})	= 0.394 in.	2.54 cm = 1 in.
	decimeter (cm)	1 dm = 0.1 m (10^{-1})	= 3.94 in.	0.254 dm = 1 in.
	meter (m)	standard unit of length	= 39.4 in.	0.0254 m = 1 in.
			= 3.28 ft	0.3048 m = 1 ft
			= 1.093 yd	0.914 m = 1 yd
	kilometer (km)	1 km = 1000 m	= 3280 ft	
			= 1093 yd	
			= 0.62 mi	1.609 km = 1 mi
Volume	microliter (μl)	1μl = 0.000001 L (10^{-6}) = 1 cubic millimeter (mm^3)		
	milliliter (ml)	1 ml = 0.001 (10^{-3}) = 1 cubic centimeter (cm^3 or cc)	= 0.0338 fl oz	5 ml = 1 tsp
				15 ml = 1 tbsp
				30 ml = 1 fl oz
	centiliter (cl)	1 cl = 0.01 L (10^{-2})	= 0.338 fl oz	2.95 cl = 1 fl oz
	deciliter (dl)	1 dl = 0.1 L (10^{-1})	= 3.38 fl oz	0.295 dl = 1 fl oz
	liter (L)	standard unit of volume	= 33.8 fl oz	0.0295 L = 1 fl oz
			2.11 pt	0.473 L = 1 pt
			1.06 qt	0.946 L = 1 qt
Mass	picogram (pg)	1 pg = 0.000000000001 g (10^{-12})		
	nanogram (ng)	1 ng = 0.000000001 g (10^{-9})	= 0.000000015 gr	66,666,666 mg = 1 gr
	microgram (μg)	1 μg = 0.000001 g (10^{-6})	= 0.000015 gr	66,666 mg = 1 gr
	milligram (mg)	1 mg = 0.001 g (10^{-3})	= 0.015 gr	66.7 mg = 1 gr
	centigram (cg)	1 cg = 0.01 g (10^{-2})	= 0.15 *gr*	6.67 cg = 1 gr
	decigram (dg)	1 dg = 0.1 g (10^{-1})	= 1.5 gr	0.667 cg = 1 gr
	gram (g)	standard unit of mass	= 0.035 oz	= 28.4 g = 1 oz
			= 0.0022 lb	= 454 g = 1 lb
	dekagram (dag)	1 dag = 10 g		
	hectogram (hg)	1 hg = 100g		
	kilogram (kg)	1 kg = 1000 g	= 2.21 lb	0.454 kg = 1 lb
	metric ton (kt)	1 mt = 1000 kg		
			= 2205 lb	0.907 kt = 1 t

Temperature	**Centigrade**	**Fahrenheit**
Freezing point of pure water	0°	32°
Normal body temperature	36.8°	98.6°
Boiling point of pure water	100°	212°
Conversion	°C → °F: °F = (1.8 × °C) + 32	°F → °C: °C = (°F − 32) × 0.56

provide higher levels of magnification and can reveal finer details. Before the 1950s, most information was provided by *light microscopy.* A photograph taken through a *light microscope* is called a **light micrograph (LM).** Light microscopy can magnify cellular structures up to about 1000 times and can show details as fine as 0.25 μm. The symbol μm stands for **micrometer;** 1μm = 0.001 mm, or 0.00004 inches. With a light microscope, we can identify cell types, such as muscle fibers or neurons, and can see large structures within a cell. Because individual cells are relatively transparent, thin sections cut through a cell are treated with dyes that stain specific structures to make them easier to see.

Although special staining techniques can show the general distribution of proteins, lipids, carbohydrates, and nucleic acids in the cell, many fine details of intracellular structure remained a mystery until investigators began using *electron microscopy.* This technique uses a focused beam of electrons, rather than a beam of light, to examine cell structure. In *transmission electron microscopy,* electrons pass through an ultrathin section to strike a photographic plate. The result is a **transmission electron micrograph (TEM).** Transmission electron microscopy shows the fine structure of cell membranes and intracellular structures. In *scanning electron microscopy,* electrons bouncing off exposed surfaces create a **scanning   electron   micrograph   (SEM).** Although it cannot achieve as much magnification as transmission microscopy, scanning microscopy provides a three-dimensional perspective of cell structure.

Appendix III

Periodic Table

The **periodic table** presents the known elements in order of their atomic weights. Each horizontal row represents a single electron shell. The number of elements in that row is determined by the maximum number of electrons that can be stored at that energy level. The element at the left end of each row contains a single electron in its outermost electron shell; the element at the right end of the row has a filled outer electron shell. Organizing the elements in this fashion highlights similarities that reflect the composition of the outer electron shell. These similarities are evident when you examine the vertical columns. All the gases of the right-most column—helium, neon, argon, krypton, xenon, and radon—have full electron shells; each is a gas at normal atmospheric temperature and pressure, and none reacts readily with other elements. These elements, highlighted in blue, are known as the *noble,* or *inert, gases.* In contrast, the elements of the leftmost column below hydrogen—lithium, sodium, potassium, rubidium, cesium, and francium—are silvery, soft metals that are so highly reactive that pure forms cannot be found in nature. The fourth and fifth electron levels can hold up to 18 electrons. Table inserts are used for the so-called *lanthanide* and *actinide series* to save space, as higher levels can store up to 32 electrons. Elements of particular importance to our discussion of human anatomy and physiology are highlighted in pink.

Periodic Table of the Elements

Legend:
Atomic number — 1 H — Chemical symbol
Hydrogen — Element name
Atomic weight — 1.01

Group 1	2	3	4	5	6	7	8	9	10	11	12	13	14	15	16	17	18
1 H Hydrogen 1.01																	2 He Helium 4.00
3 Li Lithium 6.94	4 Be Beryllium 9.01											5 B Boron 10.81	6 C Carbon 12.01	7 N Nitrogen 14.01	8 O Oxygen 16.00	9 F Fluorine 19.00	10 Ne Neon 20.18
11 Na Sodium 22.99	12 Mg Magnesium 24.31											13 Al Aluminum 26.98	14 Si Silicon 28.09	15 P Phosphorus 30.97	16 S Sulfur 32.07	17 Cl Chlorine 35.45	18 Ar Argon 39.95
19 K Potassium 39.10	20 Ca Calcium 40.08	21 Sc Scandium 44.96	22 Ti Titanium 47.88	23 V Vanadium 50.94	24 Cr Chromium 52.00	25 Mn Manganese 54.94	26 Fe Iron 55.85	27 Co Cobalt 58.93	28 Ni Nickel 58.69	29 Cu Copper 63.55	30 Zn Zinc 65.39	31 Ga Gallium 69.72	32 Ge Germanium 72.61	33 As Arsenic 74.92	34 Se Selenium 78.96	35 Br Bromine 79.90	36 Kr Krypton 83.80
37 Rb Rubidium 85.47	38 Sr Strontium 87.62	39 Y Yttrium 88.91	40 Zr Zirconium 91.22	41 Nb Niobium 92.91	42 Mo Molybdenum 95.94	43 Tc Technetium (98)	44 Ru Ruthenium 101.07	45 Rh Rhodium 102.91	46 Pd Palladium 106.42	47 Ag Silver 107.87	48 Cd Cadmium 112.41	49 In Indium 114.82	50 Sn Tin 118.71	51 Sb Antimony 121.76	52 Te Tellurium 127.60	53 I Iodine 126.90	54 Xe Xenon 131.29
55 Cs Cesium 132.91	56 Ba Barium 137.33	57 La Lanthanum 138.91 *	72 Hf Hafnium 178.49	73 Ta Tantalum 180.95	74 W Tungsten 183.85	75 Re Rhenium 186.21	76 Os Osmium 190.2	77 Ir Iridium 192.22	78 Pt Platinum 195.08	79 Au Gold 196.97	80 Hg Mercury 200.59	81 Tl Thallium 204.38	82 Pb Lead 207.2	83 Bi Bismuth 208.98	84 Po Polonium (209)	85 At Astatine (210)	86 Rn Radon (222)
87 Fr Francium (223)	88 Ra Radium 226.03	89 Ac Actinium 227.03 †	104 Rf Rutherfordium (266)	105 Db Dubnium (262)	106 Sg Seaborgium (266)	107 Bh Bohrium (264)	108 Hs Hassium (269)	109 Mt Meitnerium (268)	110 Unnamed (271)	111 Unnamed (272)	112 Unnamed (277)		114 (285)		116 (289)		118 (293)

*Lanthanide series

58 Ce Cerium 140.12	59 Pr Praseodymium 140.91	60 Nd Neodymium 144.24	61 Pm Promethium (145)	62 Sm Samarium 150.36	63 Eu Europium 151.96	64 Gd Gadolinium 157.25	65 Tb Terbium 158.93	66 Dy Dysprosium 162.50	67 Ho Holmium 164.93	68 Er Erbium 167.26	69 Tm Thulium 168.93	70 Yb Ytterbium 173.04	71 Lu Lutetium 174.97

†Actinide series

90 Th Thorium 232.04	91 Pa Protactinium 231.04	92 U Uranium 238.03	93 Np Neptunium 237.05	94 Pu Plutonium (244)	95 Am Americium (243)	96 Cm Curium (247)	97 Bk Berkelium (247)	98 Cf Californium (251)	99 Es Einsteinium (252)	100 Fm Fermium (257)	101 Md Mendelevium (258)	102 No Nobelium (259)	103 Lr Lawrencium (262)

Appendix IV

Normal Physiological Values

This table presents normal averages or ranges for the chemical composition of body fluids. These values are approximations rather than absolute values, because test results vary from laboratory to laboratory owing to differences in procedures, equipment, normal solutions, and so forth. Blanks in the tabular data appear where data are not available; sources used in the preparation of these tables follow.

Sources

Braunwauld, Eugene, Kurt J. Isselbacher, Dennis L. Kasper, Jean D. Wilson, Joseph B. Martin, and Anthony S. Fauci, eds. 1998. *Harrison's Principles of Internal Medicine,* 14th ed. New York: McGraw-Hill.

Lentner, Cornelius, ed. 1981. *Geigy Scientific Tables,* 8th ed. Basel, Switzerland: Ciba–Geigy Limited.

Halsted, James A. 1976. *The Laboratory in Clinical Medicine: Interpretation and Application.* Philadelphia: W.B. Saunders Company.

Wintrobe, Maxwell, G. Richard Lee, Dane R. Boggs, Thomas C. Bitnell, John Foerster, John W. Athens, and John N. Lukens. 1981. *Clinical Hematology,* Philadelphia: Lea and Febiger.

TABLE The Composition of Minor Body Fluids

Test	Perilymph	Endolymph	Synovial Fluid	Sweat	Saliva	Semen
pH			7.4	4–6.8	6.4*	7.19
Specific gravity			1.008–1.015	1.001–1.008	1.007	1.028
Electrolytes (mEq/L)						
Potassium	5.5–6.3	140–160	4.0	4.3–14.2	21	31.3
Sodium	143–150	12–16	136.1	0–104	14*	117
Calcium	1.3–1.6	0.05	2.3–4.7	0.2–6	3	12.4
Magnesium	1.7	0.02		0.03–4	0.6	11.5
Bicarbonate	17.8–18.6	20.4–21.4	19.3–30.6		6*	24
Chloride	121.5	107.1	107.1	34.3	17	42.8
Proteins (total) (mg /dl)	200	150	1.72 g/dl	7.7	386[†]	4.5 g/dl
Metabolites (mg/dl)						
Amino acids				47.6	40	1.26 g/dl
Glucose	104		70–110	3.0	11	224 (fructose)
Urea				26–122	20	72
Lipids (total)	12		20.9	‡	25–500[§]	188

* Increases under salivary stimulation.
† Primarily alpha-amylase, with some lysozomes.
‡ Not present in eccrine secretions.
§ Cholesterol.

Appendix V

Some Abbreviations Used in this Text

ACh	acetylcholine
AChE	acetylcholinesterase
ACTH	adrenocorticotropic hormone
ADH	antidiuretic hormone
ADP	adenosine diphosphate
AIDS	acquired immune deficiency syndrome
ALS	amyotrophic lateral sclerosis
AMP	adenosine monophosphate
ANP	atrial natriuretic peptide
ANS	autonomic nervous system
AP	arterial pressure
ARDS	adult respiratory distress syndrome
atm	atmospheric pressure
ATP	adenosine triphosphate
ATPase	adenosine triphosphatase
AV	atrioventricular
AVP	arginine vasopressin
BMR	basal metabolic rate
BCOP	blood colloid osmotic pressure
BPG	bisphosphoglycerate
bpm	beats per minute
BUN	blood urea nitrogen
C	kilocalorie; centigrade
CABG	coronary artery bypass graft
CAD	coronary artery disease
cAMP	cyclic-AMP
CAPD	continuous ambulatory peritoneal dialysis
CCK	cholecystokinin
CD	cluster of differentiation
CF	cystic fibrosis
CHF	congestive heart failure
CHP	capillary hydrostatic pressure
CsHP	capsular hydrostatic pressure
CNS	central nervous system
CO	cardiac output; carbon monoxide
CoA	coenzyme A
COMT	catechol-O-methyltransferase
COPD	chronic obstructive pulmonary disease
CP	creatine phosphate
CPK, CK	creatine phosphokinase
CPM	continuous passive motion
CPR	cardiopulmonary resuscitation
CRF	chronic renal failure
CRH	corticotropin-releasing hormone
CSF	cerebrospinal fluid; colony-stimulating factors
CT	computerized tomography; calcitonin
CVA	cerebrovascular accident
CVS	cardiovascular system
DAG	diacylglycerol
D.C.	Doctor of Chiropractic
DCT	distal convoluted tubule
DDST	Denver Developmental Screening Test
DIC	disseminated intravascular coagulation
DJD	degenerative joint disease
DMD	Duchenne's muscular dystrophy
DNA	deoxyribonucleic acid
D.O.	Doctor of Osteopathy
D.P.M.	Doctor of Podiatric Medicine
DSA	digital subtraction angiography
E	epinephrine
ECF	extracellular fluid
ECG	electrocardiogram
EDV	end-diastolic volume
EEG	electroencephalogram
EKG	electrocardiogram
ELISA	enzyme-linked immunosorbent assay
EPSP	excitatory postsynaptic potential
ERV	expiratory reserve volume
ESV	end-systolic volume
ETS	electron transport system
FAD	flavin adenine dinucleotide

FAS	fetal alcohol syndrome
FES	functional electrical stimulation
FMN	flavin mononucleotide
FRC	functional residual capacity
FSH	follicle-stimulating hormone
GABA	gamma aminobutyric acid
GAS	general adaptation syndrome
GC	glucocorticoid
GFR	glomerular filtration rate
GH	growth hormone
GH–IH	growth hormone–inhibiting hormone
GHP	glomerular hydrostatic pressure
GH–RH	growth hormone–releasing hormone
GIP	gastric inhibitory peptide
GnRH	gonadotropin-releasing hormone
GTP	guanosine triphosphate
Hb	hemoglobin
hCG	human chorionic gonadotropin
HCl	hydrochloric acid
HDL	high-density lipoprotein
HDN	hemolytic disease of the newborn
hGH	human growth hormone
HIV	human immunodeficiency virus
HLA	human leukocyte antigen
HMD	hyaline membrane disease
HP	hydrostatic pressure
hPL	human placental lactogen
HR	heart rate
Hz	Hertz
ICF	intracellular fluid
ICOP	interstitial fluid colloid osmotic pressure
IGF	insulin-like growth factor
IH	inhibiting hormone
IM	intramuscular
IP_3	inositol triphosphate
IPSP	inhibitory postsynaptic potential
IRV	inspiratory reserve volume
ISF	interstitial fluid
IUD	intrauterine device
IVC	inferior vena cava
IVF	in vitro fertilization
kc	kilocalorie
LDH	lactate dehydrogenase
LDL	low-density lipoprotein
L-DOPA	levodopa
LH	luteinizing hormone
LLQ	left lower quadrant
LM	light micrograph
LSD	lysergic acid diethylamide
LUQ	left upper quadrant
MAO	monoamine oxidase
MAP	mean arterial pressure
MC	mineralocorticoid
M.D.	Doctor of Medicine
mEq	milliequivalent
MHC	major histocompatibility complex
MI	myocardial infarction
mm Hg	millimeters of mercury
mmol	millimole
mOsm	milliosmole
MRI	magnetic resonance imaging
mRNA	messenger RNA
MS	multiple sclerosis
MSH	melanocyte-stimulating hormone
MSH–IH	melanocyte-stimulating hormone–inhibiting hormone
NAD	nicotinamide adenine dinucleotide
NE	norepinephrine
NFP	net filtration pressure
NHP	net hydrostatic pressure
NO	nitric oxide
NRDS	neonatal respiratory distress syndrome
OP	osmotic pressure
Osm	osmoles
OT	oxytocin
PAC	premature atrial contraction
PAT	paroxysmal atrial tachycardia

PCT	proximal convoluted tubule
PCV	packed cell volume
PEEP	positive end-expiratory pressure
PET	positron emission tomography
PFC	perfluorochemical emulsion
PG	prostaglandin
PID	pelvic inflammatory disease
PIH	prolactin-inhibiting hormone
PIP	phosphatidylinositol
PKC	protein kinase C
PKU	phenylketonuria
PLC	phospholipase C
PMN	polymorphonuclear leukocyte
PNS	peripheral nervous system
PR	peripheral resistance
PRF	prolactin-releasing factor
PRL	prolactin
psi	pounds per square inch
PT	prothrombin time
PTA	post-traumatic amnesia; plasma thromboplastin antecedent
PTC	phenylthiocarbamide
PTH	parathyroid hormone
PVC	premature ventricular contraction
RAS	reticular activating system
RBC	red blood cell
RDA	recommended daily allowance
RDS	respiratory distress syndrome
REM	rapid eye movement
RER	rough endoplasmic reticulum
RH	releasing hormone
RHD	rheumatic heart disease
RLQ	right lower quadrant
RNA	ribonucleic acid
rRNA	ribosomal RNA
RUQ	right upper quadrant
SA	sinoatrial
SCA	sickle cell anemia
SCID	severe combined immunodeficiency disease
SEM	scanning electron micrograph
SER	smooth endoplasmic reticulum
SGOT	serum glutamic oxaloacetic transaminase
SIADH	syndrome of inappropriate ADH secretion
SIDS	sudden infant death syndrome
SLE	systemic lupus erythematosus
SNS	somatic nervous system
STD	sexually transmitted disease
SV	stroke volume
SVC	superior vena cava
T_3	triiodothyronine
T_4	tetraiodothyronine, or thyroxine
TB	tuberculosis
TBG	thyroid-binding globulin
TEM	transmission electron micrograph
TIA	transient ischemic attack
T_m	transport (tubular) maximum
TMJ	temporomandibular joint
t-PA	tissue plasminogen activator
TRH	thyrotropin-releasing hormone
tRNA	transfer RNA
TSH	thyroid-stimulating hormone
TSS	toxic shock syndrome
TX	thyroxine
U.S.	United States
UTI	urinary tract infection
UTP	uridine triphosphate
UV	ultraviolet
$\dot{V}_A$	alveolar ventilation
V_D	anatomic dead space
$\dot{V}_E$	respiratory minute volume
V_T	tidal volume
VF	ventricular fibrillation
VLDL	very low-density lipoprotein
VPRC	volume of packed red cells
VT	ventricular tachycardia
WBC	white blood cell

629

Appendix VI

Glossary of Medical Word Parts Combining Forms, Prefixes, and Suffixes

A

a-	prefix	away from, without
ab-	prefix	away from
abdomin/o-	combining form	abdomen
ablat/o-	combining form	take away; destroy
-able	suffix	able to be
abort/o-	combining form	stop prematurely
abras/o-	combining form	scrape off
absorpt/o-	combining form	absorb or take in
-ac	suffix	pertaining to
access/o-	combining form	supplemental or contributing part
accommod/o-	combining form	to adapt
acetabul/o-	combining form	acetabulum (hip socket)
acid/o-	combining form	acid (low pH)
acous/o-	combining form	hearing, sound
acr/o-	combining form	extremity; highest point
acromi/o-	combining form	acromion
actin/o-	combining form	rays of the sun
act/o-	combining form	action
acu/o-	combining form	needle; sharpness
-acusis	suffix	hearing
acus/o-	combining form	the sense of hearing
ad-	prefix	toward
-ad	suffix	toward, in the direction of
addict/o-	combining form	surrender to; be controlled by
-ade	suffix	action; process
aden/o-	combining form	gland
adhes/o-	combining form	to stick to
adip/o-	combining form	fat
adjuv/o-	combining form	giving help or assistance
adnex/o-	combining form	accessory connecting parts
adolesc/o-	combining form	the beginning of being an adult
adrenal/o-	combining form	adrenal gland
adren/o-	combining form	adrenal gland
affect/o-	combining form	state of mind; mood; to have an influence on
affer/o-	combining form	bring toward the center
agglutin/o-	combining form	clumping, sticking
aggreg/o-	combining form	crowding together
ag/o-	combining form	to lead to
agon/o-	combining form	causing action
agor/a-	combining form	open area or space
-al	suffix	pertaining to
albin/o-	combining form	white
albumin/o-	combining form	albumin
alges/o-	combining form	sensation of pain
-algia	suffix	painful condition
alg/o-	combining form	pain
align/o-	combining form	arranged in a straight line
aliment/o-	combining form	food, nourishment
-alis	suffix	pertaining to
alkal/o-	combining form	base (high pH)
allerg/o-	combining form	allergy
all/o-	combining form	other; strange
alveol/o-	combining form	alveolus (air sac)
ambly/o-	combining form	dimness
ambulat/o-	combining form	walking
amnes/o-	combining form	forgetfulness
amni/o-	combining form	amnion (fetal membrane)
-amnios	suffix	amniotic fluid
amputat/o-	combining form	to cut off
amput/o-	combining form	to cut off
amygdal/o-	combining form	almond shape
amyl/o-	combining form	carbohydrate, starch
an-	prefix	without, not
-an	suffix	pertaining to
ana-	prefix	apart from; excessive
anabol/o-	combining form	building up
analy/o-	combining form	to separate
anastom/o-	combining form	unite two tubular structures
-ance	suffix	state of
ancill/o-	combining form	servant, accessory
-ancy	suffix	state of
andr/o-	combining form	male
aneurysm/o-	combining form	aneurysm (dilation)
angin/o-	combining form	angina
angi/o-	combining form	blood vessel; lymphatic vessel
anis/o-	combining form	unequal
ankyl/o-	combining form	fused together, stiff
an/o-	combining form	anus
ant-	prefix	against
-ant	suffix	pertaining to
antagon/o-	combining form	oppose or work against
ante-	prefix	forward, before
anter/o-	combining form	before; front part

anthrac/o-	combining form	coal
anti-	prefix	against
anxi/o-	combining form	fear, worry
aort/o-	combining form	aorta
apher/o-	combining form	withdrawal
aphth/o-	combining form	ulcer
apic/o-	combining form	apex (tip)
apo-	prefix	away from
appendic/o-	combining form	appendix
appendicul/o-	combining form	limb; small attached part
append/o-	combining form	small structure hanging from a larger structure; appendix
appercept/o-	combining form	fully perceived
aque/o-	combining form	watery substance
-ar	suffix	pertaining to
arachn/o-	combining form	spider, spider web
-arche	suffix	a beginning
areol/o-	combining form	small area around the nipple
-arian	suffix	pertaining to a person
-aris	suffix	pertaining to
arteri/o-	combining form	artery
arter/o-	combining form	artery
arteriol/o-	combining form	arteriole
arthr/o-	combining form	joint
articul/o-	combining form	joint
-ary	suffix	pertaining to
asbest/o-	combining form	asbestos
ascit/o-	combining form	ascites
-ase	suffix	enzyme
aspir/o-	combining form	to breathe in; to suck in
asthm/o-	combining form	asthma
astr/o-	combining form	starlike structure
-ate	suffix	composed of; pertaining to
-ated	suffix	pertaining to a condition; composed of
atel/o-	combining form	incomplete
ather/o-	combining form	soft, fatty substance
atheromat/o-	combining form	fatty deposit or mass
athet/o-	combining form	without position or place
-atic	suffix	pertaining to
-ation	suffix	a process; being or having
-ative	suffix	pertaining to
-ator	suffix	person or thing that produces or does
-atory	suffix	pertaining to
atri/o-	combining form	atrium (upper heart chamber)
attenu/o-	combining form	weakened
-ature	suffix	system composed of
audi/o-	combining form	the sense of hearing
audit/o-	combining form	the sense of hearing
augment/o-	combining form	increase in size or degree

aur/i-	combining form	ear
auricul/o-	combining form	ear
auscult/o-	combining form	listening
auto-	prefix	self
autonom/o-	combining form	independent, self-governing
axill/o-	combining form	axilla (armpit)
axi/o-	combining form	axis

B

bacteri/o-	combining form	bacterium
balan/o-	combining form	glans penis
bar/o-	combining form	weight
basil/o-	combining form	base of an organ
bas/o-	combining form	base of a structure
bas/o-	combining form	basic (alkaline)
behav/o-	combining form	activity or manner of acting
bi-	prefix	two
bil/i-	combining form	bile, gall
bilirubin/o-	combining form	bilirubin
bi/o-	combining form	life; living organisms; living tissue
-blast	suffix	immature cell
blast/o-	combining form	immature; embryonic
blephar/o-	combining form	eyelid
-body	suffix	a structure or thing
botul/o-	combining form	sausage
brachi/o-	combining form	arm
brachy-	prefix	short
brady-	prefix	slow
bronchi/o-	combining form	bronchus
bronchiol/o-	combining form	bronchiole
bronch/o-	combining form	bronchus
brux/o-	combined form	to grind the teeth
buccinat/o-	combining form	cheek
bucc/o-	combining form	cheek
bulb/o-	combining form	like a bulb
bunion/o-	combining form	bunion
burs/o-	combining form	bursa

C

cac/o-	combining form	bad, poor
calcane/o-	combining form	calcaneus (heel bone)
calcific/o-	combining form	hard from calcium
calci/o-	combining form	calcium
calc/o-	combining form	calcium
calcul/o-	combining form	stone
calic/o-	combining form	calix
cali/o-	combining form	calix
calor/o-	combining form	heat
cancell/o-	combining form	lattice structure
cancer/o-	combining form	cancer
candid/o-	combining form	Candida (a yeast)
can/o-	combining form	resembling a dog
capill/o-	combining form	hairlike structure
capn/o-	combining form	carbon dioxide
capsul/o-	combining form	capsule (enveloping structure)

carb/o-	combining form	carbon atoms
carbox/y-	combining form	carbon dioxide
carcin/o-	combining form	cancer
card/i-	combining form	heart
cardi/o-	combining form	heart
cari/o-	combining form	caries (tooth decay)
carot/o-	combining form	stupor, sleep
carp/o-	combining form	wrist
cartilagin/o-	combining form	cartilage
cata-	prefix	down
catabol/o-	combining form	breaking down
catheter/o-	combining form	catheter
caud/o-	combining form	tailbone; lower part of the body
caus/o-	combining form	burning
cavit/o-	combining form	hollow space
cav/o-	combining form	hollow space
cec/o-	combining form	cecum (first part of large intestine)
-cele	suffix	hernia
celi/o-	combining form	abdomen
cellul/o-	combining form	cell
-centesis	suffix	procedure to puncture
centr/o-	combining form	center; dominant part
cephal/o-	combining form	head
-cephalus	suffix	head
-ceps	suffix	head
-cere	suffix	waxy substance
cerebell/o-	combining form	cerebellum (posterior part of the brain)
cerebr/o-	combining form	cerebrum (largest part of the brain)
cervic/o-	combining form	neck; cervix
cheil/o-	combining form	lip
chem/o-	combining form	chemical, drug
chez/o-	combining form	to pass stool
chir/o-	combining form	hand
chlor/o-	combining form	chloride
cholangi/o-	combining form	bile duct
chol/e-	combining form	bile, gall
cholecyst/o-	combining form	gallbladder
choledoch/o-	combining form	common bile duct
cholesterol/o-	combining form	cholesterol
chol/o-	combining form	bile, gall
chondri/o-	combining form	little granule
chondr/o-	combining form	cartilage
chori/o-	combining form	chorion (fetal membrane)
chorion/o-	combining form	chorion (fetal membrane)
choroid/o-	combining form	choroid (middle layer around the eye)
chrom/o-	combining form	color
chron/o-	combining form	time
cid/o-	combining form	killing
cili/o-	combining form	hairlike structure
cin/e-	combining form	movement
circa-	prefix	about
circulat/o-	combining form	movement in an circular route
circul/o-	combining form	circle
circum-	prefix	around
cirrh/o-	combining form	yellow
cis/o-	combining form	to cut
-clast	suffix	cell that breaks down substances
claudicat/o-	combining form	limping pain
claustr/o-	combining form	enclosed space
clavicul/o-	combining form	clavicle (collar bone)
clav/o-	combining form	clavicle (collar bone)
-cle	suffix	small thing
cleid/o-	combining form	clavicle (collar bone)
clinic/o-	combining form	medicine
clon/o-	combining form	rapid contracting and relaxing
clon/o-	combining form	identical group derived from one
-clonus	suffix	condition of rapid contracting and relaxing
-cnemius	combining form	leg
coagul/o-	combining form	clotting
coarct/o-	combining form	pressed together
cocc/o-	combining form	spherical bacterium
-coccus	suffix	spherical bacterium
coccyg/o-	combining form	coccyx (tail bone)
cochle/o-	combining form	cochlea (of the inner ear)
cognit/o-	combining form	thinking
coit/o-	combining form	sexual intercourse
coll/a-	combining form	fibers that hold together
-collis	suffix	condition of the neck
col/o-	combining form	colon (part of large intestine)
colon/o-	combining form	colon (part of large intestine)
colp/o-	combining form	vagina
comat/o-	combining form	deep unconsciousness
comminut/o-	combining form	break into minute pieces
communic/o-	combining form	impart, transmit
compens/o-	combining form	counterbalance; compensate
compress/o-	combining form	press together
compromis/o-	combining form	exposed to danger
compuls/o-	combining form	drive or compel
con-	prefix	with
concept/o-	combining form	to conceive or form
concuss/o-	combining form	violent shaking or jarring
conduct/o-	combining form	carrying, conveying
conform/o-	combining form	having the same scale or angle
congenit/o-	combining form	present at birth
congest/o-	combining form	accumulation of fluid
coni/o-	combining form	dust
conjug/o-	combining form	joined together
conjunctiv/o-	combining form	conjunctiva
con/o-	combining form	cone
constip/o-	combining form	compacted stool
constrict/o-	combining form	drawn together, narrowed

construct/o-	combining form	to build
contin/o-	combining form	hold together
contra-	prefix	against
contract/o-	combining form	pull together
contus/o-	combining form	bruising
converg/o-	combining form	coming together
convuls/o-	combining form	seizure
copr/o-	combining form	feces, stool
corne/o-	combining form	cornea
cor/o-	combining form	pupil
coron/o-	combining form	encircling structure
corpor/o-	combining form	body
cortic/o-	combining form	cortex (outer region)
cosmet/o-	combining form	attractive, adorned
cost/o-	combining form	rib
crani/o-	combining form	cranium (skull)
-crasia	suffix	a mixing
-crine	suffix	a thing that secretes
crin/o-	combining form	secrete
-crit	suffix	separation of
cry/o-	combining form	cold
crypt/o-	combining form	hidden
cubit/o-	combining form	elbow
culd/o-	combining form	cul-de-sac
cusp/o-	combining form	projection, point
cutane/o-	combining form	skin
cut/i-	combining form	skin
cyan/o-	combining form	blue
cycl/o-	combining form	ciliary body of the eye; cycle
cycl/o-	combining form	cycle; circle
cyst/o-	combining form	bladder; fluid-filled sac; semisolid cyst
cyt/o-	combining form	cell
-cyte	suffix	cell

D

dacry/o-	combining form	lacrimal sac; tears
-dactyly	suffix	condition of fingers or toes
de-	prefix	reversal of; without
dec/i-	combining form	one tenth
decidu/o-	combining form	falling off
defici/o-	combining form	lacking, inadequate
degluti/o-	combining form	swallowing
delt/o-	combining form	triangle
delus/o-	combining form	false belief
dem/o-	combining form	people; population
dendr/o-	combining form	branching structure
densit/o-	combining form	density
dent/i-	combining form	tooth
dentit/o-	combining form	eruption of teeth
dent/o-	combining form	tooth
depend/o-	combining form	to hang onto
depress/o-	combining form	press down
derm/a-	combining form	skin
-derma	suffix	skin
dermat/o-	combining form	skin
derm/o-	combining form	skin

desicc/o-	combining form	to dry up
-desis	suffix	procedure to fuse together
dextr/o-	combining form	right
dextr/o-	combining form	sugar
di-	prefix	two
dia-	prefix	complete; completely through
diabet/o-	combining form	diabetes
diaphragmat/o-	combining form	diaphragm
diaphor/o-	combining form	sweating
diaphys/o-	combining form	shaft of a bone
diastol/o-	combining form	dilating
-didymis	suffix	testes (twin structures)
didym/o-	combining form	testes (twin structures)
dietet/o-	combining form	foods, diet
diet/o-	combining form	foods, diet
differentiat/o-	combining form	being distinct or specialized
different/o-	combining form	being distinct, different
digest/o-	combining form	break down food; digest
digit/o-	combining form	digit (finger or toe)
dilat/o-	combining form	dilate, widen
dipl/o-	combining form	double
dips/o-	combining form	thirst
dis-	prefix	away from
disk/o-	combining form	disk
dissect/o-	combining form	to cut apart
dissemin/o-	combining form	widely scattered throughout the body
distent/o-	combining form	distended, stretched
dist/o-	combining form	away from the center or point of origin
diverticul/o-	combining form	diverticulum
donat/o-	combining form	give as a gift
dors/o-	combining form	back; dorsum; uppermost part
-dose	suffix	measured quantity
dos/i-	combining form	dose
-drome	suffix	a running
duc/o-	combining form	bring or move
-duct	suffix	duct (tube)
duct/o-	combining form	bring or move; a duct
du/o-	combining form	two
duoden/o-	combining form	duodenum (first part of small intestine)
dur/o-	combining form	dura mater
dynam/o-	combining form	power; movement
dyn/o-	combining form	pain
dys-	prefix	painful, difficult, abnormal

E

e-	prefix	without, out
-eal	suffix	pertaining to
ec-	prefix	out, outward
ecchym/o-	combining form	blood in the tissues
ech/o-	combining form	echo (sound wave)

eclamps/o-	combining form	a seizure
-ectasis	suffix	condition of dilation
ectat/o-	combining form	dilation
ecto-	prefix	outermost, outside
ectop/o-	combining form	outside of a place
-ectomy	suffix	surgical excision
-ed	suffix	pertaining to
-edema	suffix	swelling
edentul/o-	combining form	without teeth
-ee	suffix	person who is the object of an action
efface/o-	combining form	do away with; obliterate
effer/o-	combining form	go out from the center
effus/o-	combining form	a pouring out
ejaculat/o-	combining form	to expel suddenly
electr/o-	combining form	electricity
-elasma	suffix	platelike structure
elast/o-	combining form	flexing, stretching
elimin/o-	combining form	expel, remove
-elle	suffix	little thing
em-	prefix	in
-ema	suffix	condition
emaci/o-	combining form	to make thin
embol/o-	combining form	embolus (occluding plug)
embryon/o-	combining form	embryo; immature form
-emesis	suffix	vomiting
emet/o-	combining form	to vomit
-emia	suffix	condition of the blood; substance in the blood
-emic	suffix	pertaining to blood or a substance in the blood
emiss/o-	combining form	to send out
emot/o-	combining form	moving, stirring up
emulsific/o-	combining form	droplets of fat suspended in a liquid; particles suspended in a solution
en-	prefix	in, within, inward
-ence	suffix	state of
encephal/o-	combining form	brain
-encephaly	suffix	condition of the brain
-ency	prefix	condition of being
endo-	prefix	innermost, within
-ent	suffix	pertaining to
enter/o-	combining form	intestine
-entery	suffix	condition of the intestine
enucle/o-	combining form	to remove the kernal or nucleus
enur/o-	combining form	to urinate in
-eon	suffix	one who performs
eosin/o-	combining form	eosin (acidic red dye)
ependym/o-	combining form	lining membrane
epi-	prefix	upon, above
epilept/o-	combining form	seizure
epiphys/o-	combining form	growth area on the end of a bone

episi/o-	combining form	vulva (female external genitalia)
-er	suffix	person or thing that produces or does
erect/o-	combining form	to stand up
erg/o-	combining form	activity; work
-ergy	suffix	activity; process of working
erupt/o-	combining form	breaking out
-ery	suffix	process of
erythemat/o-	combining form	redness
erythr/o-	combining form	red
-esis	suffix	condition
es/o-	combining form	inward
esophag/o-	combining form	esophagus
esthes/o-	combining form	sensation, feeling
esthet/o-	combining form	sensation, feeling
estr/a-	combining form	female
estr/o-	combining form	female
ethm/o-	combining form	sieve
-etic	suffix	pertaining to
eti/o-	combining form	cause of disease
-ety	suffix	condition, state
etym/o-	combining form	word origin
eu-	prefix	normal, good
ex-	prefix	out, away from
exacerb/o-	combining form	increase; provoke
excis/o-	combining form	to cut out
excori/o-	combining form	to take out skin
excret/o-	combining form	removing from the body
exhibit/o-	combining form	showing
exo-	prefix	away from, external, outward
explorat/o-	combining form	to search out
express/o-	combining form	communicate
extens/o-	combining form	straightening
extern/o-	combining form	outside
extra-	prefix	outside of
extrins/o-	combining form	on the outside
exud/o-	combining form	oozing fluid

F

faci/o-	combining form	face
factiti/o-	combining form	artificial, contrived
fallopi/o-	combining form	fallopian tube
fasci/o-	combining form	fascia
fec/a-	combining form	feces, stool
fec/o-	combining form	feces, stool
femor/o-	combining form	femur (thigh bone)
fer/o-	combining form	to bear
ferrit/o-	combining form	iron
ferr/o-	combining form	iron
fertil/o-	combining form	able to conceive a child
fet/o-	combining form	fetus
fibrill/o-	combining form	muscle fiber; nerve fiber
fibrin/o-	combining form	fibrin

fibr/o-	combining form	fiber
fibul/o-	combining form	fibula (lower leg bone)
filtrat/o-	combining form	filtering; straining
filtr/o-	combining form	filter
fiss/o-	combining form	splitting
fixat/o-	combining form	to make stable or still
flatul/o-	combining form	flatus
flex/o-	combining form	bending
fluor/o-	combining form	fluorescence
-flux	suffix	flow
foc/o-	combining form	point of activity
foli/o-	combining form	leaf
follicul/o-	combining form	follicle (small sac)
foramin/o-	combining form	foramen (opening into a cavity or channel)
forens/o-	combining form	court proceedings in criminal law
-form	suffix	having the form of
format/o-	combining form	structure; arrangement
fove/o-	combining form	small, depressed area
fract/o-	combining form	break up
fratern/o-	combining form	close association or relationship
-frice	suffix	thing that produces friction
front/o-	combining form	front
fruct/o-	combining form	fruit
fulgur/o-	combining form	spark of electricity
fund/o-	combining form	fundus (part farthest from the opening)
fundu/o-	combining form	fundus (part farthest from the opening)
fung/o-	combining form	fungus
fus/o-	combining form	pouring

G

galact/o-	combining form	milk
ganglion/o-	combining form	ganglion
gangren/o-	combining form	gangrene
gastr/o-	combining form	stomach
gemin/o-	combining form	twins; set or group
-gen	suffix	that which produces
-gene	suffix	gene
gene/o-	combining form	gene
gener/o-	combining form	production; creation
genit/o-	combining form	genitalia
gen/o-	combining form	arising from; produced by
germin/o-	combining form	embryonic tissue
ger/o-	combining form	old age
gest/o-	combining form	from conception to birth
gestat/o-	combining form	from conception to birth
gigant/o-	combining form	giant
gingiv/o-	combining form	gums
glandul/o-	combining form	gland
glen/o-	combining form	socket of a joint
-glia	suffix	substance that holds things together

gli/o-	combining form	substance that holds things together
glob/o-	combining form	shaped like a globe; comprehensive
globul/o-	combining form	shaped like a globe
glomerul/o-	combining form	glomerulus
gloss/o-	combining form	tongue
glott/o-	combining form	glottis (of the larynx)
gluc/o-	combining form	glucose (sugar)
glycer/o-	combining form	glycerol (sugar alcohol)
glyc/o-	combining form	glucose (sugar)
glycos/o-	combining form	glucose (sugar)
gnos/o-	combining form	knowledge
gonad/o-	combining form	gonads (ovaries and testes)
goni/o-	combining form	angle
gon/o-	combining form	seed (ovum or spermatozoon)
-grade	suffix	going
-graft	suffix	tissue for implant or transplant
-gram	suffix	a record or picture
granul/o-	combining form	granule
-graph	suffix	instrument used to record
graph/o-	combining form	record
-graphy	suffix	process of recording
-gravida	suffix	pregnancy
gustat/o-	combining form	the sense of taste
gynec/o-	combining form	female, woman

H

habilitat/o-	combining form	give ability
halit/o-	combining form	breath
hallucin/o-	combining form	imagined perception
hal/o-	combining form	breathe
hebe/o-	combining form	youth
hec/o-	combining form	habitual condition of the body
hedon/o-	combining form	pleasure
helic/o-	combining form	a coil
hemat/o-	combining form	blood
hemi-	prefix	one half
hem/o-	combining form	blood
hemoglobin/o-	combining form	hemoglobin
hemorrh/o-	combining form	a flowing of blood
hemorrhoid/o-	combining form	hemorrhoid
hepat/o-	combining form	liver
heredit/o-	combining form	genetic influence
hered/o-	combining form	genetic inheritance
herni/o-	combining form	hernia
heter/o-	combining form	other
hex/o-	combining form	habitual condition of the body
hidr/o-	combining form	sweat
hil/o-	combining form	hilum (indentation in an organ)
hirsut/o-	combining form	hairy
histi/o-	combining form	tissue
home/o-	combining form	same

hom/i-	combining form	man
horizont/o-	combining form	boundary between the earth and sky
hormon/o-	combining form	hormone
humer/o-	combining form	humerus (upper arm bone)
hyal/o-	combining form	clear glasslike substance
hydatidi/o-	combining form	fluid-filled vesicles
hydr/o-	combining form	water; fluid
hygien/o-	combining form	health
hy/o-	combining form	U-shaped structure
hyper-	prefix	above; more than normal
hypn/o-	combining form	sleep
hypo-	prefix	below; deficient
hypophys/o-	combining form	pituitary gland
hyster/o-	combining form	uterus (womb)

I

-ia	suffix	condition, state, thing
-iac	suffix	pertaining to
-ial	suffix	pertaining to
-ian	suffix	pertaining to
-ias	suffix	condition
-iasis	suffix	state of; process of
-iatic	suffix	pertaining to a state or process
iatr/o-	combining form	physician; medical treatment
-iatry	suffix	medical treatment
-ic	suffix	pertaining to
-ical	suffix	pertaining to
-ician	suffix	a skilled professional or expert
-ics	suffix	knowledge, practice
icter/o-	combining form	jaundice
ict/o-	combining form	seizure
-id	suffix	resembling; source or origin
-ide	suffix	chemically modified structure
idi/o-	combining form	unknown; individual
-ie	suffix	a thing
-il	suffix	a thing
-ile	suffix	pertaining to
ile/o-	combining form	ileum (third part of small intestine)
ili/o-	combining form	ilium (hip bone)
-ility	suffix	having the quality of
illus/o-	combining form	false perception
im-	prefix	not
-immune	suffix	immune response
immun/o-	combining form	immune response
impact/o-	combining form	wedged in
implant/o-	combining form	placed within
in-	prefix	in; within; not
-in	suffix	a substance
incarcer/o-	combining form	to imprison

incis/o-	combining form	to cut into
incud/o-	combining form	incus (anvil-shaped bone)
induct/o-	combining form	a leading in
-ine	suffix	pertaining to
infarct/o-	combining form	area of dead tissue
infect/o-	combining form	disease within
infer/o-	combining form	below
inflammat/o-	combining form	redness and warmth
infra-	prefix	below, beneath
-ing	suffix	doing
inguin/o-	combining form	groin
inhibit/o-	combining form	block; hold back
inject/o-	combining form	insert or put in
insemin/o-	combining form	plant a seed
insert/o-	combining form	to put in or introduce
inspect/o-	combining form	looking at
insulin/o-	combining form	insulin
insul/o-	combining form	island
integument/o-	combining form	skin
integu/o-	combining form	to cover
inter-	prefix	between
intern/o-	combining form	inside
interstiti/o-	combining form	spaces within tissue
intestin/o-	combining form	intestine
intra-	prefix	within
intrins/o-	combining form	on the inside
intussuscep/o-	combining form	to receive within
invas/o-	combining form	to go into
involut/o-	combining form	enlarged organ returns to normal size
iodin/o-	combining form	iodine
iod/o-	combining form	iodine
-ion	suffix	action; condition
-ior	suffix	pertaining to
-ious	suffix	pertaining to
irid/o-	combining form	iris (colored part of the eye)
ir/o-	combining form	iris (colored part of the eye)
ischi/o-	combining form	ischium (hip bone)
isch/o-	combining form	keep back; block
-ism	suffix	process; disease from a specific cause
-ist	suffix	one who specializes in
-istic	suffix	pertaining to
-istry	suffix	process related to the specialty of
-isy	suffix	condition of inflammation
-ite	suffix	thing that pertains to
-itian	suffix	a skilled professional or expert
-itic	suffix	pertaining to
-ition	suffix	a process; being or having
-itis	suffix	inflammation of
-ity	suffix	state; condition
-ium	suffix	a chemical element
-ive	suffix	pertaining to

-ix	suffix	a structure
-ization	suffix	process of making, creating, or inserting
-ize	suffix	affecting in a particular way
-izer	suffix	thing that affects in a particular way

J

jejun/o-	combining form	jejunum (middle part of small intestine)
jugul/o-	combining form	jugular (throat)

K

kal/i-	combining form	potassium
kary/o-	combining form	nucleus
kel/o-	combining form	tumor
kerat/o-	combining form	cornea
kerat/o-	combining form	hard, fibrous protein
ket/o-	combining form	ketones
keton/o-	combining form	ketones
-kinesis	suffix	condition of movement
kines/o-	combining form	movement
-kine	suffix	movement
kin/o-	combining form	movement
klept/o-	combining form	to steal
kyph/o-	combining form	bent; humpbacked

L

labi/o-	combining form	lip; labium
laborat/o-	combining form	workplace; testing place
labyrinth/o-	combining form	labyrinth (in the inner ear)
lacer/o-	combining form	a tearing
lacrim/o-	combining form	tears
lact/i-	combining form	milk
lact/o-	combining form	milk
-lalia	suffix	condition of speech
lamin/o-	combining form	lamina (flat area on the vertebra)
lapar/o-	combining form	abdomen
laryng/o-	combining form	larynx (voice box)
later/o-	combining form	side
lei/o-	combining form	smooth
lenticul/o-	combining form	lens
lent/o-	combining form	lens of the eye
-lepsy	suffix	seizure
leuk/o-	combining form	white
levo-	prefix	left
lex/o-	combining form	word
ligament/o-	combining form	ligament
ligat/o-	combining form	to tie up or bind
limb/o-	combining form	edge, border
lingu/o-	combining form	tongue
lipid/o-	combining form	lipid (fat)
lip/o-	combining form	lipid (fat)
-listhesis		see *-olisthesis*

-lith	suffix	stone
lith/o-	combining form	stone
lob/o-	combining form	lobe of an organ
locat/o-	combining form	a place
loc/o-	combining form	in one place
log/o-	combining form	word; the study of
-logy	suffix	the study of
lord/o-	combining form	swayback
luc/o-	combining form	clear and shining
lumb/o-	combining form	lower back; area between the ribs and pelvis
lumin/o-	combining form	lumen (opening)
lun/o-	combining form	moon
-ly	suffix	going toward
lymph/o-	combining form	lymph; lymphatic system
ly/o-	combining form	break down, separate, dissolve
-lysis	suffix	abnormal condition or process of breaking down or dissolving
lys/o-	combining form	break down or dissolve
-lyte	suffix	dissolved substance

M

macr/o-	combining form	large
macul/o-	combining form	small area or spot
magnet/o-	combining form	magnet
mal-	prefix	bad, inadequate
-malacia	suffix	condition of softening
malac/o-	combining form	softening
malign/o-	combining form	intentionally causing harm; cancer
malle/o-	combining form	malleus (hammer-shaped bone)
malleol/o-	combining form	malleolus
mamm/a-	combining form	breast
mamm/o-	combining form	breast
mandibul/o-	combining form	mandible (lower jaw)
-mania	suffix	condition of frenzy
man/o-	combining form	thin
manu/o-	combining form	hand
masset/o-	combined form	chewing
mastic/o-	combining form	chewing
mast/o-	combining form	breast; mastoid process
mastoid/o-	combining form	mastoid process
matur/o-	combining form	mature
maxill/o-	combining form	maxilla (upper jaw)
mediastin/o-	combining form	mediastinum
medic/o-	combining form	physician; medicine
medi/o-	combining form	middle
medull/o-	combining form	medulla (inner region)
meg/a-	combining form	large
megal/o-	combining form	large
-megaly	suffix	enlargement
melan/o-	combining form	black
melen/o-	combining form	black
meningi/o-	combining form	meninges

mening/o-	combining form	meninges
menisc/o-	combining form	meniscus (crescent-shaped cartilage)
men/o-	combining form	month
menstru/o-	combining form	monthly discharge of blood
-ment	suffix	action; state
ment/o-	combining form	mind; chin
mesenter/o-	combining form	mesentery
mesi/o-	combining form	middle
meso-	prefix	middle
meta-	prefix	after; subsequent to; transition; change
metabol/o-	combining form	change, transformation
-meter	suffix	instrument used to measure
metri/o-	combining form	uterus (womb)
metr/o-	combining form	measurement
metr/o-	combining form	uterus (womb)
-metry	suffix	process of measuring
micr/o-	combining form	small
micr/o-	combining form	one millionth
mictur/o-	combining form	making urine
mid-	prefix	middle
-mileusis	suffix	process of carving
mineral/o-	combining form	mineral; electrolyte
mi/o-	combining form	lessening
mit/o-	combining form	threadlike structure
mitr/o-	combining form	structure like a miter (tall hat with 2 points)
mitt/o-	combining form	to send
mon/o-	combining form	one, single
morbid/o-	combining form	disease
morb/o-	combining form	disease
morph/o-	combining form	shape
mort/o-	combining form	death
mot/o-	combining form	movement
-motor	suffix	thing that produces movement
muc/o-	combining form	mucus
mucos/o-	combining form	mucous membrane
mult/i-	combining form	many
muscul/o-	combining form	muscle
mutat/o-	combining form	to change
myc/o-	combining form	fungus
mydr/o-	combining form	widening
myelin/o-	combining form	myelin
myel/o-	combining form	bone marrow; spinal cord; myelin
myring/o-	combining form	tympanic membrane (eardrum)
my/o-	combining form	muscle
myos/o-	combining form	muscle
myx/o-	combining form	mucus-like substance

N

narc/o-	combining form	stupor, sleep
nas/o-	combining form	nose
-nate	suffix	born

nat/o-	combining form	birth
nause/o-	combining form	nausea
necr/o-	combining form	death
ne/o-	combining form	new
nephr/o-	combining form	kidney; nephron
nerv/o-	combining form	nerve
neur/o-	combining form	nerve
neutr/o-	combining form	not taking part
nid/o-	combining form	nest; focus
-nine	suffix	pertaining to a single chemical substance
noct/o-	combining form	night
nod/o-	combining form	node (knob of tissue)
nodul/o-	combining form	small knobby mass
non-	prefix	not
norm/o-	combining form	normal, usual
nuch/o-	combining form	neck; nape of neck
nucle/o-	combining form	nucleus (of a cell or an atom)
nucleol/o-	combining form	nucleolus
null/i-	prefix	none
nutri/o-	combining form	nourishment
nutriti/o-	combining form	nourishment

O

obes/o-	combining form	fat
obsess/o-	combining form	besieged by thoughts
obstetr/o-	combining form	pregnancy and childbirth
obstip/o-	combining form	severe constipation
obstruct/o-	combining form	blocked by a barrier
occipit/o-	combining form	occiput (back of the head)
occlus/o-	combining form	close against
ocul/o-	combining form	eye
odont/o-	combining form	tooth
odyn/o-	combining form	pain
-oid	suffix	resembling
-ol	suffix	chemical substance
olfact/o-	combining form	the sense of smell
olig/o-	combining form	scanty
-olisthesis	suffix	abnormal condition and process of slipping
-oma	suffix	tumor, mass
-omatosis	suffix	abnormal condition of multiple tumors or masses
oment/o-	combining form	omentum
om/o-	combining form	tumor, mass
omphal/o-	combining form	umbilicus, navel
-on	suffix	substance; structure
onc/o-	combining form	tumor, mass
-one	suffix	chemical substance
onych/o-	combining form	nail
o/o-	combining form	ovum (egg)
oophor/o-	combining form	ovary
operat/o-	combining form	perform a procedure; surgery
ophid/o-	combining form	snake

ophthalm/o-	combining form	eye
-opia	suffix	condition of vision
opportun/o-	combining form	well timed, taking advantage of an opportunity
oppos/o-	combining form	forceful resistance
-opsy	suffix	process of viewing
optic/o-	combining form	lenses; properties of light
opt/o-	combining form	eye; vision
-or	suffix	person or thing that produces or does
orbicul/o-	combining form	small circle
orbit/o-	combining form	orbit (eye socket)
orchi/o-	combining form	testis
orch/o-	combining form	testis
orex/o-	combining form	appetite
organ/o-	combining form	organ
or/o-	combining form	mouth
orth/o-	combining form	straight
-ory	suffix	having the function of
-ose	suffix	full of
-osing	suffix	a condition of doing
-osis	suffix	condition; abnormal condition; process
osm/o-	combining form	the sense of smell
osse/o-	combining form	bone
ossicul/o-	combining form	ossicle (little bone)
ossificat/o-	combining form	changing into bone
oste/o-	combining form	bone
ot/o-	combining form	ear
oure/o-	combining form	urine
-ous	suffix	pertaining to
ovari/o-	combining form	ovary
ov/i-	combining form	ovum (egg)
ov/o-	combining form	ovum (egg)
ovul/o-	combining form	ovum (egg)
ox/i-	combining form	oxygen
ox/o-	combining form	oxygen
ox/y-	combining form	oxygen; quick

P

palat/o-	combining form	palate
palliat/o-	combining form	reduce the severity of
palpat/o-	combining form	touching, feeling
palpit/o-	combining form	to throb
pan-	prefix	all
pancreat/o-	combining form	pancreas
papill/o-	combining form	elevated structure
par-	prefix	beside
para-	prefix	beside, apart from; two parts of a pair; abnormal
parenchym/o-	combining form	parenchyma (functional cells of an organ
-paresis	suffix	weakness
pareun/o-	combining form	sexual intercourse
pariet/o-	combining form	wall of a cavity
par/o-	combining form	birth

paroxysm/o-	combining form	sudden, sharp attack
part/o-	combining form	childbirth
-partum	suffix	childbirth
parurit/o-	combining form	to be in labor
patell/o-	combining form	patella (kneecap)
pat/o-	combining form	to lie open
-path	suffix	disease, suffering
pathet/o-	combining form	suffering
path/o-	combining form	disease, suffering
-pathy	suffix	disease, suffering
-pause	suffix	cessation
paus/o-	combining form	cessation
pect/o-	combining form	stiff
pector/o-	combining form	chest
pedicul/o-	combining form	lice
ped/o-	combining form	child
pelv/i-	combining form	pelvis (hip bone; renal pelvis)
pelv/o-	combining form	pelvis (hip bone; renal pelvis)
pendul/o-	combining form	hanging down
-penia	suffix	condition of deficiency
pen/o-	combining form	penis
pepsin/o-	combining form	pepsin
peps/o-	combining form	digestion
peptid/o-	combining form	peptide (two amino acids)
pept/o-	combining form	digestion
per-	prefix	through, throughout
percuss/o-	combining form	tapping
perfor/o-	combining form	to have an opening
peri-	prefix	around
perine/o-	combining form	perineum
peripher/o-	combining form	outer aspects
peritone/o-	combining form	peritoneum
periton/o-	combining form	peritoneum
perone/o-	combining form	fibula (lower leg bone)
person/o-	combining form	person
petechi/o-	combining form	petechiae
-pexy	suffix	process of surgically fixing in place
phac/o-	combining form	lens of the eye
-phage	suffix	thing that eats
phag/o-	combining form	eating, swallowing
phak/o-	combining form	lens of the eye
phalang/o-	combining form	phalanx (finger or toe)
pharmaceutic/o-	combining form	medicine, drug
pharmac/o-	combining form	medicine, drug
pharyng/o-	combining form	pharynx (throat)
-pharynx	suffix	pharynx (throat)
phas/o-	combining form	speech
phe/o-	combining form	gray
-phil	suffix	attraction to, fondness for
-phile	suffix	person who is attracted to or fond of
phil/o-	combining form	attraction to, fondness for
phleb/o-	combining form	vein
phob/o-	combining form	fear or avoidance

phor/o-	combining form	to bear, to carry
phor/o-	combining form	range
phosph/o-	combining form	phosphorus
phot/o-	combining form	light
phren/o-	combining form	diaphragm; mind
phylact/o-	combining form	guarding or protecting
-phylaxis	suffix	condition of guarding or protecting
-phyma	combining form	tumor, growth
physic/o-	combining form	body
physi/o-	combining form	physical function
-physis	suffix	state of growing
phys/o-	combining form	inflate or distend; grow
-phyte	suffix	growth
pigment/o-	combining form	pigment
pil/o-	combining form	hair
pituitar/o-	combining form	pituitary gland
pituit/o-	combining form	pituitary gland
placent/o-	combining form	placenta
plak/o-	combining form	plaque
-plasm	suffix	growth; formed substance
plasm/o-	combining form	plasma; formed substance
-plant	suffix	procedure to transfer or graft
plas/o-	combining form	growth, formation
plast/o-	combining form	growth, formation
-plasty	suffix	process of reshaping by surgery
-plegia	suffix	condition of paralysis
pleg/o-	combining form	paralysis
pleur/o-	combining form	pleura (lung membrane)
-plex	suffix	parts
-pnea	suffix	breathing
pne/o-	combining form	breathing
pneum/o-	combining form	lung; air
pneumon/o-	combining form	lung; air
pod/o-	combining form	foot
-poiesis	suffix	condition of formation
-poietin	suffix	a substance that forms
poikil/o-	combining form	irregular
pol/o-	combining form	pole
polar/o-	combining form	two opposite poles
poly-	prefix	many, much
polyp/o-	combining form	polyp
poplite/o-	combining form	back of the knee
por/o-	combining form	small openings; pores
port/o-	combining form	point of entry
post-	prefix	after, behind
poster/o-	combining form	back part
potent/o-	combining form	being capable of doing
pract/o-	combining form	medical practice
pre-	prefix	before; in front of
pregn/o-	combining form	being with child
presby/o-	combining form	old age
press/o-	combining form	pressure
prevent/o-	combining form	prevent
preventat/o-	combining form	prevent

prim/i-	combining form	first
pro-	prefix	before
-probe	suffix	rodlike instrument
proct/o-	combining form	rectum and anus
product/o-	combining form	produce
project/o-	combining form	throw forward
pronat/o-	combining form	lying face down
prostat/o-	combining form	prostate gland
prosthet/o-	combining form	artificial part
protein/o-	combining form	protein
prote/o-	combining form	protein
proxim/o-	combining form	near the center or point of origin
prurit/o-	combining form	itching
psor/o-	combining form	itching
psych/o-	combining form	mind
-ptosis	suffix	state of prolapse or drooping; falling
-ptysis	suffix	abnormal condition of coughing up
puber/o-	combining form	growing up
pub/o-	combining form	pubis (hip bone)
pulmon/o-	combining form	lung
pulsat/o-	combining form	rhythmic throbbing
punct/o-	combining form	hole, perforation
pupill/o-	combining form	pupil of the eye
purul/o-	combining form	pus
pyel/o-	combining form	renal pelvis
pylor/o-	combining form	pylorus
py/o-	combining form	pus
pyret/o-	combining form	fever
pyr/o-	combining form	fire; burning

Q

quadri-	prefix	four
quantitat/o-	combining form	quantity or amount

R

radic/o-	combining form	all parts including the root
radicul/o-	combining form	spinal nerve root
radi/o-	combining form	radius (forearm bone); x-rays; radiation
rap/o-	combining form	to seize and drag away
re-	prefix	again and again; backward; unable to
react/o-	combining form	reverse movement
recept/o-	combining form	receive
recess/o-	combining form	to move back
rect/o-	combining form	rectum
recuper/o-	combining form	recover
reduct/o-	combining form	to bring back; decrease
refract/o-	combining form	bend or deflect
regurgitat/o-	combining form	flow backward
relax/o-	combining form	relax
remiss/o-	combining form	send back
ren/o-	combining form	kidney
repress/o-	combining form	press back
resect/o-	combining form	to cut out and remove

resist/o-	combining form	withstand the effect of
resuscit/o-	combining form	revive or raise up again
retard/o-	combining form	to slow down or delay
retent/o-	combining form	keep, hold back
reticul/o-	combining form	small network
retin/o-	combining form	retina (of the eye)
retro-	prefix	behind, backward
rex/o-		see *orex/o-*
rhabd/o-	combining form	rod shaped
rheumat/o-	combining form	watery discharge
rhin/o-	combining form	nose
rhiz/o-	combining form	spinal nerve root
rhytid/o-	combining form	wrinkle
rib/o-	combining form	ribonucleic acid
roentgen/o-	combining form	x-ray; radiation
rotat/o-	combining form	rotate
-rrhage	suffix	excessive flow or discharge
rrhag/o-	combining form	excessive flow or discharge
-rrhaphy	suffix	procedure of suturing
-rrhea	suffix	flow, discharge
rrhe/o-	combining form	flow, discharge
rrhythm/o-	combining form	rhythm
-rubin	suffix	red substance
rub/o-	combining form	red
rug/o-	combining form	ruga (fold)

S

sacchar/o-	combining form	sugar
sacr/o-	combining form	sacrum
sagitt/o-	combining form	going from front to back
saliv/o-	combining form	saliva
salping/o-	combining form	fallopian tube
-salpinx	suffix	fallopian tube
saphen/o-	combining form	standing
sarc/o-	combining form	connective tissue
satur/o-	combining form	filled up
scal/o-	combining form	series of graduated steps
scaph/o-	combining form	boat shaped
scapul/o-	combining form	scapula (shoulder blade)
schiz/o-	combining form	split
scient/o-	combining form	science; knowledge
scint/i-	combining form	point of light
scintill/o-	combining form	point of light
scler/o-	combining form	hard; sclera (white of the eye)
scoli/o-	combining form	curved, crooked
-scope	suffix	instrument used to examine
scop/o-	combining form	examine with an instrument
-scopy	suffix	process of using an instrument to examine
scot/o-	combining form	darkness

script/o-	combining form	write
scrot/o-	combining form	a bag; scrotum
sebace/o-	combining form	sebum (oil)
seb/o-	combining form	sebum (oil)
secret/o-	combining form	produce; secrete
sect/o-	combining form	to cut
sedat/o-	combining form	to calm agitation
semi-	prefix	half; partly
semin/i-	combining form	spermatozoon; sperm
semin/o-	combining form	spermatozoon; semen
sen/o-	combining form	old age
sensitiv/o-	combining form	affected by, sensitive to
sensit/o-	combining form	affected by , sensitive to
sens/o-	combining form	sensation
sensor/i-	combining form	sensory
septic/o-	combining form	infection
sept/o-	combining form	septum (dividing wall)
ser/o-	combining form	serum of the blood; serumlike fluid
sex/o-	combining form	sex
sial/o-	combining form	saliva; salivary gland
sigmoid/o-	combining form	sigmoid colon
sin/o-	combining form	hollow cavity; channel
sinus/o-	combining form	sinus
-sis	combining form	condition; abnormal condition
skelet/o-	combining form	skeleton
soci/o-	combining form	human beings; community
somat/o-	combining form	body
-some	suffix	a body
somn/o-	combining form	sleep
som/o-	combining form	a body
son/o-	combining form	sound
sorb/o-	combining form	to suck up
-spasm	suffix	sudden, involuntary muscle contraction
spasm/o-	combining form	spasm
spasmod/o-	combining form	spasm
spast/o-	combining form	spasm
spermat/o-	combining form	spermatozoon; sperm
sperm/o-	combining form	spermatozoon; sperm
sphen/o-	combining form	wedge shape
sphenoid/o-	combining form	sphenoid bone or sinus
-sphere	suffix	sphere or ball
spher/o-	combining form	sphere or ball
sphincter/o-	combining form	sphincter
sphygm/o-	combining form	pulse
spin/o-	combining form	spine; backbone
spir/o-	combining form	breathe
spir/o-	combining form	a coil
splen/o-	combining form	spleen
spondyl/o-	combining form	vertebra
squam/o-	combining form	scalelike cell
stal/o-	combining form	contraction
-stalsis	suffix	process of contraction
staped/o-	combining form	stapes (stirrup-shaped bone)

-stasis	suffix	condition of standing still; staying in one place
stas/o-	combining form	standing still; staying in one place
stat/o-	combining form	standing still; staying in one place
steat/o-	combining form	fat
sten/o-	combining form	narrowness, constriction
stere/o-	combining form	three dimensions
stern/o-	combining form	sternum (breast bone)
-steroid	suffix	steroid
steroid/o-	combining form	steroid
-sterol	suffix	lipid-containing compound
steth/o-	combining form	chest
sthen/o-	combining form	strength
stigmat/o-	combining form	point, mark
stimul/o-	combining form	exciting, strengthening
stom/o-	combining form	surgically created opening or mouth
stomat/o-	combining form	mouth
-stomy	suffix	surgically created opening
strangul/o-	combining form	to constrict
strept/o-	combining form	curved
stress/o-	combining form	disturbing stimulus
styl/o-	combining form	stake
sub-	prefix	below; underneath; less than
sucr/o-	combining form	sugar (cane sugar)
suct/o-	combining form	to suck
sudor/i-	combining form	sweat
su/i-	combining form	self
super-	prefix	above, beyond
superfici/o-	combining form	on or near the surface
super/o-	combining form	above
supinat/o-	combining form	lying on the back
supposit/o-	combining form	placed beneath
suppress/o-	combining form	press down
suppur/o-	combining form	pus formation
supra-	prefix	above
surg/o-	combining form	operative procedure
suspens/o-	combining form	hanging
sym-	prefix	together, with
symptomat/o-	combining form	collection of symptoms
syn-	prefix	together
syncop/o-	combining form	fainting
synovi/o-	combining form	synovium (membrane)
synov/o-	combining form	synovium (membrane)
system/o-	combining form	the body as a whole
-systole	suffix	contracting
systol/o-	combining form	contracting

T

tachy-	prefix	fast
tact/o-	combining form	touch

tampon/o-	combining form	stop up
tard/o-	combining form	late, slow
tars/o-	combining form	ankle
tax/o-	combining form	coordination
techn/o-	combining form	technical skill
tele/o-	combining form	distance
tempor/o-	combining form	temple (side of the head)
tendin/o-	combining form	tendon
tendon/o-	combining form	tendon
ten/o-	combining form	tendon
tens/o-	combining form	pressure, tension
terat/o-	combining form	bizarre form
termin/o-	combining form	end; boundary
testicul/o-	combining form	testis; testicle
tetr/a-	combining form	four
thalam/o-	combining form	thalamus
thanat/o-	combining form	death
thec/o-	combining form	sheath or layers of membranes
theli/o-	combining form	cellular layer
therapeut/o-	combining form	treatment
therap/o-	combining form	treatment
-therapy	suffix	treatment
therm/o-	combining form	heat
thorac/o-	combining form	thorax (chest)
-thorax	suffix	thorax (chest)
thromb/o-	combining form	thrombus (blood clot)
thym/o-	combining form	thymus; rage
thyr/o-	combining form	shield-shaped structure (thyroid gland)
thyroid/o-	combining form	thyroid gland
tibi/o-	combining form	tibia (shin bone)
-tic	suffix	pertaining to
till/o-	combining form	to pull out
-tion	suffix	a process; being or having
toc/o-	combining form	labor and childbirth
toler/o-	combining form	to become accustomed to
-tome	suffix	instrument used to cut; an area with distinct edges
tom/o-	combining form	a cut, slice, or layer
-tomy	suffix	process of cutting or making an incision
ton/o-	combining form	pressure; tone
tonsill/o-	combining form	tonsil
-tope	suffix	place, position
topic/o-	combining form	a specific area
tort/i-	combining form	twisted position
-tous	suffix	pertaining to
toxic/o-	combining form	poison, toxin
tox/o-	combining form	poison
trabecul/o-	combining form	trabecula (mesh)
trache/o-	combining form	trachea (windpipe)
trac/o-	combining form	visible path
tract/o-	combining form	pulling
tranquil/o-	combining form	calm
trans-	prefix	across, through

transit/o-	combining form	changing over from one thing to another
transplant/o-	combining form	move something to another place
traumat/o-	combining form	injury
tremul/o-	combining form	shaking
-tresia	suffix	opening or hole
tri-	prefix	three
trich/o-	combining form	hair
trigemin/o-	combining form	threefold
triglycerid/o-	combining form	triglyceride
-tripsy	suffix	the process of crushing
-triptor	suffix	thing that crushes
trochanter/o-	combining form	trochanter
trochle/o-	combining form	structure shaped like a pulley
-tron	suffix	instrument
troph/o-	combining form	development
-trophy	suffix	process of development
trop/o-	combining form	having an affinity for; stimulating; turning
tubercul/o-	combining form	nodule; tuberculosis
tuber/o-	combining form	nodule
tuberos/o-	combining form	knoblike projection
tub/o-	combining form	tube
tubul/o-	combining form	tube, small tube
turbin/o-	combining form	scroll-like structure; turbinate
tuss/o-	combining form	cough
-ty	suffix	quality or state
tympan/o-	combining form	tympanic membrane (eardrum)
-type	suffix	particular kind of; a model of

U

-ual	suffix	pertaining to
-ula	suffix	small thing
-ular	suffix	pertaining to something small
ulcerat/o-	combining form	ulcer
-ule	suffix	small thing
uln/o-	combining form	ulna (forearm bone)
ultra-	prefix	beyond; higher
-um	suffix	a structure
umbilic/o-	combining form	umbilicus, navel
un-	prefix	not
ungu/o-	combining form	nail
uni-	prefix	single, not paired
-ure	suffix	system; result of
ureter/o-	combining form	ureter
urethr/o-	combining form	urethra
urin/o-	combining form	urine; urinary system
ur/o-	combining form	urine; urinary system
uter/o-	combining form	uterus (womb)
uve/o-	combining form	uvea of the eye

V

vaccin/o-	combining form	giving a vaccine
vagin/o-	combining form	vagina
vag/o-	combining form	vagus nerve
valv/o-	combining form	valve
valvul/o-	combining form	valve
varic/o-	combining form	varix; varicose vein
vascul/o-	combining form	blood vessel
vas/o-	combining form	blood vessel; vas deferens
veget/o-	combining form	vegetable
vegetat/o-	combining form	growth
venere/o-	combining form	sexual intercourse
ven/i-	combining form	vein
ven/o-	combining form	vein
ventil/o-	combining form	movement of air
vent/o-	combining form	a coming
ventricul/o-	combining form	ventricle (lower heart chamber; chamber in the brain)
ventr/o-	combining form	front; abdomen
verd/o-	combining form	green
-verse	suffix	to travel; to turn
vers/o-	combining form	to travel; to turn
vertebr/o-	combining form	vertebra
vert/o-	combining form	to travel; to turn
vesic/o-	combining form	bladder; fluid-filled sac
vesicul/o-	combining form	bladder; fluid-filled sac
vestibul/o-	combining form	vestibule (entrance)
vest/o-	combining form	to dress
viril/o-	combining form	masculine
vir/o-	combining form	virus
viscer/o-	combining form	viscera (internal organs)
viscos/o-	combining form	thickness
vis/o-	combining form	sight; vision
vitre/o-	combining form	vitreous humor; transparent substance
voc/o-	combining form	voice
volunt/o-	combining form	done by one's own free will
vuls/o-	combining from	to tear away
vulv/o-	combining form	vulva

X

xanth/o-	combining form	yellow
xen/o-	combining form	foreign
xer/o-	combining form	dry
xiph/o-	combining form	sword

Z

-zoon	suffix	animal; living thing
zygomat/o-	combining form	zygoma (cheek bone)

Glossary

Pronunciations in the text and this glossary use the following rules:

1. Accent marks follow stressed syllables. The primary stress is shown by ′ and the secondary stress by ″.

2. Unless otherwise noted, assume that vowels at the ends of syllables are long and vowels followed by consonants are short. Exceptions to this rule are indicated by a bar (ˉ) over the vowel, which indicates a long vowel, or a breve sign (˘) over the vowel, indicating that the vowel is short.

Abdominopelvic cavity (p. 16) the portion of the ventral body cavity that contains abdominal and pelvic subdivisions; also contains the peritoneal cavity.

Abduct (p. 139) *ab-dukt′* to move away from the midline of the body.

Abortion (p. 603) *ah-bor′shun* termination of a pregnancy before the embryo or fetus is viable outside the uterus.

Abscess (p. 430) a localized collection of pus within a damaged tissue.

Absorption (p. 498) *ab-sorp′shun* passage of a substance into or across a blood vessel or membrane.

Accommodation (p. 295) (1) adaptation in response to differences or changing needs; (2) adjustment of the eye for seeing objects at close range.

Acetabulum (p. 127) *as″ĕ-tab′u-lum* the cuplike cavity on the lateral surface of the hip bone that receives the head of the femur.

Acetylcholine (p. 216) *as″ĕ-til-ko′lēn* a chemical transmitter substance released by certain nerve endings.

Acetylcholinesterase (AChE) (p. 153) an enzyme found in the synaptic cleft, bound to the postsynaptic membrane, and in tissue fluids; breaks down and inactivates acetylcholine molecules.

Acetyl-CoA (p. 516) an acetyl group bound to coenzyme A, a participant in the anabolic and catabolic pathways for carbohydrates, lipids, and many amino acids.

Achilles tendon (p. 189) *ah-kil′ēz ten′don* the tendon that attaches the calf muscles to the calcaneus, or heel bone; also called the calcaneal tendon.

Acid (p. 220) a substance that liberates hydrogen ions when in an aqueous solution; compare with *base*.

Acidosis (p. 524) *as″ĭ-do′sis* a condition in which the blood has an excess hydrogen ion concentration and a decreased pH.

Acquired immune deficiency syndrome (AIDS) (p. 446) a disease caused by the human immunodeficiency virus (HIV); characterized by the destruction of helper T cells and a resulting severe impairment of the immune response.

Acromegaly (p. 324) a condition caused by the overproduction of growth hormone in adults, characterized by a thickening of bones and an enlargement of cartilages and other soft tissues.

Acromion (p. 122) *ah-kro′me-on* the outer projection of the spine of the scapula; the highest point of the shoulder.

Acrosome (p. 586) *ak′ro-sōm* an enzyme—containing structure covering the nucleus of the sperm.

Actin (p. 150) *ak′tin* a contractile protein of muscle.

Action potential (p. 153) an electrical event occurring when a stimulus of sufficient intensity is applied to a neuron or muscle cell, allowing sodium ions to move into the cell and reverse the polarity.

Active immunity (p. 434) immunity produced by an encounter with an antigen; provides immunologic memory.

Active transport (p. 65) net movement of a substance across a membrane against a concentration or electrical gradient; requires release and use of cellular energy.

Acute (p. 140) sudden in onset, severe in intensity, and brief in duration.

Addison's disease (p. 334) a condition resulting from the hyposecretion of glucocorticoids; characterized by lethargy, weakness, hypotension, and increased skin pigmentation.

Adduct (p. 139) *ah-dukt′* to move toward the midline of the body.

Adenine (p. 48) a purine; one of the nitrogenous bases in the nucleic acids RNA and DNA.

Adenoids (p. 424) the pharyngeal tonsil.

Adenosine triphosphate (ATP) (p. 49) a high-energy compound consisting of adenosine with three phosphate groups attached; the third is attached by a high-energy bond.

Adenylate cyclase (p. 319) an enzyme bound to the inner surfaces of cell membranes that can convert ATP to cyclic-AMP; also called *adenylyl cyclase*.

Adhesion (p. 74) the fusion of two mesenterial layers after damage or irritation of their opposing surfaces; this process restricts relative movement of the organs involved; the binding of a phagocyte to its target.

Adipocyte (p. 75) a fat cell.

Adipose tissue (p. 75) loose connective tissue dominated by adipocytes.

Adrenal cortex (p. 332) the superficial portion of the adrenal gland that produces steroid hormones.

Adrenal glands (p. 331) *ah-dre′nal glanz* hormone-producing glands located superior to the kidneys; each consists of a medulla and cortex -areas.

Adrenal medulla (p. 334) the core of the adrenal gland; a modified sympathetic ganglion that secretes catecholamines into the blood during sympathetic activation

Adrenergic (p. 271) a synaptic terminal that, when stimulated, releases norepinephrine.

Adventitia (p. 492) the superficial layer of connective tissue surrounding an internal organ; fibers are continuous with those of surrounding tissues, providing support and stabilization.

Aerobic metabolism (p. 521) the complete breakdown of organic substrates into carbon dioxide and water, via pyruvic acid; a process that yields large amounts of ATP but requires mitochondria and oxygen.

Aerobic respiration (p. 168) respiration in which oxygen is consumed and glucose is broken down entirely; water, carbon dioxide, and large amounts of ATP are the final products.

Aerobic (p. 170) *a-er-o′bik* requiring oxygen to live or grow.

Afferent arteriole (p. 542) an arteriole that carries blood to a glomerulus of the kidney.

Afferent fiber (p. 199) an axon that carries sensory information to the central nervous system.

Afferent neurons (p. 204) *nu′ronz* nerve cells that carry impulses toward the central nervous system.

Afferent (p. 199) *af′er-ent* carrying to or toward a center.

Agglutination (p. 356) *ah-gloo″tin-a′shun* clump- ing of (foreign) cells, induced by cross-linking of antigen-antibody complexes.

Agglutinins (p. 356) *ah-gloo′tĭ-ninz* antibodies in blood plasma that cause clumping of corpuscles or bacteria.

Agglutinogens (p. 356) *ag″loo-tin′o-jenz* antigens that stimulate the formation of a specific agglutinin; antigens found on red blood cells that are responsible for determining the ABO blood group classification.

AIDS (p. 446) see **acquired immune deficiency syndrome**.

Albuginea (p. 580) white.

Albumin (p. 346) *al-bu′min* a protein found in virtually all animals; the most abundant plasma protein.

Albuminuria (p. 558) *al′bu-mĭ-nu′re-ah* presence of albumin in the urine.

Aldosterone (p. 565) a mineralocorticoid produced by the zona glomerulosa of the adrenal cortex; stimulates sodium and water conservation at the kidneys; secreted in response to the presence of angiotensin II.

Alimentary (p. 482) *al′ĭ-men′tar-e* pertaining to the digestive organs.

Alkalosis (p. 346) *al′kah-lo′sis* a condition in which the blood has a lower hydrogen ion concentration than normal, and an increased pH.

Allergy (p. 445) *al'er-je* overzealous immune response to an otherwise harmless antigen; also called hypersensitivity.

Alveolus (p. 395) *al-ve'o-lus* a general term referring to a small cavity or depression; an air sac in the lungs.

Amino acid (p. 43) *ah-me'no* an organic compound containing nitrogen, carbon, hydrogen, and oxygen; the building block of protein.

Amnion (p. 602) *am'ne-on* the fetal membrane that forms a fluid-filled sac around the embryo.

Amniotic fluid (p. 606) fluid that fills the amniotic cavity; cushions and supports the embryo or fetus.

Amphiarthrosis (p. 130) an articulation that permits a small degree of independent movement; *see* **interosseious membrane** and **pubic symphysis**.

Anabolism (p. 517) *an-nab'o-lizm* the energy-requiring building phase of metabolism in which simpler substances are combined to form more complex substances.

Anaerobic (p. 170) *an-a'-er-ōb-ik* not requiring oxygen.

Analgesic (p. 220) a substance that relieves pain.

Anastomosis (p. 375) the joining of two tubes, usually referring to a connection between two peripheral vessels without an intervening capillary bed.

Anatomical position (p. 11) an anatomical reference position; the body viewed from the anterior surface with the palms facing forward.

Anatomy (p. 2) the science of the structure of living organisms.

Androgen (p. 341) a steroid sex hormone primarily produced by the interstitial cells of the testis and manufactured in small quantities by the adrenal cortex in either gender.

Anemia (p. 348) *ah-ne'me-ah* reduced oxygen-car-rying capacity of the blood caused by a decreased number of erythrocytes or decreased percentage of hemoglobin in the blood.

Angina pectoris (p. 375) *an-ji'nah pek'tor-is* severe, suffocating chest pain caused by brief lack of oxygen supply to heart muscle.

Angiotensin I (p. 409) the hormone produced by the activation of angiotensinogen by renin; angiotensin-converting enzyme converts angiotensin I into angiotensin II in lung capillaries.

Angiotensin II (p. 408) a hormone that causes an elevation in systemic blood pressure, stimulates the secretion of aldosterone, promotes thirst, and causes the release of antidiuretic hormone; angiotensin-converting enzyme in lung capillaries converts angiotensin I into angiotensin II.

Angiotensinogen (p. 548) the blood protein produced by the liver that is converted to angiotensin I by the enzyme renin.

Anion (p. 27) an ion bearing a negative charge.

Antagonists (p. 177) *an-tag'o-nists* muscles or hormones that act in opposition to an agonist or prime mover.

Anterior (p. 248) *an-ter'e-er* the front of an organism, organ, or part; the ventral surface.

Antibody-mediated immunity (p. 431) the form of immunity resulting from the presence of circulating antibodies produced by plasma cells; also called *humoral immunity*.

Antidiuretic hormone (ADH) (p. 329) a hormone synthesized in the hypothalamus and secreted at the posterior lobe of the pituitary gland; causes water retention at the kidneys and an elevation of blood pressure.

Antigen (p. 356) *an'tĭ˘-jen* any substance—including toxins, foreign proteins, or bacteria—that, when introduced to the body, is recognized as foreign and activates the immune system.

Antrum (p. 592) a chamber or pocket.

Anus (p. 493) *a'nus* the distal end of the digestive tract; the outlet of the rectum.

Aorta (p. 364) *a-or'tah* the major systemic artery; arises from the left ventricle of the heart.

Aponeurosis (p. 146) *ap'o-nu-ro'sis* fibrous or membranous sheet connecting a muscle and the part it moves.

Appendicular skeleton (p. 122) *ap'en-dik'u-lar* bones of the limbs and limb girdles that are attached to the axial skeleton.

Appendicular (p. 98) pertaining to the upper or lower limbs.

Appendix (p. 492) *ah-pen'diks* a worm-like extension of the large intestine.

Appositional growth (p. 101) the enlargement of a bone by the addition of cartilage or bony matrix at its surface.

Aqueous humor (p. 293) *a'kwe-us hu'mer* the watery fluid in the anterior chambers of the eye.

Arachnoid (p. 241) *ah-rak'noid* weblike; specifically, the weblike middle layer of the three meninges.

Arcuate (p. 539) *AR-kū-āt* curving.

Areola (p. 75) *ah-re'o-lah* the circular, pigmented area surrounding the nipple.

Areolar tissue (p. 75) loose connective tissue with an open framework.

Areolar (p. 75) containing minute spaces, as in areolar tissue.

Arrector pili (p. 94) *ah-rek'tor pi'li* tiny, smooth muscles attached to hair follicles, which cause the hair to stand upright when activated.

Arteriole (p. 385) *ar-tēr'e-ol* minute artery.

Arteriosclerosis (p. 279) *ar-tēr'e-o-skler-o'sis* any of a number of proliferative and degenerative changes in the arteries leading to their decreased elasticity.

Artery (p. 374) a vessel that carries blood away from the heart.

Arthritis (p. 140) *ar-thri'tis* inflammation of the joints.

Articular cartilage (p. 99) the cartilage pad that covers the surface of a bone inside a joint cavity.

Articulation (p. 129) joint; point where two bones meet.

Ascending tract (p. 248) a tract carrying information from the spinal cord to the brain.

Association neuron (p. 205) *see* **interneurons**.

Astigmatism (p. 298) *ah-stig'mah-tizm* a visual defect resulting from irregularity in the lens or cornea of the eye causing the image to be out of focus.

Astrocyte (p. 200) one of the four types of neuroglia in the central nervous system; responsible for maintaining the blood-brain barrier by the stimulation of endothelial cells.

Atherosclerosis (p. 413) *d'ther-o''skler-o'sis* changes in the walls of large arteries consisting of lipid deposits on the artery walls. The early stage of arteriosclerosis and increased rigidity.

Atlas (p. 118) the first cervical vertebra; articulates with the occipital bone of the skull and the second cervical vertebra (axis).

Atom (p. 2) *at'um* the smallest part of an element; indivisible by ordinary chemical means.

Atomic mass number (p. 25) the sum of the number of protons and neutrons in the nucleus of an atom.

Atomic number (p. 25) the number of protons in an atom.

Atomic symbol (p. 22) a one- or two-letter symbol indicating a particular element.

Atomic weight (p. 25) average of the mass numbers of all of the isotopes of an element.

Atria (p. 363) thin-walled chambers of the heart that receive venous blood from the pulmonary or systemic circuit atrial natruretic peptide (ANP): See **natruretic peptides.**

Atrial natriuretic peptide (ANP) (p. 409) see natriuretic peptides.

Atrial reflex (p. 385) the reflexive increase in heart rate after an increase in venous return; due to mechanical and neural factors; also called *Bainbridge reflex.*

Atrioventricular (AV) node (p. 377) specialized cardiocytes that relay the contractile stimulus to the bundle of His, the bundle branches, the Purkinje fibers, and the ventricular myocardium; located at the boundary between the atria and ventricles.

Atrium (p. 363) *a'tre-um* a chamber of the heart receiving blood from the veins; superior heart chamber.

Atrophy (p. 82) *at'ro-fe* a reduction in size or wasting away of an organ or cell resulting from disease or lack of use.

Auditory tube (p. 300) a passageway that connects the nasopharynx with the middle ear cavity; also called *Eustachian tube* or *pharyngotympanic tube.*

Auricle (p. 299) a broad, flattened process that resembles the external ear; in the ear, the expanded, projecting portion that surrounds the external auditory canal, also called *pinna*; in the heart, the externally visible flap formed by the collapse of the outer wall of a relaxed atrium .

Autonomic nervous system (p. 263) the division of the nervous system that functions involuntarily; innervates cardiac muscle, smooth muscle, and glands.

Autonomic (p. 199, 263) *au″to-nom′ik* self-directed; self-regulating; independent.

Autoregulation (p. 402) changes in activity that maintain homeostasis in direct response to changes in the local environment; does not require neural or endocrine control.

Avascular (p. 70) without blood vessels.

Axial skeleton (p. 98) *ak′se-al* the bones of the skull, vertebral column, thorax, and sternum.

Axilla (p. 11) *ak-sih′lah* armpit.

Axis (p. 118) (1) the second cervical vertebra; has a vertical projection called the dens around which the atlas rotates; (2) the imaginary line about which a joint or structure revolves.

Axon hillock (p. 201) in a multipolar neuron, the portion of the cell body adjacent to the initial segment.

Axon (p. 201) *ak′son* neuron process that carries impulses away from the nerve cell body; efferent process; the conducting portion of a nerve cell.

B cells (p. 432) lymphocytes that oversee humoral immunity; their descendants differentiate into antibody-producing plasma cells; also called B lymphocytes.

Bainbridge reflex (p. 385) *see* **atrial reflex**.

Baroreceptor reflex (p. 405) a reflexive change in cardiac activity in response to changes in blood pressure.

Baroreceptors (p. 286) the receptors responsible for baroreception.

Basal metabolic rate (p. 527) *met′ah-bol′ik* the rate at which energy is expended (heat produced) by the body per unit time under controlled (basal) conditions: 12 hours after a meal, at rest.

Basal nuclei (p. 239) *nu′kle-i* gray matter areas deep within the white matter of the cerebral hemispheres; also called basal ganglia.

Base (p. 37) a substance that accepts hydrogen ions; proton acceptor; compare with *acid*.

Basement membrane (p. 70) a thin layer of extracellular material to which epithelial cells are attached in mucosal surfaces.

Basophils (p. 352) *ba′zo-filz* white blood cells whose granules stain deep blue with basic dye; have a relatively pale nucleus and granular—appearing cytoplasm.

Benign (p. 83) *be-nīn′* not malignant.

Beta cells (p. 38) cells of the pancreatic islets that secrete insulin in response to elevated blood sugar concentrations.

Bicarbonate ions (p. 468) HCO_3^-; anion components of the carbonic acid—bicarbonate buffer system.

Biceps (p. 188) *bi′seps* two-headed, especially applied to certain muscles.

Bicuspid (p. 366) *bi-kus′pid* having two points or cusps.

Bile salts (p. 41) steroid derivatives in bile; responsible for the emulsification of ingested lipids.

Bile (p. 496) a greenish-yellow or brownish fluid produced in and secreted by the liver, stored in the gallbladder, and released into the small intestine.

Bilirubin (p. 571) a pigment that is the by-product of hemoglobin catabolism.

Blastocyst (p. 600) *blas′to-sist* a stage of early embryonic development.

Blood pressure (p. 400) a force exerted against vessel walls by the blood in the vessels, due to the push exerted by cardiac contraction and the elasticity of the vessel walls; usually measured along one of the muscular arteries, with systolic pressure measured during ventricular systole and diastolic pressure during ventricular diastole.

Blood-brain barrier (p. 246) a mechanism that inhibits passage of materials from the blood into brain tissues.

Bohr effect (p. 472) the increased oxygen release by hemoglobin in the presence of elevated carbon dioxide levels.

Bolus (p. 492) *bo′lus* a rounded mass of food prepared by the mouth for swallowing.

Bony thorax (p. 120) *bōn′e tho′raks* bones of the thorax, including ribs, sternum, and thoracic vertebrae.

Brachial (p. 11) *bra′ke-al* pertaining to the arm.

Bradycardia (p. 379) an abnormally slow heart rate, usually below 50 bpm.

Brain stem (p. 233) the portion of the brain consisting of the medulla, pons, and midbrain.

Brevis (p. 188) short.

Broca's area (p. 238) the speech center of the brain, normally located on the neural cortex of the left cerebral hemisphere.

Bronchodilation (p. 477) the dilation of the bronchial passages; can be caused by sympathetic stimulation.

Buccal (p. 11) *buk′al* pertaining to the cheek.

Buffer (p. 37) a substance or substances that help to stabilize the pH of a solution.

Bulbourethral glands (p. 583) mucous glands at the base of the penis that secrete into the penile urethra; the equivalent of the greater vestibular glands of females; also called *Cowper's glands.*

Bundle branches (p. 377) specialized conducting cells in the ventricles that carry the contractile stimulus from the bundle of His to the Purkinje fibers.

Bundle of His (p. 377) specialized conducting cells in the interventricular septum that carry the contracting stimulus from the AV node to bundle branches and then to Purkinje fibers.

Bursa (p. 134) *ber′sah* a small sac filled with fluid and located at friction points, especially joints.

Calcaneal tendon (p. 189) the large tendon that inserts on the calcaneus; tension on this tendon produces extension (plantar flexion) of the foot; also called *Achilles tendon.*

Calcification (p. 105) the deposition of calcium salts within a tissue.

Calcitonin (p. 109) the hormone secreted by C cells of the thyroid when calcium ion concentrations are abnormally high; restores homeostasis by increasing the rate of bone deposition and the rate of calcium loss at the kidneys.

Calorie (p. 514) *kal′o-re* unit of heat; the large calorie (spelled with a capital letter C) is the amount of heat required to raise 1 kg of water 1°C; also used in metabolic and nutrition studies as the unit to measure the energy value of foods.

Canaliculi (p. 101) microscopic passageways between cells; bile canaliculi carry bile to bile ducts in the liver; in bone, canaliculi permit the diffusion of nutrients and wastes to and from osteocytes.

Cancer (p. 83) a malignant, invasive cellular neoplasm that has the capability of spreading throughout the body or body parts.

Capitulum (p. 122) a general term for a small, elevated articular process; refers to the rounded distal surface of the humerus that articulates with the head of the radius.

Carbohydrase (p. 508) an enzyme that breaks down carbohydrate molecules.

Carbohydrate (p. 38) *kar″bo-hi′drāt* organic compound composed of carbon, hydrogen, and oxygen; includes starches, sugars, cellulose.

Carbon dioxide (p. 29) CO_2; a compound produced by the decarboxylation reactions of aerobic metabolism.

Carbonic anhydrase (p. 569) an enzyme that catalyzes the reaction $H_2O + CO_2 \rightarrow H_2CO_3$; important in carbon dioxide transport, gastric acid secretion, and renal pH regulation.

Carcinogen (p. 83) *kar-sin′o-jen* cancer-causing agent.

Cardiac (p. 148) *kar′de-ak* pertaining to the heart.

Cardiac cycle (p. 380) sequence of events encompassing one complete contraction and relaxation of the atria and ventricles of the heart.

Cardiac muscle (p. 80) specialized muscle of the heart.

Cardiac output (p. 381) the blood volume (in liters) ejected per minute by the left ventricle.

Cardiovascular centers (p. 407) poorly localized centers in the reticular formation of the medulla oblongata of the brain; includes cardioacceleratory, cardioinhibitory, and vasomotor centers.

Cardiovascular system (p. 4) organ system that distributes blood to all parts of the body.

Cardiovascular (p. 404) pertaining to the heart, blood, and blood vessels.

Carotene (p. 90) a yellow-orange pigment, found in carrots and in green and orange leafy vegetables, that the body can convert to vitamin A.

Carotid artery (p. 110) the principal artery of the neck, servicing cervical and cranial structures; one branch, the internal carotid, provides a major blood supply to the brain.

Carotid (p. 389) *kah-rot′id* the main artery in the neck.

Carotid sinus (p. 286) *si'nus* a dilation of a common carotid artery; involved in regulation of systemic blood pressure.

Carpal (p. 11) *kar'pal* one of the eight bones of the wrist.

Cartilage (p. 75) *kar'ti-lij* white, semiopaque connective tissue.

Cartilaginous joint (p. 132) *kar''ti-laj'ĭ-nus* bones united by cartilage; no joint cavity is present.

Catabolism (p. 517) *kah-tab'o-lizm* the process in which living cells break down substances into simpler substances; destructive metabolism.

Catalyst (p. 32) a substance that accelerates a specific chemical reaction but that is not altered by the reaction.

Cataract (p. 293) *kat'ah-rakt* partial or complete loss of transparency of the crystalline lens of the eye.

Catecholamines (p. 334) *kat'ĕ-kol'ah-menz* epinephrine and norepinephrine.

Catheter (p. 561) a tube surgically inserted into a body cavity or along a blood vessel or excretory passageway for the collection of body fluids, monitoring of blood pressure, or introduction of medications or radiographic dyes.

Cation (p. 27) an ion that bears a positive charge.

Cauda equina (p. 248) spinal nerve roots distal to the tip of the adult spinal cord; they extend caudally inside the vertebral canal en route to lumbar and sacral segments.

Cecum (p. 492) *se'kum* the blind-end pouch at the beginning of the large intestine.

Cell (p. 2) the basic biological unit of living organisms, containing a nucleus and a variety of organelles enclosed by a limiting membrane.

Cell body (p. 201) body; the body of a neuron; also called *soma*.

Cellular respiration (p. 518) metabolic processes in which ATP is produced.

Cementum (p. 496) *se-men'tum* the bony connective tissue that covers the root of a tooth.

Central nervous system (CNS) (p. 198) the brain and the spinal cord.

Centriole (p. 58) *sen'tre-ōl* a minute body found near the nucleus of the cell composed of microtubules; active in cell division.

Cephalic (p. 12) pertaining to the head.

Cerebellum (p. 233) *ser''ĕ-bel'um* part of the hindbrain; involved in producing smoothly coordinated skeletal muscle activity.

Cerebral aqueduct (p. 240) *ser'ĕ-bral ak'we-dukt'* the slender cavity of the midbrain that connects the third and fourth ventricles; also called the aqueduct of Sylvius.

Cerebral cortex (p. 238) an extensive area of neural cortex covering the surfaces of the cerebral hemispheres.

Cerebral hemispheres (p. 232) a pair of expanded portions of the cerebrum covered in neural cortex.

Cerebrospinal fluid (CSF) (p. 235) fluid bathing the internal and external surfaces of the central nervous system; secreted by the choroid plexus.

Cerebrum (p. 232) *ser'ĕ-brum* the largest part of the brain; consists of right and left cerebral hemispheres.

Cerumen (p. 299) *sĕ-roo'men* earwax.

Cervical (p. 11) *ser'vĭ-kal* refers to the neck or the necklike portion of an organ or structure.

Cervix (p. 589) *ser'viks* the inferior necklike portion of the uterus leading to the vagina.

Chemical bond (p. 26) an energy relationship holding atoms together; involves the interaction of electrons.

Chemical energy (p. 22) energy form stored in chemical bonds.

Chemical reaction (p. 26) process in which molecules are formed, changed, or broken down.

Chemoreceptors (p. 306) *ke'mo-re-sep'torz* receptors sensitive to various chemicals in solution.

Chemotaxis (p. 428) the attraction of phagocytic cells to the source of abnormal chemicals in tissue fluids.

Chiasma (p. 295) *ki-as'mah* a crossing or intersection of two structures, such as the optic nerves.

Cholecystokinin (p. 505) *ko''le-sis'to-kin'in* an intestinal hormone that stimulates gallbladder contraction and pancreatic juice release.

Cholesterol (p. 43) *ko-les'ter-ol* a steroid found in animal fats as well as in most body tissues; made by the liver.

Choline (p. 218) a breakdown product or precursor of acetylcholine.

Cholinergic synapse (p. 217) a synapse where the presynaptic membrane releases acetylcholine on stimulation.

Cholinesterase (p. 155) *ko-lin-es-ter-as* the enzyme that breaks down and inactivates acetylcholine.

Chondrocyte (p. 101) *kon'dro-sīt* a mature cartilage cell.

Chondroitin (p. 101) *kon-dro-i-tin* **sulfate** the predominant proteoglycan in cartilage, responsible for the gelatinous consistency of the matrix.

Chordae tendineae (p. 366) fibrous cords that stabilize the position of the AV valves in the heart, preventing backflow during ventricular systole.

Chorion (p. 600) *ko're-on* the outermost fetal membrane; helps form the placenta.

Choroid plexus (p. 240) the vascular complex in the roof of the third and fourth ventricles of the brain, responsible for the production of cerebrospinal fluid.

Choroid (p. 290) *ko'roid* the pigmented nutritive layer of the eye.

Chromatin (p. 53) *kro'mah-tin* the structures in the nucleus that carry the hereditary factors (genes).

Chromosomes (p. 53) dense structures, composed of tightly coiled DNA strands and associated histones, that become visible in the nucleus when a cell prepares to undergo mitosis or meiosis; normal human somatic cells contain 46 chromosomes apiece.

Chylomicrons (p. 511) relatively large droplets that may contain triglycerides, phospholipids, and cholesterol in association with proteins; synthesized and released by intestinal cells and transported to the venous blood by the lymphatic system.

Chyme (p. 488) *kīm* the semifluid stomach contents consisting of partially digested food and gastric secretions.

Cilia (p. 588) *sil'e-ah* tiny, hairlike projections on cell surfaces that move in a wavelike manner.

Ciliary body (p. 292) a thickened region of the choroid that encircles the lens of the eye; includes the ciliary muscle and the ciliary processes that support the suspensory ligaments of the lens.

Ciliary zonule (p. 290) suspensory ligament that attaches the lens to the ciliary body in the anterior eye.

Circumduction (p. 137) *ser'kum-duk'shun* circular movement of a body part.

Circumvallate papilla (p. 307) one of the large, dome-shaped papillae on the superior surface of the tongue that form a V, separating the body of the tongue from the root.

Cirrhosis (p. 496) *sĭ-ro'sis* a chronic disease of the liver, characterized by an overgrowth of connective tissue or fibrosis.

Cleavage (p. 600) *klēv'ij* an early embryonic phase consisting of rapid cell divisions without intervening growth periods.

Clitoris (p. 590) *kli'to-ris* a small, erectile structure in the female, homologous to the penis in the male.

Clonal selection (p. 434) *klo'nul* the process during which a B cell or T cell becomes sensitized through binding contact with an antigen.

Clone (p. 434) descendants of a single cell.

Clot (p. 353) a network of fibrin fibers and trapped blood cells; also called a *thrombus* if it occurs within the cardiovascular system.

Clotting factors (p. 356) plasma proteins, synthesized by the liver, that are essential to the clotting response.

Coagulation (p. 353) clotting (of blood).

Coccyx (p. 120) the terminal portion of the spinal column, consisting of relatively tiny, fused vertebrae.

Cochlea (p. 301) *kok'le-ah* a cavity of the inner ear resembling a snail shell; houses the hearing receptor.

Cochlear duct (p. 303) the central membranous tube within the cochlea that is filled with endolymph and contains the organ of Corti; also called *scala media*.

Coenzymes (p. 516) complex organic cofactors; most are structurally related to vitamins.

Coitus (p. 598) *ko'ĭ-tus* sexual intercourse.

Collagen (p. 75) a strong, insoluble protein fiber common in connective tissues.

Collateral ganglion (p. 270) a sympathetic ganglion situated anterior to the spinal column and separate from the sympathetic chain.

Coma (p. 336) *ko' mah* unconsciousness from which the person cannot be aroused.

Compact bone (p. 98) dense bone that contains parallel osteons.

Complement (p. 430) a group of plasma proteins that normally circulate in inactive forms; when activated by complement fixation, causes lysis of foreign cells and enhances phagocytosis and inflammation.

Compound (p. 26) substance composed of two or more different elements, the atoms of which are chemically united.

Concave (p. 487) *kon' kāv* having a curved or depressed surface.

Concentration gradient (p. 62) regional differences in the concentration of a particular substance.

Concentration (p. 37) the amount (in grams) or number of atoms, ions, or molecules (in moles) per unit volume.

Concha/conchae (p. 116) three pairs of thin, scroll-like bones that project into the nasal cavities; the superior and medial conchae are part of the ethmoid, and the inferior conchae are separate bones.

Conductivity (p. 214) *kon" duk-tiv' ĭ-te* ability to transmit an electrical impulse.

Condyle (p. 127) *kon' dĭl* a rounded projection at the end of a bone that articulates with another bone.

Cones (p. 291) one of the two types of photoreceptor cells in the retina of the eye. Provides for color vision.

Congenital (p. 117) *kon-jen' ĭ-tal* existing at birth.

Congestive heart failure (CHF) (p. 385) condition in which the pumping efficiency of the heart is depressed so that circulation is inadequate to meet tissue needs.

Conjunctiva (p. 287) *kon' junk-ti' vah* the thin, protective mucous membrane lining the eyelids and covering the anterior surface of the eyeball.

Connective tissue (p. 74) a primary tissue; form and function vary extensively. Functions include support, storage, and protection.

Contraception (p. 608) *kon' trah-sep' shun* the prevention of conception; birth control.

Contraction (p. 146) *kon-trak' shun* to shorten or develop tension, an ability highly developed in muscle cells.

Convergence (p. 227) *kon-ver' jens* turning toward a common point from different directions.

Convoluted (p. 542) *kon' vo-lūted* rolled, coiled, or twisted.

Coracoid process (p. 122) a hook-shaped process of the scapula that projects above the anterior surface of the capsule of the shoulder joint.

Cornea (p. 290) *kor' ne-ah* the transparent anterior portion of the eyeball.

Coronoid (p. 122) hooked or curved.

Corpora quadrigemina (p. 240) the superior and inferior colliculi of the mesencephalic tectum (roof) in the brain.

Corpus callosum (p. 239) the bundle of axons that links centers in the left and right cerebral hemispheres.

Corpus luteum (p. 341) the progestin-secreting mass of follicle cells that develops in the ovary after ovulation.

Corpus/corpora (p. 239) body.

Cortex (p. 232) *kor' teks* the outer surface layer of an organ.

Corticobulbar tracts (p. 255) descending tracts that carry information or commands from the cerebral cortex to nuclei and centers in the brain stem.

Corticosteroid (p. 332) a steroid hormone produced by the adrenal cortex.

Cortisol (p. 333) a corticosteroid secreted by the zona fasciculata of the adrenal cortex; a glucocorticoid.

Costal (p. 121) *kos' tal* pertaining to the ribs.

Cotransport (p. 511) the membrane transport of a nutrient, such as glucose, in company with the movement of an ion, normally sodium; transport requires a carrier protein but does not involve direct ATP expenditure and can occur regardless of the concentration gradient for the nutrient.

Countercurrent multiplication (p. 551) active transport between two limbs of a loop that contains a fluid moving in one direction; responsible for the concentration of urine in the kidney tubules.

Covalent bond (p. 27) *ko-va' lent* a bond involving the sharing of electrons between atoms.

Coxal (p. 11) pertaining to the hip.

Cranial nerves (p. 262) the 12 pairs of nerves that arise from the brain.

Cranial (p. 198) *kra' ne-al* pertaining to the skull.

Cranium (p. 110) the braincase; the skull bones that surround and protect the brain.

Creatine (p. 547) a nitrogenous compound, synthesized in the body, that can form a high-energy bond by connecting to a phosphate group and that serves as an energy reserve.

Creatine phosphate (p. 168) a high-energy compound in muscle cells; during muscle activity, the phosphate group is donated to ADP, regenerating ATP; also called *phosphorylcreatine*.

Creatinine (p. 543) a breakdown product of creatine metabolism.

Cross-bridge (p. 155) a myosin head that projects from the surface of a thick filament and that can bind to an active site of a thin filament in the presence of calcium ions.

Cryptorchidism (p. 612) *krip-tor' kĭ-dizm* a developmental defect in which the testes fail (or one testis fails) to descend into the scrotum.

Cuneiform cartilages (p. 102) a pair of small cartilages in the larynx.

Cupula (p. 302) *ku' pu-lah* a domelike structure.

Cushing's disease (p. 335) a condition caused by the oversecretion of adrenal steroids.

Cutaneous membrane (p. 86) the epidermis and papillary layer of the dermis.

Cutaneous (p. 90) *ku-ta' ne-us* pertaining to the skin.

Cuticle (p. 94) the layer of dead, keratinized cells that surrounds the shaft of a hair.

Cyanosis (p. 90) *si" ah-no' sis* a bluish coloration of the mucous membranes and skin caused by deficient oxygenation of the blood.

Cystic duct (p. 496) a duct that carries bile between the gallbladder and the common bile duct.

Cytoplasm (p. 54) *si' to-plazm* the substance of a cell other than that of the nucleus.

Cytosine (p. 48) a pyrimidine; one of the nitrogenous bases in the nucleic acids RNA and DNA.

Cytoskeleton (p. 57) a network of microtubules and microfilaments in the cytoplasm.

Cytosol (p. 59) the fluid portion of the cytoplasm.

Cytotoxic (p. 440) poisonous to cells.

Cytotoxic T cells (p. 440) lymphocytes involved in cell-mediated immunity that kill target cells by direct contact or by the secretion of lymphotoxins; also called *killer T cells* and T_c *cells*.

Deamination (p. 570) the removal of an amino group from an amino acid.

Deciduous (p. 494) *de-sid' u-us* temporary.

Decomposition reaction (p. 30) a destructive chemical reaction in which complex substances are broken down into simpler ones.

Decussate (p. 255) to cross over to the opposite side, usually referring to the crossover of the descending tracts of the corticospinal pathway on the ventral surface of the medulla oblongata.

Defecation (p. 498) *def" ih-ka' shun* the elimination of the contents of the bowels (feces).

Deglutition (p. 500) *deg' loo-tish' un* the act of swallowing.

Dehydration synthesis (p. 39) process by which a larger molecule is synthesized from smaller ones by removal of a water molecule at each site of bond formation.

Dendrites (p. 201) *den' drīts* the branching extensions of neurons that carry electrical signals to the cell body; the receptive portion of a nerve cell.

Dentin (p. 496) *den' tin* the calcified tissue forming the major part of a tooth; deep to the enamel.

Deoxyribonucleic acid (DNA) (p. 52) a nucleic acid consisting of a chain of nucleotides that contain the sugar deoxyribose and the nitrogenous bases adenine, guanine, cytosine, and thymine.

Depolarization (p. 213) *de-po" lar-i-za' shun* the loss of a state of polarity; the loss of a negative charge inside the plasma membrane.

Depression (p. 140) inferior (downward) movement of a body part.

Dermis (p. 88) *der' mis* the deep layer of the skin; composed of dense, irregular connective tissue.

Detrusor muscle (p. 559) a smooth muscle in the wall of the urinary bladder.

Detumescence (p. 599) the loss of a penile erection.

Development (p. 104) growth and the acquisition of increasing structural and functional complexity; includes the period from conception to maturity.

Diabetes insipidus (p. 565) polyuria due to inadequate production of antidiuretic hormone.

Diabetes mellitus (p. 336) *di"ah-be' tēz mel-li' tus* a disease caused by deficient insulin release or inadequate responsiveness to insulin, leading to inability of the body cells to use carbohydrates at a normal rate.

Diapedesis (p. 349) *di"ah-pě-de' sis* the passage of blood cells through intact vessel walls into the tissues.

Diaphragm (p. 16) *di' ah-fram* (1) any partition or wall separating one area from another; (2) a muscle that separates the thoracic cavity from the abdominopelvic cavity.

Diaphysis (p. 99) *di-af' ĭ-sis* elongated shaft of a long bone.

Diastole (p. 380) *di-as' to-le* a period (between contractions) of relaxation of the heart during which it fills with blood.

Diastolic pressure (p. 401) pressure measured in the walls of a muscular artery when the left ventricle is in diastole.

Diencephalon (p. 240) *di"en-sef' ah-lon* that part of the forebrain between the cerebral hemispheres and the midbrain including the thalamus, the third ventricle, and the hypothalamus.

Diffusion (p. 62) *dĭ-fu' zhun* the spreading of particles in a gas or solution with a movement toward uniform distribution of particles.

Digestion (p. 7) *di-jest' jun* the bodily process of breaking down foods chemically and mechanically.

Digestive system (p. 4) system that processes food into absorbable units and eliminates indigestible wastes.

Digital (p. 11) pertaining to the digits; fingers, toes.

Disaccharide (p. 39) *di-sak' ĭ-rīd* literally, double sugar; examples include sucrose and lactose.

Distal convoluted tubule (DCT) (p. 542) the portion of the nephron closest to the connecting tubules and collecting duct; an important site of active secretion.

Distal (p. 14) *dis' tal* farthest from the point of attachment of a limb or origin of a structure.

Diuresis (p. 565) fluid loss at the kidneys; the production of urine.

Diuretics (p. 558) drugs or foods that promote loss of water.

Divergence (p. 227) in neural tissue, the spread of information from one neuron to many neurons; an organizational pattern common along sensory pathways of the central nervous system.

Dopamine (p. 219) an important neurotransmitter in the central nervous system.

Dorsal root ganglion (p. 248) a peripheral nervous system ganglion containing the cell bodies of sensory neurons.

Dorsal (p. 248) *dor' sal* pertaining to the back; posterior.

Dorsiflexion (p. 140, 174) the elevation of the superior surface of the foot through flexion at the ankle.

Duct (p. 582) *dukt* a canal or passageway.

Ductus arteriosus (p. 398) a vascular connection between the pulmonary trunk and the aorta that functions throughout fetal life; normally closes at birth or shortly thereafter and persists as the ligamentum arteriosum.

Ductus deferens (p. 582) a passageway that carries spermatozoa from the epididymis to the ejaculatory duct.

Duodenal papilla (p. 488) a conical projection from the inner surface of the duodenum that contains the opening of the duodenal ampulla.

Duodenum (p. 488) *du' o-de' num* the first part of the small intestine.

Dura mater (p. 241) *du' rah ma' ter* the outermost and toughest of the three membranes (meninges) covering the brain and spinal cord.

Dynamic equilibrium (p. 302) sense that reports on angular or rotatory movements of the head in space.

Eccrine glands (p. 91) sweat glands of the skin that produce a watery secretion.

Ectoderm (p. 601) one of the three primary germ layers; covers the surface of the embryo and gives rise to the nervous system, the epidermis and associated glands, and a variety of other structures.

Edema (p. 75) *ě-de' mah* an abnormal accumulation of fluid in body parts or tissues; causes swelling.

Effector (p. 9) *ef-fek' tor* an organ, gland, or muscle capable of being activated by nerve endings.

Efferent arteriole (p. 542) an arteriole carrying blood away from a glomerulus of the kidney.

Efferent neurons (p. 205) neurons that conduct impulses away from the central nervous system.

Efferent (p. 199) *ef' er-ent* carrying away or away from.

Ejaculation (p. 584, 599) *e-jak' u-la' shun* the sudden ejection of semen from the penis.

Ejaculatory ducts (p. 582) short ducts that pass within the walls of the prostate gland and connect the ductus deferens with the prostatic urethra.

Elastase (p. 512) a pancreatic enzyme that breaks down elastin fibers.

Electrocardiogram (ECG, EKG) (p. 378) a graphic record of the electrical activities of the heart, as monitored at specific locations on the body surface.

Electroencephalogram (EEG) (p. 275) a graphic record of the electrical activities of the brain.

Electrolyte (p. 52) *e-lek' tro-līt* a substance that breaks down into ions when in solution and is capable of conducting an electric current.

Electron (p. 24) negatively charged subatomic particle; orbits the atomic nucleus.

Electron transport chain (p. 520) metabolic pathway within the mitochondria in which energy harvested from high-energy hydrogen atoms is used to make ATP. Final delivery of H to molecular oxygen produces water.

Element (p. 22) *el' ĕ-ment* any of the building blocks of matter; oxygen, hydrogen, carbon, for example.

Elevation (p. 140) movement in a superior, or upward, direction.

Elimination (p. 498) the ejection of wastes from the body through urination or defecation.

Embolus (p. 355) an air bubble, fat globule, or blood clot drifting in the bloodstream.

Embryo (p. 600) *em' bre-o* an organism in its early stages of development; in humans, the first 2 months after conception.

Emesis (p. 505) *em' ě-sis* vomiting.

Emmetropia (p. 298) the eye that focuses images correctly on the retina is said to have this "harmonious vision."

Enamel (p. 495) the hard, calcified substance that covers the crown of a tooth.

Emulsify (p. 496) physically breaking down large fat molecules into smaller ones.

Endocarditis (p. 367) *en' do-kar-di' tis* an inflammation of the inner lining of the heart.

Endocardium (p. 362) *en' do-kar' de-um* the endothelial membrane lining the interior of the heart.

Endocardium (p. 362) the simple squamous epithelium that lines the heart and is continuous with the endothelium of the great vessels.

Endochondral ossification (p. 105) the conversion of a cartilaginous model to bone; the characteristic mode of formation for skeletal elements other than the bones of the cranium, the clavicles, and sesamoid bones.

Endocrine glands (p. 4, 71) *en' do-krin* ductless glands that empty their hormonal products directly into the blood.

Endocrine system (p. 315) body system that includes internal organs that secrete hormones.

Endocytosis (p. 67) the movement of relatively large volumes of extracellular material into the cytoplasm via the formation of a membranous vesicle at the cell surface; includes pinocytosis and phagocytosis.

Endoderm (p. 601) one of the three primary germ layers; the layer on the undersurface of the embryonic disc; gives rise to the epithelia and glands of the digestive system, the respiratory system, and portions of the urinary system.

Endolymph (p. 301) the fluid contents of the membranous labyrinth (the saccule, utricle, semicircular ducts, and cochlear duct) of the inner ear.

Endometrium (p. 589) *en-do-me' tre-um* the mucous membrane lining of the uterus.

Endomysium (p. 146) *en″do-mis′e-um* the thin connective tissue surrounding each muscle cell.

Endoneurium (p. 262) a delicate network of connective tissue fibers that surrounds individual nerve fibers.

Endoplasmic reticulum (p. 55) a network of membranous channels in the cytoplasm of a cell that function in intracellular transport, synthesis, storage, packaging, and secretion.

Endorphins (p. 220) neuromodulators, produced in the central nervous system, that inhibit activity along pain pathways.

Endothelium (p. 386) *en′do-the′le-um* the single layer of simple squamous cells that line the walls of the heart and the vessels that carry blood and lymph.

Energy (p. 22) the ability to do work.

Enkephalins (p. 220) neuromodulators, produced in the central nervous system, that inhibit activity along pain pathways.

Enteroendocrine cells (p. 489) endocrine cells scattered among the epithelial cells that line the digestive tract.

Enterokinase (p. 509) an enzyme in the lumen of the small intestine that activates the proenzymes secreted by the pancreas.

Enzyme (p. 32) *en′zīm* a substance formed by living cells that acts as a catalyst in bodily chemical reactions.

Eosinophils (p. 352) *e′o-sin′o-filz* granular white blood cells whose granules readily take up a stain called eosin.

Ependyma (p. 201) the layer of cells lining the ventricles and central canal of the central nervous system.

Epicardium (p. 362) a serous membrane that tightly hugs the external surface of the heart and is actually part of the heart wall; also called visceral pericardium.

Epididymis (p. 580) *ep″ĭ-did′ĭ-mis* that portion of the male duct system in which sperm mature. Empties into the ductus, or vas, deferens.

Epiglottis (p. 454) *ep′ĭ-glot′is* the elastic cartilage at the back of the throat; covers the glottis during swallowing.

Epimysium (p. 146) *ep″ĭ-mis′e-um* the sheath of fibrous connective tissue surrounding a muscle.

Epineurium (p. 262) a dense layer of collagen fibers that surrounds a peripheral nerve.

Epiphyseal cartilage (p. 106) the cartilaginous region between the epiphysis and diaphysis of a growing bone.

Epiphysis (p. 99) *ĕ-pif′ĭ-sis* the end of a long bone.

Epithelium (p. 69) *ep′ĭ-the′le-um* one of the primary tissues; covers the surface of the body and lines the body cavities, ducts, and vessels.

Equilibrium (p. 285) *e′kwĭ-lib′re-um* balance; a state when opposite reactions or forces counteract each other exactly.

Erection (p. 598) the stiffening of the penis due to the engorgement of the erectile tissues of the corpora cavernosa and corpus spongiosum.

Erythema (p. 90) redness and inflammation at the surface of the skin.

Erythrocyte (p. 68) a red blood cell; has no nucleus and contains large quantities of hemoglobin.

Erythrocytes (p. 348) *ĕ-rith′ro-sīts* red blood cells.

Erythropoietin (p. 353) a hormone released by tissues, especially the kidneys, exposed to low oxygen concentrations; stimulates erythropoiesis (red blood cell formation) in bone marrow.

Escherichia coli (p. 576) a normal bacterial resident of the large intestine.

Esophagus (p. 484) a muscular tube that connects the pharynx to the stomach.

Essential amino acids (p. 524) amino acids that cannot be synthesized in the body in adequate amounts and must be obtained from the diet.

Estrogens (p. 334) *es′tro-jenz* hormones that stimulate female secondary sex characteristics; female sex hormones.

Eupnea (p. 472) *ūp-ne′ah* easy, normal breathing.

Evaporation (p. 530) a movement of molecules from the liquid state to the gaseous state.

Eversion (p. 177) special movement of the foot achieved by turning the sole laterally.

Exchange reaction (p. 31) a chemical reaction in which bonds are both made and broken; atoms become combined with different atoms.

Excitatory postsynaptic potential (EPSP) (p. 221) the depolarization of a post-synaptic membrane by a chemical neurotransmitter released by the presynaptic cell.

Excretion (p. 8) *ek-skre′shun* the elimination of waste products from the body.

Exocrine glands (p. 90) *ek′so-krin* glands that have ducts through which their secretions are carried to a body surface (skin or mucosa).

Exocytosis (p. 66) the ejection of cytoplasmic materials by the fusion of a membranous vesicle with the cell membrane.

Expiration (p. 460) *eks″pĭ-ra′shun* the act of expelling air from the lungs; exhalation.

Extension (p. 174) movement that increases the angle of a joint; e.g., straightening a flexed knee.

External ear (p. 299) the auricle, external acoustic canal, and tympanic membrane.

External respiration (p. 462) the actual exchange of gases between the alveoli and the blood (pulmonary gas exchange).

Exteroceptors (p. 283) general sensory receptors in the skin, mucous membranes, and special sense organs that provide information about the external environment and about our position within it.

Extracellular fluid (p. 561) all body fluids other than that contained within cells; includes plasma and interstitial fluid.

Extracellular matrix (p. 74) nonliving material in connective tissue consisting of ground substance and fibers that separate the living cells.

Facilitated diffusion (p. 63) the passive movement of a substance across a cell membrane by means of a protein carrier.

Facilitated (p. 226) brought closer to threshold, as in the depolarization of a nerve cell membrane toward threshold; making the cell more sensitive to depolarizing stimuli.

Falx (p. 241) sickle-shaped.

Fascicle (p. 146) *fas′ĭ-kul* a bundle of nerve or muscle fibers bound together by connective tissue.

Fasciculus (p. 249) a small bundle; usually refers to a collection of nerve axons or muscle fibers.

Fatty acid (p. 40) a building block of fats.

Feces (p. 507) *fe′sēz* material discharged from the bowel composed of food residue, secretions, and bacteria.

Femoral (p. 11) pertaining to the thigh.

Fenestra (p. 396) an opening.

Fertilization (p. 600) *fer′tĭ-lĭ-za′shun* fusion of the nuclear material of an egg and a sperm.

Fetus (p. 602) *fe′tus* the unborn young; in humans the period from the third month of development until birth.

Fibrin (p. 354) *fi′brin* the fibrous insoluble protein formed during the clotting of blood.

Fibrinogen (p. 354) *fi-brin′o-jen* a blood protein that is converted to fibrin during blood clotting.

Fibroblasts (p. 75) cells of connective tissue proper that are responsible for the production of extracellular fibers and the secretion of the organic compounds of the extracellular matrix.

Fibrocartilage (p. 75) cartilage containing an abundance of collagen fibers; located around the edges of joints, in the intervertebral discs, the menisci of the knee, and so on.

Fibrous joint (p. 132) bones joined by fibrous tissue; no joint cavity is present.

Fibrous protein (p. 44) a strandlike protein that appears most often in body structures. They are very important in binding structures together and for providing strength in certain body tissues.

Fibrous tunic (p. 290) the outermost layer of the eye, composed of the sclera and cornea.

Fibula (p. 128) the lateral, slender bone of the leg.

Fibular (p. 11) pertaining to the area of the fibula, the lateral bone of the leg.

Filtration pressure (p. 547) the hydrostatic pressure responsible for filtration.

Filtration (p. 63) *fil-tra′shun* the passage of a solvent and dissolved substances through a membrane or filter.

Filtration (p. 63) the movement of a fluid across a membrane whose pores restrict the passage of solutes on the basis of size.

Fimbriae (p. 588) fringes; the fingerlike processes that surround the entrance to the uterine tube.

Fissure (p. 236) *fis′zher* (1) a groove or cleft; (2) the deepest depressions or inward folds on the brain.

Fixators (p. 177) *fiks-a′torz* muscles acting to immobilize a joint or a bone; fixes the origin of a muscle so that muscle action can be exerted at the insertion.

Flaccid (p. 170) *flak'sid* soft; flabby; relaxed.

Flagellum/flagella (p. 58) an organelle that is structurally similar to a cilium but is used to propel a cell through a fluid.

Flatus (p. 507) intestinal gas.

Flexion (p. 137) *flek'shun* bending; the movement that decreases the angle between bones.

Follicle (p. 587) *fol'lĭ-kul* (1) structure in an ovary consisting of a developing egg surrounded by follicle cells; (2) colloid-containing structure in the thyroid gland.

Follicle-stimulating hormone (FSH) (p. 325) a hormone secreted by the anterior pituitary; stimulates oogenesis (female) and spermatogenesis (male).

Foramen/foramina (p. 127) an opening or passage through a bone.

Forearm (p. 122) the distal portion of the upper limb between the elbow and wrist.

Formed elements (p. 348) cellular portion of blood.

Fossa (p. 240) *fos'ah* a depression; often an articular surface.

Fourth ventricle (p. 291) an elongate ventricle of the metencephalon (pons and cerebellum) and the myelencephalon (medulla oblongata) of the brain; the roof contains a region of choroid plexus.

Fovea (p. 291) *fo-ve'ah* a pit.

Frenulum (p. 482) a bridle;usually referring to a band of tissue that restricts movement, e.g. *lingual frenulum.*

Fructose (p. 582) a hexose (six-carbon simple sugar) in foods and in semen.

Fundus (p. 295) *fun'dus* the base of an organ; that part farthest from the opening of the organ.

Gallbladder (p. 496) the sac beneath the right lobe of the liver used for bile storage.

Gamete (p. 580) *gam'ĕt* male or female sex cell (sperm/egg).

Gamma aminobutyric acid (GABA) (p. 220) a neurotransmitter of the central nervous system whose effects are generally inhibitory.

Ganglion/ganglia (p. 203) a collection of neuron cell bodies outside the central nervous system.

Gap junctions (p. 54) connections between cells that permit electrical coupling.

Gastric glands (p. 488) the tubular glands of the stomach whose cells produce acid, enzymes, intrinsic factor, and hormones.

Gastric (p. 501) pertaining to the stomach.

Gastrin (p. 501) *gas'trin* a hormone that stimulates gastric secretion, especially hydrochloric acid release.

Gastrointestinal (GI) tract (p. 482) *see* **digestive tract**.

General senses (p. 282) sensitivity to temperature, pain, touch, pressure, vibrations and proprioception.

Genitalia (p. 582) *jen'ĭ-ta'le-ah* the external sex organs.

Germinal centers (p. 422) pale regions in the interior of lymphoid tissues or nodules, where cell divisions are under way.

Gingiva (p. 495) *jin-ji'vah* the gums.

Gland (p. 71) an organ specialized to secrete or excrete substances for further use in the body or for elimination.

Glaucoma (p. 295) *glaw-ko'mah* an abnormal increase of the pressure within the eye.

Glenoid cavity (p. 122) a rounded depression that forms the articular surface of the scapula at the shoulder joint.

Globular protein (p. 44) a protein whose functional structure is basically spherical. Also referred to as functional protein; includes hemoglobin enzymes and some hormones.

Glomerular capsule (p. 542) *glo-mer'yoo-ler* double walled cuplike end of a renal tubule; encloses a glomerulus; also called Bowman's capsule.

Glomerular filtration rate (p. 547) the rate of filtrate formation at the glomerulus.

Glomerulus (p. 540) *glo-mer'u-lus* a knot of coiled capillaries in the kidney; forms filtrate.

Glottis (p. 454) *glot'is* the opening between the vocal cords in the larynx.

Glucagon (p. 335) a hormone secreted by the alpha cells of the pancreatic islets; elevates blood glucose concentrations.

Glucocorticoids (p. 333) hormones secreted by the zona fasciculata of the adrenal cortex to modify glucose metabolism; cortisol and corticosterone are important examples.

Gluconeogenesis (p. 525) the synthesis of glucose from protein or lipid precursors.

Glucose (p. 518) *gloo'kōs* the principal sugar in the blood; a monosaccharide.

Glycerides (p. 40) lipids composed of glycerol bound to fatty acids.

Glycerol (p. 498) *glis'er-ol* a sugar alcohol; one of the building blocks of fats.

Glycogen (p. 525) *gli'ko-jen* the main carbohydrate stored in animal cells; a polysaccharide.

Glycogenesis (p. 525) *gli'ko-jen'ĕ-sis* formation of glycogen from glucose.

Glycogenolysis (p. 525) *gli'ko-jĕ-nol'ĭ-sis* break-down of glycogen to glucose.

Glycolysis (p. 520) *gli-kol'ĭ-sis* breakdown of glucose to pyruvic acid; an anaerobic process.

Glycoprotein (p. 59) a compound containing a relatively small carbohydrate group attached to a large protein.

Glycosuria (p. 551) the presence of glucose in urine.

Goblet cells (p. 71) individual cells (simple glands) that produce mucus.

Goiter (p. 329) *goi'ter* a benign enlargement of the thyroid gland.

Golgi apparatus (p. 56) a cellular organelle consisting of a series of membranous plates that give rise to lysosomes and secretory vesicles.

Gonads (p. 580) *go'nadz* organs producing gametes; ovaries or testes.

Graded potential (p. 213) a local change in membrane potential that varies directly with the strength of the stimulus, declines with distance.

Granulocytes (p. 350) white blood cells containing granules that are visible with the light microscope; includes eosinophils, basophils, and neutrophils; also called *granular leukocytes.*

Gray matter (p. 203) the gray area of the central nervous system; contains unmyelinated nerve fibers and nerve cell bodies.

Greater omentum (p. 487) a large fold of the dorsal mesentery of the stomach; hangs anterior to the intestines.

Gross anatomy (p. 99) the study of the structural features of the body without the aid of a microscope.

Growth hormone (GH) (p. 324) an anterior pituitary hormone that stimulates tissue growth and anabolism when nutrients are abundant and restricts tissue glucose dependence when nutrients are in short supply.

Gyrus (p. 232) *ji'rus* an outward fold of the surface of the cerebral cortex.

Hair cells (p. 303) sensory cells of the inner ear.

Hair follicle (p. 93) an accessory structure of the integument; a tube lined by a stratified squamous epithelium that begins at the surface of the skin and ends at the hair papilla.

Hair (p. 92) a keratinous strand produced by epithelial cells of the hair follicle.

Hard palate (p. 482) the bony roof of the oral cavity, formed by the maxillary and palatine bones.

Heat stroke (p. 530) the failure of the heat-regulating ability of an individual under heat stress.

Helper T cells (p. 440) lymphocytes whose secretions and other activities coordinate cell-mediated and antibody-mediated immunities; also called T_H cells.

Hematocrit (p. 346) the percentage of the volume of whole blood contributed by cells; also called *volume of packed red cells (VPRC)* or *packed cell volume (PCV).*

Hematoma (p. 90) a tumor or swelling filled with blood. (AM)

Hematopoiesis (p. 352) *he'mato-poi-e'sis* formation of blood cells.

Hematuria (p. 550) the presence of abnormal numbers of red blood cells in urine.

Heme (p. 470) a porphyrin ring containing a central iron atom that can reversibly bind oxygen molecules; a component of the hemoglobin molecule.

Hemocytoblasts (p. 352) stem cells whose divisions produce each of the various populations of blood cells.

Hemoglobin (p. 348) *he'mo-glo'bin* the oxygen-transporting pigment of erythrocytes.

Hemolysis (p. 357) *he-mol'ĭ-sis* the rupture of eryth-rocytes.

Hemophilia (p. 356) *hē' mo-fil' e-ah* an inherited clotting defect caused by absence of a blood-clotting factor.

Hemorrhage (p. 400) *hem' or-ij* the loss of blood from the vessels by flow through ruptured walls; bleeding.

Hemostasis (p. 353) the cessation of bleeding.

Heparin (p. 356) An anticoagulant released by activated basophils and mast cells.

Hepatic duct (p. 496) the duct that carries bile away from the liver lobes and toward the union with the cystic duct.

Hepatic portal vein (p. 391) the vessel that carries blood between the intestinal capillaries and the sinusoids of the liver.

Hepatitis (p. 496) *hep' ah-ti' tis* inflammation of the liver.

Hiatus (p. 120) a gap, cleft, or opening.

High-density lipoprotein (HDL) (p. 526) a lipoprotein with a relatively small lipid content; thought to be responsible for the movement of cholesterol from peripheral tissues to the liver.

Hilum/hilus (p. 423) a localized region where blood vessels, lymphatic vessels, nerves, and/or other anatomical structures are attached to an organ.

Histamine (p. 427) *his' tah-mēn* a substance that causes vasodilation and increased vascular permeability.

Homeostasis (p. 9) *ho' me-o-sta' sis* a state of body equilibrium or stable internal environment of the body.

Hormones (p. 324) *hor' mōnz* chemical messengers secreted by endocrine glands; responsible for specific regulatory effects on certain parts or organs.

Human chorionic gonadotropin (hCG) (p. 600) the placental hormone that maintains the corpus luteum for the first 3 months of pregnancy.

Human immunodeficiency virus (HIV) (p. 448) the infectious agent that causes acquired immune deficiency syndrome (AIDS).

Human placental lactogen (hPL) (p. 342) the placental hormone that stimulates the functional development of the mammary glands.

Hyaline (p. 75) *hi' ah-lin* glassy; transparent.

Hydrochloric acid (p. 425, 488) *hi' dro-klo' rik* HCl; aids protein digestion in the stomach; produced by parietal cells.

Hydrogen bond (p. 29) weak bond in which a hydrogen atom forms a bridge between two electron-hungry atoms; an important intramo-lecular bond.

Hydrolysis (p. 29) *hi-drol' ĭ-sis* the process in which water is used to split a substance into smaller particles.

Hydrophilic (p. 35) freely associating with water; readily entering into solution.

Hydrophobic (p. 35) incapable of freely associating with water molecules; insoluble.

Hydrostatic pressure (p. 546) fluid pressure.

Hyperopia (p. 298) *hi"per-o' pe-ah* far-sightedness.

Hypertension (p. 511) *hi"per-ten' shun* an abnormally high blood pressure.

Hypertonic (p. 65) *hi"per-ton' ik* excessive, above normal, tone or tension.

Hypertrophy (p. 167) *hi-per' tro-fe* an increase in the size of a tissue or organ independent of the body's general growth.

Hypotension (p. 410) low blood pressure.

Hypothalamus (p. 233) the floor of the diencephalon; the region of the brain containing centers involved with the subconscious regulation of visceral functions, emotions, drives, and the coordination of neural and endocrine functions.

Hypothermia (p. 528) an abnormally low body temperature.

Hypotonic (p. 65) *hi-po-ton' ik* below normal tone or tension.

Hypoxia (p. 468) *hi-pok' se-ah* a condition in which inadequate oxygen is available to tissues.

Ileum (p. 488) *il' e-um* the terminal part of the small intestine; between the jejunum and the cecum of the large intestine.

Ilium (p. 125) the largest of the three bones whose fusion creates an os coxae.

Immune response (p. 431) antigen-specific defenses mounted by activated lymphocytes (T cells and B cells).

Immunity (p. 425) *ĭ-mu' nĭ-te* the ability of the body to resist many agents (both living and nonliving) that can cause disease; resistance to disease.

Immunoglobulin (p. 436) *im' mu-no-glob' u-lin* a protein molecule, released by plasma cells, that mediates humoral immunity; an antibody.

Implantation (p. 589) the erosion of a blastocyst into the uterine wall.

Inclusions (p. 55) aggregations of insoluble pigments, nutrients, or other materials in cytoplasm.

Incus (p. 301) the central auditory ossicle, situated between the malleus and the stapes in the middle ear cavity.

Infarct (p. 379) an area of dead cells that results from an interruption of blood flow.

Inferior (caudal) (p. 14) pertaining to a position near the tail end of the long axis of the body.

Inferior vena cava (p. 368) the vein that carries blood from the parts of the body inferior to the heart to the right atrium.

Inferior (p. 391) below, in reference to a particular structure, with the body in the anatomical position.

Infundibulum (p. 223) a tapering, funnel-shaped structure; in the brain, the connection between the pituitary gland and the hypothalamus; in the uterine tube, the entrance bounded by fimbriae that receives the oocytes at ovulation.

Ingestion (p. 497) the introduction of materials into the digestive tract by way of the mouth.

Inguinal region (p. 16) the area near the junction of the trunk and the thighs that contains the external genitalia; a.k.a. groin.

Inguinal (p. 11) *ing' gwĭ-nal* pertaining to the groin region.

Inhibin (p. 596) a hormone, produced by sustentacular cells of the testes and follicular cells of the ovaries, that inhibits the secretion of follicle-stimulating hormone by the anterior lobe of the pituitary gland.

Inhibitory postsynaptic potential (IPSP) (p. 221) a hyperpolarization of the postsynaptic membrane after the arrival of a neurotransmitter.

Initial segment (p. 221) the proximal portion of the axon where an action potential first appears.

Inner cell mass (p. 600) a cluster of cells in the blastocyst from which the embryo develops.

Inorganic compound (p. 32) a compound that lacks carbon; for example, water.

Insertion (p. 172) *in-ser' shun* the movable attachment of a muscle as opposed to its origin.

Inspiration (p. 460) *in' spĭ-ra' shun* the drawing of air into the lungs; inhalation.

Insulin (p. 335) a hormone secreted by the beta cells of the pancreatic islets; causes a reduction in plasma glucose concentrations.

Integument (p. 86) the skin.

Integumentary system (p. 2) *in-teg-u-men' tar-e* the skin and its accessory organs.

Intercalated discs (p. 367) regions where adjacent cardiocytes interlock and where gap junctions permit electrical coupling between the cells.

Intercellular (p. 313) *in' ter-sel' u-lar* between the body cells.

Interferons (p. 430) peptides released by virus infected cells, especially lymphocytes, that slow viral replication and make other cells more resistant to viral infection.

Internal respiration (p. 469) the use of oxygen by body cells; also called *cellular respiration*.

Interneurons (p. 205) complete the pathway between afferent and efferent neurons; also called *association neurons*.

Interoceptors (p. 283) sensory receptors monitoring the functions and status of internal organs and systems.

Intersegmental reflex (p. 231) a reflex that involves several segments of the spinal cord.

Interstitial fluid (p. 52, 61) *in" ter-stish' al* the fluid between the cells.

Interstitial growth (p. 101) a form of cartilage growth through the growth, mitosis, and secretion of chondrocytes in the matrix.

Intervertebral discs (p. 117) *in" ter-ver' tĕ-bral* the discs of fibrocartilage between the vertebrae.

Intracellular fluid (p. 61) fluid within a cell.

Intramembranous ossification (p. 105) the formation of bone within a connective tissue without the prior development of a cartilaginous model.

Inversion (p. 140) a turning inward.

Involuntary (p. 148) not under conscious control.

Ion (p. 27) *i' on* an atom with a positive or negative electric charge.

Ionic bond (p. 27) bond formed by the complete transfer of electron(s) from one atom to another (or others). The resulting charged atoms, or ions, are oppositely charged and attract each other.

Ionization (p. 33) dissociation; the breakdown of a molecule in solution to form ions.

Iris (p. 290) *i' ris* the pigmented, involuntary muscle that acts as the diaphragm of the eye.

Irritability (p. 7) *ir"ĭ-tah-bil'ĭ-te* ability to respond to a stimulus.

Ischemia (p. 375) *is-ke' me-ah* a local decrease in blood supply.

Islets of Langerhans (p. 335) *see* **pancreatic islets**.

Isometric (p. 158) *ĭ"so-met' rik* of the same length.

Isotonic (p. 64) *ĭ"so-ton' ik* having a uniform tension; of the same tone.

Isotope (p. 25) *i' sĭ-tōp* different atomic form of the same element. Isotopes vary only in the number of neutrons they contain.

Jaundice (p. 90) *jawn' dis* an accumulation of bile pigments in the blood producing a yellow color of the skin.

Jejunum (p. 488) the middle part of the small intestine.

Joint (p. 129) the junction of two or more bones; an articulation.

Juxtaglomerular apparatus (p. 548) the macula densa and the juxtaglomerular cells; a complex responsible for the release of renin and erythropoietin.

Keratin (p. 44) *ker' ah-tin* a tough, insoluble protein found in tissues such as hair, nails, and epidermis of the skin.

Ketoacidosis (p. 516) a reduction in the pH of body fluids due to the presence of large numbers of ketone bodies.

Ketone bodies (p. 516) keto acids produced during the catabolism of lipids and ketogenic amino acids; specifically, acetone, acetoacetate, and beta-hydroxybutyrate.

Kidney (p. 538) a component of the urinary system; an organ functioning in the regulation of plasma composition, including the excretion of wastes and the maintenance of normal fluid and electrolyte balances.

Killer T cell (p. 440) effector T cell that directly kills foreign cells; also called a cytotoxic T cell.

Kilocalories (kcal) (p. 514) unit used to measure the energy value of food.

Kinetic energy (p. 62) energy of motion.

Kinins (p. 427) *ki' ninz* group of polypeptides that dilate arterioles, increase vascular permeability, and induce pain.

Krebs cycle (p. 520) the aerobic pathway occurring within the mitochondria, in which energy is liberated during metabolism of carbohydrates, fats, and amino acids and CO_2 is produced.

Labia (p. 482) *la' be-ah* lips.

Labyrinth (p. 301) bony cavities and membranes of the inner ear that house the hearing and equilibrium receptors.

Lacrimal gland (p. 288) a tear gland on the dorsolateral surface of the eye.

Lacrimal (p. 116) *lak' rĭ-mal* pertaining to tears.

Lactase (p. 510) an enzyme that breaks down milk proteins.

Lactation (p. 341) *lak-ta' shun* the production and secretion of milk.

Lacteal (p. 489) *lak' te-al* special lymphatic capillaries of the small intestine that take up lipids.

Lactic acid (p. 168) *lak' tik* the product of anaerobic metabolism, especially in muscle.

Lacuna (p. 101) *lah-ku' nah* a little depression or space; in bone or cartilage, lacunae are occupied by cells.

Lamellae (p. 101) concentric layers; the concentric layers of bone within an osteon.

Lamellated corpuscle (p. 284) a receptor sensitive to vibration.

Lamina propria (p. 75) the reticular tissue that underlies a mucous epithelium and forms part of a mucous membrane.

Large intestine (p. 492) the terminal portions of the intestinal tract, consisting of the colon, the rectum, and the anal canal.

Laryngopharynx (p. 454) the division of the pharynx that is inferior to the epiglottis and superior to the esophagus.

Larynx (p. 454) *lar' inks* the cartilaginous organ located between the trachea and the pharynx; voice box.

Latent period (p. 162) the time between the stimulation of a muscle and the start of the contraction phase.

Lateral ventricle (p. 234) a fluid-filled chamber within a cerebral hemisphere.

Lateral (p. 14) *lat' er-al* away from the midline of the body.

Lens (p. 290) the elastic, doubly convex structure in the eye that focuses the light entering the eye on the retina.

Lesser omentum (p. 487) a small pocket in the mesentery that connects the lesser curvature of the stomach to the liver.

Leukemia (p. 350) *lu-ke' me-ah* a cancerous condition in which there is an excessive production of immature leukocytes.

Leukocyte (p. 349) *lu' ko-sīt* white blood cell.

Ligament (p. 75) *lig' ah-ment* a cord of fibrous tissue that connects bones.

Ligamentum arteriosum (p. 398) the fibrous strand in adults that is the remnant of the ductus arteriosus of the fetal stage.

Limbic system (p. 240) the group of nuclei and centers in the cerebrum and diencephalon that are involved with emotional states, memories, and behavioral drives.

Lipid (p. 40) *lip' id* organic compound formed of carbon, hydrogen, and oxygen; examples are fats and cholesterol.

Lipolysis (p. 525) the catabolism of lipids as a source of energy.

Lipoprotein (p. 526) a compound containing a relatively small lipid bound to a protein.

Liver (p. 496) an organ of the digestive system that has varied and vital functions, including the production of plasma proteins,

the excretion of bile, the storage of energy reserves, the detoxification of poisons, and the interconversion of nutrients.

Lobule (p. 597) histologically, the basic organizational unit of the liver.

Loop of Henle (p. 542) the portion of the nephron that creates the concentration gradient in the renal medulla.

Loose connective tissue (p. 75) a loosely organized, easily distorted connective tissue that contains several fiber types, a varied population of cells, and a viscous ground substance.

Lumbar (p. 12) pertaining to the lower back.

Lumen (p. 484) *lu' men* the space inside a tube, blood vessel, or hollow organ.

Lungs (p. 455) the paired organs of respiration, situated in the pleural cavities.

Luteinizing hormone (LH) (p. 586) also called *lutropin*; a hormone produced by the anterior lobe of the pituitary gland. In females, it assists FSH in follicle stimulation, triggers ovulation, and promotes the maintenance and secretion of endometrial glands. In males, it was formerly called *interstitial cell-stimulating hormone* because it stimulates testosterone secretion by the interstitial cells of the testes.

Lymph node (p. 421) a mass of lymphatic tissue.

Lymphatic system (p. 4) *lim-fat' ik* a system of lymphatic vessels, lymph nodes, and other lymphoid organs and tissues.

lymphatic vessels (p. 420) the vessels of the lymphatic system; also called *lymphatics*.

Lymphocytes (p. 352) *lim' fo-sītz* agranular white blood cells formed in the bone marrow that mature in the lymphoid tissue.

Lymphoid organs (p. 423) refers to organs in the lymphatic system including lymphatic vessels, lymph nodes, spleen, and tonsils; see *Lymphatic system.*

Lymphokines (p. 440) *lim' fo-kīnz* proteins involved in cell-mediated immune responses that enhance the immune and inflammatory responses.

Lysosomes (p. 57) *li' so-sōmz* organelles that originate from the Golgi apparatus and contain strong digestive enzymes.

Lysozyme (p. 288) *li' so-zīm* an enzyme found in sweat, saliva, and tears that is capable of destroying certain kinds of bacteria.

Macrophage (p. 422) a phagocytic cell of the monocyte-macrophage system.

Macula (p. 301) a receptor complex, located in the saccule or utricle of the inner ear, that responds to linear acceleration or gravity.

Macula densa (p. 548) a group of specialized secretory cells that is located in a portion of the distal convoluted tubule, adjacent to the glomerulus and the juxtaglomerular cells; a component of the juxtaglomerular apparatus.

Malleus (p. 301) the first auditory ossicle, bound to the tympanic membrane and the incus.

Mammary glands (p. 595) *mam' mer-e* milk-pro-ducing glands of the breasts.

Marrow (p. 100) a tissue that fills the internal cavities in bone; dominated by hemopoietic cells (red bone marrow) or by adipose tissue (yellow bone marrow).

Mast cell (p. 445) a connective tissue cell that, when stimulated, releases histamine, serotonin, and heparin, initiating the inflammatory response.

Matrix (p. 74) the extracellular fibers and ground substance of a connective tissue.

Matter (p. 22) anything that occupies space and has mass.

Meatus (p. 299) *me-a'tus* the external opening of a canal.

Mechanical energy (p. 22) energy form directly involved in putting matter into motion.

Mechanoreceptors (p. 283) *mek'ah-no-re-sep'terz* receptors sensitive to mechanical pressures such as touch, sound, or contractions.

Medial (p. 287) *me'de-al* toward the midline of the body.

Mediastinum (p. 362) *me'de-as-ti'num* the region of the thoracic cavity between the lungs.

Medulla oblongata (p. 240) the most caudal of the brain regions, also called the *myelencephalon.*

Medulla (p. 423) *me-dul'ah* the central portion of certain organs.

Medullary cavity (p. 100) the space within a bone that contains the marrow.

Meiosis (p. 584) *mi-o'sis* the two successive cell divisions in gamete formation producing nuclei with half the full number of chromosomes (haploid).

Melanin (p. 88) *mel'ah-nin* the dark pigment synthesized by melanocytes; responsible for skin color.

Melanocyte (p. 88) a cell that produces melanin.

Melatonin (p. 337) a hormone secreted by the pineal gland; inhibits secretion of MSH and GnRH.

Membrane (p. 53) any sheet or partition; a layer consisting of an epithelium and the underlying connective tissue.

Membrane potential (p. 206) *see* **transmembrane potential**.

Membranous labyrinth (p. 301) endolymph-filled tubes that enclose the receptors of the inner ear.

Memory cell (p. 434) member of T cell and B cell clones that provides for immunologic memory.

Memory (p. 431) the ability to recall information or sensations; can be divided into short-term and long-term memories.

Menarche (p. 612) *me-nar'ke* establishment of men-strual function; the first menstrual period.

Meninges (p. 241) three membranes that surround the surfaces of the central nervous system; the dura mater, the pia mater, and the arachnoid.

Meningitis (p. 246) *men'in-ji'tis* inflammation of the meninges of the brain or spinal cord.

Menopause (p. 613) *men'o-pawz* the physiological end of menstrual cycles.

Menses (p. 595) *men'sez* monthly discharge of blood from the uterus. Menstruation.

Menstruation (p. 589) *men''stroo-a'shun* the periodic, cyclic discharge of blood, secretions, tissue, and mucus from the mature female uterus in the absence of pregnancy.

Mesencephalon (p. 233) the midbrain; the region between the diencephalon and pons.

Mesentery (p. 485) *mes'en-ter''e* the double-layered membrane of the peritoneum that supports most organs in the abdominal cavity.

Mesoderm (p. 601) the middle germ layer, between the ectoderm and endoderm of the embryo.

Metabolic rate (p. 527) *met'ah-bol'ik* the energy expended by the body per unit time.

Metabolism (p. 517) *me-tab'o-lizm* the sum total of the chemical reactions that occur in the body.

Metabolites (p. 32) compounds produced in the body as a result of metabolic reactions.

Metabolize (p. 516) *me-tab'o-liz* to transform sub-stances into energy or materials the body can use or store by means of anabolism or catabolism.

Metacarpal (p. 125) *met'ah-kar'pal* one of the five bones of the palm of the hand.

Metastasis (p. 83) *me-tas'tah-sis* the spread of cancer from one body part or organ into another not directly connected to it.

Metatarsal (p. 128) *met'ah-tar'sal* one of the five bones between the tarsus and the phalanges of the foot.

Metencephalon (p. 234) the pons and cerebellum of the brain.

Micelle (p. 511) a droplet with hydrophilic portions on the outside; a spherical aggregation of bile salts, monoglycerides, and fatty acids in the lumen of the intestinal tract.

Microfilaments (p. 57) fine protein filaments visible with the electron microscope; components of the cytoskeleton.

Microglia (p. 201) phagocytic neuroglia in the central nervous system.

Microtubules (p. 57) microscopic tubules that are part of the cytoskeleton and are a component in cilia, flagella, the centrioles, and spindle fibers.

Microvilli (p. 54) *mi''kro-vil'i* the tiny projections on the free surfaces of some epithelial cells; increase surface area for absorption.

Micturition (p. 560) *mik'tu-rish'un* urination, or voiding; emptying the bladder.

Midbrain (p. 240) the mesencephalon.

Middle ear (p. 300) the space between the external and internal ears that contains auditory ossicles.

Mineralocorticoid (p. 332) corticosteroids produced by the zona glomerulosa of the adrenal cortex; steroids such as aldosterone that affect mineral metabolism.

Minerals (p. 516) the inorganic chemical compounds found in nature.

Mitochondria (p. 55) *mi''to-kon'dre-ah* the rodlike cytoplasmic organelles responsible for ATP generation.

Mitosis (p. 80) *mi-to'sis* the division of the cell nucleus; often followed by division of the cytoplasm of a cell.

Mixed nerve (p. 262) a peripheral nerve that contains sensory and motor fibers.

Molecule (p. 2) *mol'e-kyool* particle consisting of two or more atoms held together by chemical bonds.

Monoclonal antibodies (p. 436) *mon''o-klon'ul* pure preparations of identical antibodies that exhibit specificity for a single antigen.

Monocyte (p. 352) *mon'o-sit* large single-nucleus white blood cell; agranular leukocyte.

Monoglyceride (p. 511) a lipid consisting of a single fatty acid bound to a molecule of glycerol.

Monokines (p. 434) secretions released by activated cells of the monocyte-macrophage system to coordinate various aspects of the immune response.

Monosaccharide (p. 39) *mon''o-sak'i-rid* literally, one sugar; the building block of carbohydrates; examples include glucose and fructose.

Monosynaptic reflex (p. 230) a reflex in which the sensory afferent neuron synapses directly on the motor efferent neuron.

Motor nervous system (p. 199) carries impulses from the central nervous system to effector organs muscles and glands.

Motor unit (p. 164) all of the muscle cells controlled by a single motor neuron.

Mucosa (p. 71) a mucous membrane; the epithelium plus the lamina propria.

Mucous membrane (mucosa) (p. 71) membrane that forms the linings of body cavities open to the exterior (digestive, respiratory, urinary, and reproductive tracts).

Mucus (noun) (p. 56) a lubricating fluid that is composed of water and mucins and is produced by unicellular and multicellular glands along the digestive, respiratory, urinary, and reproductive tracts.

Multipolar neuron (p. 205) a neuron with many dendrites and a single axon; the typical form of a motor neuron.

Muscle fibers (p. 146) muscle cells.

Muscle spindle (p. 286) encapsulated sensory receptor found in skeletal muscle that is sensitive to stretch.

Muscle tissue (p. 78) a tissue characterized by the presence of cells capable of contraction; includes skeletal, cardiac, and smooth muscle tissues.

Muscle tone (p. 170) sustained partial contraction of a muscle in response to stretch receptor inputs; keeps the muscle healthy and ready to react.

Muscle twitch (p. 161) a single rapid contraction of a muscle followed by relaxation.

Muscle (p. 146) a contractile organ composed of muscle tissue, blood vessels, nerves, connective tissues, and lymphatic vessels.

Muscular system (p. 2) organ system consisting of skeletal muscles and their connective tissue attachments.

Muscularis externa (p. 485) concentric layers of smooth muscle responsible for peristalsis.

Muscularis mucosae (p. 491) the layer of smooth muscle beneath the lamina propria; responsible for moving the mucosal surface.

Myelin (p. 201) *mi'ĕ-lin* a white, fatty lipid substance.

Myelination (p. 279) the formation of myelin.

Myocardial infarction (p. 416) *mi''o-kar'de-al-in-fark'shun* a condition characterized by dead tissue areas in the myocardium caused by interruption of blood supply to the area.

Myocardium (p. 362) *mi''o-kar'de-um* the cardiac muscle layer of the heart wall.

Myofibrils (p. 150) *mi''o-fi'brilz* contractile organelles found in the cytoplasm of muscle cells.

Myofilament (p. 150) *mi''o-fil'ah-ment* filaments composing the myofibrils. Of two types actin and myosin.

Myoglobin (p. 165) an oxygen-binding pigment that is especially common in slow skeletal muscle fibers and cardiac muscle cells.

Myometrium (p. 590) *mi''o-me'tri-um* the thick uterine musculature.

Myopia (p. 298) *mi-ō'pe-ah* nearsightedness.

Myosin (p. 150) *mi'o-sin* one of the principal contractile proteins found in muscle.

Nail (p. 94) a keratinous structure produced by epithelial cells of the nail root.

Nares, external (p. 451) the entrance from the exterior to the nasal cavity.

Nares, internal (p. 453) the entrance from the nasal cavity to the nasopharynx.

Nasal cavity (p. 451) a chamber in the skull that is bounded by the internal and external nares.

Nasal (p. 451) pertaining to the nose.

Nasolacrimal duct (p. 288) the passageway that transports tears from the nasolacrimal sac to the nasal cavity.

Nasopharynx (p. 453) a region that is posterior to the internal nares and superior to the soft palate and ends at the oropharynx.

Natriuretic peptides (NP) (p. 40) hormones released by specialized cardiocytes when they are stretched by an abnormally large venous return; promotes fluid loss and reductions in blood pressure and in venous return. Includes atrial natural peptide (ANP) and brain natriuretic (BNP).

Negative feedback (p. 9) a corrective mechanism that opposes or negates a variation from normal limits.

Neoplasm (p. 81) *ne'o-plazm* an abnormal growth of cells; sometimes cancerous.

Nephrons (p. 540) *nef'ronz* structural and functional units of the kidney.

Nerve (p. 198) bundle of neuronal processes (axons) outside the central nervous system.

Nerve impulse (p. 213) a self-propagating wave of depolarization; also called an *action potential*.

Nervous system (p. 3) fast-acting control system that employs nerve impulses to trigger muscle contraction or gland secretion.

Neural cortex (p. 232) an area of gray matter at the surface of the central nervous system.

Neurilemma (p. 201) the outer surface of a neuroglia that encircles an axon.

Neurofibrils (p. 201) microfibrils in the cytoplasm of a neuron.

Neuroglia (p. 200) cells of the central nervous system and peripheral nervous system that support and protect neurons; also called *glial cells*.

Neuromodulator (p. 220) a compound, released by a neuron, that adjusts the sensitivities of another neuron to specific neurotransmitters.

Neuromuscular junction (p. 152) *nu''ro-mus'ku-lar* the region where a motor neuron comes into close contact with a skeletal muscle cell.

Neuron or **neurone** (p. 201) a cell in neural tissue that is specialized for intercellular communication through changes in membrane potential and synaptic connections.

Neurotransmitter (p. 201) chemical released by neurons that may, upon binding to receptors of neurons or effector cells, stimulate or inhibit them.

Neutralization (p. 37, 438) *nu'tral-i-za'shun* (1) a chemical reaction that occurs between an acid and a base; (2) blockage of the harmful effects of bacterial exotoxins or viruses by the binding of antibodies to their functional sites.

Neutron (p. 24) a fundamental particle that does not carry a positive or a negative charge.

Neutrophil (p. 352) a microphage that is very numerous and normally the first of the mobile phagocytic cells to arrive at an area of injury or infection.

Nipple (p. 597) an elevated epithelial projection on the surface of the breast; contains the openings of the lactiferous sinuses.

Nitrogenous wastes (p. 543) organic waste products of metabolism that contain nitrogen, such as urea, uric acid, and creatinine.

Norepinephrine (NE) (p. 219) a catecholamine neurotransmitter in the peripheral nervous system and central nervous system, released at most sympathetic neuromuscular and neuroglandular junctions, and a hormone secreted by the adrenal medulla; also called *noradrenaline*.

Nucleic acid (p. 46) a polymer of nucleotides that contains a pentose sugar, a phosphate group, and one of four nitrogenous bases that regulate the synthesis of proteins and make up the genetic material in cells.

Nucleoli (p. 53) *nu-kle'o-li* small spherical bodies in the cell nucleus; function in ribosome synthesis.

Nucleoplasm (p. 53) the fluid content of the nucleus.

Nucleotide (p. 46) a compound consisting of a nitrogenous base, a simple sugar, and a phosphate group.

Nucleus (p. 52) a cellular organelle that contains DNA, RNA, and proteins; in the central nervous system, a mass of gray matter.

Nutrient (p. 8) an inorganic or organic compound that can be broken down in the body to produce energy.

Obesity (p. 532) body weight 10–20 percent above standard values as a result of body fat accumulation.

Olfaction (p. 122) *ol-fak'shun* smell.

Oligodendrocytes (p. 201) central nervous system neuroglia that maintain cellular organization within gray matter and provide a myelin sheath in areas of white matter.

Oocyte (p. 69) a cell whose meiotic divisions will produce a single ovum and three polar bodies.

Oogenesis (p. 591) *o''o-jen'ĕ-sis* the process of formation of the ova.

Opposition (p. 177) the action by which the thumb is used to touch the tips of the other fingers on the same hand. This unique action makes the human hand such a fine tool for grasping and manipulating things.

Opsonization (p. 430) an effect of coating an object with antibodies; the attraction and enhancement of phagocytosis.

Optic chiasm (p. 295) the crossing point of the optic nerves.

Optic nerve (p. 291) the second cranial nerve (II), which carries signals from the retina of the eye to the optic chiasm.

Optic tract (p. 296) the tract over which nerve impulses from the retina are transmitted between the optic chiasm and the thalamus.

Oral (p. 11) relating to the mouth.

Orbital (p. 11) eye area.

Organ (p. 2) a part of the body formed of two or more tissues that performs a specialized function.

Organ system (p. 2) a group of organs that work together to perform a vital body function; e.g., nervous system.

Organelles (p. 54) *or''gan-elz'* specialized structures in a cell that perform specific metabolic functions.

Organic compound (p. 32) a compound containing carbon; examples include proteins, carbohydrates, and fats.

Organism (p. 2) an individual living thing.

Organs (p. 2) combinations of tissues that perform complex functions.

Origin (p. 172) attachment of a muscle that remains relatively fixed during muscular contraction.

Oropharynx (p. 454) the middle portion of the pharynx, bounded superiorly by the nasopharynx, anteriorly by the oral cavity, and inferiorly by the laryngopharynx.

Osmolarity (p. 512) the total concentration of dissolved materials in a solution, regardless of their specific identities, expressed in moles; also called *osmotic concentration*.

Osmoreceptor (p. 565) *oz''mo-re-cep'tor* a structure sensitive to osmotic pressure or concentration of a solution.

Osmosis (p. 62) *oz-mo'sis* the diffusion of a solvent through a membrane from a dilute solution into a more concentrated one.

Osmotic pressure (p. 412) the force of osmotic water movement; the pressure that must be applied to prevent osmosis across a membrane.

Ossicles (p. 301) *os'sĭ-kulz* the three bones of the middle ear: hammer, anvil, and stirrup.

Ossification (p. 105) the formation of bone.

Osteoblasts (p. 105) *os'te-o-blasts''* bone-forming cells.

Osteocyte (p. 101) a bone cell responsible for the maintenance and turnover of the mineral content of the surrounding bone.

Osteon (p. 101) *os'te-on* a system of interconnecting canals in the microscopic structure of adult compact bone; unit of bone.

Otolith (p. 301) *o'to-lith* one of the small calcified masses in the utricle and saccule of the inner ear.

Oval window (p. 300) an opening in the bony labyrinth where the stapes attaches to the membranous wall of the vestibular duct.

Ovarian cycle (p. 592) *o-va're-an* the monthly cycle of follicle development, ovulation, and corpus luteum formation in an ovary.

Ovary (p. 587) *o'var-e* the female sex organ in which ova (eggs) are produced.

Ovulation (p. 587) *ov''u-la'shun* the release of an ovum (or oocyte) from the ovary.

Ovum/ova (p. 580) the functional product of meiosis II, produced after the fertilization of a secondary oocyte.

Oxidation (p. 520) *ok'sĭ-da'shun* the process of substances combining with oxygen or the removal of hydrogen.

Oxygen debt (p. 169) *ok'sĭ-jen* the volume of oxygen required after exercise to oxidize the lactic acid formed during exercise.

Oxyhemoglobin (p. 468) *ok''sĭ-he''mo-glo'bin* hemoglobin combined with oxygen.

Oxytocin (p. 327) a hormone produced by hypothalamic cells and secreted into capillaries at the posterior lobe of the pituitary gland; stimulates smooth muscle contractions of the uterus or mammary glands in females and the prostate gland in males.

Pacemaker cells (p. 378) cells of the sinoatrial node that set the pace of cardiac contraction.

Palate (p. 452) *pal'at* roof of the mouth.

Palatine (p. 114) pertaining to the palate.

Palpate (p. 452) to examine by touch.

Pancreas (p. 496) *pan'kre-as* gland posterior to the stomach, between the spleen and the duodenum; produces both endocrine and exocrine secretions.

Pancreatic duct (p. 488) a tubular duct that carries pancreatic juice from the pancreas to the duodenum.

Pancreatic islets (p. 335) aggregations of endocrine cells in the pancreas; also called *islets of Langerhans.*

Pancreatic juice (p. 505) *pan''kre-at'ik* a secretion of the pancreas containing enzymes for digestion of all food categories.

Papilla (p. 307) *pah-pil'ah* small nipple-like projection.

Papillary muscles (p. 371) *pap'ĭ-ler''e* cone-shaped muscles found in the heart ventricles.

Paranasal sinuses (p. 116) bony chambers, lined by respiratory epithelium, that open into the nasal cavity; the frontal, ethmoidal, sphenoidal, and maxillary sinuses.

Parasympathetic division (p. 270) *par''ah-sim''pah-thet'ik* a division of the autonomic nervous system; also referred to as the craniosacral division.

Parathyroid glands (p. 331) *par''ah-thi'roid* small endocrine glands located on the posterior aspect of the thyroid gland.

Parathyroid hormone (PTH) (p. 108) hormone released by the parathyroid glands that regulates blood calcium level.

Parturition (p. 605) childbirth or process of birthing a child.

Parietal cells (p. 488) cells of the gastric glands that secrete hydrochloric acid and intrinsic factor.

Passive immunity (p. 435) short-lived immunity resulting from the introduction of "borrowed antibodies" obtained from an immune animal or human donor; immunological memory is not established.

Passive transport (p. 62) membrane transport processes that do not require cellular energy (ATP); e.g., diffusion, which is driven by kinetic energy.

Patella (p. 99) the sesamoid bone of the kneecap.

Pathogen (p. 425) disease-causing microorganism (e.g., some bacteria, fungi, viruses, etc.).

Peduncle (p. 240) *pe-dung'kul* a stalk of fibers, especially that connecting the cerebellum to the pons, midbrain, and medulla oblongata.

Pelvic cavity (p. 16) the inferior subdivision of the abdominopelvic cavity; encloses the urinary bladder, the sigmoid colon and rectum, and male or female reproductive organs.

Pelvic girdle (p. 125) incomplete bony basin formed by the two coxal bones that secures the lower limbs to the sacrum of the axial skeleton.

Pelvis (p. 125) *pel'vis* a basin-shaped structure; lower portion of the skeleton of the body trunk.

Penis (p. 583) *pe'nis* the male organ of copulation and urination.

Pepsin (p. 488) an enzyme capable of digesting proteins in an acid pH.

Peptide bond (p. 512) a covalent bond between the amino group of one amino acid and the carboxyl group of another.

Peptide (p. 333) a chain of amino acids linked by peptide bonds.

Perception (p. 282) the conscious awareness of a sensation

Pericardial cavity (p. 455) the space between the parietal pericardium and the epicardium (visceral pericardium) that covers the outer surface of the heart.

Pericardium (p. 362) *per''ĭ-kar'de-um* the membranous sac enveloping the heart.

Perichondrium (p. 101) the layer that surrounds a cartilage, consisting of an outer fibrous region and an inner cellular region.

Perilymph (p. 301) a fluid similar in composition to cerebrospinal fluid; located in the spaces between the bony labyrinth and the membranous labyrinth of the inner ear.

Perimysium (p. 146) a connective tissue partition that separates adjacent fasciculi in a skeletal muscle.

Perineum (p. 590) *per''i-ne'um* that region of the body extending from the anus to the scrotum in males and from the anus to the vulva in females.

Periosteum (p. 99) *per''e-os'te-um* double-layered connective tissue that covers and nourishes the bone.

Peripheral nervous system (PNS) (p. 262) *pĕ-rif'er-al* a system of nerves that connects the outlying parts of the body with the central nervous system.

Peripheral resistance (p. 401) the resistance to blood flow offered by the systemic blood vessels; a measure of the amount of friction encountered by blood.

Peristalsis (p. 492) *per''ĭ-stal'sis* the waves of contraction seen in tubelike organs; propels substances along the tract.

Peritoneum (p. 485) *per''ĭ-to-ne'um* the serous membrane lining the interior of the abdominal cavity and covering the surfaces of the abdominal organs.

Peritonitis (p. 487) *per''ĭ-to-ni'tis* an inflammation of the peritoneum.

Peritubular capillaries (p. 542) a network of capillaries that surrounds the proximal and distal convoluted tubules of the kidneys.

pH (p. 36) the symbol for hydrogen ion concentration; a measure of the relative acidity or alkalinity of a solution.

Phagocyte (p. 425) *fag'o-sīt* a cell capable of engulfing and digesting particles or cells harmful to the body.

Phagocytosis (p. 67) *fag'o-si-to'sis* the ingestion of solid particles by cells.

Phalanges (p. 125) *fah-lan'jēz* the bones of the finger or toe.

Pharynx (p. 453) *far'inks* the muscular tube extending from the posterior of the nasal cavities to the esophagus.

Phospholipid (p. 40) *fos'fo-lip'id* a modified triglyceride containing phosphorus.

Phosphorylation (p. 319) the addition of a high-energy phosphate group to a molecule.

Photoreceptors (p. 291) *fo''to-re-sep'torz* specialized receptor cells that respond to light energy.

Physiology (p. 2) *fiz''e-ol'o-je* the science of the functioning of living organisms.

Pia mater (p. 241) the tough, outer meningeal layer that surrounds the central nervous system.

Pineal gland (p. 337) neural tissue in the posterior portion of the roof of the diencephalon; secretes melatonin.

Pinocytosis (p. 67) *pi''no-si-to'sis* the engulfing of extracellular fluid by cells.

Pituitary gland (p. 233) *pĭ-tu'ĭ-tār''e* the neuroendocrine gland located beneath the brain that serves a variety of functions including regulation of the gonads, thyroid, adrenal cortex, water balance, and lactation.

Placenta (p. 342) *plah-sen' tah* the temporary organ that provides nutrients and oxygen to the developing fetus, carries away wastes, and produces the hormones of pregnancy.

Plantar flexion (p. 140) ankle extension.

Plantar (p. 13) *plan' tar* pertaining to the sole of the foot.

Plasma cell (p. 422) member of a B cell clone; specialized to produce and release antibodies.

Plasma membrane (p. 53) membrane that encloses cell contents; outer limiting membrane.

Plasma (p. 346) *plaz' mah* the fluid portion of the blood.

Platelet (p. 352) *plāt' let* one of the irregular cell fragments of blood; involved in clotting.

Pleura (p. 457) *ploor' ah* the serous membrane covering the lungs and lining the thoracic cavity.

Plexus (p. 240) *plek' sus* a network of interlacing nerves, blood vessels, or lymphatics.

Polar body (p. 592) a minute cell produced during meiosis in the ovary.

Polar molecules (p. 33) nonsymmetrical molecules that contain electrically unbalanced atoms.

Polarized (p. 213) *po' lar-īzd* the state of an unstimulated neuron or muscle cell in which the inside of the cell is relatively negative in comparison to the outside; the resting state.

Polycythemia (p. 349) *pol" e-si-the' me-ah* presence of an abnormally large number of erythrocytes in the blood.

Polypeptide (p. 43) *pol" e-pep' tīd* a chain of amino acids.

Polysaccharide (p. 39) *pol" e-sak' ĭ-rīd* literally, many sugars; a polymer of linked monosaccharides; examples include starch and glycogen.

Polysynaptic reflex (p. 230) a reflex in which interneurons are interposed between the sensory fiber and the motor neuron(s).

Pons (p. 240) the portion of the metencephalon that is anterior to the cerebellum.

Popliteal (p. 12) pertaining to the back of the knee.

Positive feedback (p. 10) feedback that tends to cause a variable to change in the same direction as the initial change; enhances the stimulus.

Posterior (p. 14) toward the back; dorsal.

Potential difference (p. 206) the separation of opposite charges; requires a barrier that prevents ion migration.

Precipitation (p. 438) formation of insoluble complexes that settle out of solution.

Pressure gradient (p. 63) difference in hydrostatic (fluid) pressure that drives filtration.

Presynaptic membrane (p. 220) the synaptic surface where neurotransmitter release occurs.

Prime mover (p. 177) muscle whose contractions are primarily responsible for a particular movement; agonist.

Progesterone (p. 341) the most important progestin secreted by the corpus luteum after ovulation.

Progestins (p. 596) steroid hormones structurally related to cholesterol; progesterone is an example.

Projection fibers (p. 307) axons carrying information from the thalamus to the cerebral cortex.

Prolactin (p. 325) the hormone that stimulates functional development of the mammary gland in females; a secretion of the anterior lobe of the pituitary gland.

Pronation (p. 140) *pro-na' shun* the inward rotation of the forearm causing the radius to cross diagonally over the ulna—palms face posteriorly.

Proprioception (p. 283) the awareness of the positions of bones, joints, and muscles.

Proprioceptor (p. 204) *pro" pre-oh-sep' tor* a receptor located in a muscle or tendon; concerned with locomotion, posture, and muscle tone.

Prostaglandin (p. 312) a fatty acid secreted by one cell that alters the metabolic activities or sensitivities of adjacent cells; also called *local hormone*.

Prostate gland (p. 582) an accessory gland of the male reproductive tract, contributing roughly one-third of the volume of semen.

Proteoglycan (p. 101) a compound containing a large polysaccharide complex attached to a relatively small protein; examples include hyaluronan and chondroitin sulfate.

Proton (p. 24) *pro' ton* subatomic particle that bears a positive charge; located in the atomic nucleus.

Protraction (p. 140) movement anteriorly in the horizontal plane.

Proximal convoluted tubule (PCT) (p. 542) the portion of the nephron that is situated between Bowman's capsule and the loop of Henle; the major site of active reabsorption from filtrate.

Proximal (p. 14) *prok' sĭ-mal* toward the attached end of a limb or the origin of a structure.

Puberty (p. 612) *pu' ber-te* the period at which reproductive organs become functional.

Pubic symphysis (p. 127) the fibrocartilaginous amphiarthrosis between the pubic bones of the ossa coxae.

Pubic (p. 11) pertaining to the genital region.

Pubis (p. 127) the anterior, inferior component of the os coxae.

Pulmonary (p. 366) *pul' mo-ner" e* pertaining to the lungs.

Pulmonary circuit (p. 396) blood vessels between the pulmonary semilunar valve of the right ventricle and the entrance to the left atrium; the blood flow through the lungs.

Pulmonary circulation (p. 364) system of blood vessels that carry blood to and from the lungs for gas exchange.

Pulmonary edema (p. 385) *ĕ-de' mah* a leakage of fluid into the air sacs and tissue of the lungs.

Pulmonary ventilation (p. 458) breathing; consists of inspiration and expiration.

Pulse (p. 400) the rhythmic expansion and recoil of arteries resulting from heart contraction; can be felt from the outside of the body.

Pupil (p. 290) an opening in the center of the iris through which light enters the eye.

Purkinje fibers (p. 378) *pur-kin' je* the modified cardiac muscle fibers of the conduction system of the heart.

Pus (p. 429) an accumulation of debris, fluid, dead and dying cells, and necrotic tissue.

Pyelonephritis (p. 558) *pi" ĕ-lo-nĕ-fri' tis* an inflammation of the kidney pelvis and surrounding kidney tissues.

Pyloric sphincter (p. 487) a sphincter of smooth muscle that regulates the passage of chyme from the stomach to the duodenum.

Pylorus (p. 487) the gastric region between the body of the stomach and the duodenum; includes the pyloric sphincter.

Pyramid (p. 255) any cone-shaped structure of an organ.

Pyrogen (p. 431) *pi' ro-jen* an agent or chemical substance that induces fever.

Pyruvic acid (p. 521) a three-carbon compound produced by glycolysis.

Radioisotope (p. 25) *ra" de-o-i' sĭ-tōp* isotope that exhibits radioactive behavior.

Ramus (p. 112) *ra' mus* a branch of a nerve, artery, vein, or bone.

Ramus/rami (p. 116) a branch.

Receptive field (p. 282) the area monitored by a single sensory receptor.

Rectum (p. 493) the inferior 15 cm (6 in.) of the digestive tract.

Rectus (p. 177) straight.

Red blood cell (RBC) (p. 348) *see* **erythrocyte**.

Reduction (p. 134) restoring broken bone ends (or a dislocated bone) to its original position.

Reflex arc (p. 228) neural pathway for reflexes.

Reflex (p. 228) automatic reaction to a stimulus.

Refract (p. 295) bend; usually refers to light.

Relaxation phase (p. 163) the period after a contraction when the tension in the muscle fiber returns to resting levels.

Relaxin (p. 603) a hormone that loosens the pubic symphysis; secreted by the placenta.

Renal calculus (p. 599) *re' nal kal' ku-lus* a kidney stone.

Renal corpuscle (p. 572) the initial portion of the nephron, consisting of an expanded chamber that encloses the glomerulus.

Renin (p. 333) *re' nin* a substance released by the kidneys that is involved with raising blood pressure.

Rennin (p. 504) a gastric enzyme that breaks down milk proteins.

Repolarization (p. 213) restoration of the membrane potential to the initial resting (polarized) state.

Reproductive system (p. 4) organ system that functions to produce offspring.

Respiration (p. 458) the exchange of gases between cells and the environment; includes pulmonary ventilation, external respiration, internal respiration, and cellular respiration.

Respiratory pump (p. 386) a mechanism by which changes in the intrapleural pressures during the respiratory cycle assist the venous return to the heart; also called *thoracoabdominal pump.*

Respiratory system (p. 4) organ system that carries out gas exchange; includes the nose, pharynx, larynx, trachea, bronchi, and lungs.

Responsiveness (p. 7) the ability to sense changes (stimuli) in the environment and then to react to them; see also **Irritability**.

Resting potential (p. 206) the transmembrane potential of a normal cell under homeostatic conditions.

Rete (p. 580) an interwoven network of blood vessels or passageways.

Reticular activating system (RAS) (p. 241) the mesencephalic portion of the reticular formation; responsible for arousal and the maintenance of consciousness.

Reticular formation (p. 240) a diffuse network of gray matter that extends the entire length of the brain stem.

Reticulospinal tracts (p. 258) Descending tracts of the medial pathway that carry involuntary motor commands issued by neurons of the reticular formation.

Reticulum (p. 55) *rĕ-tik′ u-lum* a fine network.

Retina (p. 291) *ret′ ĭ-nah* light sensitive layer of the eye; contains rods and cones.

Retinal (p. 294) a visual pigment derived from vitamin A.

Retraction (p. 140) movement posteriorly in the horizontal plane.

Retroperitoneal (p. 496) behind or outside the peritoneal cavity.

Reverberation (p. 227) a positive feedback along a chain of neurons such that they remain active once stimulated.

Rhodopsin (p. 294) the visual pigment in the membrane disks of the distal segments of rods.

Rhythmicity center (p. 475) a medullary center responsible for the pace of respiration; includes inspiratory and expiratory centers.

Ribonucleic acid (RNA) (p. 48) *ri″ bo-nu-kle′ ic* the nucleic acid that contains ribose; acts in protein synthesis.

Ribose (p. 39) a five-carbon sugar that is a structural component of RNA.

Ribosomes (p. 55) *ri′ bo-sōmz* cytoplasmic organelles at which proteins are synthesized.

Rods (p. 291) one of the two types of photosensitive cells in the retina.

Rugae (p. 487) mucosal folds in the lining of the empty stomach that disappear as gastric distension occurs; folds in the urinary bladder.

Sacral (p. 12) *sa′ kral* the lower portion of the back, just superior to the buttocks.

Sagittal section (plane) (p. 236) *sa′ jih-tul* a longitudinal (vertical) plane that divides the body or any of its parts into right and left portions.

Saliva (p. 493) *sah-li′ vah* the secretion of salivary gland which is ducted into the mouth.

Salt (p. 27) ionic compound that dissociates into charged particles (other than hydrogen or hydroxyl ions) when dissolved in water.

Sarcolemma (p. 150) the cell membrane of a muscle cell.

Sarcomere (p. 150) *sar′ ko-mēr* the smallest contractile unit of muscle; extends from one Z disc to the next.

Sarcoplasm (p. 146) the cytoplasm of a muscle cell.

Schwann cells (p. 201) neuroglia responsible for the neurilemma that surrounds axons in the peripheral nervous system.

Sciatic nerve (p. 187) a nerve innervating the posteromedial portions of the thigh and leg.

Sclera (p. 290) *skle′ rah* the firm white fibrous outer layer of the eyeball; protects and maintains eyeball shape.

Scrotum (p. 583) the loose-fitting, fleshy pouch that encloses the testes of the male.

Sebum (p. 91) *se′ bum* the oily secretion of sebaceous glands.

Second messenger (p. 614) intracellular molecule generated by binding of a chemical to a membrane receptor; mediates intracellular responses.

Secondary sex characteristics (p. 586) anatomical features that develop under influence of sex hormones (male or female pattern of muscle development, bone growth, body hair, etc.) that are not directly involved in the reproductive process.

Secretin (p. 505) a hormone, secreted by the duodenum, that stimulates the production of buffers by the pancreas and inhibits gastric activity.

Secretion (p. 71) *se-kre′ shun* the passage of material formed by a cell to its exterior; cell product that is transported to the cell exterior.

Sensation (p. 282) information received by the sensory receptors.

Semen (p. 583) *se′ men* fluid mixture produced by male reproductive structures; contains sperm, nutrients, and mucus.

Semilunar valves (p. 366) *sem″ e-lu′ nar* valves that prevent blood return to the ventricles after contraction.

Seminal vesicles (p. 582) glands of the male reproductive tract that produce roughly 60 percent of the volume of semen.

Seminiferous tubules (p. 586) *se′ mi-nif′ er-us* highly convoluted tubes within the testes that form sperm.

Serosa (p. 70) *see* **Serous membrane**.

Serotonin (p. 219) a neurotransmitter in the central nervous system; a compound that enhances inflammation and is released by activated mast cells and basophils.

Serous membrane (p. 70) membrane that lines a cavity without an opening to the outside of the body (except for joint cavities); serosa.

Serum (p. 354) the ground substance of blood plasma from which clotting agents have been removed.

Sex chromosomes (p. 611) chromosomes that determine genetic sex; the X and Y chromosomes.

Shoulder girdle (p. 122) composite of two bones, scapula and clavicle, that attach the upper limb to the axial skeleton; also called the pectoral girdle.

Sigmoid colon (p. 493) the S-shaped 18-cm-long portion of the colon between the descending colon and the rectum.

Simple epithelium (p. 70) an epithelium containing a single layer of cells above the basal lamina.

Sinoatrial (SA) node (p. 377) the natural pacemaker of the heart; situated in the wall of the right atrium.

Skeletal muscle tissue (p. 146) a contractile tissue dominated by skeletal muscle fibers; characterized as striated, voluntary muscle.

Skeletal muscle (p. 146) muscle composed of cylindrical multinucleate cells with obvious striations; the muscle(s) attached to the body's skeleton; also called *voluntary muscle.*

Skeletal system (p. 2) system of protection and support composed primarily of bone and cartilage.

Skull (p. 110) bony enclosure for the brain.

Sliding filament theory (p. 150) the concept that a sarcomere shortens as the thick and thin filaments slide past one another.

Small intestine (p. 488) the duodenum, jejunum, and ileum; the digestive tract between the stomach and the large intestine.

Smooth endoplasmic reticulum (SER) (p. 152) a membranous organelle in which lipid and carbohydrate synthesis and storage occur.

Smooth muscle tissue (p. 80) muscle tissue in the walls of many visceral organs; characterized as nonstriated, involuntary muscle.

Smooth muscle (p. 80) muscle consisting of spindle-shaped, unstriped (nonstriated) muscle cells; involuntary muscle.

Soft palate (p. 452) the fleshy posterior extension of the hard palate, separating the nasopharynx from the oral cavity.

Solution (p. 33) a homogenous mixture of two or more components.

Solvent (p. 33) the fluid component of a solution.

Somatic nervous system (p. 254) *so-mat′ ik* a division of the peripheral nervous system; also called the voluntary nervous system.

Spermatocyte (p. 584) a cell of the seminiferous tubules that is engaged in meiosis.

Spermatogenesis (p. 584) *sper″ mah-to-jen′ ĕ-sis* the process of sperm production in the male; involves meiosis.

Spinal nerve (p. 263) one of 31 pairs of nerves that originate on the spinal cord from anterior and posterior roots.

Spinal nerves (p. 263) the 31 pairs of nerves that arise from the spinal cord.

Spinothalamic tracts (p. 251) ascending tracts that carry poorly localized touch, pressure, pain, vibration, and temperature sensations to the thalamus.

Spinous process (p. 118) the prominent posterior projection of a vertebra; formed by the fusion of two laminae.

Spleen (p. 423) a lymphoid organ important for the phagocytosis of red blood cells, the immune response, and lymphocyte production.

Squamous epithelium (p. 70) an epithelium whose superficial cells are flattened and platelike.

Squamous (p. 71) *skwa'mus* flat, scale-like; pertaining to flat, thin cells that form the free surface of some epithelial tissues.

Stapes (p. 301) the auditory ossicle attached to the tympanic membrane.

Static equilibrium (p. 301) *stat'ik e'kwĭ-lib're-um* balance concerned with changes in the position of the head.

Sternal (p. 11) breastbone area.

Steroids (p. 312) *stĕ'roidz* a specific group of chemical substances including certain hormones and cholesterol.

Stimulus (p. 9) *stim'u-lus* an excitant or irritant; a change in the environment producing a response.

Stratified (p. 70) containing several layers. (4, epithelium, for example)

Stratum (p. 87) *stra'tum* a layer.

Stroke volume (p. 381) a volume of blood ejected by a ventricle during systole.

Stroke (p. 75) a condition in which brain tissue is deprived of a blood supply, as in blockage of a cerebral blood vessel.

Stroma (p. 75) the connective tissue framework of an organ; distinguished from the functional cells (parenchyma) of that organ.

Subarachnoid space (p. 241) a meningeal space containing cerebrospinal fluid; the area between the arachnoid membrane and the pia mater.

Subclavian (p. 389) pertaining to the region immediately posterior and inferior to the clavicle.

Subcutaneous (p. 87) *sub'ku-ta'ne-us* beneath the skin.

Submucosa (p. 491) the region between the muscularis mucosae and the muscularis externa.

Substrate (p. 236) a participant (product or reactant) in an enzyme-catalyzed reaction.

Sulcus (p. 238) *sul'kus* a furrow on the brain, less deep than a fissure.

Summation (p. 225) *sum-ma'shun* the accumulation of effects, especially those of muscular, sensory, or mental stimuli.

Superficial (external) (p. 14) located close to or on the body surface.

Superior vena cava (SVC) (p. 391) the vein that carries blood to the right atrium from parts of the body that are superior to the heart.

Superior (p. 14) refers to the head or upper body regions.

Supination (p. 177) *su'pĭ-na'shun* the outward rotation of the forearm causing palms to face anteriorly.

Suppressor T cells (p. 441) regulatory T lymphocytes that suppress the immune response.

Surfactant (p. 478) *sur-fak'tant* a chemical substance coating the pulmonary alveoli walls that reduces surface tension, thus preventing collapse of the alveoli after expiration.

Sutures (p. 110) *soo'churz* immovable fibrous joints that connect the bones of the adult skull.

Sweat glands (p. 91) the glands that produce a saline solution called sweat; also called sudoriferous glands.

Sympathetic division (p. 271) a division of the autonomic nervous system; opposes parasympathetic functions; called the fight-or-flight division.

Symphysis (p. 127) a fibrous amphiarthrosis, such as that between adjacent vertebrae or between the pubic bones of the ossa coxae.

Synapse (p. 201) *sin'aps* the region of communication between neurons.

Synaptic cleft (p. 153) *sĭ-nap'tik* the fluid-filled space at a synapse between neurons.

Synaptic delay (p. 218) the period between the arrival of an impulse at the presynaptic membrane and the initiation of an action potential in the postsynaptic membrane.

Syndrome (p. 240) a discrete set of symptoms that occur together.

Synergist (p. 177) a muscle that assists a prime mover in performing its primary action.

Synergists (p. 177) *sin'er-jists* muscles cooperating with another muscle or muscle group to produce a desired movement.

Synovial fluid (p. 135) *sĭ-no've-al* a fluid secreted by the synovial membrane; lubricates joint surfaces and nourishes articular cartilages.

Synovial joint (p. 134) freely movable joint exhibiting a joint cavity enclosed by an articular (fibrous) capsule lined with synovial membrane.

Synovial membrane (p. 134) membrane that lines the capsule of a synovial joint.

Synthesis reaction (p. 30) chemical reaction in which larger molecules are formed from simpler ones.

System (p. 2) a group of organs that function cooperatively to accomplish a common purpose; there are eleven major systems in the human body.

Systemic circulation (p. 364) system of blood vessels that carries nutrient and oxygen-rich blood to all body organs.

Systemic edema (p. 420) *e˘-de'mah* an accumulation of fluid in body organs or tissues.

Systole (p. 380) *sis'to-le* the contraction phase of heart activity.

Systolic pressure (p. 394) *sis-tol'ik* the pressure generated by the left ventricle during systole.

T cells (p. 432) lymphocytes that mediate cellular immunity; include helper, killer, suppressor, and memory cells. Also called T lymphocytes.

Tachycardia (p. 379) *tak'e-kar'de-ah* an abnormal, excessively rapid heart rate; over 100 beats per minute.

Tactile (p. 283) pertaining to the sense of touch.

Target cells (p. 314) specific cells that possess the receptors needed to find and "read" the hormonal messages as they arrive.

Tarsal bones (p. 128) the bones of the ankle (the talus, calcaneus, navicular, and cuneiform bones).

Taste buds (p. 306) receptors for taste on the tongue, roof of mouth, pharynx, and larynx.

TCA (tricarboxylic acid) cycle (p. 520) the aerobic reaction sequence that occurs in the matrix of mitochondria; in the process, organic molecules are broken down, carbon dioxide molecules are released, and hydrogen molecules are transferred to coenzymes that deliver them to the electron transport system; also called *citric acid cycle* or *Krebs cycle.*

Tectospinal tracts (p. 258) descending tracts of the medial pathway that carry involuntary motor commands issued by the colliculi.

Telodendria (p. 204) terminal axonal branches that end in synaptic knobs.

Temporal (p. 110) pertaining to time (temporal summation) or to the temples (temporal bone).

Tendon (p. 134) *ten'dun* cord of dense fibrous tissue attaching a muscle to a bone.

Terminal (p. 152) toward the end.

Testis (p. 580) *tes'tis* the male primary sex organ that produces sperm.

Testosterone (p. 586) *tes-tos'tĕ-rŏn* male sex hormone produced by the testes; during puberty promotes virilization and is necessary for normal sperm production.

Tetanus (p. 163) *tet'ah-nus* the tense, contracted state of a muscle; an infectious disease.

Thalamus (p. 233) *tha'luh-mis* a mass of gray matter in the diencephalon of the brain.

Thermoreceptor (p. 283) *ther'mo-re-sep'ter* a receptor sensitive to temperature changes.

Thick filament (p. 150) a cytoskeletal filament in a skeletal or cardiac muscle cell; composed of myosin, with a core of titin.

Thin filament (p. 150) a cytoskeletal filament in a skeletal or cardiac muscle cell; consists of actin, troponin, and tropomyosin.

Thoracic (p. 11) *tho-ras'ik* refers to the chest.

Thorax (p. 120) *tho'raks* that portion of the body trunk above the diaphragm and below the neck.

Thrombin (p. 354) *throm'bin* an enzyme that induces clotting by converting fibrinogen to fibrin.

Thrombus (p. 355) *throm'bus* a fixed clot that develops and persists in an unbroken blood vessel.

Thymosins (p. 341) thymic hormones essential to the development and differentiation of T cells.

Thymus gland (p. 341) *thi'mus* an endocrine gland active in the immune response.

Thymus (p. 341) a lymphoid organ, the site of T cell formation.

Thyroid gland (p. 329) *thi'roid* one of the largest of the body's endocrine glands; straddles the anterior trachea.

Thyroid hormones (p. 329) thyroxine and triiodothyronine   hormones of the thyroid gland; stimulate tissue metabolism, energy utilization, and growth.

Thyroxine (p. 329) a thyroid hormone; also called or *tetraiodothyronine*.

Tidal volume (p. 460) amount of air inhaled or exhaled with a normal breath.

Tissue (p. 2) a group of similar cells specialized to perform a specific function; primary tissue types are epithelial, connective, muscle, and nervous tissues.

Tonsil (p. 424) a lymphoid nodule in the wall of the pharynx; the palatine, pharyngeal, and lingual tonsils.

Total metabolic rate (p. 528) total amount of kilocalories the body must consume in order to fuel all ongoing activities.

Trabecula (p. 422) a connective tissue partition that subdivides an organ.

Trachea (p. 454) *tra′ke-ah* the windpipe; the respiratory tube extending from larynx to bronchi.

Tract (p. 203) a collection of nerve fibers in the CNS having the same origin, termination, and function.

Transmembrane potential (p. 207) the potential difference, measured across a cell membrane and expressed in millivolts, that results from the uneven distribution of positive and negative ions across the cell membrane.

Tricuspid valve (p. 366) the right atrioventricular valve, which prevents the backflow of blood into the right atrium during ventricular systole.

Triglycerides (p. 40) *tri-glis′ er-īdz* compounds composed of fatty acids and glycerol; fats and oils; also called neutral fats.

Trochanter (p. 127) *tro-kan′ ter* a large, somewhat blunt process.

Trochlea (p. 122) a pulley; the spool-shaped medial portion of the condyle of the humerus.

Tropic hormone (p. 325) *trōp′ ik* a hormone that regulates the function of another endocrine organ.

Trunk (p. 182) the thoracic and abdominopelvic regions; a major arterial branch.

Tubercle (p. 122) *tu′ ber-kul* a nodule or small rounded process.

Tuberosity (p. 112) a large, roughened elevation on a bony surface.

Tumor (p. 83) a tissue mass formed by the abnormal growth and replication of cells.

Tunica (p. 386) *too′ nĭ-kah* a covering or tissue coat; layer.

Twitch (p. 162) a single stimulus-contraction-relaxation cycle in a skeletal muscle.

Ulcer (p. 502) *ul′ ser* a lesion or erosion of the mucous membrane, such as gastric ulcer of stomach.

Umbilical cord (p. 602) *um-bĭ′ lĭ-kul* a structure bearing arteries and veins connecting the placenta and the fetus.

Unipolar neuron (p. 206) a sensory neuron whose cell body is in a dorsal root ganglion or a sensory ganglion of a cranial nerve.

Urea (p. 524) *u-re′ ah* the main nitrogen-containing waste excreted in the urine.

Ureters (p. 558) *u-re′ terz* tubes that carry urine from kidney to bladder.

Urethra (p. 560) *u-re′ thrah* the canal through which urine passes from the bladder to the outside of the body.

Urinary bladder (p. 559) the muscular, distensible sac that stores urine prior to micturition.

Urinary system (p. 4) system primarily responsible for water, electrolyte, and acid-base balance and the removal of nitrogenous wastes from the blood.

Urine (p. 540) filtrate containing waste and excess ions excreted by the kidneys.

Uterine tube (p. 588) the oviduct. The tube through which the ovum is transported to the uterus; also called fallopian tube.

Uterus (p. 589) the muscular organ of the female reproductive tract in which implantation, placenta formation, and fetal development occur.

Uvula (p. 482) *u′ vu-lah* tissue tag hanging from soft palate.

Vagina (p. 590) a muscular tube extending between the uterus and the vestibule.

Vasectomy (p. 582) cutting of the deferens to keep sperm from reaching the exterior of the body and allowing fertilization to take place.

Vasoconstriction (p. 528) *vas″o-kon-strik′ shun* narrowing of blood vessels.

Vasomotor center (p. 404) the center in the medulla oblongata whose stimulation produces vasoconstriction and an elevation of peripheral resistance.

Vein (p. 375) *vān* a vessel carrying blood away from the tissues toward the heart.

Ventilation (p. 458) air movement into and out of the lungs.

Ventral (p. 16) anterior or front.

Ventricles (p. 234) *ven′ trĭ-kulz* discharging cham-bers of the heart; cavities within the brain.

Venule (p. 385) *ven′ ūl* a small vein.

Vertebral column (p. 116) the spine, formed of a number of individual bones called vertebrae and two composite bones (sacrum and coccyx).

Villus/villi (p. 488) a slender projection of the mucous membrane of the small intestine.

Visceral (p. 148) *vis′ er-al* pertaining to the internal part of a structure or the internal organs.

Viscosity (p. 401) *vis-kos′ ĭ-te* the state of being sticky or thick.

Visual acuity (p. 291) *ah-ku′ ĭ-te* the ability of the eye to distinguish detail.

Vital capacity (p. 462) the volume of air that can be expelled from the lungs by forcible expiration after the deepest inspiration; total exchangeable air.

Vitamins (p. 513) organic compounds required by the body in minute amounts for physiological maintenance and growth.

Vitreous humor (p. 293) a gel-like substance that helps prevent the eyeball from collapsing inward by reinforcing it internally.

Voluntary muscle (p. 146) muscle under control of the will; skeletal muscle.

Voluntary (p. 148) controlled by conscious thought processes.

Vulva (p. 590) *vul′ va* female external genitalia.

White blood cells (WBCs) (p. 422) the granulocytes and agranulocytes of blood.

White matter (p. 203) white substance of the central nervous system; the myelinated nerve fibers.

Xiphoid process (p. 120) the slender, inferior extension of the sternum.

Zygote (p. 600) *zi′ gōt* the fertilized ovum; produced by union of two gametes.

Index